T0329114

Nanomaterials for Medical Applications

Nanomaterials for Medical Applications

Zoraida P. Aguilar

Director of Research and Development
Ocean NanoTech
Springdale, AR

AMSTERDAM • BOSTON • HEIDELBERG • LONDON
NEW YORK • OXFORD • PARIS • SAN DIEGO
SAN FRANCISCO • SYDNEY • TOKYO

ELSEVIER

Elsevier
225 Wyman Street, Waltham, MA 02451, USA
The Boulevard, Langford Lane, Kidlington, Oxford, OX5 1GB, UK
Radarweg 29, PO Box 211, 1000 AE Amsterdam, The Netherlands

Notice
No responsibility is assumed by the publisher for any injury and/or damage to persons or
property as a matter of products liability, negligence or otherwise, or from any use or operation
of any methods, products, instructions or ideas contained in the material herein

British Library Cataloguing in Publication Data
A catalogue record for this book is available from the British Library

Library of Congress Cataloging-in-Publication Data
Aguilar, Zoraida.
  Nanomaterials for medical applications / Zoraida Aguilar.
    p. ; cm.
  Includes bibliographical references and index.
  ISBN 978-0-12-385089-8
  I. Title.
  [DNLM: 1. Nanostructures--diagnostic use. 2. Nanostructures--therapeutic use.
3. Biocompatible Materials--chemical synthesis. 4. Biosensing Techniques. QT 36.5]

  610.28′4--dc23
                    2012028617

ISBN: 978-0-12-385089-8

For information on all Elsevier publications
visit our web site at store.elsevier.com

Printed and bound in the USA
12 13 14 15 16   10 9 8 7 6 5 4 3 2 1

Contents

Foreword

The encompassing contents and approach of this book on the medical applications of nanomaterials are unique. Reviewing the various contents of this book, it is apparent that the primary intent is to provide a reference to people in all walks of life especially scientists, engineers, medical professionals, law makers, patent lawyers, students, and common people to inspire new innovations. The author, Dr Zoraida P. Aguilar, PhD, has put together her experiences in biotechnology, nanotechnology, devices, molecular biology, and medical sensors and devices to describe the current status of nanomaterials for medical applications and to move existing applications toward the realization of the great potential of nanoscale science and technology in medicine. She has described nanomaterials in medicine all the way from their synthesis to the eventual enormous health and economic impact they will have worldwide. The author ingeniously interconnected the various aspects of an emerging technology and detailed its properties all the way to the existing and future commercial products.

While nanotechnology has wide and far-reaching applications in various industries, its relevance in medicine is beyond doubt. This is because the nanoscale phenomena is not only applicable to nanomaterials in nanotechnology but more so to enzyme action, cell cycle, cell signaling, cell damage, cell repair, and the metabolic products within the living system. Nanomaterials have structural features and properties in between those of single atoms/molecules and continuous bulk materials just like the various biomolecules in the human body. The only difference is that the nanoscale dimensions of nanomaterials enable unique optical, electronic, magnetic, and catalytic properties that are distinct from those of atoms/molecules or bulk/macroscale materials. Proper control of the growth, size, shape, size/shape distribution, as well as the encompassing ligand technologies of these nanomaterials will allow the full exploitation of their unique nanoscale properties enabling the creation of new products, devices and technologies as well as the improvement of existing ones.

The author successfully presents the most current levels of nanomaterials in medical research, commercialized products, as well as products in clinical trials. She describes nano-enabled medical products that have entered the market to date as well as potential applications in complicated diseases such as cancer, cardiovascular, neurodegenerative disorders, infection, tissue engineering, and as components of medical implants. Her presentation of the market trends and the patent landscape provide an overview of commercial and intellectual status of nanomaterials today.

Aside from the various medical uses of nanomaterials, the author has also given attention to their potential harmful effects. With any new material, it is necessary to fully understand the potential toxic effects it may have, especially nanomaterials since their size and bio-accessibility leads to the potential for quick incorporation into organisms. The author's presentation of nanotoxicology shows a clear balance between the possible advantageous aspects of nanomaterials versus their potential harmful effects to humans. This book's views on Nanotoxicology address the toxicity profiles of nanomaterials which are known to differ from their bulk/larger forms; this has led to the creation and drafting of various government guidelines worldwide.

As in any new and emerging technology, the current state of intellectual property related to nanotechnology is growing tremendously. The author presents a section on current patent status that is vital for the attaining of its promising potential beyond academic research. The author has very ingenuously touched on all the important aspects of nanomaterials to realize their far-reaching applications in medicine. NO other book in the market has covered such a wide scope in its presentation of the medical applications of nanomaterials.

Signed:

David P. Battaglia, PhD
PhD in Physical Chemistry with a focus in Nanoscale Materials Science

Preface

Nanotechnology, the 21st century's cutting edge technology, seeks to discover, describe, and manipulate the unique properties of matter at the nanoscale to develop new capabilities with potential applications across all fields of science, engineering, technology, and medicine. Various potential applications of nanomaterials and nanotechnology have been touted in scientific and layman press for the promises of the ability of nanoscale technology to revolutionize life into a fiction that once was found only in books. Outside of enormous speculations and hype, current applications of nanomaterials and nanodevices that already impact global commerce are living proofs of the nanotechology revolution.

From its beginning since the late 20th century to its current status in the early 21st century, nanotechnology is continuing to show that it is an evolving technology that has influenced various areas of research and industry. It has shown its pivotal and encompassing role and impact on nearly all-industrial sectors. At the same time, nanotechnology and biotechnology have converged giving rise to various prospective biomedical applications. Moreover, unlike any other existing technology, the nanoscale nature of nanomaterials and nanodevices exhibits potential applications in the sub-cellular scales with near perfect accuracy in targeting cellular and tissue-specific clinical applications with maximum therapeutic effects and with minimal or no bad effects.

During the past decade, increase in awareness and understanding of the factors that govern growth and properties of nanomaterials gave rise to novel structures and functionalities that showed applications in electronic industry, biomedical field, computer information technology, and other fields. This brought a downpour of financial support from various governments worldwide. Projections of trillions of dollars' worth of growth in the global nanotechnology market have led to a scenario guided by competition among the leading players lead by the US. There are currently a handful (in the hundreds) of nanomaterials that have reached commercial productions and applications. These include those that are used in medicine in the form of drug nanocarriers, imaging contrast agents, implants, and other applications. These nano-enabled products show advantages over their conventional counterparts.

Many more nanomaterials are currently being tested for various sensitive and accurate medical diagnostics as well as for effective therapeutics. Nanomaterials have become very attractive for drug delivery purposes due to their unique capabilities and their negligible side effects in cancer therapy and in the treatment of other ailments. While some nanomaterials are fast advancing in their medical applications such as chitosan, liposomes, and polymers, a few others are trailing behind. However, a few of the inorganic nanoparticles have also advanced faster than others such as the gold, iron oxide, hydroxyapatite, and gadolinium nanoparticles.

Various instruments that are useful for NMs characterization were discussed. For clearer and better understanding of nanomaterials and their interactions with biological systems for medical applications, novel high-resolution imaging and analysis tools which allow for easy sample preparation and in situ monitoring are needed. These instruments are also relevant in the desire to regulate and monitor exposure levels or environmental release of nanomaterials.

It is important to emphasize the role of NMs for drug delivery in cancer, tumor, and other types of diseases because of the enormous negative impact of chemotherapy for these diseases. Engineered nanomaterials have the potential to deliver the chemotherapeutic drugs at the site of the disease to optimize the effect of drugs while reducing toxic side effects which damage healthy cells. Nanomaterials can effectively deliver drugs to the tumor bearing organ but these have to be carefully and meticulously engineered before they can perform the functions they are designed for. Proper engineering of the nanomaterials must bring about a desired size, biocompatibility, biodegradability, and must avoid opsonization for prolonged circulation time so that the drug payload can be released over an extended period of time. The ability of nano-enabled drugs that are currently available in the market to minimize the side effects that are normally observed in conventional drugs open up doors for safer alternatives to drug delivery.

Just like any new technology or new drug that are intended for human consumption, nanomaterials for medical applications needs scrutiny in terms of biodistribution, organ accumulation, degradation and/or toxicity, damage of cellular structures or inflammatory effects, and genetic damage. Although the use of nanomaterials in medicine is still its infancy, studies on absorption, distribution, metabolism and elimination (ADME), and drug metabolism and pharmacokinetics (DMPK) require intense studies. The pharmacokinetics of various NMs used as drug delivery systems demand exhaustive research including the path that the nano-enabled drugs take after entry into the living system. One advantage of a few of the NMs is that they have unique optical and magnetic properties that may be used while elucidating the ADME and PK in nanodrug delivery systems.

Thus, as suggested by Richard Feynman at an American Physical Society meeting at Caltech on December 29, 1959 where he focused on a process which involved the ability to manipulate down to the individual atoms and molecules using a set of precise tools to build and operate another proportionally smaller set is now beginning to come to reality. It was in the early 2000s that the use of nanotechnology in commercial products began. To date concerted efforts between academia, government, and industry ascertain the development and discovery of many new materials with novel properties and new applications. Various approaches in nanofabrication and nanomaterials synthesis are continuing to grow with the goal of developing more efficient, less expensive, and more reproducible large scale manufacturing techniques. More sophisticated instrumentation for the characterization, detection, and quantification of various NMs will provide the needed level of analysis to reach molecular and sub-molecular level applications. It is no longer fiction in nature but a reality that new and improved biocompatible NMs and nanomechanical components are now being tested for implants, artificial organs, and greatly improved mechanical, visual, auditory, and other prosthetic devices. With continued support for research and development efforts from the various sectors, this may be closer to reality than we can imagine at this point in time.

The author offers this book as a guide to various important aspects of nanomaterials in order to hasten the realization of its far-reaching applications in medicine. No other book in the market has covered such a wide scope in its presentation and approach on the medical applications of nanomaterials.

Acknowledgements

First and foremost I thank God for allowing me to have the knowledge and courage to undertake a huge project such as this book. Without my faith, the demise of my beloved mother, the car accident, and the many challenges that I had to overcome while working on this book, I would have given up and quit writing. However, I persevered and pushed my limits and with the help of my family and friends, this book has finally seen the press and now you are about to read it.

My deepest gratitude goes next to my mom and dad who pushed me into the field of chemistry. I would not have been what I am now had I pursued my choice then, which was a career in fine arts. Today, I paint on canvass during my few leisure moments.

Endless thanks to my mentors, Dr. Paul, Dr. William R. Heineman, and Dr. Ingrid Fritsch who guided me towards my current maturity in the sciences. They took time out of their daily busy schedules to provide nurturing academic advice that paved the way for my path in my professional career especially in my writing skills.

Sincere thanks goes to Dr. Coy Batoy, Dr. David Battaglia, and Dr. Ruben Morawicki. You all who have always been there when I needed someone no matter for what reason, someone to brainstorm with, and someone to hold on to. Coy is the sweetest darling who searched and provided me with the references that I could not acquire. Ruben took me out to dinner or a drink when I was too physically and mentally exhausted and I needed a break. David picked up the phone whenever I needed someone to hear me on the other line and his wife Tara, was there to listen to me too. These are friends and professional soul mates that gave me all the support and encouragement I needed at any time.

Thanks are owed to Dr. Hong Xu, Dr. Hengyi Xu, and Dr. Nick Wu. They supported me in writing this book with photos, references, and their papers. Although located in different parts of the country and the world, they were but one email and one phone call away at all times. Without question or hesitation, they gave me their wholehearted support and provided what I needed.

Special thanks go to Dr. Susan Grisham Banerjee. She spent hours discussing various aspects of nanomaterials and their medical and toxicity applications which are her areas of interest.

There are more people to thank and they are at Ocean NanoTech. Dr. Andrew Wang, the president of the company provided an all-out support when he learned that I accepted the challenge to write this book. He offered anything and everything that I needed from Ocean NanoTech. The Vice president of the company, Alice Bu provided the photos and the catalog which contained the various products of the company. Just like Andrew, Alice fully supported this book as if it was one of Ocean's products. John Dixon, the production scientist provided me with all the TEM of the various nanomaterials and other photos that he had on his file so that I may be able to choose the best ones to use. Toni Mohrhauser provided the disk for the photos and packed the nanomaterials that I needed when I took some photographs for my on-going projects and for this book. Jenny Alarcon took a load of photographs especially for the purpose of use in this book. And Dr. Hong Xu provided the gel electrophoresis photos and fluorescent microscope images that I used.

My appreciation goes to my son, Ysmael Aguilar, and my niece Christna Aguilar, who were thrilled that I was writing this book. They sometimes cooked dinner when I was too engrossed to take a bite. My brother Tony Boy who provided me advice and encouragement after my mom passed away, my sister Tess with her constant and continued text messages, and my sister Lyn with her loving facebook messages.

Many others contributed their heart and soul for me to complete this book. These are all my friends who are too many to mention but Dr. Marites Sales deserves a special mention, Mr Albert Morales who has provided me with encouraging words, Mrs. Edna Pacia Pestano who is the picture of a genuine altruist, Ms Mayett Maling Cope whose words of wisdom are a daily inspiration, Mrs Marilou Ramos Szabo whose faith is endless, Mrs Jeneva Canlas Takasawa who never forgets to call me when I do, my uncle Dr. Vianmar Pascual who does not forget to send text messages, and my brother Freddie Aguilar with his big brother words of advice.

To all of you, my sincerest gratitude from the deepest recesses of my soul for all the support that you have provided me. I hope you all will still be there for me even after I publish this book. To my publisher, Graham Nisbet and to Louisa Hutchins, thank you for giving me the opportunity to write and publish this book.

Very sincerely,
Zoraida P. Aguilar, PhD

Introduction

This chapter serves as an introduction to nanotechnology and focuses on nanomaterials (NMs) in particular. It will introduce the various potential applications of nanotechnology in general and the various medical applications of NMs in particular. The chapter will also present a market analysis of nanotechnology and will converge into the market analysis of NMs specifically in medical applications. A summary of the various chapters of the book will be presented individually to have a glimpse of the contents of each chapter. In addition, this chapter will focus on the market analysis of nanotechnology and of NMs as well as the regulatory status and the historical perspectives. The author's view of the future of nanotechnology in medicine will be described.

1.1 NANOTECHNOLOGY POTENTIAL APPLICATIONS AND MARKET ANALYSIS

Nanotechnology seeks to discover, describe, and manipulate the unique properties of matter at the nanoscale in order to develop new capabilities with potential applications across all fields of science, engineering, technology, and medicine. In the United States, the National Nanotechnology Initiative (NNI) was established to support the advances in nanoscale science and technology that are predicted to have an enormous potential economic impact. Various potential applications of NMs and nanotechnology have been touted in scientific and layman press for the promises of the ability of nanoscale technology to revolutionize life as we know it. Outside enormous speculations and hype, the NNI can point to current applications of NMs and nanodevices that are already impacting our nation's commerce as well as advances that are mature enough to promise impacts in the near future.

Nanomaterials for Medical Applications. http://dx.doi.org/10.1016/B978-0-12-385089-8.00001-7

Nanotechnology is continuing to show that it is an evolving technology that has influenced various areas of research and industry. It has shown a trend toward a pivotal role in various industry segments in the coming years. The economic activities from nanotech are wide in scope and are anticipated to have a huge impact on nearly all-industrial sectors and will enter the consumer market in large quantities.[1] The convergence of nanotechnology and biotechnology has given rise to various prospective biomedical applications.[1] The nanoscale nature of NMs and nanodevices allows applications at the subcellular scales with higher accuracy in targeting cellular and tissue-specific clinical applications that can yield maximum therapeutic effects with minimal or no bad effects.

In the last 10 years, increase in awareness and understanding of the factors that govern growth and properties of NMs has led to a number of novel structures and functionalities.[2–9] These nanostructures include nanofibers, nanotubes, amphiphilic protein scaffolds, and nanowires that have potential applications in the electronic industry, biomedical field, computer information technology, etc.[2–17] Knowing the potential economic impact of NMs, various governments worldwide showed support for nanotechnology. In 2004, support for nanotechnology was $989 M from US (federal), $815 from Japan, $402 from EU, $318 M from Germany, $205M from France, $114 from the UK, $$90 M from China, $188M from South Korea, and $3.9M from India.[18]

In the US, the NNI is the body coordinating Federal programs and investment in research and development (R&D) activities in nanoscale science, engineering, technology, and related efforts across 25 agencies and programs.[19] The NNI is regularly reviewed by the President's Council of Advisors on Science and Technology (PCAST) since the council was designated in 2004. Based on the NNI PCAST review report,[20] the US Federal Government has proposed a budget of $1.8 billion in fiscal year (FY) 2013 for 15 agencies with budgets dedicated to nanotechnology R&D.[20] This 2013 budget request represents a total funding of $18 billion from 2004 to 2013.

According to a newly released report by the RNCOS industry Research Solutions in April 2012,[21] the US nanotechnology market has significant R&D activities on the initial phase of emerging products. Based on this report,[1] the leading areas of development are in nanobio, NMs, surfaces, electronics, and IT and instrumentation. The NM segment is by far the most lucrative and marketable segment in the US especially in California and Massachusetts where a well-established nanotechnology community exists. This growth is supported by the NNI that proposed an investment around US$ 2.13 billion in nanotechnology.[21]

As has been predicted by various experts, the past few years have seen a significant growth rate in global nanotechnology market that created new opportunities for improving the characterization of NMs, monitoring capabilities, minimizing contaminations in the environment, emergence of new NMs, and many more. The RNCOS report predicts that the US and Europe will likely remain as the major geographic markets for nanotechnology until 2014[1] and the market share of Asia Pacific region is expected to grow significantly in the nanotechnology market. According to RNCOS, with increasing usage of nanotechnology in various applications, global nanotechnology market is projected to reach US$ 26 billion by the end of 2014, growing at a compound annual growth rate (CAGR) of around 20% since 2011.

1.2 NMS FOR MEDICAL APPLICATIONS

This book is focused in one particular area of nanotechnology, which is the NMs. NMs are smaller than or comparable to a virus (20–450 nm), a protein (5–50 nm), or a gene (2-nm wide and 10–100 nm long), and it is bigger than the molecule of water but smaller than a bacteria (1 μm) or a pollen (100 μm) (Figure 1.1). In addition to the size, specific NMs can be manipulated under an external magnetic field or can be observed instrumentally to exhibit bright stable fluorescence, Raman active, or other unique characteristics that lead to their various applications in the medical field.[22–32] In addition, properly engineered NMs are stable and allow attachment of multiple kinds of biomolecules leading to their highly efficient use in medicine.[5,9,23,24,33–78]

NMs have structural features and properties in between those of single atoms/molecules and continuous bulk materials and have at least one dimension in the nanometer range (1 nm = 1×10^{-9} m). They include clusters,[1,2] nanoparticles (NPs),[2–10,79–96] quantum dots (QDs),[9,97–100] nanotubes,[7,101] as well as the collection or organization of these individual structures into two- and three-dimensional assemblies. The nanoscale dimensions of NMs bring optical,

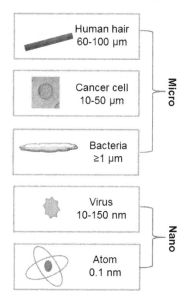

Human hair
60-100 μm

Cancer cell
10-50 μm

Bacteria
≥1 μm

Micro

Virus
10-150 nm

Atom
0.1 nm

Nano

FIGURE 1.1 Comparative sizes of various micro- and nanoparticles. *(For color version of this figure, the reader is referred to the online version of this book)*

electronic, magnetic, catalytic, and other properties that are distinct from those of atoms/molecules or bulk materials. In order to exploit the special properties that arise due to the nanoscale dimensions of materials, researchers must control and manipulate the size, shape, and surface functional groups of NMs, and structure them into periodically ordered assemblies to create new products, devices, and technologies or improve existing ones.[102–109] The science of controlling, manipulating, or engineering the properties and utilizing these NMs for the purpose of building microscopic machinery is termed as nanotechnology. The control and manipulation process can be done using the "top-down" or "bottom-up" approach. In the "top-down" approach, large chunks of materials are broken down into nanostructures by lithography or any other outside force that impose order on NMs.[110]

NMs are directly relevant to medicine because of the role of nanoscale phenomena, such as enzyme action, cell cycle, cell signaling, and damage repair. NMs can be used to create tools for analyzing the structure of cells and tissues from the atomic and cellular levels and to design and create biocompatible materials at the nanoscale for therapies, diagnostics, and replacements. NMs can be used to create precisely targeted drugs that are engineered to locate and sit on specific proteins and nucleic acids associated with the disease and/or disorders. These NMs can also be used to deliver small organic molecules and peptides at effective sites of action to carry out their function more effectively, protected from degradation, immune attack, and shielded to pass through barriers that block the passage of large molecules.

At present, NMs are being tested for various biomedical applications to learn if they can help facilitate sensitive and accurate medical diagnostics as well as for effective therapeutics. More specifically for drug delivery purposes, the use of NMs is attracting increasing attention due to their unique capabilities and their negligible side effects not only in cancer therapy but also in the treatment of other ailments. Among all types of NMs, biocompatible superparamagnetic iron oxide NMs or nanoparticles (SPIONs) with proper surface architecture and conjugated targeting ligands/proteins have attracted a great deal of attention for drug delivery applications.

Several biological applications of NMs appear to be a few years away from producing practical products. One example is nanosized semiconductor crystals called QDs that are being developed for the analysis of biological systems. In the presence of a light source, these QDs emit specific colors of light depending upon their size. QDs of different sizes can be attached to biological molecules allowing researchers to follow these molecules simultaneously during biological processes with a single screening tool. When used as disease screening tool, these QDs offer quicker, less laborious DNA and antibody screening compared with more traditional methods.[111] Use of nanoscale particles and coatings is also being pursued for drug delivery systems to achieve improved timed release of the active ingredients or delivery to specific organs or cell types. New developments in nanotechnology have led to optical nanosensor systems with nanoscale dimensions that are suitable for intracellular measurements. The use of such nanosensors for monitoring in vivo biological processes in single living cells could greatly improve current knowledge of cellular functions. Biosensors with optical transduction can involve fiber optics for chemical sensors and biosensors.[112–114]

One of the most active areas of research for NM applications is in medicine. Nanosized liposomes have been used to encapsulate anticancer drugs for the treatment of various diseases.[115–134] A number of studies using magnetic NPs in the analyses of blood, urine, and other body fluids to speed up separation and improve selectivity are ongoing.[15,16,23–26,32,33,36,51,52,59,108,109,135–153] Several scientists at academic and industrial institutions have developed engineered fluorescent NMs that form the basis for new detection technologies.[9,25,33,35,49,66,68,78,100,135,154–173] These biocompatible NMs are used in new devices and systems for infectious and genetic disease diagnosis, treatment, and for drug discovery.[15–17,139,174] Recent studies show that NMs can be effective in delivering a variety of vaccine antigens/epitopes with enhancements of antibody and/or cellular responses.[30,108,109,135,154,175–177,178] Chitosan, in particular, is a novel nasal delivery system for vaccines and inorganic particles[38,179] with sizes varying from 40 nm to <1 μm. Parenteral injection routes (SC/IM/IP) with NM-based vaccines showed efficacy in the range of 40–800 nm NMs.[180–182] A well-recognized obstacle with the use of NMs in biomolecule delivery is that they are too rapidly cleared from the body.[30,123,183–185] However, NMs larger than 10 nm will avoid single pass renal clearance and the presence of negative charge minimizes nonspecific interaction with proteins and cells to achieve pharmacokinetic (PK) manipulations.[30] These NMs can be highly effective when readily taken up by antigen-presenting cells.

It has been shown that the remarkable recognition capabilities of biomolecules when combined with the unique properties of NMs can lead to novel tissue substitutes, biological electronics such as biosensors, sensitive diagnostic systems, and controlled drug delivery systems with significantly improved performances. In this light, NMs can be divided into three major categories according to their geometry, such as equiaxed, one-dimensional (or fibrous), and two-dimensional (or lamellar) forms. Selected examples and typical applications of such NMs and their use in biomedical applications are highlighted in Table 1.1.

Many nano-enabled medical products have entered the market to date and as the applications grow and infiltrate complicated diseases such as all kinds of cancer, cardiac, and neurodegenerative disorders, infection, tissue engineering, etc., the market is predicted to reach considerable growth in the near future.[1] This has been shown in the application of NMs in biomedical sciences that posted a year-on-year growth of over 37% in 2009.[1] In 2013, this area is expected to close at US$750 M with a CAGR of over 30% since 2010. The US leads the nanotechnology market and accounts for an estimated share of around 35% of the global nanotechnology market.[1]

TABLE 1.1 Medical Applications of some NMs

NMs	Medical applications	References
Gold	Pregnancy test	Gourley[186]
Gold	Diagnosis of various diseases	Wagner et al.,[26] Nakamura et al.,[187] Sabuncu et al.,[188] Ambrosi et al.[189]
Gold	Biosensors	Ambrosi et al.,[189] Doering et al.,[43] El-Sayed et al.,[46] Li et al.[190–192]
Iron oxide	Magnetic resonance imaging	Bulte and Kraitchman,[193] Yang et al.[108]
Iron oxide	Drug and vaccine delivery	Aguilar et al.,[33,154] Hans and Lowman,[194] Mahmoudi et al.,[15] Sajja et al.,[175] Yang et al.[108]
Iron oxide	Cell separation	Xu et al.,[32] Aguilar et al.[33]
Iron oxide	Tissue regeneration	Bulte et al.[138]
Hydroxyapatite	Tissue regeneration	Hong et al.,[195,197] Freed et al.,[196] Webster et al.,[10] Shuai et al.[198]
Titanium oxide	Protein adsorption	Topoglidis et al.[71]
Titanium and ceramics	Implants	Albrektsson and Wennerberg,[199] Att et al.,[200] Ben-Nissan and Choi,[201] Cochran et al.,[202] Kim et al.[203]
Titanium	Biosensor	Topoglidis et al.[71]
QDs	Fluorescence, IR imaging	Aguilar et al.,[35] Byers and Hitchman,[157] Cai et al.,[158] Xu et al.,[78,172] Surendiran et al.,[25] Gao et al.,[160] Michalet et al.[29]
QDs	Vaccine delivery	Aguilar et al.[154], Pusic[30]
QDs	Biosensors	Aguilar et al.,[33] Geiber et al.,[49] Lidke et al.,[163] Smith et al.,[167] Xu et al.,[173] Thuurer et al.[204]
Chitosan	Drug and gene delivery	Calvo et al.,[205] Hu et al.,[206] Illum et al.,[207] Aspden et al.,[208] Erbacher et al.,[209] Pille et al.[210]
PLGA	Drug delivery	Govender et al.,[211] Panyam et al.,[212,213] Wang et al.[214]
Liposome	Drug delivery	Allen,[115] Drummond,[118] Fetterly and Straubinger,[119] Jin and Ye,[122] Moghimi and Szebeni[125]

(Continued)

TABLE 1.1 Medical Applications of some NMs—Cont'd

NMs	Medical applications	References
Carbon nanotubes	Tissue regeneration	Tran et al.,[215] Bakry et al.[216]
Carbon nanotubes	Biosensors	Wang et al.[217]
Polymers	Gene delivery	Dang and Leong,[218] Govender et al.[211]
Polymers	Drug delivery	Ge et al.,[219] Gelperina et al.,[220] Lindhart,[221] Kreuter[222]
Polymers and nanocomposites	Tissue engineering	Armentano et al.,[223] Koegler and Griffith[224]

In January 2012, Cientifica[225] tracked the growth of government funding to a total of $67.5 billion from 2000 to 2011. They have indicated that nano-enabled drug delivery therapeutics will grow from a current value of $2.3 billion to $136 billion by the year 2021 and will represent approximately 15% of the global nanotechnology market in 2021. It is the healthcare sector that offers the greatest opportunity to add value to NMs with China as the fastest-growing market sector[225]. The CEO of Cientifica, Tim Harper, stated that drug delivery with NMs offers higher margins than other uses of NMs and allows manufacturers to harness more value than supplying materials for paint or sunscreen[225]. The drug and pharmaceutical industry benefits from the formulation of nano-enabled drugs because this enables the extension of patents maintaining if not increasing their existing revenue sources. By 2021, the global growth in the drug delivery market will be led by Asia with a CAGR of 32.5%. The largest Asian market for nano-based drug delivery systems will be China that will have a worth more than $18 billion and representing 43% of the Asian market.[225] In other countries, France is forecast to surpass Japan as a drug delivery market within 10 years.

BCC research, on the other hand, reported that the global nanomedicine market reached $63.8 billion in 2010 and $72.8 billion in 2011.[226] They predicted that the market is expected to grow to $130.9 billion by 2016 at a CAGR of 12.5% in 2011–2016.[226] They reported that the central nervous system (CNS) products market reached $11.7 billion in 2010 and $14.0 billion in 2011 and expect this market to grow to $29.5 billion by 2016 with a CAGR of 16.1% in 2011–2016 while the anticancer products market reached $25.2 billion in 2010 and $28.0 billion in 2011[226]. It is expected to reach $46.7 billion by 2016 at a CAGR of 10.8% in 2011–2016, they said in the report (Figure 1.2).

Chapter 2 of this book provides an overview of the various NMs that are currently very useful in nanomedicine. A few of the sNMs were provided with

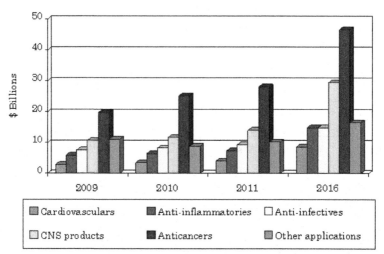

FIGURE 1.2 Summary of nanomedical global sales by therapeutic in 2009–2016 ($ billions). *From BCC[226] publisher of technology market research reports based in Wellesley, Mass, 19 May 2012. (For color version of this figure, the reader is referred to the online version of this book)*

protocols for synthesis while others that are more well documented in some other references were given an overview. There are NMs at their infancy and require much more testing before their full potential in medicine can be realized. For this reason, only a selected group of NMs that are well advanced in their medical applications was given much attention. In addition, selected current NM characterization techniques were included to provide an overview of how the properties of NMs are established. Again, there are many other techniques at their infancy of development that were not included in this chapter. Instruments that are useful for NM topography, chemical composition, size, and shape analysis techniques of particular benefit to NM characterization were discussed. For clearer and better understanding of NMs and their interactions with biological systems for medical applications, novel high-resolution imaging and analysis tools, which allow for easy sample preparation and in situ monitoring, are still needed.[28]

In Chapter 3, the focus is on the synthesis and conversion of NMs into biocompatible forms in order that the physical, electronic, chemical, and optical properties of NMs can be exploited to benefit biomolecules that are useful in medicine. The novel and unique quantum mechanical effects leading to varied and unexpected physicochemical properties enable nanotechnology to provide promising solutions for nanomedicine. The NMs that have been exploited in medicine are usually produced in organic solvents making them hydrophobic and incompatible to biological molecules. Alongside the organic synthesis of NMs, conversion methods into the water-soluble form to make them biocompatible have also emerged. Various techniques such as ligand exchange, encapsulation, and polymer coating have been developed

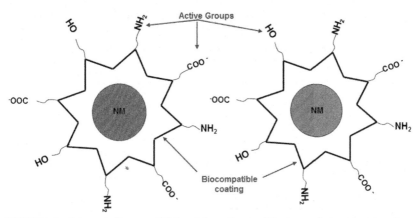

FIGURE 1.3 Schematic diagram of NMs and the surface modification to allow conjugation of various molecules of medical relevance (green sphere—fluorescent NMs; gray sphere—nonfluorescent NM). *(For color version of this figure, the reader is referred to the online version of this book)*

and used in the preparation of water soluble NMs. The water-soluble NMs that are now currently commercially available contain functional groups on their surfaces making them easy to manipulate for various medical applications. Functional groups anchored to the surface of NMs during synthesis or modification into their water soluble forms provide reactive sites for subsequent bioconjugation reactions. These active functional groups often involve sulfhydryl –SH, carboxyl –COOH, amine –NH_2, hydroxyl –OH, and others that allow attachment of biomolecules through various bioconjugation or crosslinking chemistry (Figure 1.3). Linkers for these NMs are carbodiimide, succinimide, maleidiimide, and bifunctional crosslinkers through direct attachment (hydrophobic or electrostatic interactions) and sometimes through biodin–avidin system. These various methods have their unique qualities and applications along with inherent disadvantages, such as possible low yield and loss of functionality after conjugation, which researches are actively studying to solve and improve. NMs that are found in biosensors offer high sensitivity and high stability that are easier to use, faster, and more inexpensive as compared with conventional diagnostics methods. In addition, inexpensive instrumentation that accompanies these NM-based biosensors are also currently being developed. These novel biosensors use the small dimensions of NMs which allow their assembly into barcodes and high density arrays to detect multiple analytes using miniature hand held sensing devices that may only need light emitting diodes as power source.

Nanotechnology has also opened up new perspectives in the development of biosensors that are applied to medicine, food, agriculture, industry, and environmental monitoring. The nanotechnological innovations promise to improve the sensitivity, accuracy, and flexibility for the analysis of chemical and biochemical compounds. In addition, NMs allow a cost-effective production of miniaturized devices with the opportunity of using disposables in various fields of application for faster, automated, and less subjective or error prone. In addition, the nano-enabled biosensors allow for the analysis of genetic structures and their influence on cellular functions and this shifts the medicine focus from diagnosis and treatment to identification and prevention. By combining nano-enabled diagnosis and therapeutics, nanotechnology is predicted to eventually lead to production of individually tailored patient-specific treatments and therapies.

Inorganic semiconductor QDs have emerged as novel fluorescent labels in biosensing and imaging, and are substituting the conventional organic fluorophores. This is ascribed to great advantages of inorganic nanocrystals over the conventional organic dyes. Semiconductor QDs exhibit broad excitation profiles, narrow and symmetric emission spectra, high photostability and high quantum efficiency, and excellent multiplexed detection capability.[62,227] For example, QDs with different emission wavelengths can be excited by a single excitation source, while organic dyes with different emission wavelengths must be excited by multiple excitation sources. Demand of simultaneous detection of more targets in single assay drives the development of inorganic nanocrystal-based fluorescent probes to replace organic fluorophores.[49,158,163,228,229]

Most of past research on the nanostructured biosensors was the proof-of-concept work that demonstrated the advantages of NMs and nanostructures. In the future, more efforts need to be made to move the proof-of-concept studies to the applications of biosensors to the real-world samples. One trend of future research is the integration of nanostructured sensors with microfluidics to form lab-on-chip devices. Furthermore, more studies need to be performed to integrate the nanostructured sensors with signal-processing instruments to build portable devices for on-site measurement of analytes to meet the need for on-time (real-time) monitoring of the targets of interest and rapid assessment of risks. One of the resulting examples is the point-of-care device that has an increasing need in the commercial market.

Reports on the development and application of submicron-sized fiberoptic chemical sensors with distal diameters between 20 and 500 nm have been used with submicron spatial resolution that is achievable using near-field scanning optical microscopy (NSOM).[29] It is worth noting that, different from the traditional separation between transducers and molecular recognition probes, a novel tactic is to integrate transducers with molecular recognition probes to form nano-transducers that recognize the binding events and actively transduce sensing signals simultaneously.[230]

In Chapter 5, the role of NMs for drug delivery in cancer, tumor, and other types of diseases is discussed including a few examples of drug delivery systems (Figure 1.4) for optimizing the effect of drugs and reducing toxic side effects. Several nanotechnologies, mostly based on NMs can facilitate drug delivery to tumors but these have to be carefully and meticulously engineered before they can perform

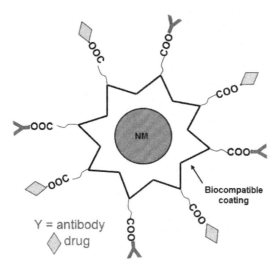

Y = antibody
◇ drug

FIGURE 1.4   Schematic diagram of NMs that are used for targeted drug delivery (green sphere—fluorescent NMs; gray sphere—nonfluorescent NM). *(For interpretation of the references to color in this figure legend, the reader is referred to the online version of this book)*

the functions they are designed for. Excellent candidates for drug delivery purposes must be small (less than 100 nm), nontoxic, biodegradable, biocompatible, does not aggregate, avoids the reticulo-endothelial system (RES) uptake, and escapes opsonization, noninflammatory, with prolonged circulation time making the drug more efficient for therapy and, therefore, more cost effective. Many drugs in the market that are now available for human use are already nano-enabled. The ability of these drugs to minimize the side effects that are normally observed in conventional drugs opens up doors for applications of NMs as safer alternatives to drug delivery. Aside from the requirements of size, charge, shape, surface modifications, loading, and other chemical properties to effectively deliver drugs using the NM carrier systems other challenges need further attention. These studies need to focus on the interaction of NMs and their hosts in terms of biodistribution, organ accumulation, degradation and/or toxicity, damage of cellular structures or inflammatory foreign body effects, and genetic damage. It is essential to investigate the possible adverse effects or toxicity of nanocarriers.[231–233] But, the NM drug delivery system is still in its infancy. Research protocols like absorption, distribution, metabolism, and elimination (ADME), and drug metabolism and pharmacokinetics (DMPKs) will definitely be part of further studies on NM drug delivery systems in the future[184,234,235]. The PKs and excretion routes of the various NMs used as drug delivery systems demand exhaustive research. The path that the nano-enabled drugs take after entry into the living system depends on many factors. The NM properties that allow its in vivo imaging may be the most useful property for elucidating the ADME and PK in nanodrug delivery systems.

NMs have also now been used for drug formulations. A few of these examples are discussed in this chapter and more on targeted drug delivery is discussed in Chapter 5. Drugs that are formulated with polymer coated NMs and iron oxide NMs coated with dextran have emerged as very sensitive contrast agents for magnetic resonance imaging (MRI). Additionally, cancer drugs have also been loaded in NPs for ease of delivery. More studies are underway for the specific targeting of these drugs so that effect on healthy cells can be minimized while focusing the unloading of the drugs on the sick cells such as cancer cells. Other studies have also focused on the use of NMs for eradicating viral infections, which have been one of the most difficult challenges of the human population during the last century and into the millennium. Several studies have also been focused on the use of NMs for the delivery of vaccines especially those diseases that have no existing vaccines in the market. Thus, transforming the NMs into their water-soluble forms opened seemingly endless possibilities of their applications in medicine. Such applications go from detection to treatment of various diseases that may be molecular in nature or may be caused by infective materials. More studies toward improving success in attachment of biomolecules on the NM surfaces or for loading of molecules into the NMs are necessary to ensure successful incorporation of relevant and important molecules for medical applications. The succeeding chapters will focus more seriously on the various applications that have been introduced and partly discussed in this chapter.

Chapter 6 focuses on the new nano-enabled medical devices that are used in various medical applications. The medical area of nanotechnology has been growing and has been progressively assimilated into a variety of disciplines including neurosurgery, but this area of application is less well characterized compared to other organ systems.[162] Recently, nanotechnology has offered promising potential for a wide range of utilities including new therapeutic options for glioblastoma multiforme, neurprotection against oxidative stress, nerve nanorepair, nanodiagnosis of Alzheimer's disease, nanoimaging with NPs and QDs, nanomanipulation of CNS with surgical nanobots, and nanoneuromodulation with nanofibres and nanowires.[162] The applications of NMs as components or as additives for various medical devices have led to improved biocompatibility and functionality as nanorobots, novel nanochips, and nanoimplants serving as tissue substitutes, tissue regeneration, prostheses, tissue engineering, and cell repair. Although a majority of these applications of NMs in medicine are still in the laboratory, a few are already in full blast clinical use. More prototypes and more research are necessary to harness the full potential of NMs as medical devices.

In Chapter 7, the area of focus is the application of NMs for Pharmacology, which has definitely been revolutionized by the coming of the nanotechnology era that has seen a boost at the end of the twentieth century and toward the beginning of the twenty-first century. NMs R&D continue to engineer various types of NMs to diagnose disease and health conditions; to recognize pathogenic infections; to locate, attach, and penetrate target tissue or structures or pathogens; and dispense the payload of drugs or biological compound to the targeted regions of the body. This is the area now known as nanopharmacology. This chapter discusses various NMs for nanopharmacology and the issues that may become an outcome of the applications of NMs in pharmaceuticals.

Chapter 8 is one of the most important chapters of this book because it focuses on the safety and toxicity of the various NMs. To date, various governments have become more aware of the possible benefits as well as the dangers of exposure to NMs in various consumer products. This awareness has led to various guidelines worldwide.[236–239] The need for proper characterization of the various properties of the NMs has also been recognized as essential for the evaluation of the possible effects on health and environmental safety. However, limitations in the risk assessment of NMs are still preventing proper evaluations, and probably, also the possible adoption of strict regulations. The lack of high quality exposure and dose-related data for humans and the environment is one of the major drawbacks in adopting regulations for use and applications of NMs. There is also the difficulty in how to quantify the presence of NMs reproducibly on a routine basis in various substrates, which is due to the lack of reliable and standardized measurement techniques. These difficulties must first be overcome before regulations for screening/monitoring of nanoscale particles in sensitive work areas can be implemented. The biggest challenges lie in the measurement of NMs in the air, water, and land. This consequently holds as well for food and food products that come from water and land. Currently, the information on the presence of NMs relies on information provided by manufacturers. The detection of NMs in consumer products suffers from the difficulty in discriminating between background signals and added NMs. This is also complicated by the coating proteins and other biomolecules on NMs exposed to biological matrices. In addition, exposure estimation is also hampered by lack of information on product use and use of multiple products containing NMs. Better instrumentation, toxicological techniques suited to NMs, and regulation standards are necessary to pre-empt possible short-term or long-term harmful effects if there are any.

1.3 HISTORICAL AND FUTURE PERSPECTIVE

The beginning of the concept of nanotechnology without the word itself was in a talk given by physicist Richard Feynman at an American Physical Society meeting at Caltech on 29 December 1959.[240–243] In this talk entitled "There's Plenty of Room at the Bottom", Feynman focused on a process which involved the ability to manipulate down to the individual atoms and molecules using a set of precise tools to build and operate another proportionally smaller set, and so on down to the smallest needed scale.[242]

Feynman suggested that in principle, it should be possible to make tiny machines that can specifically arrange atoms as needed and mechanically manipulate chemical synthesis. In his talk, he presented the idea of building a tiny, swallowable surgical robot by developing a set of one-quarter-scale manipulator hands slaved to the operator's hands to build one-quarter-scale machine tools analogous to those found in any machine shop. This set of small tools would then be used by the small hands to build and operate 10 sets of one-sixteenth-scale hands and tools, and so forth, culminating in perhaps a billion tiny factories to achieve multiple equivalent operations, which was coincidentally anticipated earlier by science fiction author, Robert A. Heinlein in his story called "Waldo" in 1942.[244]

Feynman also suggested the idea to shrink computing devices down their physical limits, where "wires should be 10 or 100 atoms in diameter".[242] In 2009, Samsung announced large-scale production of devices built with 30 nm technology as envisioned by Feynman.[242] Feynman also suggested that focused electron beams could write nanoscale features on a surface, which we now call e-beam lithography.[242] He gave out the idea of the possibilities of improved microscopes that could visualize objects that are much smaller than is possible with scanning electron microscopes. These ideas are now in the form of scanning tunneling microscope (STM), transmission electron microscope (TEM), atomic force microscope (AFM), and other examples of probe microscopy. He discussed complex, active, nanoscale biological mechanisms that have now become the basis of biotechnology, which has delivered what are in some ways the most advanced type of nanotechnologies.[242]

Thus, Feynman basically envisioned a path to the atomically precise world from the top to the smallest detail by building smaller and smaller machines, and ultimately using these to build machines the smallest possible scale by "manipulating atom by atom".[242] At this talk, Feynman offered a prize of $1000 for the first individuals to solve challenges. In November 1960, the first challenge which involved the construction of a tiny motor was achieved by William McLellan to Feynman's surprise.[242] McLellan was a meticulous craftsman that developed the first tiny motor using conventional tools without advancing the art. In the second challenge, the letters were to be scaled down small enough so as to be able to fit the entire Encyclopedia Britannica on the head of a pin, by writing the information from a book page on a surface 1/25,000 smaller in linear scale.[242] A Stanford graduate student, Tom Newman, successfully reduced the first paragraph of A Tale of Two Cities by 1/25,000, and collected the second Feynman prize in 1985.[245]

It was not until 1974 that the term "nanotechnology" was defined by Tokyo Science University Professor Norio Taniguchi in a paper:[246] "Nanotechnology mainly consists of the processing of, separation, consolidation, and deformation of materials by one atom or by one molecule." The significance of this concept was popularized in depth by Dr K. Eric Drexler, who promoted the technological significance of nanoscale phenomena and devices through conferences, speeches, and his books entitled *Engines of Creation: The Coming Era of Nanotechnology* in 1986[240] and *Nanosystems: Molecular Machinery, Manufacturing, and Computation.*[243] Drexler's book, the *Engines of Creation: The Coming Era of Nanotechnology* is considered the first book on nanotechnology. The first publication of a cover article in nanotechnology over 20 years back, swept into the minds of a large, science-aware public quite abruptly, in November 1986, when nearly a million readers encountered the cover story of a leading general-audience, science-oriented magazine of that time, OMNI while a month before then, the term and concept had been known to very few earliest readers of *Engines of Creation.*[247] Feynman's speeches, his stature as a Nobel laureate, and as an iconic figure in twentieth century science helped advocates of nanotechnology and provided a valuable intellectual link to the past but it was Drexler who popularized the concept of nanotechnology.[248]

Major developments in instrumentation started nanotechnology and the nanoscience in the early 1980s: cluster science and the invention of the STM.[249] This development led to the discovery of fullerenes in 1985 and carbon nanotubes a few years later. Don Eigler from IBM was the first to manipulate atoms using an STM in 1989.[250] He used 35 xenon atoms to spell out the IBM logo for which he shared the 2010 Kavli Prize in Nanoscience.[251] The study of the synthesis and properties of semiconductor nanocrystals emerged and led to a rapid increase in the number of metal and metal oxide NPs and QDs. The atomic force microscope (AFM or SFM) was invented six years after the STM was invented. The AFM has a very high resolution on the order of fractions of a nanometer that is >1000 times better than the optical diffraction limit. The first commercially available AFM was introduced in 1989, which became the instrument of choice for imaging, measuring, and manipulating objects at the nanoscale.

In the early 1990s Huffman and Kraetschmer, of the University of Arizona, discovered and published how to synthesize and purify large quantities of fullerenes.[252] They described the material as a new form of pure, solid carbon consisting of a somewhat disordered hexagonal close packing of soccer-ball-shaped C_{60} molecules. The molecules were characterized by infrared spectra and X-ray diffraction as well as by mass spectroscopy. This publication was followed by an upsurge of characterization and functionalization by investigators in various laboratories. In 1992, Dr T. Ebbesen published the large-scale synthesis of carbon nanotubes.[253] In his method, a variant of the standard arc-discharge technique for fullerene synthesis under a helium atmosphere was used to produce bulk nanotube material with conductivity of about 100 S/cm[11].

In 2004, the Royal Society and Royal Academy of Engineering reported on the implications of nanoscience and nanotechnologies,[254] which was a result of Prince Charles' concerns about nanotechnology and molecular manufacturing. The report covers possible risks such as NP toxicology and provides an overview of several nanoscale fields.

It was in the early 2000s that the use of nanotechnology in commercial products began. To this date, there are non-nanotechnology-specific regulatory agencies that cover nano-enabled products. Some products and processes are controlled under existing regulations but there are insufficient regulations of the NMs, which enable some nano-enabled products to be released without coverage by any regulations. This is particularly the case for titanium dioxide (TiO$_2$) that is used in sunscreen. [255,256] The US FDA reviewed the immediate health effects of exposure but did not review its impacts for aquatic ecosystems when the sunscreen rubs off, nor did the EPA, or any other agency.[257] In similar context, the Australian Therapeutic Goods Administration (TGA)[258] approved the use of NMs in sunscreens (without inclusion in the package label) on the basis that although NMs TiO$_2$ and zinc oxide (ZnO) produce free radicals and oxidative DNA damage in vitro, these were unlikely to pass into the stratum corneum of human skin. This decision was short sighted because it did not consider prolonged use especially on children with cut skin, the elderly with thin skin, people with diseased skin, or use over other skin imperfections. [259] A more thorough investigation of the long-term effects of NMs on the skin shows that the uncoated anatase form of TiO$_2$ undergoes a photocatalytic reaction that degraded the surface of newly installed prepainted steel roofs in areas that came in contact with sunscreen coated hands of workers.[260] The rapid growth in nanotechnology and the fast upsurge of commercial products in the international market are more than likely to create more gaps in regulation such as these. Aside from titanium dioxide and zinc oxide NPs which are found in sunscreen, cosmetics, and some food products, silver NPs are also found in food packaging, clothing, disinfectants, and household appliances such as Silver Nano.[261,262]

In the US, foresight on the potential of nanotechnology was immediately picked up resulting in the creation of the National Nanotechnology, which is a federal nanotechnology R&D program.[19] The goals of NNI are to advance a world-class nanotechnology R&D program, foster the transfer of new technologies into products for commercial and public benefit, develop and sustain educational resources, a skilled workforce, and the supporting infrastructure and tools to advance nanotechnology, as well as to support responsible development of nanotechnology.[19] The NNI was initially proposed by Mihail Roco to the Office of Science and Technology Policy to President Bill Clinton in 1999, who advocated nanotechnology development. In 2003, President George W. Bush further increased funding for nanotechnology and signed the Twenty-First Century Nanotechnology Research and Development Act into law,[263] which authorized expenditures totaling US$3.63 billion over four years for five of the participating agencies.

1.4 THE FUTURE OF NANOTECHNOLOGY

Various efforts in the different sectors of nanotechnology ascertain the development and discovery of many new materials with novel properties and new applications. Different approaches in research related to nanofabrication and NM synthesis are continuing to grow with the goal of developing more efficient, less expensive, and more reproducible large-scale manufacturing techniques. These manufacturing techniques are expected to combine the best aspects of top-down processes, such as microlithography, with bottom-up processes based on self-assembly and self-organization processes allowing two- and three-dimensional devices and NM fabrication to create diverse molecular and nanoscale materials. In addition, these large-scale manufacturing techniques would allow many of the new and promising nanostructures, such as carbon nanotubes, magnetic NMs, inorganic and organic nanostructures, polymers, and QDs, to be rapidly assembled into more complex structures for various applications. New devices will have efficient and improved electronic capabilities and new NMs will have better performance properties. The large-scale manufacturing techniques will lead to better and less expensive nanopowders, NPs, and nanocomposites for a wide variety of applications.

Aside from improved large-scale manufacturing, the future holds promise toward the development of improved instrumentation for the characterization, detection, and quantification of various NMs. Although existing instrumentation provides the needed analysis of NMs for the current applications, more sophisticated instruments are needed to reach the ultimate application of NMs at the molecular level. To date, instruments are capable of detecting NMs at the nano-Molar concentration levels, which are still too high as observed in the current various applications. Future instruments need to detect down to the pico-Molar or even down to the atto- and zepto-Molar levels to further use the single molecule capabilities of NMs. These ultra low levels are useful for in vivo drug delivery, vaccine delivery, and imaging, where the NMs are given to an animal or to a human. At the same time, more sophisticated instruments are needed to detect levels of NMs in the workplace, the environment, in air, water, and in soil in order to be able to monitor levels that may be toxic to living things.

Different possible applications of NMs in the future abound. For instance, metabolic processes in the living systems can be studied through tiny nanorobots that can be equipped with various probes before these are deployed. Targeting molecules that are designed to find specific receptors in the living system will allow the nanorobot to go where it has to go and stay for the period of time designated in order to gather sufficient data for the analysis. Thus, new and improved NMs can be used for molecular level diagnostics in living systems.

A combination approach is also more than likely for the future of NMs in medicine. To date, many NMs have been modified with two or more biomolecular components in order to allow diagnostics and therapeutic capabilities, a new emerging area today called nanotheranostics. Nanotheranostics is envisioned to be able to provide the impossible today during cancer therapy. This involves, precise targeting of the cancer tissue/cells and diagnosis of therapeutic effects of drugs given to patients in a single event. With engineered NMs, it will be possible to modify the NMs to target only the liver if the cancer or the disease is in the liver, or wherever the disease is, by precise control and manipulation of the NMs so that they will bring the drug or drugs only to the disease-affected tissue or cells and release it there as well. By precise targeting, harmful side effects of drugs can potentially be minimized if not eliminated completely. In addition, aside from precise delivery of the drug load, the NMs can be used to detect the degree of treatment. This is what nanotheranostic offers: a combination of efficient treatment and precise diagnosis.

It is within the realm of possibilities to make implantable, in vivo diagnostic and monitoring devices that approach the size of cells using NMs. New and improved biocompatible NMs and nanomechanical components could lead to fabrication of new materials and components for implants, artificial organs, and greatly improved mechanical, visual, auditory, and other prosthetic devices. With continued support for R&D efforts from the various sectors, this may be closer to reality than we can imagine at this point in time.

The current status of nanotechnology resembles that of semiconductor and electronics technology in 1947 during the development of the first transistor that welcomed the Information Age, which bloomed in the 1990s. The lessons learned from the history of the semiconductor industry teach us that the invention of individual devices does not immediately unleash the power of the technology but takes time until the fabrication costs are controlled down to low levels; and the devices are assembled, connected to the outside, and controlled to perform a certain function that is of benefit to a large population. Similarly, success in nanotechnology will require an era of advances in the development of processes to integrate nanoscale components into devices at a repeatable, reliable, and at a low-cost process. Large-scale techniques for manufacturing fault-tolerant devices and equivalent lots of NMs will have to be invented. At the current widespread application of nanotechnology, we expect that its societal impact may be many times greater than that of the microelectronics and computer revolution.

The potential of nanomedicine may emerge in the very near future, 5–10 years from now, when the design to construct artificial nanorobots with nanometer-scale parts like molecular gears and bearings is completed.[241] These nanorobots will be composed of autonomous subsystems including onboard sensors, motors, manipulators, power supplies, and molecular computers. The trick to achieving this structure is a molecular or atomic level manufacturing technique that can build a molecular structure through level-by-level positional assembly. The process will involve repetitious part-by-part and level-by-level assembly until the final product is fully assembled. Such a process is yet to be developed and reported in the near future. To date, only a few molecular level manufacturing techniques have been seen and majority of these apply to NM synthesis, many of which are still at a small-scale level. A few more years are predicted before large-scale processes for QDs, iron oxide, and other NMs can be mastered to reproducibly fabricate stable, uniform, and inexpensive NMs that can cause the costs to appreciably go down. The lower costs of NMs will be followed by more research and faster development in the applications of NMs for medicine.

The succeeding chapters of this book focus on the various current statuses of R&D in NMs and their medical applications. A few processes and protocols are included in each chapter that can be used and followed by those who are interested in starting their own research in the areas of nanomedicine. The author envisions that the students, scientists, engineers, and the professionals will gain much needed awareness in NMs and their various applications in nanomedicine. At the same time, this book also provides sufficient information to apply the concepts discussed and the processes presented to improve on existing processes or to begin new R&Ds to develop new applications of NMs in medicine and/or to develop novel biocompatible NMs for medical applications. It is the author's vision to inspire more interest in the medical applications of NMs.

REFERENCES

1. RNCOS *Nanotechnology Market Forecast to 2014*. 2012.
2. Ahmad, M. B.; Shameli, K.; Darroudi, M.; Yunus, W.; Ibrahim, N. A. Synthesis and Characterization of Silver/Clay Nanocomposites by Chemical Reduction Method. *Am. J. Appl. Sciences* **2009,** *6,* 1909–1914.
3. Borum-Nicholas, L.; Wilson, J. O. C. Surface Modification of Hydroxyapatite. Part I. Dodecyl Alcohol. *Biomaterials* **2003,** *24,* 367–369.
4. Carbó-Argibay, E.; Rodríguez-González, B.; Pastoriza-Santos, I.; Pérez-Juste, J.; Liz-Marán, L. M. Growth of Pentatwinned Gold Nanorods into Truncated Decahedra. *Nanoscale* **2010,** *2,* 2377–2383.
5. Huang, C.; Zusing Yang, Z.; Lee, K.; Chang, H. Synthesis of Highly Fluorescent Gold Nanoparticles for Sensing Mercury(II). *Angew. Chem. Int. Ed.* **2007,** *46,* 6824–6828.
6. Li, J.; Lu, X. L.; Zheng, Y. F. Effect of Surface Modified Hydroxyapatite on the Tensile Property Improvement of HA/PLA Composite. *Appl. Surf. Sci.* **2008,** *255,* 494–497.
7. Nasibulin, A. G.; Moisala, A.; Jiang, H.; Kauppinen, E. I. Carbon Nanotube Synthesis by a Novel Aerosol Method. *J. Nanopart. Res.* **2006,** *8,* 465–475.
8. Sau, T. K.; Murphy, C. J. Room Temperature, High-Yield Synthesis of Multiple Shapes of Gold Nanoparticles in Aqueous Solution. *J. Am. Chem. Soc.* **2004,** *126,* 8648–8649.
9. Su, H.; Xu, H.; Gao, S.; Dixon, J.; Aguilar, Z. P.; Wang, A., et al. Microwave Synthesis of Nearly Monodisperse Core/Multishell Quantum Dots with Cell Imaging Applications. *Nanoscale. Res. Lett.* **2010,** *5,* 625–630.
10. Webster, T. J.; Ergun, C. D.; Siegel, R. W.; Bizios, R. Enhanced Functions of Osteoclast-Like Cells on Nanophase Ceramics. *Biomaterials* **2001,** *22,* 1327–1333.
11. Barrett, T.; Ravizzini, G.; Choyke, P.; Kobayashi, H. Dendrimers in Medical Nanotechnology. *IEEE. Eng. Med. Biol. Mag.* **2009,** *28,* 12–22.
12. Bharali, D.; Khalil, M.; Gurbuz, M.; Simone, T.; Mousa, S. Nanoparticles and Cancer Therapy: A Concise Review with Emphasis on Dendrimers. *Int. J. Nanomedicine.* **2009,** *4,* 1–7.
13. Langer, R.; Vacanti, J. P. Tissue Engineering. *Science* **1993,** *260,* 9220–9926.
14. Li-Na, M.; Dian-Jun, L.; Zhen-Xin, W. Synthesis and Applications of Gold Nanoparticle Probes. *Chinese J. Anal. Chem.* **2010,** *38,* 1–7.
15. Mahmoudi, M.; Sant, S.; Wang, B.; Laurent, S.; Sen, T. Superparamagnetic Iron Oxide Nanoparticles (SPIONs): Development, Surface Modification and Applications in Chemotherapy. *Adv. Drug Deliv. Rev.* **2011,** *63,* 24–46.
16. Wilhelm, C.; Gazeau, F. Universal Cell Labelling with Anionic Magnetic Nanoparticles. *Biomaterials* **2008,** *29,* 3161–3174.
17. Xie, J.; Peng, S.; Brower, N.; Pourmand, N.; Wang, S. X.; Sun, S. One-Pot Synthesis of Monodisperse Iron Oxide Nanoparticles for Potential Biomedical Applications. *Pure. Applied Chem.* **2006,** *78,* 1003–1014.

18. Jia, L. Global Government Investments in Nanotechnologies. *Curr. Nanosci.* **2005,** *1,* 263–266.

19. NNI *National Nanotechnology Initiative.* 2012, Available from: www.nano.gov.

20. USPCAST *The Fourth Assessment of the National Nanotechnology Initiative.* 2012, Available from: http://nano.gov/sites/default/files/pub_resource/pcast_4th_review_2012_final_for_upload.pdf.

21. RNCOS *US Nanotechnology Market Leading Globally from "Nanotechnology Forecast to 2014".* 2012, Available from: http://www.rncos.com/Report/IM376.htm.

22. Brigger, I.; Dubernet, C.; Couvreur, P. Nanoparticles in Cancer Therapy and Diagnosis. *Adv. Drug Del. Rev.* **2002,** *54,* 631–651.

23. Gong, J.; Liang, Y.; Huang, Y.; Chen, J.; Jiang, J.; Shen, G., et al. Ag/SiO(2) Core-Shell Nanoparticle-Based Surface-Enhanced Raman Probes for Immunoassay of Cancer Marker using Silica-Coated Magnetic Nanoparticles as Separation Tools. *Biosens. Bioelectron.* **2006,** *22,* 1501–1507.

24. Osterfeld, S. J.; Yu, H.; Gaster, R. S.; Caramuta, S.; Xu, L.; Han, S., et al. Multiplex Protein Assays based on Real-Time Magnetic Nanotag Sensing. *PNAS* **2008,** *105,* 20637–20640.

25. Surendiran, A.; Sandhiya, S.; Pradhan, S. C.; Adithan, C. Novel Applications of Nanotechnology in Medicine. *Indian J. Med. Res.* **2009,** *130,* 689–701.

26. Wagner, W.; Dullaart, A.; Bock, A. K.; Zweck, A. The Emerging Nanomedicine Landscape. *Nat. Biotechnol.* **2006,** *24,* 1211–1217.

27. Yun, Y.; Eteshola, E.; Bhattacharya, A.; Dong, Z.; Shim, J.; Conforti, L., et al. Tiny Medicine: Nanomaterial-Based Biosensors. *Sensors* **2009,** *9,* 9275–9299.

28. Liu, H.; Webster, T. J. Review: Nanomedicine for Implants: A Review of Studies and Necessary Experimental Tools, Cellular and Molecular Biology Techniques for Biomaterials Evaluation. *Biomaterials* **2007,** *28,* 354–369.

29. Michalet, X.; Pinaud, F. F.; Bentolila, L. A.; Tsay, J. M.; Doose, S.; Li, J. J.,Sundaresan, G.; Wu, A. M.; Gambhir, S. S.; Weiss, S. et al. Quantum dots for live cells, *in vivo* imaging, and diagnostics. *Science* **2005,** *307,* 538–544.

30. Pusic, K.; Xu, H.; Stridiron, A.; Aguilar, Z.; Wang, A. Hui, G. Blood Stage Merozoite Surface Protein Conjugated to Nanoparticles Induce Potent Parasite Inhibitory Antibodies. *Vaccine* **2011,** *29,* 8898–8908.

31. Xu, H.; Aguilar, Z.; Wei, H.; Wang, A. Development of Semiconductor Nanomaterial Whole Cell Imaging Sensor on Silanized Microscope Slides. *Front Biosci. (Elite Ed.)* **2011,** *E3,* 1013–1024.

32. Xu, H.; Aguilar, Z. P.; Yang, L.; Kuang, M.; Duan, H.; Xiong, Y., et al. Antibody Conjugated Magnetic Iron Oxide Nanoparticles for Cancer Cell Separation in Fresh Whole Blood. *Biomaterials* **2011,** *32,* 9758–9765.

33. Aguilar, Z.; Aguilar, Y.; Xu, H.; Jones, B.; Dixon, J.; Xu, H., et al. Nanomaterials in Medicine. *Electrochem. Soc. Trans.* **2010,** *33,* 69–74.

34. Aguilar, Z.; Xu, H.; Dixon, J.; Wang, A. Blocking Non-Specific Uptake of Engineered Nanomaterials. *Electrochem. Soc. Trans.* **2010,** *25,* 37–48.

35. Aguilar, Z.; Xu, H.; Jones, B.; Dixon, J.; Wang, A. Semi Conductor Quantum Dots for Cell Imaging. *Mater. Res. Soc. Proc.* **2010,** , 1237, TT1206-1201.

36. Chen, G.; Shen, B.; Zhang, F.; Wu, J.; Xu, Y.; He, P., et al. A New Electrochemically Active-Inactive Switching Aptamer Molecular Beacon to Detect Thrombin Directly in Solution. *Biosens. Bioelectron.* **2010,** *25,* 2265–2269.

37. Chu, X.; Duan, D.; Shen, G.; Yu, R. Amperometric Glucose Biosensor Based on Electrodeposition of Platinum Nanoparticles onto Covalently Immobilized Carbon Nanotube Electrode. *Talanta.* **2007,** *71,* 2040–2047.
38. Clapp, A.; Medintz, I.; Mauro, J.; Fisher, B.; Bawendi, M; Mattoussi, H. Fluorescence Resonance Energy Transfer between Quantum Dot Donors and Dye-Labeled Protein Acceptors. *J. Am. Chem. Soc.* **2004,** *126,* 301–310.
39. Demers, L.; Mirkin, C.; Mucic, R.; Reynolds, R.; Letsinger, R.; Elghanian, R., et al. A Fluorescence-Based Method for Determining the Surface Coverage and Hybridization Efficiency of Thiol-Capped Oligonucleotides Bound to Gold Thin Films and Nanoparticles. *Anal. Chem.* **2000,** *72,* 5535–5541.
40. Diessel, E.; Grothe, K.; Siebert, H. M.; Warner, B. D.; Burmeister, J. Online Resistance Monitoring during Autometallographic Enhancement of Colloidal Au Labels for DNA Analysis. *Biosens. Bioelectron.* **2004,** *19,* 1229–1235.
41. Dinega, D. P.; Bawendi, M. G. A Solution-Phase Chemical Approach to a New Crystal Structure of Cobalt. *Angew. Chem.* **1999,** 1906–1909.
42. Dixit, S.; Goicochea, N.; Daniel, M.; Murali, A.; Bronstein, L.; De, M., et al. Quantum Dot Encapsulation in Viral Capsids. *Nano. Lett.* **2006,** *6,* 1993–1999.
43. Doering, W. E.; Piotti, M. E.; Natan, M. J.; Freeman, R. G. SERS as a Foundation for Nanoscale, Optically Detected Biological Labels. *Adv. Mater.* **2007,** *19,* 3100–3108.
44. Du, P.; Li, H.; Mei, Z.; Liu, S. Electrochemical DNA Biosensor for the Detection of DNA Hybridization with the Amplification of Au Nanoparticles and CdS Nanoparticles. *Bioelectrochemistry* **2009,** *75,* 37–43.
45. Dyadyusha, L.; Yin, H.; Jaiswal, S.; Brown, T.; Baumberg, J.; Booye, F., et al. Quenching of CdSe Quantum Dot Emission, a New Approach for Biosensing. *Chem. Commun.* **2005,** 3201–3203.
46. El-Sayed, I. H.; Huang, X.; El-Sayed, M. A. Surface Plasmon Resonance Scattering and Absorption of Anti-EGFR Antibody Conjugated Gold Nanoparticles in Cancer Diagnostics: Applications in Oral Cancer. *Nano. Lett.* **2005,** *5,* 829–834.
47. Escosura-Miniz, A. D.; Diaz-Freitas, B.; Sanchez-ESpinel, C.; Gonzalez-Fernandez, A.; Merkoci, A. Rapid Identification and Quantification of Tumour Cells using a Novel Electrocatalytic Method Based in Gold Nanoparticles. *Anal. Chem.* **2009,** *81,* 10268–10274.
48. Fujiwara, M.; Yamamoto, F.; Okamoto, K.; Shiokawa, K.; Nomura, R. Adsorption of Duplex DNA on Mesoporous Silicas: Possibility of Inclusion of DNA into their Mesopores. *Anal. Chem.* **2005,** *77,* 8138–8145.
49. Geiber, D.; Charbonnière, L. J.; Ziessel, R. F.; Butlin, N. G.; Löhmannsröben, H.; Hildebrandt, N. Quantum Dot Biosensors for Ultrasensitive Multiplexed Diagnostics. *Angew. Chem. Int. Ed.* **2010,** *49,* 1–6.
50. Gill, R.; Willner, I.; Shweky, I.; Banin, U. Fluorescence Resonance Energy Transfer in CdSe/ZnS-DNA Conjugates: Probing Hybridization and DNA Cleavage. *J. Phys. Chem. B.* **2005,** *109,* 23715–23719.
51. Haun, J. B.; Yoon, T.; Lee, H. J.; Weissleder, R. Magnetic Nanoparticle Biosensors. *Wiley. Interdiscip. Rev. Nanomed. Nanobiotechnol.* **2010,** *2,* 291–304.
52. Herr, J. K.; Smith, J. E.; Medley, C. D.; Shangguan, D.; Tan, W. Aptamer-Conjuagted Nanoparticles for Selective Collection and Detection of Cancer Cells. *Anal. Chem.* **2007,** *78,* 2918–2924.
53. Hutter, E.; Pileni, M. P. Detection of DNA Hybridization by Gold Nanoparticle Enhanced Transmission Surface Plasmon Resonance Spectroscopy. *J. Phys. Chen. B.* **2003,** *107,* 6497–6499.

54. Jaffrezic-Renault, N.; Martelet, C.; Chevolot, Y.; Cloarec, J. Biosensors and Bio-Bar Code Assays Based on Biofunctionalized Magnetic Microbeads. *Sesors* **2007,** *7,* 589–614.

55. Jiang, W.; Mardyani, S.; Fischer, H.; Chan, W. Design and Characterization of Lysine Cross-Linked Mercapto-Acid Biocompatible Quantum Dots. *Chem. Mater.* **2006,** *18,* 872–878.

56. Joyce, J. A.; Pollard, J. W. Microenvironmental Regulation of Metastasis. *Nat. Rev.* **2009,** *9,* 239–252.

57. Khanna, V. K. New-Generation Nano-Engineered Biosensors, Enabling Nanotechnologies and Nanomaterials. *Sens. Rev.* **2008,** *28,* 39–45.

58. Le Ru, E. C.; Etchegoin, P. G. *Principles of Surface-Enhanced Raman Spectroscopy and Related Plasmonic Effects*; Elsevier, 2009.

59. Lee, H.; Yoon, T.; Figueiredo, J.; Swirski, F. K.; Weissleder, R. Rapid Detection and Profiling of Cancer Cells in Fine-Needle Aspirates. *PNAS* **2009,** *106,* 12459–12464.

60. Li, J.; Zhao, X.; Zhao, Y.; Gu, Z. Quantum-Dot-Coated Encoded Silica Colloidal Crystals Beads for Multiplex Coding. *Chem. Commun.* **2009,** , 2329–2331.

61. Liu, J.; Lu, Y. A Colorimetric Lead Biosensor using DNAzyme-Directed Assembly of Gold Nanoparticles. *J. Am. Chem. Soc.* **2003,** *125,* 6642–6643.

62. Medintz, I.; Clapp, A.; Mattoussi, H.; Goldman, E.; Fisher, B.; Mauro, J. Self-Assembled Nanoscale Biosensors Based on Quantum Dot FRET Donors. *Nat. Mater.* **2003,** *2,* 630–638.

63. Merkoci, A. Nanoparticles-Based Strategies for DNA, Protein and cell Sensors. *Biosens. Bioelectron.* **2010,** *26,* 1164–1177.

64. Neely, A.; Perry, C.; Varisli, B.; Singh, A.; Arbneshi, T.; Senapati, D., et al. Ultrasensitive and Highly Selective Detection of Alzheimer's Disease Biomarker using Two-Photon Rayleigh Scattering Properties of Gold Nanoparticle. *ACS. Nano.* **2009,** *3,* 2834–2840.

65. Roy, R.; Hohng, S.; Ha, T. A Practical Guide to Single-Molecule FRET. *Nat. Methods* **2008,** *5,* 507–516.

66. Somers, R.; Bawendi, M.; Nocera, D. CdSe Nanocrystal based Chem-/Bio- Sensors. *Chem. Soc. Rev.* **2007,** *36,* 579–591.

67. Sun, L. F.; Liu, Z. Q.; Ma, X. C.; Zhong, Z. Y.; Tang, S. B.; Xiong, Z. T., et al. Growth of Carbon Nanotube Arrays using the Existing Array as a Substrate and their Raman Characterization. *Chem. Phys. Lett.* **2001,** *340,* 222–226.

68. Susumu, K.; Uyeda, H.; Medintz, I.; Pons, T.; Delehanty, J.; Mattoussi, H. Enhancing the Stability and Biological Functionalities of Quantum Dots via Compact Multifunctional Ligands. *J. Am. Chem. Soc.* **2007,** *129,* 13987–13996.

69. Tang, D.; Yuan, R.; Chai, Y.; Liu, Y.; Dai, J.; Zhong, X. Novel Potentiometric Immunosensor for Diphtheria Antigen based on Compound Nanoparticles and Bilayer Two Dimensional Sol-Gel as Matrices. *Anal. Bioanal. Chem.* **2005,** *381,* 674–680.

70. Tang, H.; Chen, J.; Yao, S.; Nie, L.; Deng, G.; Kuang, Y. Amperometric Glucose Biosensor based on Adsorption of Glucose Oxidase at Platinum Nanoparticle-Modified Carbon Nanotube Electrode. *Anal. Biochem.* **2004,** *331,* 89–97.

71. Topoglidis, E. A.; Cass, E., et al. Protein Adsorption on Nanocrystalline TiO_2 Films: an Immobilization Strategy for Bioanalytical Devices. *Anal. Chem.* **1998,** *70,* 5111–5113.

72. Vaidya, S.; Gilchrist, M.; Maldarelli, C.; Couzis, A. Spectral Bar Coding of Polystyrene Microbeads using Multicolored Quantum Dots. *Anal. Chem.* **2007,** *79,* 8520–8530.

73. Vaseashta, A.; Dimova-Malinovska, D. Nanostructured and Nanoscale Devices, Sensors and Detectors. *Sci. Technol. Adv. Mat.* **2005,** *6,* 312–318.

74. Wang, J. Nanomaterial-Based Electrochemical Biosensors. *Analyst.* **2005,** *130,* 421–426.

75. Wang, Z.; Levy, R.; Fernig, D.; Brust, M. Kinase-Catalyzed Modification of Gold Nanoparticles: A New Approach to Colorimetric Kinase Activity Screening. *J. Am. Chem. Soc.* **2006,** *128,* 2214–2215.

76. Weizmann, Y.; Patolsky, F.; Willner, I. Amplified Detection of DNA and Analysis of Single-Base Mismatches by the Catalyzed Deposition of Gold on Au-Nanoparticles. *Analyst.* **2001,** *126,* 1502–1504.

77. Xiao, Y.; Patolsky, F, et al. Plugging into Enzymes: Nanowiring of Redox Enzymes by a Gold Nanoparticle. *Science* **2003,** *299,* 1877–1881.

78. Xu, H.; Aguilar, Z.; Dixon, J.; Jones, B.; Wang, A.; Wei, H. Breast Cancer Cell Imaging using Semiconductor Quantum Dots. *Electrochemical Society Transactions* **2009,** *25,* 69–77.

79. Balasubramanian, S. K.; Yang, L.; Yung, L. Y. L.; Ong, C. N.; Ong, W. Y.; Yu, L. E. Characterization, Purification, and Stability of Gold Nanoparticles. *Biomaterials* **2010,** *31,* 9023–9030.

80. Frens, G. Controlled Nucleation for the Regulation of the Particle Size in Monodisperse Gold Suspensions. *Nat. Phys. Sci.* **1973,** *241,* 20–22.

81. Gole, A.; Murphy, C. J. Seed-Mediated Synthesis of Gold Nanorods: Role of the Size and Nature of the Seed. *Chem. Mater.* **2004,** *16,* 3633–3640.

82. Handley, D. A. Methods for Synthesis of Colloidal Gold. In *Colloidal Gold: Principles, Methods, and Applications*; Hayat, M. A., Ed.; Academic Press: New York, NY, 1989.

83. Hazarika, P.; Giorgi, T.; Reibner, M.; Ceyhan, B.; Neimeyer, C. Synthesis and Characterization of Deoxyribonucleic Acid-Conjugated Gold Nanoparticles. In *Bioconjugation Protocols: Strategies and Methods*; Niemeyer, C., Ed.; Humana Press: New Jersey, 2004.

84. Katz, E.; Willner, I. Integrated Nanoparticle-Biomolecule Hybrid Systems: Synthesis, Properties, and Applications. *Angew. Chem. Int. Ed.* **2004,** *43,* 6018–6042.

85. Kimlong, J.; Maier, M.; Okenve, B.; Kotaidis, V.; Ballot, H.; Turkevich, P. A. Method for Gold Nanoparticle Synthesis Revisited. *J. Phys. Chem. B.* **2006,** *110,* 15700–15707.

86. LizMarzan, L. M.; Giersig, M.; Mulvaney, P. Synthesis of nanosized goldsilica coreshell particles. *Langmuir* **1996,** *12,* 4329–4335.

87. Liu, C.; Yang, X.; Yuan, H.; Zhou, Z.; Xiao, D. Preparation of Silver Nanoparticle and its Application to the Determination of ct-DNA. *Sensors* **2007,** *7,* 708–718.

88. Murray, C. B.; Kagan, C. R.; Bawendi, M. G. Synthesis and Characterization of Monodisperse Nanocrystals and Close-Packed Nanocrystal Assemblies. *Ann. Rev. Mater. Sci.* **2000,** *30,* 545–610.

89. Murray, C. B.; Sun, S.; Gaschler, W.; Doyle, H.; Betley, T. A.; Kagan, C. R. Colloidal Synthesis of Nanocrystals and Nanocrystal Superlattices. *IBM. J. Res. Dev.* **2001,** *45,* 47–56.

90. NanoTech, O. *Preparation of Uniform Size and Size Tunable Iron Oxide Magnetic Nanocrystals.* Available from: http://www.oceannanotech.com/nav.php?qid=6. [February 5, 2012].

91. Nickel, U.; Castell, A. Z.; Poppl, K.; Schneider, S. A Silver Colloid Produced by Reduction with Hydrazine as support for Highly Sensitive Surface-Enhanced Raman Spectroscopy. *Langmuir* **2000,** *16,* 9087–9091.

92. Tao, A.; Sinsermsuksaku, P.; Yang, P. Polyhedral Silver Nanocrystals with Distinct Scattering Signatures. *Angew. Chem. Int. Ed.* **2006,** *45,* 4597–4601.

93. Tartaj, P.; Sema, C. J. Synthesis of Monodisperse Superparamagnetic Fe/silica Nanospherical Composites. *J. Am. Chem. Soc.* **2003,** *125,* 15754–15755.

94. Teja, A. S.; Koh, P. Y. Synthesis, Properties, and Applications of Magnetic Iron Oxide Nanoparticles. *Prog. Cryst. Growth. Characterization Mater.* **2009,** *55,* 22–45.

95. Turkevich, J.; Stevenson, P. C.; Hillier, J. A Study of the Nucleation and Growth Processes in the Synthesis of Colloidal Gold. *Discuss. Faraday. Soc.* **1951,** *11,* 55–75.

96. Wiley, B.; Sun, Y.; Mayers, B.; Xia, Y. Shape-Controlled Synthesis of Metal Nanostructures: The Case of Silver. *Chem-Eur. J.* **2005,** *11,* 454–463.

97. Dabbousi, B. O.; Rodríguez-Viejo, J.; Mikulec, F. V.; Heine, J. R.; Mattoussi, H.; Ober, R., et al. (CdSe)ZnS Core–Shell Quantum Dots: Synthesis and Characterization of a Size Series of Highly Luminescent Nanocrystallites. *J. Phys. Chem. B.* **1997,** *101,* 9463–9475.

98. Manna, L.; Scher, E.; Alivisatos, A. Synthesis of Soluble and Processable Rod-, Arrow-, Teardrop-, and Tetrapod-Shaped CdSe Nanocrystals. *JACS* **2000,** *122,* 12700–12706.

99. Murray, C.; Norris, D.; Bawendi, M. Synthesis and Characterization of Nearly Monodisperse CdE (E = Sulfur, Selenium, Tellurium) Semiconductor Nanocrystallites. *JACS* **1993,** *115,* 8706–8715.

100. Pradhan, N.; Battaglia, D. M.; Liu, Y.; Peng, X. Efficient, Stable, Small, and Water Soluble Doped ZnSe Nanocrystal Emitters as Non-Cadmium Based Biomedical Labels. *Nano. Lett.* **2007,** *7,* 312–317.

101. Gao, X. P.; Qin, X.; Wu, F.; Liu, H.; Lan, Y.; Fan, S. S., et al. Synthesis of Carbon Nanotubes by Catalytic Decomposition of Methane using LaNi5 Hydrogen Storage Alloy as Catalyst. *Chem. Phys. Lett.* **2000,** *327,* 271–276.

102. Baranov, D.; Fiore, A.; van Huis, M.; Giannini, C.; Falqui, A.; Lafont, U., et al. Assembly of Colloidal Semiconductor Nanorods in Solution by Depletion Attraction. *Nano. Lett.* **2010,** *10,* 743–749.

103. Carbone, L.; Kudera, S.; Carlino, E.; Parak, W. J.; Giannini, C.; Cingolani, R., et al. Multiple Wurtzite twinning in CdTe Nanocrystals induced by Methylphosphonic Acid. *J. Am. Chem. Soc.* **2006,** *128,* 748–755.

104. Casavola, M.; Grillo, V.; Carlino, E.; Giannini, C.; Gozzo, F.; Pinel, E. F., et al. Topologically Controlled Growth of Magnetic-Metal-Functionalized Semiconductor Oxide Nanorods. *Nano. Lett.* **2007,** *7,* 1386–1395.

105. Cozzoli, P. D.; Manna, L.; Curri, M. L.; Kudera, S.; Giannini, C.; Striccoli, M., et al. Shape and Phase Control of Colloidal ZnSe Nanocrystals. *Chem. Mater.* **2005,** *17,* 1296–1306.

106. Deka, S.; Falqui, A.; Bertoni, G.; Sangregorio, C.; Poneti, G.; Morello, G., et al. Fluorescent Asymmetrically Cobalt-Tipped CdSe@CdS core@shell Nanorod Heterostructures Exhibiting Room-Temperature Ferromagnetic Behavior. *J. Am. Chem. Soc.* **2009,** *131,* 12817–12828.

107. Zeng, C. H. Synthetic Architecture of Interior Space for Inorganic Nanostructures. *J. Mater. Chem.* **2006,** *16,* 649–662.

108. Yang, L.; Cao, Z.; Sajja, H.; Mao, H.; Wang, L.; Geng, H., et al. Development of Receptor Targeted Iron Oxide Nanoparticles for Efficient Drug Delivery and Tumor Imaging. *J. Biomed. Nanotech.* **2008,** *4,* 1–11.

109. Yang, L.; Peng, X.; Wang, Y.; Wang, X.; Cao, Z.; Ni, C., et al. Receptor-Targeted Nanoparticles for in Vivo Imaging of Breast Cancer. *Clin. Cancer. Res.* **2009,** *15,* 4722–4732.

110. Kubik, T.; Bogunia-Kubik, K.; Sugisaka, M. Nanotechnology on Duty in Medical Applications. *Curr. Pharm. Biotechnol.* **2005,** *6,* 17–33.

111. Han, M.; Gao, X.; Su, J.; Nie, S. Quantum Dot Tagged Microbead for Multiplexed Coding of Biomolecules. *Nat. Biotechnol.* **2001,** *19,* 631–635.

112. Didenko, Y.; Suslick, K. Chemical Aerosol Flow Synthesis of Semiconductor Nanoparticles. *J. Am. Chem. Soc.* **2005,** *127,* 12196–12197.

113. Kumar, S.; Nann, T. Shape Control of II–VI Semiconductor Nanomaterials. *Small* **2006,** *2,* 316.

114. Vo Dinh, T.; Kasili, P.; Wabuyele, M. Nanoprobes and Nanobiosensors for Monitoring and Imaging Individual Living Cells. *Nanomedicine* **2006,** *2,* 22–30.

115. Allen, T. M.; Mumbengegwi, D. R.; Charrois, G. J. Anti-CD19-Targeted Liposomal Doxorubicin Improves the Therapeutic Efficacy in Murine B-Cell Lymphoma and Ameliorates the Toxicity of Liposomes with Varying Drug Release Rates. *Clin. Cancer. Res.* **2005**, *11*, 3567–3573.

116. Chonn, A.; Semple, S. C.; Cullis, P. R. Association of Blood Proteins with Large Unilamellar Liposomes in Vivo. Relation to Circulation Lifetimes. *J. Biol. Chem.* **1992**, *267*, 18759–18765.

117. Dagar, S.; Sekosan, M.; Lee, B. S.; Rubinstein, I.; Onyuksel, H. VIP Receptors as Molecular Targets of Breast Cancer: Implications for Targeted Imaging and Drug Delivery. *J. Controlled Release* **2001**, *74*, 129–134.

118. Drummond, D. C.; Meyer, O.; Hong, K.; Kirpotin, D. B.; Papahadjopoulos, D. Optimizing Liposomes for Delivery of Chemotherapeutic Agents to Solid Tumors. *Pharmacol. Rev.* **1999**, *51*, 691–743.

119. Fetterly, G. J.; Straubinger, R. M. Pharmacokinetics of Paclitaxel-Containing Liposomes in Rats. *AAPS. PharmSci.* **2003**, *5*, 1–11.

120. Heath, J. R.; Davis, M. E. Nanotechnology and Cancer. *Annu. Med. Rev.* **2008**, *59*, 251–265.

121. Hoarau, D.; Delmas, P.; David, S.; Roux, E.; Leroux, J. C. Novel Long Circulating Lipid Nanocapsules. *Pharm. Res.* **2004**, *21*, 1783–1789.

122. Jin, S.; Ye, K. Nanoparticle-Mediated Drug Delivery and Gene Therapy. *Biotechnol. Prog.* **2007**, *23*, 32–41.

123. Kamps, J. A.; Scherphof, G. L. Receptor Versus Non-Receptor Mediated Clearance of Liposomes. *Adv. Drug. Deliv. Rev.* **1998**, *32*, 81–97.

124. Mattiasson, B.; Borrebaeck, C. In *Enzyme Immunoassay*; Maggio, E. T., Ed.; CRC Press, Inc.: Boca Raton, 1980; pp 295.

125. Moghimi, S. M.; Szebeni, J. Stealth Liposomes and Long Circulating Nanoparticles: Critical Issues in Pharmacokinetics, Opsonization and Protein-Binding Properties. *Prog. Lipid. Res.* **2003**, *42*, 463–478.

126. Morgen, M.; Lu, G. W.; Dub, D.; Stehle, R.; Lembke, F.; Cervantes, J., et al. Targeted Delivery of a Poorly Water-Soluble Compound to Hair Follicles using Polymeric Nanoparticle Suspensions. *Int. J. Pharm.* **2011**, In Press.

127. Papahadjopoulos, D.; Jacobson, K.; Nir, S.; Isac, T. Phase Transitions in Phospholipid Vesicles. Fluorescence Polarization and Permeability Measurements Concerning the Effect of Temperature and Cholesterol. *Biochim. Biophys. Acta.* **1973**, *311*, 330–348.

128. Pastorino, F.; Brignole, C.; Marimpietri, D.; Sapra, P.; Moase, E. H.; Allen, T. M., et al. Doxorubicin-Loaded Fab' Fragments of Anti-Disialoganglioside Immunoliposomes Selectively Inhibit the Growth and Dissemination of Human Neuroblastoma in Nude Mice. *Cancer Res.* **2003**, *63*, 86–92.

129. Tiwari, S. B.; Amiji, M. M. A Review of Nanocarrier-Based CNS Delivery Systems. *Curr. Drug. Del.* **2006**, *3*, 219–232.

130. Tobio, M.; Sanchez, A.; Vila, A.; Soriano, I.; Evora, C.; Vila-Jato, J. L., et al. Investigation of Lectin-Modified Insulin Liposomes as Carriers for Oral Administration. *Colloids Surf B.: Biointerfaces* **2000**, *18*, 315–323.

131. Torchilin, V. P.; Shtilman, M. I.; Trubetskoy, V. S.; Whiteman, K.; Milstein, A. M. Amphiphilic Vinyl Polymers Effectively Prolong Liposome Circulation Time in Vivo. *Biochim. Biophys. Acta.* **1994**, *1195*, 181–184.

132. Yan, X.; Kuipers, F.; Havekes, L. M.; Havinga, R.; Dontje, B.; Poelstra, K., et al. The Role of Apolipoprotein E in the Elimination of Liposomes from Blood by Hepatocytes in the Mouse. *Biochem. Biophys. Res. Commun.* **2005**, *328*, 57–62.

133. Zhang, J. A.; Anyarambhatla, G.; Ma, L.; Ugwu, S.; Xuan, T.; Sardone, T., et al. Development and Characterization of a Novel Cremophor® EL Free Liposome-Based Paclitaxel (LEP-ETU) Formulation. *Eur. J. Pharm. Biopharm.* **2005,** *59,* 177–187.

134. Zhang, N.; Ping, Q. N.; Huang, G. H.; Xu, W. F. Investigation of Lectin-Modified Insulin Liposomes as Carriers for Oral Administration. *Int. J. Pharm.* **2005,** *294,* 247–259.

135. Aguilar, Z. P.; Xu, H.; Dixon, J. D.; Wang, A. W. *Nanomaterials for Enhanced Antibody Production*; Small business innovations research for the National Science Foundation, 2012.

136. Arruebo, M.; Fernandez-Pacheco, R.; Ricardo-Ibarra, M.; Santamaria, J. Magnetic Nanoparticles for Drug Delivery. *Nanotoday* **2007,** *2,* 22–32.

137. Brzeska, M.; Panhorst, M.; Kamp, P. B.; Schotter, J.; Reiss, G.; Pühler, A., et al. Detection and Manipulation of Biomolecules by Magnetic Carriers. *J. Biotechnol.* **2004,** *112,* 25.

138. Bulte, J. W.; Douglas, T.; Witwer, B.; Zhang, S. C.; Strable, E.; Lewis, B. K., et al. Magnetodendrimers Allow Endosomal Magnetic Labeling and in Vivo Tracking of Stem Cells. *Nat. Biotechnol.* **2001,** *19,* 1141–1147.

139. Gaster, R. S.; Hall, D. A.; Nielsen, C. H.; Osterfeld, S. J.; Yu, H.; Mach, K. E.; Wilson, R. J.; Murmann, B.; Liao, J. C.; Gambhir, S. S.; Wang, S. X. Matrix-insensitive protein assays push the limits of biosensors in medicine. *Nat Medicine* **2009,** *15,* 1327–1332.

140. Ge, Y.; Zhang, Y.; He, S.; Nie, F.; Teng, G.; Gu, N. Fluorescence Modified Chitosan-Coated Magnetic Nanoparticles for High-Efficient Cellular Imaging. *Nanoscale. Res. Lett.* **2009,** *4,* 287–295.

141. Kim, J.; Piao, T.; Hyeon, T. Multifunctional Nanostructured Materials for Multimodal Imaging, and Simultaneous Imaging and Therapy. *Chem. Soc. Rev.* **2009,** *38,* 372–390.

142. Kularatne, B.; Lorigan, P.; Browne, S.; Suvarna, S.; Smith, M.; Lawry, J. Monitoring Tumour Cells in the Peripheral Blood of Small Cell Lung Cancer Patients. *Cytometry* **2002,** *50,* 160–167.

143. Lee, H.; Lee, E. J.; Kim, D. K.; Jang, N. K.; Jeong, Y. Y.; Jon, S. Antibiofouling Polymer-Coated Superparamagnetic Iron Oxide Nanoparticles as Potential Magnetic Resonance Contrast Agents for in Vivo Cancer Imaging. *J. Am. Chem. Soc.* **2006,** *128,* 7383–7389.

144. Mahmoudi, M.; Simchi, A.; Imani, M.; Milani, A. S.; Stroeve, P. An in Vitro Study of Bare and Poly(Ethylene Glycol)-*co*-Fumarate-Coated Superparamagnetic Iron Oxide Nanoparticles: A New Toxicity Identification Procedure. *Nanotechnology* **2009,** *20,* 40–47.

145. Mejias, R.; Perez-Yague, S.; Gutierez, L.; Cabrera, L. I.; Spada, R.; Acedo, P., et al. Dimercaptosuccinic Acid-Coated Magnetite Nanoparticles for Magnetically Guided in Vivo Delivery of Interferon Gamma for Cancer Immunotherapy. *Biomaterials* **2011,** *32,* 2938–2952.

146. Osaka, T.; Nakanishi, T.; Shanmugam, S.; Takahama, S.; Zhang, H. Effect of Surface Charge of Magnetite Nanoparticles on their Internalization into Breast Cancer and Umbilical Vein Endothelial Cells. *Colloids and Surfaces. B.: Biointerfaces* **2009,** *71,* 325–330.

147. Perez, F. G.; Mascini, M. T.; Turner, I. E.; Anthony, P. F. Immunomagnetic Separation with Mediated Flow Injection Analysis Amperometric Detection of Viable *Escherichia coli* 0157. 228; *Anal. Chem.* **1998,** *70,* 2380–2386.

148. Philipse, A. P.; Vanbruggen, M. P. B.; Pathmamanoharan, C. Magnetic Silica Dispersions—Preparation and Stability of Surface-Modified Silica Particles with a Magnetic Core. *Langmuir* **1994,** *10,* 92–99.

149. Sekhon, B.; Kamboj, S. Inorganic Nanomedicine: part 1. *Nanomedicine: Nanotechnoloy, Biology, and Medicine* **2010,** *6,* 516–522.

150. Shubayev, V. I.; Pisanic, T. R.; Jin, S. Magnetic Nanoparticles for Theragnostics. *Adv. Drug. Delivery Rev.* **2009,** *61,* 467–477.

151. Splettstoesser, W. D.; Grunow, R.; Rahalison, L.; Brooks, T. J.; Chanteau, S.; Neubauer, H. Serodiagnosis of Human Plague by Combination of Immunomagnetic Separation and Flow Cytometry. *Cytometry Part A.* **2003,** *53A,* 88–96.

152. Xiao, L.; Alderisio, K.; Limor, J.; Royer, M.; Lal, A. A. Identification of Species and Sources of *Cryptosporidium Oocysts* in Storm Waters with a Small-Subunit rRNA-Based Diagnostic and Genotyping Tool. 320; *Appl. Environ. Microbiol.* **2000,** *66,* 5492–5498.

153. Zhao, X.; Harris, J. M. Novel Degradable Poly(Ethylene Glycol) Hydrogels for Controlled Release of Protein. *J. Pharm. Sci.* **1998,** *87,* 1450–1458.

154. Aguilar, Z. P.; Wang, Y. A.; Xu, H.; Hui, G.; Pusic, K. M. Nanoparticle based immunological stimulation 2012. [January 19 2012, US Patent App: 13/350,849].

155. Akerman, M. E.; Chan, W. C.; Laakkonen, P.; Bhatia, S. N.; Ruoslahti, E. Nanocrystal Targeting in Vivo. *PNAS. U.S.A.* **2002,** *99,* 12617–12621.

156. Ballou, B.; Lagerholm, B. C.; Ernst, L. A.; Bruchez, M. P.; Waggoner, A. S. Noninvasive Imaging of Quantum Dots in Mice. *Bioconjug. Chem.* **2004,** *15,* 79–86.

157. Byers, R.; Hitchman, E. Quantum Dots Brighten Biological Imaging. *Prog. Histochem. Cytochem.* **2011,** *45,* 201–237.

158. Cai, W.; Shin, D.; Chen, K.; Gheysens, O.; Cao, Q.; Wang, S. X., et al. Peptide-Labeled Near-Infrared Quantum Dots for Imaging Tumor Vasculature in Living Subjects. *Nano. Lett.* **2006,** *6,* 669–676.

159. Dennis, A. M.; Bao, G. Quantum Dot-Fluorescent Protein Pairs as Novel Fluorescence Resonance Energy Transfer Probes. *Nano. Lett.* **2008,** *8,* 1439–1445.

160. Gao, X.; Cui, Y.; Levenson, R. M.; Chung, L. W. K.; Nie, S. In Vivo Cancer Targeting and Imaging with Semiconductor Quantum Dots. *Nat. Biotechnol.* **2004,** *22,* 969–976.

161. Juzenas, P.; Chen, W.; Sun, Y. P.; Coelho, M. A. N.; Genralov, R.; Genralova, N.; et al Quantum Dots and Nanoparticles for Photodynamic and Radiation Therapies of Cancer. *Adv. Drug. Delivery. Revs.* **2008,** *60.*

162. Khawaja, A. M. Review: The Legacy of Nanotechnology: Revolution and Prospects in Neurosurgery. *Int. J. Surgery.* **2011,** IN Press.

163. Lidke, D. S.; Nagy, P.; Heintzmann, R.; Arndt-Jovin, D. J.; Post, J. N.; Grecco, H. E., et al. Quantum Dot Ligands Provide New Insights into erbB/HER Receptor-Mediated Signal Transduction. *Nat. Biotechnol.* **2004,** *22,* 198–203.

164. Parak, W. J.; Pellegrino, T.; Plank, C. Labelling of Cells with Quantum Dots. *Nanotechnology* **2005,** *16,* R9–R25.

165. Resch-Genger, U.; Grabolle, M.; Cavaliere-Jaricot, S.; Nitschke, R.; Nann, T. Quantum Dots Versus Organic Dyes as Fluorescent Labels. *Nat. Methods* **2008,** *5,* 763–775.

166. Smith, A. M.; Duan, H.; Mohs, A. M. Bioconjugated Quantum Dots for in Vivo Molecular and Cellular Imaging. *Adv. Drug. Delivery. Revs.* **2008,** *60.*

167. Smith, A. M.; Gao, X.; Nie, S. Quantum Dot Nanocrystals for in Vivo Molecular and Cellular Imaging. *Photochem. Photobiol.* **2004,** *80,* 377–385.

168. Su, Y. Y.; Peng, F.; Jiang, Z. Y.; Zhong, Y. L.; Lu, Y. M., et al. In Vivo Distribution, Pharmacokinetics, and Toxicity of Aqueous Synthesized Cadmium-Containing Quantum Dots. *Biomaterials* **2011,** *32,* 5855–5862.

169. Tada, H.; Higuchi, H.; Wanatabe, T. M.; Ohuchi, N. In vivo Real-Time Tracking of Single Quantum Dots Conjugated with Monoclonal Anti-HER2 Antibody in Tumors of Mice. *Cancer Res.* **2007,** *67,* 1138–1144.

170. Willard, D.; Carillo, L.; Jung, J.; van Orden, A. CdSe-ZnS Quantum Dots as Resonance Energy Transfer Donors in a Model Protein-Protein Binding Assay. *Nano. Lett.* **2001,** *1.*

171. Wolcott, A.; Gerion, D.; Visconte, M.; Sun, J.; Schwartzberg, A.; Chen, S., et al. Silica-Coated CdTe Quantum Dots Functionalized with Thiols for Bioconjugation to IgG Proteins. *J. Phys. Chem. B.* **2006**, *110*, 5779–5789.

172. Xu, H.; Aguilar, Z.; Waldron, J.; Wei, H.; Wang, Y. Application of Semiconductor Quantum Dots for Breast Cancer Cell Sensing, 2009 Biomedical Engineering and Informatics. *IEEE Computer Society BMEI* **2009**, *1*, 516–520.

173. Xu, H.; Aguilar, Z.; Wang, A. Quantum Dot-Based Sensors for Proteins. *ECS. Trans.* **2010**, *25*, 1–10.

174. Mathieu, J. B.; Martel, S.; Yahia, L.; Soulez, G.; Beaudoin, G. Preliminary Investigation of the Feasibility of Magnetic Propulsion for Future Microdevices in Blood Vessels. *Biomed. Mater. Eng.* **2002**, *15*, 367–374.

175. Sajja, H.; East, M.; Mao, H.; Wang, Y.; Nie, S.; Yang, L. Development of Multifunctional Nanoparticles for Targeted Drug Delivery and Noninvasive Imaging of Therapeutic Effect. *Curr. Drug. Discov. Technol.* **2009**, *6*, 43–51.

176. Sajja, H. K.; East, M. P.; Mao, H.; Wang, A. Y.; Nie, S.; Yang, L. Development of Multifunctional Nanoparticles for Targeted Drug Delivery and Non-Invasive Imaging of Therapeutic Effect. *Curr. Drug. Discov. Technol.* <http://www.ncbi.nlm.nih.gov/entrez/eutils/elink.fcgi?dbfrom=pubmed&retmode=ref&cmd=prlinks&id=19275541>.

177. Xiang, S. D.; Scalzo-Inguanti, K.; Minigo, G.; Park, A.; Hardy, C. L.; Plebanski, M. Promising Particle-Based Vaccines in Cancer Therapy. *Expert. Rev. Vaccines.* **2008**, *7*, 1103–1119.

178. Akagi, T.; Wang, X.; Uto, T.; Baba, M.; Akashi, M. Protein Direct Delivery to Dendritic Cells Using Nanoparticles based on Amphiphilic Poly(Amino Acid) Derivatives. *Biomaterials* **2007**, *28*, 3427–3436.

179. Ueno, Y.; Futagawa, H.; Takagi, Y.; Ueno, A.; Mizuzshima, Y. Drug-Incorporating Calcium Carbonate Nanoparticles for a New Delivery System. *J. Controlled Release* **2005**, *103*, 93–98.

180. Fifis, T.; Gamvrellis, A.; Crimeen-Irwin, B.; Pietersz, G. A.; Li, J.; Mottram, P. L., et al. Size-Dependent Immunogenicity: Therapeutic and Protective Properties of Nano-Vaccines against Tumors. *J. Immunol.* **2004**, *173*, 3148–3154.

181. Mingo, G.; Scholzen, A.; Tang, C. K.; Hanley, J. C.; Kalkainidis, M.; Pietersz, G. A., et al. Poly-L-lysine-Coated Nanoparticles: A Potent Delivery System to Enhance DNA Vaccine Efficacy. *Vaccine* **2007**, *25*, 1316–1327.

182. Mottram, P. L.; Leong, D.; Crimeen-Irwin, B.; Gloster, S.; Xiang, S. D.; Meanger, J., et al. Type 1 and 2 Immunity following Vaccination is Influenced by Nanoparticle Size: Formulation of a Model Vaccine for Respiratory Syncytial Virus. *Mol. Pharm.* **2007**, *4*, 73–84.

183. Cherukuri, P.; Bachilo, S. M.; Litovsky, S. H.; Weisman, R. B. Weisman, Near-Infrared Fluorescence Microscopy of Single-Walled Carbon Nanotubes in Phagocytic Cells. *J. Am. Chem. Soc.* **2004**, *126*, 15638–15639.

184. Kreyling, W. G.; Möller, W.; Semmler-Behnke, M.; Oberdörster, G. In *Particle Toxicology*; Born, D. K., Ed.; CRC Press: Boca Raton, 2007.

185. Moghimi, S. M.; Hunter, A. C.; Murray, J. C. Nanomedicine: Current Status and Future Prospects. *FASEB* **2005**, *19*, 311–330.

186. Gourley, P. L. Brief Overview of BioMicroNano Technologies. *Biotechnol. Prog.* **2005**, *21*, 2–10.

187. Nakamura, T.; Sakaeda, T.; Takahashi, M.; Hashimoto, K.; Gemma, N.; Moriya, Y., et al. Simultaneous Determination of Single Nucleotide Polymorphisms of MDR1 Genes by Electrochemical DNA Chip. *Drug. Metab. Pharmacokinet.* **2005**, *20*, 219–225.

188. Sabuncu, A. C.; Grubbs, J.; Qian, S.; Abdel-Fattah, T. M.; Stacey, M. W.; Beskok, A. Probing Nanoparticle Interaction in Cell Culture Media. *Colloids and Surfaces B.: Biointerfaces* **2012,** *95,* 96–102.

189. Ambrosi, A.; Castaneda, M.; Killard, A.; Smyth, M.; Alegret, S.; Merkoci, A. Double-Codified Gold Nanolabels for Enhanced Immunoanalysis. *Anal. Chem.* **2007,** *79,* 5232–5240.

190. Li, M.; Cushing, S. K.; Zhang, J.; Lankford, J.; Aguilar, Z. P.; Ma, D., et al. Shape-Dependent Surface-Enhanced Raman Scattering in Gold-Raman-Probe-Silica Sandwiched Nanoparticles for Biocompatible Applications. *Nanotechnology* **2012,** *23,* 115501–115511.

191. Li, M.; Li, R.; Li, C. M.; Wu, N. Electrochemical and Optical Biosonesors Based on Nanomaterials and Nanostructures: A Review. *Front. Biosci.* **2011,** *S3,* 1308–1331.

192. Li, M.; Zhang, J.; Suri, S.; Sooter, L. J.; Ma, D.; Wu, N. Detection of Adenosine Triphosphate with and Aptamer Biosensor Based on the Surface-Enhanced Raman Scattering. *Anal. Chem.* **2012,** *84,* 2837–2842.

193. Bulte, J. W.; Kraitchman, D. L. Iron Oxide MR Contrast Agents for Molecular and Cellular Imaging. *NMR. Biomed.* **2004,** *17,* 484–499.

194. Hans, M. L.; Lowman, A. M. Biodegradable Nanoparticles for Drug Delivery and Targeting. *Curr. Opin. Solid. State. Mater. Sci.* **2002,** *6,* 319–327.

195. Hong, Z. K.; Zhang, P.; He, C.; Qiu, X.; Liu, A.; Chen, L., et al. Nano-Composite of Poly (L-lactide) and Surface Grafted Hydroxyapatite: Mechanical Properties and Biocompatibility. *Biomaterials* **2005,** *26,* 6296–6304.

196. Freed, L. E.; Novakovic, G. V.; Biron, R. J.; Eagles, D. B.; Lesnoy, D. C.; Barlow, S. K., et al. Biodegradable Polymer Scaffolds for Tissue Engineering. *Biotechnology* **1994,** *12,* 689–693.

197. Hong, Z. K.; Qui, X. Y.; Sun, J. R.; Deng, M. X.; Chen, X. S.; Jing, X. B. Grafting Polymerization of L-Lactide on the Surface of Hydroxyapatite Nano-Crystal. *Polymer* **2004,** *45,* 6705–6713.

198. Shuai, C.; Gao, C.; Nie, Y.; Hu, H.; Zhou, Y.; Peng, S. Structure and Properties of Nano-Hydroxyapatite Scaffolds for Bone Tissue Engineering with a Selective Laser Sintering System. *Nanotechnology* **2011,** *22,* 285703.

199. Albrektsson, T.; Wennerberg, A. Oral Implant Surfaces: Part 1—Review Focusing on Topographic and Chemical Properties of Different Surfaces and in Vivo Responses to them. *Int. J. Prosthodont.* **2004,** *7,* 536–543.

200. Att, W.; Kurun, S.; Gerds, T.; Strub, J. R. Fracture Resistance of Single-Tooth Implant-Supported All-Ceramic Restorations: An in Vitro Study. *J. Prosthet. Dent.* **2006,** *95,* 111–116.

201. Ben-Nissan, B.; Choi, A. H. Sol-Gel Production of Bioactive Nanocoatings for Medical Applications. Part 1: An Introduction. *Nanomedicine* **2006,** *1,* 311–319.

202. Cochran, D.; Oates, T.; Morton, D.; Jones, A.; Buser, D.; Peters, F. Clinical Field Trial Examining an Implant with a Sand-Blasted, Acid-Etched Surface. *J. Periodontol.* **2007,** *78,* 974–982.

203. Kim, H. W.; Koh, Y. H.; Li, L. H.; Lee, S.; Kim, H. E. Hydroxyapatite Coating on Titanium Substrate with Titania Buffer Layer Processed by Sol-Gel Method. *Biomaterials* **2004,** *25,* 2533–2538.

204. Thuurer, R.; Vigassy, T.; Hirayaman, M.; Wang, J.; Bakker, E.; Pretsch, E. Potentiometric Immunoassay with Quantum Dots. *Anal. Chem.* **2008,** *80,* 707–712.

205. Calvo, P.; Remuñán-López, C.; Vila-Jato, J. L.; Alonso, M. J. Chitosan and Chitosan/Ethylene Oxide-Propylene Oxide Block Copolymer Nanoparticles as Novel Carriers for Proteins and Vaccines. *Pharm. Res.* **1997,** *14,* 1431–1436.

206. Hu, Y.; Jiang, X.; Ding, Y.; Ge, H.; Yuan, Y.; Yang, C. Synthesis and Characterization of Chitosan–Poly(Acrylic Acid) Nanoparticles. *Biomaterials* **2002,** *23,* 3193–3201.

207. Illum, L.; Farraj, N. F.; Davis, S. S. Chitosan as a Novel Nasal Delivery System for Peptide Drugs. *Pharm. Res.* **1994,** *11,* 1186–1189.
208. Aspden, T. J.; Mason, J. D.; Jones, N. S. Chitosan as a Nasal Delivery System: The Effect of Chitosan Solutions on in Vitro and in Vivo Mucociliary Transport Rates in Human Turbinates and volunteers. *J. Pharm. Sci.* **1997,** *86,* 509–513.
209. Erbacher, P.; Zou, S.; Bettinger, T.; Steffan, A. M.; Remy, J. S. Chitosan-Based Vector/DNA Complexes for Gene Delivery: Biophysical Characteristics and Transfection Ability. *Pharm. Res.* **1998,** *15,* 1332–1339.
210. Pille, J. Y.; Li, H.; Blot, E.; Bertrand, J. R.; Pritchard, L. L.; Opolon, P., et al. Intravenous Delivery of Anti-RhoA Small Interfering NA Loaded in Nanoparticles of Chitosan in Mice: Safety and Efficacy in Xenografted Aggressive Breast Cancer. *Hum. Gene. Ther.* **2006,** *17,* 1019–1026.
211. Govender, T.; Stolnik, S.; Garnett, M. C.; Illum, L.; Davis, S. S. PLGA Nanoparticles Prepared by Nanoprecipitation: Drug Loading and Release Studies of a Water Soluble Drug. *J. Controlled. Release.* **1999,** *57,* 171–185.
212. Panyam, J.; Sahoo, S. K.; Prabha, S.; Bargar, T.; Labhasetwar, V. Fluorescence and Electron Microscopy Probes for Cellular and Tissue Uptake of polyD L -lactide-*co*-glycolide) Nanoparticles. *Int. J. Pharm.* **2003,** *262,* 1–11.
213. Panyam, J.; Williams, D.; Dash, A.; Leslie-Pelecky, D.; Labhasetwar, V. Solid-State Solubility Influences Encapsulation and Release of Hydrophobic Drugs from PLGA/PLA Nanoparticles. *J. Pharm. Sci.* **2004,** *93,* 1804–1814.
214. Wang, Y. -C.; Wu, Y. -T.; Huang, H. -Y.; Lin, H. -I.; Lo, L. -W.; Tzeng, S. -F., et al. Sustained Intraspinal Delivery of Neurotrophic Factor Encapsulated in Biodegradable Nanoparticles following Contusive Spinal Cord Injury. *Biomaterials* **2008,** *29,* 4546–4553.
215. Tran, P. A.; Zhang, L.; Webster, T. J. Carbon Nanofibers and Carbon Nanotubes in Regenerative Medicine. *Adv. Drug. Deliv. Rev.* **2009,** *61,* 1097–1114.
216. Bakry, R.; Vallant, R. M.; Najam-ul-hag, M.; Rainer, M.; Szabo, Z.; Huck, C. W., et al. Medicinal Applications of Fullerenes. *Int. J. Nanomed.* **2007,** *2,* 639–649.
217. Wang, J.; Musameh, M.; Lin, Y. Solubilization of Carbon Nanotubes by Nafion Toward the Preparation of Amperometric Biosensors. *J. Am. Chem. Soc.* **2003,** *125,* 2408–2409.
218. Dang, J. M.; Leong, K. W. Natural Polymers for Gene Delivery and Tissue Engineering. *Adv. Drug. Deliv. Rev.* **2006,** *58,* 487–499.
219. Ge, H.; Hu, Y.; Jiang, X.; Cheng, D.; Yuan, Y.; Bi, H., et al. Preparation, Characterization, and Drug Release Behaviors of Drug Nimodipine-Loaded Poly(Epsilon-Caprolactone)-Poly(Ethylene Oxide)-Poly(Epsilon-Caprolactone) Amphiphilic Triblock Copolymer Micelles. *J. Pharm. Sci.* **2002,** *91,* 1463–1473.
220. Gelperina, S. E.; Khalansky, A. S.; Skidan, I. N.; Smirnova, Z. S.; Bobruskin, A. I.; Severin, S. E., et al. Toxicological Studies of Doxorubicin Bound to Polysorbate 80-Coated Poly(Butyl Cyanoacrylate) Nanoparticles in Healthy Rats and Rats with Intracranial Glioblastoma. *Toxicol. Lett.* **2002,** *126,* 131–141.
221. Linhardt, R. J. In *Controlled Release of Drugs*; Rosoff, M., Ed.; VCH Publishers: New York, NY, 1989; pp 53–95.
222. Kreuter, J. *Nanoparticles*; M. Dekker: New York, NY, 1994.
223. Armentano, I.; Dottori, M.; Fortunati, E.; Mattioli, S.; Kenny, J. M. Biodegradable Polymer Matrix Nanocomposites for Tissue Engineering: A Review. *Polym. Degrad. Stab.* **2010,** *95,* 2126–2146.
224. Koegler, W. S.; Griffith, L. G. Osteoblast Response to PLGA Tissue Engineering Scaffolds with PEO Modified Surface Chemistries and Demonstration of Patterned Cell Response. *Biomaterials* **2004,** *25,* 2819–2830.

225. Cientifica *Nanotech Drug Delivery*. 2012, Available from: http://www.pitchengine.com/cientificaltd/nanotech-drug-delivery-will-be-15-of-global-nanotechnology-market-by-2021.
226. BCC Research *Nanotechnology in Medical Applications*. 2012, Available from: http://www.bccresearch.com/report/nanotechnology-medical-applications-global-market-hlc069b.html.
227. Bruchez, M., Jr.; Moronne, M.; Gin, P.; Weiss, S.; Alivisatos, A. P. Semiconductor nanocrystals as fluorescent biological labels. *Science* **1998**, *281*, 2013–2016.
228. Chan, C.; Nie, S. Quantum Dot Bioconjugates for Ultrasensitive Nonisotopic Detection. *Science* **1998**, *281*, 2016–2018.
229. Freeman, R.; Tali Finder, T.; Bahshi, L.; Willner, I. β-Cyclodextrin-Modified CdSe/ZnS Quantum Dots for Sensing and Chiroselective Analysis. *Nano. Lett.* **2009**, *9*, 2073–2076.
230. Grieshaber, D.; MacKenzie, R.; Voros, J.; Reimhult, E. Electrochemical Biosensors-Sensor Principles and Architectures. *Sensors* **2008**, *8*, 1400–1458.
231. Chen, X.; Schluesener, H. J. Nanosilver: A Nanoproduct in Medical Application. *Toxicol. Lett.* **2008**, *176*, 1–12.
232. Tian, F.; Cui, D.; Schwarz, H.; Estrada, G.; Kobayashic, H. Cytotoxicity of Singlewall Carbon Nanotubes on Human Fibroblasts. *Toxicol. In. Vitro.* **2006**, *20*, 1202–1212.
233. Beyerle, A.; Merkel, O.; Stoeger, T.; Kissel, T. PEGylation Affects Cytotoxicity and Cell-Compatibility of Poly(Ethylene Imine) for Lung Application: Structure–Function Relationships. *Toxicol. Appl. Pharmacol.* **2010**, *242*, 146–154.
234. Hagens, W. I.; Oomen, A. G.; de Jong, W. H.; Cassee, F. R.; Sips, A. What do we (need to) know about the Kinetic Properties of Nanoparticles in the Body? *Reg. Toxicol. Pharmacol.* **2007**, *49*, 217–229.
235. Kreyling, W. G.; Geiser, M. In *Inhalation and Health Effects*; Marijnissen, J. C., Ed.; Springer: Berlin, 2009.
236. SCENIHR; (SCCP), S. C. o. C. P., (SCHER), S. C. o. H. a. E. R., (SCENIHR), S. C. o. E. a. N. I. H. R., Eds., 2009.
237. USFDA FDA issues draft guidance on nanotechnology documents address use of nanotechnology by food and cosmetics industries 2012 Available from: http://www.fda.gov/Cosmetics/GuidanceComplianceRegulatoryInformation/GuidanceDocuments/ucm300886.htm.
238. USFDA. Cosmetics: Draft Guidance for Industry: Safety of Nanomaterials in Cosmetic Products. 2012, Available from: http://www.fda.gov/Cosmetics/GuidanceComplianceRegulatory-Information/GuidanceDocuments/ucm300886.htm.
239. USFDA. Draft Guidance for Industry: Safety of Nanomaterials in Cosmetic Products. 2012. Available from:USFDA. Draft guidance for industry: assessing the effects of significant manufacturing process changes, including emerging technologies, on the safety and regulatory status of food ingredients and food contact substances, including food ingredients that are color additives. 2012.
240. Drexler, E. *Engines of Creation: The Coming Era of Nanotechnology*; Knopf Doubleday Publishing Group, 1987.
241. Drexler, E. *Nanosystems: Molecular Machinery, Manufacturing, and Computation*; John Wiley and Sons: New York, 1992.
242. Drexler, E. *There's Plenty of Room at the Bottom (Richard Feynman, Pasadena, 29 December 1958)*. 2009, Available from: http://metamodern.com/2009/12/29/theres-plenty-of-room-at-the-bottom%E2%80%9D-feynman-1959/.
243. Drexler, E. *The Promise that Launched the Field of Nanotechnology*. 2009, Available from: http://metamodern.com/2009/12/15/when-a-million-readers-first-encountered-nanotechnology/.
244. Milburn, C. *Nanovision: Engineering the Future*; Duke University Press, 2008.

245. Feynman, R. P.; Sykes, C. *No Ordinary Genius: The Illustrated Richard Feynman*; W.W. Norton & Company, 1995.

246. Taniguchi, N. *On the Basic Concept of 'Nano-Technology*; Japan Society of Precision Engineering: Tokyo, 1974.

247. Hapgood, F. Nanotechnology: Molecular Machines that Mimic Life. *OMNI.* **1986.**

248. Tourney, C. Apostolic Succession. *Eng. Sci.* **2005,** *1,* 16–23.

249. Binnig, G.; Rohrer, H. Scanning Tunneling Microscopy. *IBM. J. R.&D.* **1986,** *30,* 4.

250. Shankland, S. IBM's 35 atoms and the rise of nanotech. 2009.

251. KAVLI Prize: Nanoscience Laureates 2010 May 19 2012

252. Kratschmer, W.; Lamb, L. D.; Fostiropoulos, K.; Huffman, D. R. C60: a New Form of Carbon. *Nature* **1990,** *347,* 345–358.

253. Ebbesen, T. W.; Ajayan, P. M. Large-Scale Synthesis of Carbon Nanotubes. *Nature* **1992,** *358,* 220–222.

254. Society, R. *Nanoscience and Nanotechnologies: Opportunities and Uncertainties.* 2004, Available from: http://www.nanotec.org.uk/finalReport.htm.

255. Imanaka, N.; Masui, T.; Hirai, H.; Adachi, G. Do Nanoparticles and Sunscreens Mix? *Chem. Mater.* **2003,** *15,* 2289–2291.

256. Brunner, T. J.; Wick, P.; Manser, P.; Spohn, P.; Grass, R. N.; Limbach, L. K., et al. In vitro Cytotoxicity of Oxide Nanoparticles: Comparison to Asbestos, Silica, and the Effect of Particle Solubility. *Environ. Sci. Technol.* **2006,** *40,* 4374–4381.

257. Bowman, D.; Hodge, G. Nanotechnology: Mapping the Wild Regulatory Frontier. *Futures* **2006,** *38,* 1060–1073.

258. TGA Safety of sunscreens containing nanoparticles of zinc oxide or titanium dioxide. 2006

259. Faunce, T. A.; Nasu, H.; Murray, K.; Bowman, D. Sunscreen Safety: The Precautionary Principle, the Australian Therapeutic Goods Administration and Nanoparticles in Sunscreens. *Nanoethics* **2008,** *2,* 231–240.

260. Barker, P. J.; Branch, A. The Interaction of Modern Sunscreen Formulations with Surface Coatings. *Progress in Organic Coatings* **2008,** *62,* 313–320.

261. *SAMSUNG Electronics Introduces Korea's First "Silver Sterilization Washing Machine".* 2003.

262. Atiyeh, B. S.; Costagliola, M.; Hayek, S. N.; Dibo, S. A. Effect of Silver on Burn Wound Infection Control and Healing: Review of the Literature. *Burns* **2007,** *33,* 139–148.

263. USA *21st Century Nanotechnology Research and Development Act (Public Law 108-153).* 2003, Available from: http://www.gpo.gov/fdsys/pkg/PLAW-108publ153/html/PLAW-108publ153.htm.

Types of Nanomaterials and Corresponding Methods of Synthesis

Chapter Outline

Nanomaterials for Medical Applications. http://dx.doi.org/10.1016/B978-0-12-385089-8.00002-9

The technology revolution in the twenty-first century is defined by the discovery and design of new materials that are systematically engineered at the atomic level to achieve unique physico-chemical properties that can be exploited for a variety of applications. Recent developments in chemistry and material science have resulted in the engineering control enabling the miniaturization trend in nanotechnology. Among the components of nanotechnology to date, various types of nanomaterials (NMs) offer the widest number of selections and the widest area of possible applications.

NMs come in different chemical compositions, different sizes, different shapes, different intrinsic properties that make them unique, and different functional groups making them even more versatile. Their preparation or synthesis processes vary as well from one chemical composition to another or even within the same composition.

Some NMs exhibit optical properties while others have magnetic properties. The optical properties may be due only to absorbance of light while others may be caused by the NMs ability to absorb and emit light. These properties of NMs are largely depended on their chemical composition and their size, shape, crystal structure, and surface characteristics. These parameters, especially the shape and size within the same chemical components, can be manipulated to alter their unique characteristics. For example, the shape of an NM controls its dimensions and reduction of its size results in the infinitesimal increase of the electronic band of semiconductor nanoparticles (NPs) leading to changes in its optical properties such as in the case of quantum dots (QDs), which are made of semiconductor elements. High quality QDs, which exhibit stable spectroscopic properties, including high photoluminescence yield, have been studied and reported extensively in the literature.[1] A narrow size distribution in a sample of NMs can minimize the broadening of spectroscopic properties that can conceal details of the size-dependent properties.[2,3] To date, NMs of different shapes and different sizes have emerged and with different properties than those which are spherical.[4–10] Various methods for the synthesis of the sophisticated shapes (e.g., nanorods, nanowires, and tetrapods) have emerged as well as for the modifications to introduce various functionalities making the NMs more versatile.[8–17] The controlled synthesis of these various NMs provides new applications.[9,10,17,18]

A long list of novel NMs forms and different compositions exhibiting unique properties have been grown over the past two to three decades involving different numerous synthetic routes of preparation. Development of novel synthetic methods for preparation of new NMs requires control of experimental parameters in order to control their various effects on the growth process. As more and more NMs emerged using different routes of synthesis, various mechanisms for controlling the size, shape, and structure have been proposed and demonstrated. These mechanisms serve as a guide for the design of new synthetic routes.

Today, there are no standard procedures to precisely engineer NMs unlike synthetic organic chemistry, which is accurately controlled and reproducible.

Synthesis of NMs is yet to be standardized and controlled to yield reproducible results. There are a few guiding parameters that can be used to control the size and the shape, which will be shown in some of the synthesis routes that are featured in this chapter. These include the crystalline phase of nucleation seeds, surface energy, and the choice of crystal growth regimes. The readers are encouraged to try some of the routes presented and make changes to the proposed methods to achieve different sizes and shapes of NMs.

2.1 INORGANIC NMs

The inorganic NMs consist of elements that belong to the inorganic groups. These can be semiconductors, conductors, single element or multielement in composition. Among the semiconductors, QDs, gold and silver, metal oxides, iron oxide magnetic NPs, and carbon nanotubes (CNTs) are the most popular.

QDs are semiconductor nanocrystals having diameters ranging between 2 and 8 nm,[19] which are characterized by broadband excitation wavelength, narrow emission wavelength, very bright fluorescence even when lighted only with a light emitting diode flashlight (Figure 2.1), and resistance to photobleaching; they have emerged as a new class of fluorescent labels with better brightness, resistance against photobleaching, and multicolor fluorescence emission.[20] These may be synthesized from atoms belonging to elements in groups II and VI (e.g., CdSe and CdTe) or groups III and V elements [e.g., indium phosphide (InP) and indium arsenide (InAs)].[21–25] QDs can be made of a semiconductor core (i.e., CdSe core) or coated with a shell (i.e., CdSe/ZnS core/shell) that improves the optical properties. To make them soluble in water, they are capped with a polymer or other materials that bring hydrophilicity to the NMs.

Among the range of available QDs, the ones composed of CdSe cores over coated with a layer of zinc sulfide (ZnS) are produced by a range of well-developed synthetic routes.[26] These QDs become highly fluorescent and exhibit attractive optical properties such as high quantum yield, large absorption

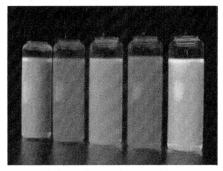

FIGURE 2.1   Digital photograph of water soluble QDs in vials under a 364-nm UV light. *By Z.P. Aguilar. (For color version of this figure, the reader is referred to the online version of this book)*

cross-section, and high photostability.[27] To be used for biological applications, different solubilization strategies for QDs have been developed over the past decades[28–30] especially for use in fluorescent imaging in vitro and in vivo. In most cases, these QDs are modified with thiol-containing compounds, such as mercaptoacetic acid (dihydrolipoic acid derivatives), or more sophisticated compounds such as alkylthiol-terminated DNA, thioalkylated oligoethylene-glycols, D,L-cysteine, poly(ethylene glycol) (PEG)-terminated dihydrolipoic acid having significant in vitro and in vivo stability.[31–33] Encapsulation in a layer of amphiphilic diblock or triblock copolymers, phospholipid micelles, silica shells, or amphiphilic polysaccharides, polymer shells, oligomeric phosphine coating, or by phytochelatin-peptides coating or histidine-rich proteins is another QD solubilization technique.[34–36] The modified water soluble QDs can be covalently linked with biorecognition molecules such as peptides, antibodies, nucleic acids, or small-molecule ligands for use as biological labels in molecular and cellular imaging.[37–41] Biological applications of QDs include fluorescence imaging, immunoassays, DNA assay, fluorescence labeling of cellular proteins, cell tracking, pathogen and toxin detection, and in vivo animal imaging.

The most extensively studied QDs are the cadmium containing NMs CdSe or CdTe core or core/shell that are encapsulated in various coatings.[42] QDs are NMs, which are semiconductor metalloid-crystal structures of approximately 2–100 nm, containing about 200–10,000 atoms.[43,44] QDs have unique optical and electronic properties including high brightness and stable fluorescence that are dependent upon their nanometer size. QDs are brighter than organic dyes and are more stable. The large surface area to volume ratio that is imparted by the small size makes QDs easy to functionalize with different biomolecules for various applications. These properties provide QDs the potential for biological imaging, cancer detection and imaging,[43] drug,[45] and vaccine delivery,[46] as well as immunotherapy and hyperthermia.[44,47] However, the cadmium content of QDs dampens the enthusiasm for its biomedical significance because little is known about the health risks of exposure to cadmium containing NMs.[42]

The most significant and also the most exploited feature of QDs is their size-tunable fluorescence. The bandgap energy, which is the minimum energy required to excite an electron to an energy level above its ground state, is a fixed entity that is unique to the nature of the semiconductor material[42,44] and fluorescence is the result of relaxation of the excited electron back to its ground state through the emission of a photon. When an incoming photon of energy that is greater than the bandgap of the material is absorbed, an electron is excited from the valence band to the conduction band, creating a hole in the valence band.[48] As the electron relaxes back down to the valence band, a photon that has energy proportional to the bandgap of the material is emitted. Unlike fluorescent organic dyes, QDs can absorb at a broad range of wavelengths of light greater than its bandgap and emit at a specific wavelength because of this process. As the size of a particle decreases to the nanoscale (less than the Bohr radius of the material), a quantum confinement effect occurs, making the bandgap energy dependent on particle size.[42] Hence, at the nanoscale level, optical properties, such as fluorescence excitation and emission, can be "tuned" by altering the size.[42]

QDs are significantly brighter and more stable than their corresponding organic fluorophores (similar emission wavelength). Unlike organic fluorophores, fluorescence of QDs is dependent on size and, therefore, a single light source can be used for excitation and emission, which is tuned via particle size to various wavelengths from the UV, visible, and near-mid infrared regions of the electromagnetic spectrum.[42] Unlike organic fluorophores, QDs have larger diameters allowing easy addition of targeting groups and small/big molecules to the surface.

Due to the high surface area of QDs, a large number of atoms are exposed at the surface.[42] These atoms have molecular orbitals that lack the full complement of electrons necessary for stability. These "defect" sites can be highly reactive, so another semiconductor with a wider bandgap is grown over the CdSe core.[49] ZnS is usually used for this purpose serving as the "shell" around the core because it enhances fluorescence efficiency[42,50] and also reduces cadmium toxicity. The ZnS shell, shown in Figure 2.2, also decreases QD oxidation and photobleaching while increasing chemical stability.[42] Other shells have also been used.[43,44,47]

Synthesis of QDs has been reviewed by Biju et al.[49] The QD core is mostly responsible for all the physical attributes such as the absorption and emission wavelengths. The shell structure protects the QD from losing its physical properties. After the QD is converted into its water-soluble form the external coating introduces its biocompatibility. The external coating is also responsible for the attachment of various molecules on the QD surface. The core is composed of

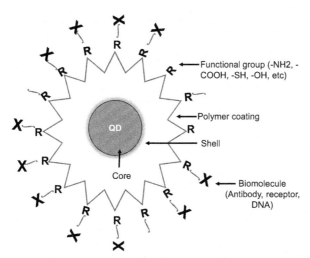

FIGURE 2.2   Schematic diagram of core/shell QDs. *(For color version of this figure, the reader is referred to the online version of this book)*

atoms from groups II to VI, with CdSe and CdTe being the most commonly used for biological applications.[43]

2.1.1 QD Core Synthesis Protocol

One of the many ways by which QDs are synthesized (Figure 2.2) uses high-temperature reaction of organometallic precursors in a mixture of trioctylphosphine/trioctylphosphine oxide (TOP/TOPO) and alkylamine.[22,24,50–52] The TOP/TOPO-capped QDs are allowed to undergo cap exchange with the newly synthesized ligands to achieve water solubility.[53–55]

The CdSe core nanocrystals are synthesized from CdO and elemental Se using a kinetic growth method, where particle size depends on reaction time.[56] To carry out this process the following protocol is followed:

(1) Prepare a stock solution of Se precursor by combining 30 mg of Se and 5 mL of 1-octadecene (90%) in a 10-mL round-bottom flask that is continuously stirred with a magnetic stirrer.
(2) Use a syringe to add 0.4 mL of TOP.
(3) Add a magnetic stir bar to stir the solution on a magnetic stir plate.
(4) Warm the solution to dissolve the Se.
(5) The stock solution can be stored at room temperature (RT) in a sealed container.
(6) This stock solution has enough Se precursor for five preparations.
(7) For each CdSe preparation, make the Cd precursor by adding 13 mg of CdO to a 25-mL round-bottom flask in a heating mantle.
(8) Add 0.6 mL of oleic acid and 10 mL of octadecene.
(9) Insert a thermometer that is capable of measuring 225 °C.
(10) Heat the setup to 225 °C and add 1 mL of the RT Se precursor.
(11) Begin the timer upon the addition of the Se precursor because the properties of the QDs are size-dependent.
(12) Use a 9-inch Pasteur pipette to quickly remove and quench about 1-mL samples at regular time intervals from the start and when a noticeable color change is detected.
(13) Obtain nine or 10 samples within 2–3 min (Figure 2.3).
(14) Record the visible absorption and emission spectra of individual samples to find the maximum wavelength peaks at an excitation wavelength of 400 nm.

Caution:[56]

(a) All synthesis must be performed inside the fume hood wearing goggles, nitrile gloves, and long sleeve lab gown covering arms.
(b) Octadecene vapor should not be inhaled, and contact with skin and eyes should be avoided.
(c) Use a syringe to transfer TOP because it is corrosive and causes burns.
(d) Oleic acid is air, light, and heat sensitive and irritates the eyes, the respiratory system, and the skin.

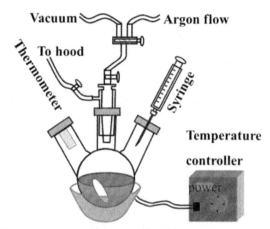

FIGURE 2.3   QD synthesis setup. *Courtesy of Ocean NanoTech. (For color version of this figure, the reader is referred to the online version of this book)*

(e) Elemental selenium is toxic by inhalation, absorption through the skin, and the effects of ingestion are cumulative.

(f) Cadmium oxide is highly toxic and cadmium compounds are human carcinogens if inhaled or swallowed.

(g) All leftover CdO, Se, and CdSe octadecene solutions should be collected in a waste container for proper disposal.

(h) All glassware must be soaked in soap and water before clean up.[57]

2.1.2 QD Core/Shell Synthesis Protocol

The ZnS precursor is prepared using tributylphosphine (TBP), diethylzinc ($ZnEt_2$), and hexamethyldisilathiane ((TMS)2S).

(1) Purge the TBP with nitrogen for 10–15 min before use.

(2) Simultaneously, purge a 50-mL round-bottom flask sealed with septa and containing a stir bar with nitrogen.

(3) Using a syringe, transfer 5.6 mL of TBP into the flask.

(4) Purge the $ZnEt_2$ with nitrogen for 5 min.

(5) Using a syringe, transfer 0.22 mL (1.04 mmol) of (TMS)2S to the flask containing the TBP.

(6) Transfer 1.42 mL (or the desired volume) of $ZnEt_2$ to the flask containing TBP and (TMS)2S using a syringe.

(7) The solution is stirred at 500 rpm, without heating, for 20 min to fully mix.

(8) Transfer this solution to a vial capped with a septum, then purge with nitrogen for 5–10 min. The solutions could be stored for up to one week without significant degradation. If the solution turned cloudy, it was a sign of degradation due to oxygen exposure, and the solution was discarded.

(9) Heat the oil bath to 160 °C and allow it to stabilize for 20 min.

(10) Place a stir bar in a 50-mL round-bottom flask capped with a septum.
(11) Transfer the desired CdSe precursor (between 3 and 20 mL) into this flask.
(12) Heat the solution to 160 °C and allow it to stabilize for 10 min while purging the ZnS precursor with N_2.
(13) Inject the desired volume of ZnS precursor solution dropwise over 2 min (according to the concentration of CdSe QDs and coating thickness[48]).
(14) Hold the temperature constant at 160 °C during reaction over 10 min.
(15) At the end of 10 min, raise the flask out of the oil bath and allow it to cool down to 60 °C.
(16) Upon reaching 60 °C, add 1 mL of butanol to avoid solidification and flocculation.
(17) Once the solution reaches RT, transfer the solution to a vial using a transfer pipette. A visible change in fluorescence should be observed under UV light.
(18) Characterize the QDs to establish their properties. The absorption and emission spectra of some QDs are given in Figure 2.4.

2.1.3 Water-Soluble QD Core/Shell Synthesis Protocol

The synthesized QDs are hydrophobic and, therefore, cannot be used for biomedical applications.[42] The core/shell QDs must be functionalized with secondary coatings or "capping" materials such as mercaptopropionic acid or PEG to improve water solubility and maintain QDs in a nonaggregated state.[42] The surface of the functionalized QD can be further conjugated with targeting molecules such as antibodies or receptor ligands as shown in the schematic diagram in Figure 2.1, which allows the QD to be attached to a specific tissue or organ.[26] Various applications of biocompatible CdSe/ZnS-QDs have been demonstrated[45] such as in vivo imaging of breast cancer in vitro[37,41] and imaging of tumor metastases in vivo in mice.[58] The CdSe/ZnS-QDs coated with targeting

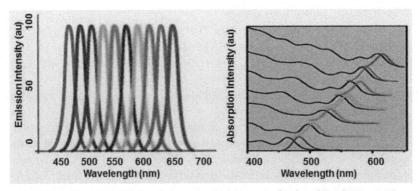

FIGURE 2.4 The emission (left) and absorption (right) spectra of various QDs. *Courtesy of Ocean NanoTech. (For color version of this figure, the reader is referred to the online version of this book)*

peptides were able to locate and track the tumors with imaging techniques in mice. Using triblock copolymer coating, QDs modified with prostate tumor targeting ligands were used to tag injected cancer cells as well as to locate tumors and in mice using a whole-body illumination system with spectral QD imaging.[59] Polyethylene glycol–phosphatidylethanolamine (PEG–PE) and PEG-phosphatidylcholine modified CdSe/ZnS-QDs were used to image Xenopus embryo development.

2.1.4 Ligand-Exchange Reaction to Make QDs Water Soluble[60]

One way to convert the hydrophobic QDs into their water-soluble form is to perform ligand exchange. The stepwise process is described as follows:

(1) The TOPO-capped QDs in toluene are precipitated with methanol and re-dispersed in $CHCl_3$.

(2) In a separate flask, dissolve 500 µL of 3-mercaptopropionic acid (3MPA) in 10 mL of $CHCl_3$.

(3) To this flask, add 1 g of the organic base tetramethylammonium hydroxide pentahydrate (TMAH, $(CH_3)4N–OH·5H_2O$). The chemical combination forms a two-phase mixture.

(4) Collect the bottom organic phase, containing deprotonated 3MPA and add 1 mL of TOPO-capped QDs (1 µM) and incubate at RT for 48 h.

(5) Remove excess 3MPA because alkyl thiols are deactivators of 1-ethyl-3-(3-dimethylaminopropyl)-carbodiimide (EDC), which is the promoter used to couple amine-modified biomolecules such as proteins, peptides, or DNA onto the QDs. This can be carried out using dialysis against a phosphate-buffered saline (PBS) buffer (10 mM, pH 7).[60]

(6) The water soluble QDs maintain their fluorescence and absorbance properties (Figure 2.5) and can be kept at 4–8 °C before conjugation with biomolecules (see Chapters 3 and 4).

2.1.5 Characterization of QDs[56]

One of the most important goal in the preparation of NMs is the production of monodisperse particles. Monodisperse pertains to the narrow size distribution of the NPs that is responsible for a narrow absorbance, which is measured through the full width at half the maximum (FWHM) absorption peak and a single emission peak (Figure 2.5). QDs exhibiting such properties are considered high quality NMs that are preferred for labeling studies where different sizes are used as different labels. Unlike fluorescent organic dyes, one excitation wavelength causes different-sized QDs to fluoresce at their respective emission peak wavelengths with narrow and nonoverlapping emission peaks enabling multiple labels to be simultaneously observed.[61,62] In general, the experimental,[48] the FWHM of the QD fluorescence curve, is a measure of the particle size dispersion in the sample. For multiple imaging applications,

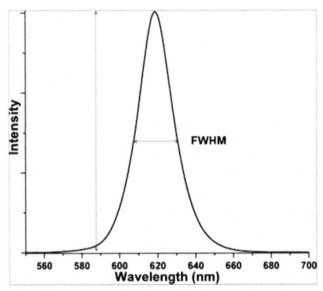

FIGURE 2.5 Emission spectrum of ~6 nm water-soluble QDs emitting at 620 nm with FWHM of ~26 nm. *Courtesy of Ocean NanoTech. (For color version of this figure, the reader is referred to the online version of this book)*

a small FWHM is necessary to detect the multiple analytes of interest. Thus, during synthesis, the absorption and emission wavelengths are measured continuously. When the QDs are not properly purified, the absorption spectra show peak maxima with additional absorption at lower wavelength due to starting materials and oleic acid polymerization.[56] The separation between the excitation and emission wavelengths is called the Stokes shift. The Stokes shift indicates the ability to separate the emission from excitation peak that is necessary in multiple analytes' labeling and detection. The presence of nearby energy labels allows semiconductor NMs to be excited by photons with greater than or equal to the minimum absorption energies. In Figure 2.4, the same excitation wavelength of 364 nm was used to observe the emission colors for all different sizes and optical colors, which indicates that a single light source can be used to excite multiple QDs of different sizes and all the labels can be excited and detected simultaneously.

2.1.6 UV Absorption and Emission

The synthesis of QDs is followed by measurements of UV absorption and emission (Figure 2.6) from the preparation of the precursor to the core/shell QD. This protocol is a step-by-step process of measuring the absorption and emission of a QD during and after synthesis.

(1) Place dilute QD in a quartz cuvette.
(2) Measure the absorbance with a UV spectrophotometer.

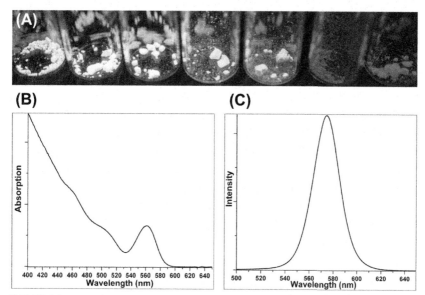

FIGURE 2.6   A) Various hydrophobic QDs (A) in powder form. (B) Absorption and (C) emission spectra of ~5 nm QDs. *Courtesy of Ocean NanoTech. (For color version of this figure, the reader is referred to the online version of this book)*

(3) Measure the emission with a fluorescence spectrophotometer.

(4) Use a QD of known excitation and emission wavelength to generate a standard curve to establish the molar absorption and molar extinction coefficient. The presence of nearby energy levels allows semiconductor NMs to be excited by photons with greater than or equal to the minimum absorption energies. In Figure 2.4, the same excitation wavelength of 364 nm was used for all samples, which indicates that a single light source can be used to excite multiple QDs of different sizes and all the labels can be excited and detected simultaneously.

2.1.7 Transmission Electron Microscopy

After synthesis, transmission electron microscopy (TEM) measurements of CdSe nanocrystals reveal their mean diameters. The following protocol can be used to perform TEM on a QD sample.

(1) Prepare the TEM sample grid by cleaning carefully with ethanol.

(2) Dip the carbon-coated copper sample grid in a 0.5 μM QD solution. Alternatively, drop 10 μL of the QD solution on the grid.[63,64]

(3) Dry the sample grid under ambient conditions.

(4) Take TEM photographs at various sections of the sample grid.

(5) Measure the diameter of at least 100 particles and record the average and the standard deviation.

2.1.8 Photostability[48]

Various applications of QDs require exposure to UV irradiation; therefore, they must remain stable over longer periods of time under UV. Most fluorescent organic dyes lose brightness after a few hours of exposure to UV. The following protocol is used to measure photostability of QDs:

(1) Place a 2 µM water soluble QD in a vial.
(2) Expose to UV lamp for 12-h recording the fluorescence every hour.
(3) Plot the fluorescence signal intensity against time.
(4) Repeat the process over three days for a total of 36-h exposure.

2.1.9 Atomic Absorption Spectroscopy

Atomic absorption spectroscopy (AAS) is another technique that can be used to characterize NMs in terms of elemental composition. For example, a known amount of CdSe/ZnS core/shell QDs can be used to determine the concentration of cadmium and zinc. The following protocol is used to determine the amount of Cd and Zn in a CdSe/ZnS core/shell:[48]

(1) Take a known mass of the organic soluble QD powder and dissolve with 16 M nitric acid in a fume hood. Sonicate for 10–15 min and allow it to dissolve overnight in the fume hood.
(2) Add a few drops of 12 M HCl to dissolve any precipitates.
(3) Dilute the solution to 25 mL with DI water (resistivity ≥ 18 MΩ-cm).
(4) Prepare standard solutions of Cd and Zn in DI water (resistivity ≥ 18 MΩ-cm) following manufacturer's recommendation.
(5) Take the signal of the blank solution (DI water, resistivity ≥ 18 MΩ-cm) in triplicate.
(6) Take the signals of the standard solutions (in triplicate) using the lamp corresponding to each element.
(7) Prepare the calibration curves for Cd and for Zn after subtracting the blank from the recorded signals.
(8) Calculate the absorption constant for each element using the Beer law equation:

$$A = abC$$

where A is the absorbance, a is the molar absorptivity constant, b is the light path length, and C is the concentration.

(9) Take the absorption of the CdSe/ZnS core/shell solution using the respective elements.
(10) Calculate the concentration of Cd from the Cd calibration curve.
(11) Similarly, calculate the concentration of Zn from the Zn calibration curve. Note: You can find the concentration of any other element in an NM with AAS following the same principle that was used above.

2.2 GOLD AND SILVER NMs

Gold nanoparticles (AuNPs) are among the first NPs in colloidal suspension, smaller than 10 nm that have been produced by chemical processes.[65,66] AuNPs are one of the most widely used engineered NMs for biomedical applications[67,68] because of facile modification with thiols, amines, and silane that allows conjugation with biomolecules such as proteins, peptides, and DNA.[69,70]

Usually, AuNPs are synthesized through reduction of Au(III) derivatives.[71] The citrate reduction process involves a simple procedure, yielding stable and reproducible production of AuNPs with narrow size distribution that was pioneered by Turkevich et al.[65] It involves the reduction of $HAuCl_4$ via trisodium citrate to produce 20-nm gold and was modified by Frens[72] to generate 16–150 nm by adjusting the ratio between the gold and citrate concentration. Excess unused reagents are removed by centrifugation,[73] ion exchange,[74] solvent extraction,[75] dialysis,[76] and filtration.[77]

2.2.1 Protocol for Citrate AuNP Synthesis

The following protocol for the synthesis of citrate AuNPs is described by Turkevich et al.[65] The process produces 20-nm AuNPs.

(1) Clean all glass thoroughly and rinse with DI water 3×.
(2) Place 5 mg of high purity tetrachloroauric acid ($HAuCl_4$) in DI water to a final volume of 95 mL.
(3) Boil for 20 min with mechanical stirring.
(4) Add 50 mg of trisodium citrate dihydrate (5 mL of 1% solution in water[78]) and boil for additional 20 min.
(5) Allow it to cool down at RT. Gold atoms that are released from the $HAuCl_4$ during the synthesis form the AuNPs that continue to grow until all the $HAuCl_4$ is reduced.
(6) Take a TEM scan to establish shape and size.

AuNPs now come in various shapes such as nanorods and nanostars [9,10,17]. Each of these differently shaped AuNPs come as a result of the synthesis protocol used. The nanospheres that are about 15 nm in diameter are synthesized using a trisodium citrate reduction method.[79]

This process involves the following protocol:

(1) Take trisodium citrate (2 mL, 1 wt%) and add to a boiling aqueous solution of $HAuCl_4 \cdot 3H_2O$ (50 mL, 0.4 mM).
(2) Continue to boil the solution for 30 min to form a wine-red solution.
(3) Cool the solution down and store at 4 °C.
(4) Establish the concentration of the nanospheres based on the UV–vis absorption spectroscopy by applying the Beer–Lambert law using a molar extinction coefficient of 1×10^8 M^{-1} cm^{-1}.[80]

An alternative process developed by Frens produces 40-nm gold particles.[72] Following this procedure, 50 mL of $HAuCl_4$ (0.01% solution w/v) is put to boil before adding 0.5 mL of 1% solution of trisodium citrate. Upon addition, the solution has a gray color which changes to lavender and with continued boiling for 1–3 min, develops wine-red color. Further heating or addition of citrate solution does not change particle diameter after the colloid is formed. A change in the proportions of components results in an increase of some 20% in the final particle size. Another process is found in a protocol published by McFarland et al.[78]

Purification to remove all components with a maximized recovery of the synthesized AuNP from solution involves centrifugation at different forces (3000, 5000, 7000, 9000, and 11,000g) and five durations (10 min, 20 min, 30 min, 45 min, and 60 min) by following a purification process that involves centrifugation and washing.[81] After centrifugation, the AuNP pellets are immediately resuspended in ultrapure water. The process can be repeated to remove all other undesirable components and to harvest stable AuNPs. The size of the resulting AuNPs can be controlled through the percentage of the citrate used in solution.

2.2.2 Citrate AuNP Characterization

Similar to the chemical analysis and elemental quantification of QDs, AuNPs can be analyzed using inductively coupled plasma mass spectrometry (ICP-MS) (Perkin Elmer, Massachusetts, USA). ICP-MS quantification is done by direct injection of samples into the ICP-MS sample holder. The presence of non-AuNP components (chloride, citrate, ketoglutarate, and acetate) in the synthesized AuNP solution can be examined with ion chromatography (IC) system[81] after passing a 1–5 mL sample of the AuNP solution through a nylon syringe filter (pore size: 0.45 mm) to remove AuNPs. Removal of the AuNPs is important to ensure that IC columns were protected from possible interference from the AuNPs. To monitor losses and instrument performance in the process, an internal standard (oxalate, 32.8 mg) needs to be spiked to the synthesized AuNP solution[81] to monitor procedural loss and instrument performance in a triplicate analysis. The total organic carbon (TOC) present in the reactant solution ($HAuCl_4$ and citrate) and in the product (synthesized AuNP) solution can be established using a TOC analyzer. Aggregation of the AuNPs can be established with a Zeta Trac Analyzer to assess stability over time and storage temperature.

2.2.3 AuNP Characterization with X-Ray Photoelectron Spectroscopy

To establish the AuNPs oxidation state, an X-ray photoelectron spectroscopy (XPS) coupled with a Kratos AXIS His spectrometer (Kratos Analytical Ltd, UK) is suggested. Preparation of sample is summarized below as previously described.[81]

(1) Freeze dry the AuNPs suspension at $-50\ °C$ and 0.05 mbar for more than 8 h.

(2) Aerosolize the AuNPs powder or suspension through an aerosol generation system and collect on 25-mm polycarbonate filters (pore size: 0.015 mm, Whatman, USA) and place on individual stages of a low-pressure impactor (Dekati, Finland).

(3) Impregnate portions of the filters loaded with AuNPs over a glass support for XPS analysis.

(4) Heat at 500 °C for 1 h in a tubular furnace (Nabertherm Furnace, Bremen, Germany), with air as carrier gas at a flow rate of 2 L/min.

(5) Perform XPS measurements in a vacuum of $10^{-7}–10^{-9}$ Torr using a mono-chromatized AlKa X-ray radiation (1486.7 eV photons), at a constant dwelling time of 100 ms and pass energy of 40 eV. Keep the anode voltage at 15 mV with a current of 10 mA. Obtain the survey scans and the core-level spectra at a photoelectron take-off angle of 90° (α with respect to the sample surface). Survey scans are recorded within a range of 0e1100 eV. All core-level spectra were referenced to the C1s hydrocarbon peak at 284.5 eV to compensate for surface charging. This process was used to record high-resolution photoelectron spectra for Au4f. Use the XPSPEAK software to interpret the binding energy of most prominent peaks based on a nonlinear least-square regression method.

$$2HAuCl_4 + 3Na_3C_6H_5O_7 \xrightarrow{AuNP} 2Au^0 + 3Na_2C_5H_6O_5 + 3NaCl +$$

tetrachloro-auric acid   trisodium citrate   sodium ketoglutarate   sodium chloride

$$5Cl^- + 5H^+ + 3CO_2$$

chloride ion   hydronium ions   carbon dioxide

(2.2)

More than 75% of citrate originally added as a reactant remains in the synthesized AuNP solution, which may help to stabilize the AuNPs.[82] Other side products found include ketoglutarate and acetate that must be eliminated before use to avoid interference.

The size of the AuNPs is established using TEM (Figure 2.7). About 250 NPs are used to measure size distribution using an imaging software (Image J). To calculate the average NP mass, density is assumed to be equivalent to that of bulk gold ($19.30\ g/cm^3$). As an example, using a particle size of 15.7 ± 1.2 nm, an average particle mass was calculated to be 2.4×10^7 g/mol.[83] By combining these data with inductively coupled plasmon atomic emission spectroscopy (ICP-AES) data and the average particle volume obtained by TEM analysis the molar concentration of gold particles in a given preparation is about ~10 nM. Using the UV–vis absorbance of AuNP solutions at the surface plasmon frequency (520 nm), the calculated molar extinction coefficient is typically $4.2 \times 10^8\ M^{-1}\ cm^{-1}$ for 15.7 ± 1.2-nm diameter.[83]

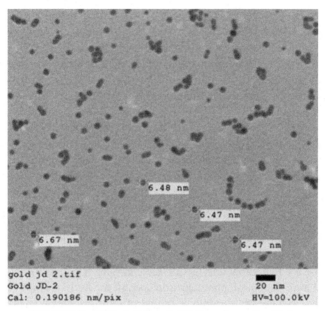

FIGURE 2.7   TEM of ~6.5 nm AuNP. *From Ocean NanoTech.*

Colloidal citrate AuNPs are made up of particles varying in diameter from ~ 5 to 150 nm. Typical diagnostic assays use gold conjugates with size ranging between 20 and 40 nm indicating a large surface area having a very high surface energy. By controlling the percentage of the trisodium citrate aqueous solution, the diameter of the resulting AuNPs may range from 15 to 150 nm. AuNPs with diameter between 6 and 15 nm are formed by reducing the $HAuCl_4$ solution with an aqueous sodium ascorbate solution. Particles with diameters smaller than 5 nm are produced by reduction with either white or yellow phosphorus in diethyl ether. Any colloidal suspension with high surface energy can lose stability when proper processing conditions are not maintained during production and use. Depending upon the ratio of the gold to citrate, the AuNPs can grow to different sizes. Colloidal AuNPs are composed of a core made of pure gold that is surrounded by a surface layer of adsorbed $AuCl^{-2}$ ions. This state confers a negative charge to the colloidal gold resulting in electrostatic repulsion that prevents particle aggregation. The introduction of electrolytes compresses the ionic double layer, thereby reducing electrostatic repulsion. This results in destabilization that causes particle aggregation that is accompanied by a color change and eventual sedimentation of the gold. Chlorides affect colloidal AuNPs more strongly than iodides.

During the synthesis of citrate AuNPs prior to the addition of the reducing agent, gold ions exist in solution. Upon the addition of the reducing agent, sodium citrate, gold atoms begin to form until the concentration reaches supersaturation that results in precipitation through nucleation. When this is reached, all the gold atoms remaining in solution continue to bind to the nucleation sites under an energy-reducing gradient until all atoms are removed from solution. The number of nucleation sites determines the number of particles that finally grow in solution. When the concentration of $HAuCl_4$ in solution is fixed, the concentration of the reducing agent controls the number of nuclei that forms: the more nuclei, the smaller the AuNPs produced. In an optimized condition, all nucleation sites will be formed instantaneously and simultaneously, resulting in the formation of AuNPs of exactly the same size (monodisperse gold).

Colloidal AuNPs display a single absorption peak in the visible range between 510 and 550 nm. As the particle size increases, the absorption maximum shifts to a longer wavelength. The width of the absorption spectra relates to the size distribution range. The colors are size-dependent such that the smallest gold colloids (2–5 nm) are yellow-orange, midrange particles (10–20 nm) are wine-red, and larger particles (30–64 nm) are blue-green.

Various strategies are suggested to attain high quality and stability in AuNPs. The first of such consideration is the use of thoroughly cleaned glassware, 0.2-μm-filtered solutions, and, ideally, triple-distilled water or nanopure water. These strategies suggest the adverse effect of trace contaminants on the preparation of colloidal AuNPs.

The order of reagent addition has also been observed as a critical parameter in controlling the quality of the gold colloid. However, the effect of adding citrate solution to the $HAuCl_4$ solution or vice versa in relation to methods of manufacturing colloidal gold suspensions has not been elucidated. In addition, the role of mixing during the process has also not been clarified.

Researchers have not exploited the role of mixing in the formation of the AuNP colloidal suspension. However, it must be noted that a large-scale operation is dependent on both the chemistry of the process and the physical parameters. Small changes in process conditions such as temperature, rate of mixing, and rate reagent addition can adversely affect the quality of the product. The following physical parameters affect the quality of the final gold suspension that is produced by the reaction of aqueous $HAuCl_4$ with an aqueous solution of trisodium citrate.

- The concentration of reactants.
- Mixing of the reactants.
- The order in which reactants are added.
- Operating temperature.
- Liquid head in the reactor.
- The reactor's material of construction.

2.2.4 Synthesis of Nanorods and Nanostars

Nanorods and nanostars can be synthesized following the seed-mediated growth method.[15,16] The protocol for the nanorods synthesis is summarized as follows:

(1) Synthesize nanorod seeds using cetyltrimethylammonium bromide (CTAB) aqueous solution, 5 mL of 0.20 M.

(2) Mix this with 5.0 mL of 0.5 mM $HAuCl_4$.

(3) Add 0.60 mL ice-cold 10 mM $NaBH_4$ solution and stir vigorously at 25 °C.

(4) Prepare the growth solution using CTAB (5 mL, 0.20 M) with 0.15 mL of 4 mM $AgNO_3$ solution at 25 °C, followed by 5.0 mL of 1 mM $HAuCl_4$ and 70 μL of 78.8 mM ascorbic acid.

(5) Add 12 μL of the seed solution to the growth solution at 27–30 °C.

(6) Keep the temperature of the growth medium constant at 27–30 °C in all preparations.

(7) Continue reaction to last for about 10 h.

(8) Centrifuge and re-disperse in pure water and store in glass bottles at RT before use.

The protocol for the synthesis of nanostars is summarized as follows:

(1) Dilute 1 mL, 1 wt% $HAuCl_4 \cdot 3H_2O$ aqueous solution with 90 mL water.

(2) Inject 2 mL of 38.8 mM trisodium citrate and add freshly prepared $NaBH_4$ solution (1 mL, 0.075 wt% in 38.8 mM trisodium citrate solution).

(3) Allow the reaction to proceed with constant stirring at RT overnight to form the seed solution.

(4) Mix 50-mL gold seed solution with 10 mM polyvinylpyrrolidone (PVP) at RT for 24 h to prepare the PVP-coated gold seed solution.

(5) Add 82 μL of 50 mM $HAuCl_4$ aqueous solution to 15 mL of 10 mM PVP in dimethylformamide (DMF), followed by the rapid addition of 43 μL of the PVP-coated gold seed solution ([Au] ≈ 4 mM) with constant stirring at RT for about 13 h.

(6) Centrifuge and re-disperse in pure water and store in glass bottles at RT before use.

Silver (Ag) has been known to have a disinfecting effect and has found applications in traditional medicines. Just like the salts of silver and their derivatives, silver nanoparticles (AgNPs) have been found to exhibit antimicrobial properties.[84] AgNPs have been reported to eliminate microorganisms on textile[85] or are used for water purification.[86]

One of the easiest ways to synthesize AgNPs is by reduction. Reduction synthesis uses silver nitrate as the raw material source of silver.

2.2.5 Protocol for Synthesis of AgNPs[87]

The AgNPs were produced by reducing silver nitrate with hydrazine in the presence of PVP.[87,88] The synthesis is carried out as follows:

(1) Dissolve 300 mg of PVP powder in 8 mL of aqueous 25-mM silver nitrate solution ($AgNO_3$).

(2) Dilute the solution with 14-mL deionized water.

(3) After 5 min at RT add 4 mL of 70-mM hydrazine ($N_2H_4 \cdot H_2O$) dropwise in stoichiometric excess to achieve complete reduction of the silver salt with continuous stirring.

(4) Purify the resulting suspension by centrifugation at 4000 rpm ($1467g$) for 10 min and by dialysis for 24 h against deionized water using a 14 kDa membrane.

(5) Determine the size distribution with dynamic light scattering (DLS). DLS is also used to establish the zeta potential.

(6) Establish the silver concentration at 450 µg/mL by inductively coupled plasma optical emission spectrometry.

(7) Like QDs, the particle size and shape is established by TEM by putting a drop of a diluted solution on a Formvar-coated copper grid.

2.2.6 Magnetic Nanoparticles

Inorganic magnetic nanoparticles (MNPs) are rapidly emerging as important NMs in medicine.[89–94] These NMs include nanowires, nanospheres, nanotubes, and magnetic thin films. Medical applications of MNPs include diagnosis (such as detection of malignant tissues in magnetic resonance imaging (MRI) and cell tracking) and therapy (such as guided drug and gene delivery, cancer therapy, tissue engineering, and bioseparation). The diagnostic and therapeutic applications of MNPs can be combined such as in MNP-mediated drug delivery and MRI imaging (i.e., theranostics).[83,89–92,95]

MNPs (5–60 nm) can be coated with dextran, phospholipids, or other compounds to inhibit aggregation and passive or active targeting agents.[96] After surface functionalization and attachment of DNA fragments, proteins, peptides, or drugs, MNPs can be used for drug delivery, magnetic separation, diagnostics, or MRI contrast enhancement.[89–93,96–105] A nonspecific labeling method based on anionic MNPs can be used to predict uptake efficiency in various cell types including tumor cells and at the same time provides sufficient magnetization for MRI detection and distal manipulation.[106,107]

MNPs represent an important class of NMs. Their magnetic properties drastically change with size as magnetic anisotropic energy (KV, where K is the magnetic anisotropic constant and V is the particle volume) becomes comparable to the thermal energy (kT) resulting in moment randomization and superparamagnetism.[108,109] Their magnetic signal stands out in the presence of biomolecules making them readily identified even in vivo.[92,110,111] The MNPs do not show net magnetic moment in the absence of external magnetic field allowing for their long-term stability in various dispersion media.[112] Their susceptibility to functionalization and manipulation under an external magnetic field provide controllable magnetic tagging of biomolecules, leading to highly efficient bioseparation–biodelivery[111] and highly sensitive biolabeling and MRI contrast enhancement.[92,97,111]

To be applicable for biomedical applications, the NMs need to be monodisperse to have uniform physical and chemical properties that are important for controlled biodistribution, bioelimination, and contrast effects.[112] The MNPs need to be water soluble and can be modified, so that they are capable of binding specifically to a biological entity. They have to be able to withstand various physiological conditions and a high magnetic moment. The chemical and magnetic stabilities of iron oxide NMs coupled with their low level toxicity in biological systems make them attractive for medical applications.[113] However, nonuniformity in size and shape has slowed down the advances in the biomedical applications of MNPs. Numerous changes in the parameters during synthesis have generated MNPs with narrow size and uniform size distribution in a large-scale production.[114]

Among the MNPs, the iron oxide magnetic nanoparticles (IOMNPs) have the greatest potential for various medical applications especially for drug delivery.[89,92,115–117] This is due to the chemical composition of IOMNPs which allow them to be biodegradable and nontoxic.[112,115,117–125] Various sizes of IOMNPs are commercially available from various sources as shown in Table 2.1. The IOMNPs come in various sizes and different surface modifications.

2.2.6.1 Protocol for IOMNP Synthesis[112]

The materials used for the synthesis were commercially available. Synthesis was carried out using clean reaction vessels and standard airless procedures.

2.2.6.1.1 Method for Fe_3O_4 Synthesis

Absolute ethanol, hexane, phenyl ether (99%), benzyl ether (99%), 1-octadecene (90%), 1,2-hexadecanediol (90%), 1,2-tetradecanediol (97%), oleic acid (90%), oleylamine (>70%), D-(+)-glucose, and HABA/avidin, iron(III) acetylacetonate [$Fe(acac)_3$], cobalt(II) acetylacetonate [$Co(acac)_2$], and manganese(II)

TABLE 2.1 Vendors of IOMNPs

Size (nm)	Surface modification	Company
5–50	Streptavidin, protein G, antibody, enzyme (HRP or alkaline phosphatase), PEG, polyethylene imine (PEI), carboxyl, amine, chitosan, lipid, dextran	Ocean NanoTech (Arkansas, USA)
5–10	PEG	Sigma (Missouri, USA)
30–50	Streptavidin, protein A, silica, vinyl, carboxyl, amine, DNA	TurboBeads (Switzerland)
50–100	Amine silane, glucuronic acid, bromoacetyl, chitosan, citric acid, starch, DEAE-starch, phosphate-starch, dextran, lipid, diphosphate, etc.	Chemicell (Berlin, Germany)
800	Biotin, streptavidin	Solulink (California, USA)

acetylacetonate   [Mn(acac)$_2$];   1,2-distearoyl-*sn*-glycero-3-phosphoethanol-amine-*N*-[biotinyl(polyethylene glycol)2000], DSPE-PEG(2000)Biotin.

(1) Under a flow of nitrogen gas, mix Fe(acac)$_3$ (2 mmol), 1,2-hexadecane-diol (10 mmol), oleic acid (6 mmol), oleyl amine (6 mmol), and benzyl ether (20 mL) with a magnetic stirrer.

(2) Heat to 200 °C for 2 h.

(3) Under a blanket of nitrogen, heat to reflux at 300 °C for 1 h. This will lead to a blackish brown mixture.

(4) Remove from heat source and cool the mixture down to RT.

(5) At ambient conditions add 40 mL ethanol.

(6) Centrifuge to separate the black residue.

(7) Dissolve the black product in hexane in the presence of oleic acid (~0.05 mL) and oleyl amine (~0.05 mL).

(8) Centrifuge at 6000 rpm for 10 min to remove any undispersed residue.

(9) Precipitate the NPs, 6 nm Fe$_3$O$_4$ with ethanol.

(10) Centrifuge at 6000 rpm for 10 min to remove the solvent and re-disperse in hexane.

The reaction of Fe(acac)$_3$ with surfactants at high temperature leads to mono-disperse Fe$_3$O$_4$ NPs.[112] The most important factor to monodispersity of the particles is to heat the mixture to 200 °C first for 2 h before raising the temperature to reflux at 265 °C in phenyl ether, or at ~300 °C in benzyl ether, or 310 °C in 1-octadecene. Avoid directly heating the mixture to reflux from RT because this would result in Fe$_3$O$_4$ NPs with a wide size distribution from 4 to 20 nm, which indicates that the formation of Fe-based nuclei at these reaction conditions is not a fast process.[112] The 2 mmol Fe(acac)$_3$ with 6 mmol of oleic acid, 6 mmol of oleylamine, and 10 mmol of 1,2-hexadecanediol reaction in 20 mL benzyl ether produced 6 nm Fe$_3$O$_4$ NPs while when phenyl ether (or 1-octadecene) was used as a solvent, 4 nm (or ~12 nm) Fe$_3$O$_4$ NPs were formed. Because the boiling point of 1-octadecene (310 °C) or benzyl ether (298 °C) is higher than that of phenyl ether (259 °C), the larger size of Fe$_3$O$_4$ NPs obtained from benzyl ether (or 1-octadecene) solution indicates that high reaction temperature facilitates the formation of large particles.

2.2.6.1.2 Method for 5 nm CoFe$_2$O$_4$ NP Synthesis[112]

(1) Mix Co(acac)$_2$ (1 mmol), Fe(acac)$_3$ (2 mmol), 1,2-hexadecanediol (10 mmol), oleic acid (6 mmol), oleyl amine (6 mmol), and benzyl ether (20 mL) with a magnetic stirrer under a flow of nitrogen.

(2) Heat the mixture to 200 °C for 2 h.

(3) Under a blanket of nitrogen, heat to reflux at ~300 °C for 1 h.

(4) Remove from heat source and cool the black mixture down to RT.

(5) Repeat steps 5–10 in the methods for Fe$_3$O$_4$.

(6) A black-brown hexane dispersion of 5 nm CoFe$_2$O$_4$ NPs is produced.

2.2.6.1.3 Method for 7 nm MnFe$_2$O$_4$ NP Synthesis[112]

(1) Mix Mn(acac)$_2$ (1 mmol), Fe(acac)$_3$ (2 mmol), 1,2-hexadecanediol (10 mmol), oleic acid (6 mmol), oleyl amine (6 mmol), and benzyl ether (20 mL) with magnetic stirrer under a flow of nitrogen.
(2) Heat the mixture to 200 °C for 2 h.
(3) Reflux at ~300 °C for 1 h under a blanket of nitrogen.
(4) Remove from heat source and cool the black mixture down to RT.
(5) Repeat steps 5–10 in the methods for Fe$_3$O$_4$.
(6) A black-brown hexane dispersion of 7 nm MnFe$_2$O$_4$ NPs is produced.

Using the above protocols, IOMNPs with various sizes were made by choosing different solvent for the reaction, or by controlling the concentration of the metal precursors and metal/surfactant ratio. The protocols produced up to 15-nm diameter NPs.

2.2.6.2 Surface Modification of the Iron Oxide NPs

The synthesis of iron oxide NPs leads to hydrophobic MNPs that are not biocompatible. The non-water soluble properties of the MNPs require further surface chemical modifications in order to ensure safety and good dispersibility in aqueous media. Various approaches have been developed for converting the MNPs into their water-soluble form. Such approaches utilize procedures that can involve (i) the exchange of the hydrophobic ligand surfactant coatings on the NP surface with more hydrophilic ligands;[53,126,127] (ii) the growth of a water soluble protecting layer material around the original NPs;[128,129] (iii) the complete encapsulation of the hydrophobic NP within an amphiphilic polymeric shell.[58,59,130,131] One protocol for the conversion of organic soluble MNPs to their water-soluble form is as follows.

2.2.6.2.1 Protocol for MNP Modification

(1) Evaporate the hexane under a flow of nitrogen gas and collect the black solid residue of iron oxide NPs.
(2) Dissolve the residue in chloroform at a concentration of 0.5 mg particles/ mL solution.
(3) Add 1 mL of chloroform solution of DSPE-PEG(2000)Biotin (10 mg/mL) to every 2 mL of the NP dispersion.
(4) Put the mixture in a shaker for 1 h and evaporate the solvent under nitrogen gas.
(5) Disperse the residue in PBS solution.
(6) Filter off undissolved residue with a 0.2-μm syringe filter.
(7) Purify using a Nanosep 100K Omega to remove unreacted DSPE-PEG(2000)Biotin or use a magnetic separator (Figure 2.8).

The most important aspect of MNPs for medical and other biological applications is biocompatibility and surface engineering. Surface engineering of MNPs allows for the introduction of (a) ligands that are used for specific cell/tissue/

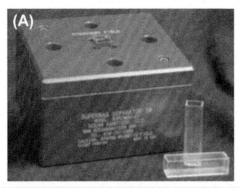

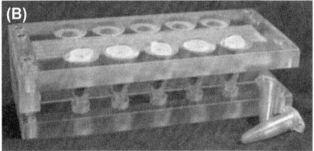

FIGURE 2.8   Small instrument for the purification of magnetic NMs: (A) Multitube Magnetic Separator™ and (B) Supermag Separator™. *From Ocean NanoTech. (For color version of this figure, the reader is referred to the online version of this book)*

organ targeting, (b) therapeutic molecules for drug delivery, and (c) other molecules such as small organic dyes for detection and other functions of NP.

2.2.6.3 MNPs Characterization

The characterization of MNPs is similar to those of the AuNPs and QDs. TEM and gel electrophoresis are used to establish size and size distribution (Figure 2.9), quantitative elemental analysis can be carried out with ICP-AES or with electron diffraction spectrum (EDS). Magnetic properties are measured with a Lakeshore 7404 high-sensitivity vibrating sample magnetometer (VSM) with fields up to 1 T at RT. The hydrodynamic diameter of the particles (core diameter plus shell thickness) in water is measured using a Malvern Zeta Sizer Nano S-90 DLS instrument. UV–vis analysis is used to establish concentration. Just like in the preparation of QDs samples for TEM, the MNP samples are prepared by drying a hexane dispersion of the particles on amorphous carbon-coated copper grids.

2.3 ORGANIC NMs

Currently, the most widely used NMs for medical applications are those that are organic in nature. These include liposomes, micelles, dendrimers, and

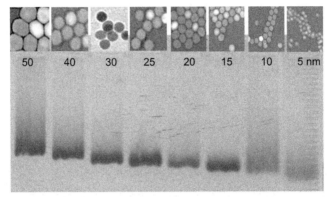

FIGURE 2.9 TEM and agarose gel electrophoresis of water soluble IOMNPs at 5–50 nm. *Courtesy of Ocean NanoTech. (For color version of this figure, the reader is referred to the online version of this book)*

even proteins and peptides. Synthesis of a few of these NMs will be discussed below.

2.3.1 Liposomes

The original models of nanoscaled drug delivery devices are the liposomes that were discovered in mid-1960s.[132] These are spherical NMs made of lipid bilayer membranes that have an aqueous interior but can be unilamellar (having a single lamella of membrane) or multilamellar (having multiple membranes). These are used as effective drug delivery systems for cancer chemotherapeutic drugs and other drugs. Potent and toxic drugs like amphotericin and hamycin when formulated as liposomal drugs exhibit improved efficacy and safety compared with conventional preparations. In these liposomes, water-soluble drugs are loaded in an aqueous compartment and lipid soluble drugs are incorporated in the liposomal membrane 2. However, the rapid degradation of liposome and clearance by the liver macrophages[133] reduces the duration of action of the drug it carries. This can be circumvented with the advent of stealth liposomes that are coated with materials like polyoxyethylene,[134] which prevents opsonization of the liposome and uptake by macrophages.[135] Other ways of prolonging the circulation time of liposomes are incorporation of substances like cholesterol,[136] PVP polyacrylamide lipids,[137] and high transition temperature phospholipids distearoyl phosphatidylcholine.[138]

Phospholipid vesicles called liposomes have been recognized in biology and medicine, as promising nanoscaled drug delivery devices.[132] Liposome preparations can lead to multilamellar vesicles (MLV) or the development of the sonicated unilamellar vesicles (SUV).[135] Both preparations show relatively low volume of entrapped aqueous space per mole of lipid restricting the ability to encapsulate large macromolecules. This can be a result of the MLV having most of the lipid in the internal lamellae, and the close apposition of the adjacent concentric bilayers restricts the internal water space. In single-compartment vesicles formed during SUV, the ratio of surface area to encapsulated volume is larger resulting in only a small aqueous volume per mole of lipid.

Various methods for the synthesis of MLVs and SUVs have been described. One of these is the ethanol injection method that produces vesicles of about the same size as SUV, while the ether infusion technique produces large unilamellar vesicles with high captured volumes per mole of lipid low encapsulation efficiency.[139]

Szoka's group produced vesicles with the following desirable properties: (i) the ability to entrap a large percentage of the aqueous material presented; (ii) a high aqueous space-to-lipid ratio; and (iii) widely variable chemistry of the lipid components.[139] They developed conditions that achieve a high percentage of encapsulation and vesicles with a large aqueous space-to-lipid ratio in a method they called the reverse-phase evaporation technique.[140]

2.3.1.1 Liposome Synthesis

There are a number of published protocols for the synthesis of different liposome NMs. In this book, we focused on the protocol pioneered by the group of Papahadjopoulos.[139–141] In their process, cholesterol, palmitic acid, phosphatidylcholine, (PtdCho), phosphatidylglycerol (PtdGro), and phosphatidylserine (PtdSer) used were isolated from egg yolk and bovine brain,[140] while phosphatidic acid and dipalmitoyl phosphatidylcholine ($Pal_2PtdCho$) were synthesized as reported.[140] These were purified with silicic acid columns and tested by thin-layer chromatography to check the purity[141] before storage in chloroform in sealed ampules under nitrogen at -50 °C until use.

Protocol for preparation of reverse-phase evaporation vesicles is given below:[139]

(1) Prepare a mixture of several phospholipids, either pure or mixed with other lipids such as cholesterol, long-chain alcohols, etc., can be used with similar results.

(2) Add the lipid mixture to a 50-mL round-bottom flask with a long extension neck, and remove the solvent by rotary evaporation under reduced pressure.

(3) Purge the system with nitrogen and redissolve the lipids in the organic phase to form the reversed phase vesicles using diethyl ether and isopropyl ether or halothane and trifluorotrichloroethane.

(4) When the lipid has low solubility in ether, add chloroform or methanol to increase their solubility (Table X from Szoka and Papahadjopoulos[139]).

(5) Add the aqueous phase and keep the system continuously under nitrogen.

(6) Briefly sonicate the resulting two-phase system (2–5 min) in a bath-type sonicator (Lab Supply T-80-80-IRS) until the mixture becomes either a clear one-phase dispersion or a homogeneous opalescent dispersion

that does not separate for at least 30 min after sonication. The degree of opalescence depends upon the solvent, phospholipid, and amount of aqueous phase in the preparation. The sonication temperature for diethyl ether and most lipids is 0–5 °C unless otherwise stated.

(7) Place the mixture on the rotary evaporator to evaporate the organic solvent at 20–25 °C, rotating at approximately 200 rpm. As the solvent is removed, the material first forms a viscous gel and subsequently (within 5–10 min) becomes an aqueous suspension.

(8) You may add water or buffer (optional) and evaporate for 15 min at 20 °C to remove traces of solvent.

(9) When lipid mixtures in the absence of cholesterol are used at low concentrations (<7.5 umol of lipid per milliliter of aqueous phase) the gel phase may not be apparent since the system rapidly reverts to a lipid-in-water suspension. In this case, either dialyze, pass through a Sepharose 4B column, or centrifuge to remove nonencapsulated material and residual organic solvent.

In general, a lipid preparation contains 33 µmol of phospholipid and 33 µmol of cholesterol in 1.0 mL of aqueous phase (PBS) and 3 mL of solvent. These ratios are optimal, but can be scaled down or up without any change in the characteristics of the resulting vesicles. To make vesicles from $Pal_2PtdCho$, an additional 3 mL chloroform or 0.8 mL of methanol is added and the vesicles are allowed to remain at 45 °C for at least 30 min after evaporation of the solvent.

Detection of the amount of encapsulated small molecules such as sodium, sucrose, or [3H]ara C can be achieved by dialyzing the vesicles overnight against 300 vol of PBS (three changes) at 4 °C. Column chromatography can be used to separate encapsulated proteins from unencapsulated proteins (Sepharose 4B, 1.5 × 42 cm). Ultracentrifugation at 100,000g for 30 min can be used to separate encapsulated [3H]poly(A) from unencapsulated material and resuspension of the pelleted vesicles in buffer (twice); the unencapsulated poly(A) remains in solution.[139]

2.3.2 Polymeric NPs[142]

Polymer-based nanoparticles (PNPs) are among the most advanced NMs when it comes to their medical applications because these can effectively carry drugs, proteins, and DNA to target cells and organs.[142] They are effective for cell membrane permeation and they exhibit stability in the blood stream. They are convenient materials for various unique molecular designs with many potential medical applications.[143]

Polymers are being studied to carry drugs (small molecules and/or proteins) and to release these when the PNPs reach the destination.[144] Their long shelf life and their minimal toxicity make them good candidates as delivery system for drugs and proteins.[144,145] In aqueous solution, amphiphilic block or graft copolymers assemble spontaneously into NPs.[142] Polymers, such as poly-lactic acid

(PLA), poly-glycolic acid (PGA), poly-lactic glycolic acid (PLGA), poly(ε-caprolactone), polyglutamic acid, and polymalic acid, and their copolymers are among the most extensively studied.[142] These polymers are usable for NP formulation, biocompatible, and have been used in surgery for 30 years and have shown biocompatibility.[146] The drug release rate that is controlled by the polymer degradation can be controlled by adjusting the molecular mass of the PNPs; in the case of copolymers, their composition and microstructure can be used to control the drug release.[147]

2.3.2.1 Synthesis of PLGA NPs[148]

A solvent diffusion method is used to prepare PLGA NPs. The protocol is as follows:[148]

(1) PLGA, 50 mg, was dissolved in 3.0 mL acetone.
(2) This PLGA solution was added to 30 mL of 0.2% poly(ethylene-*alt*-maleic anhydride (PEMA) through a syringe pump at a rate of 20 mL/h with stirring at 200 rpm in a hood to evaporate the acetone. PEMA was utilized as a surfactant to increase the number of carboxyl groups on the particles.[149]
(3) Collect the NPs by centrifugation at 15,000 rpm for 45 min.
(4) Wash the NPs with double-distilled water three times.

The sizes and zeta potentials of the PLGA NPs can be determined using a DLS system.

2.3.2.2 Synthesis of PLA NPs[150]

Materials: D,L-lactide (from Aldrich, Milwakee, USA); monomethoxy PEG (M_w 5000 Da) and stannous octoate (Sigma Chemical, St Louis, USA). Purified tetanus toxoid (TT, M_w 150,000 Da, 85–95% monomeric) dissolved at 10 mg/mL in PBS, pH 7.4 (Massachusetts Biological Laboratories, Boston, MA). Cholic acid (sodium salt, purity 99%), pepsin A from porcine stomach mucosa, and pancreatin from porcine pancreas (Sigma Quı́mica, Madrid, Spain).

The polymer NPs were prepared by the double emulsion technique as previously described.[151,152]

(1) Place 50 mL of the TT solution and emulsify in a 1-mL solution of PLA or PLA–PEG (50 mg) in ethyl acetate by sonication (Branson 250, Sonifier®) for 15 s (20 W).
(2) Add 2 mL of aqueous sodium cholate solution (1% w/v).
(3) Sonicate the emulsion for 15 s (20 W).
(4) Dilute the emulsion in 100 mL sodium cholate solution (0.3% w/v).
(5) Evaporate the solvent rapidly under vacuum (Rotavapor R-114, Buchi, Switzerland).
(6) Collect the NPs by centrifugation at 22,000g for 30 min (Avanti™ 30, Beckman, Spain).
(7) Purify by washing three times with double-distilled water.

2.3.2.3 Characterization of Polymer NMs

The particle size and zeta potential of NPs can be determined, respectively, by photon correlation spectroscopy (PCS) and laser Doppler anemometry (LDA) using a Mastersizer® (Malvern Instruments, UK). The copolymer composition and number-average molecular weight can be studied by ^{1}H NMR spectroscopy at 400 MHz using D-chloroform as a solvent.

2.3.3 Chitosan[153]

The chitosan for this methodology was first refined twice by dissolving it in dilute acetic acid solution, filtered, precipitated with aqueous NaOH, and dried in vacuum at RT[153] resulting in 90% deacetylation. The weight-average molecular weights of chitosan were 40, 80, 100, 200, and 300 kDa that were established by viscometric methods.[154] The potassium persulfate ($K_2S_2O_8$) was purified by dissolving in DI water and recrystallized water and acrylic acid (AA) was distilled under reduced pressure in nitrogen atmosphere. Silk peptide powder was used as the model drug.

2.3.3.1 Preparation of Chitosan–Poly(Acrylic Acid) (CS–PAA) NPs by Polymerization[153]

The following protocol is followed for the preparation of CS–PAA.

(1) Dissolve chitosan in 50-mL AA in the ratio of 1:1 ([aminoglucoside units]:[AA]) with magnetic stirring. (Maintain the AA in all experiments at 3 mmol).
(2) When the solution becomes clear, add 0.1 mmol of $K_2S_2O_8$.
(3) Maintain the pH at 4.0.
(4) Heat to 70 °C under a stream of nitrogen and magnetic stirring until an opalescent suspension is produced.
(5) Cool down the reaction to RT.
(6) Filter the reaction mixture with filter paper to remove any polymer aggregation.
(7) Dialyze in a buffer solution of pH 4.5 for 24 h using a dialysis membrane bag with a molecular weight cut-off of 10 kDa.

2.3.3.2 Preparation of CS–PAA NPs by Dropping Method[153]

CS–PAA NPs can also be prepared by mixing positively charged CS and negatively charged PAA using the dropping method as follows:

(1) Add 1 mL of 0.02% CS solution (CS with a molecular weight of 80 kDa dissolved in 1% (w/v)acetic acid solution) dropwise to 5 mL 0.02% PAA (M_n = 100 kDa) aqueous solution with magnetic stirring to form the opalescent suspension.

(2) Filter the obtained suspension with a filter paper and incubate in buffer solution of pH = 4.5 for 24 h using a dialysis membrane bag for characterization.

(3) Add PAA 1 mL 0.02% PAA (M_n = 100 kDa) solution dropwise to 5 mL 0.02% CS solution (CS with molecular weight 80 kDa in 1% (w/v) acetic acid solution) under magnetic stirrer.

2.3.3.3 Preparation of Drug-Loaded CS NPs[153]

For the most part, liposomes are used in drug encapsulation. The following protocol describes the preparation of drug-loaded NPs:

(1) Dissolve 50 mg of SP in 50-mL CS–PAA NPs that were prepared by polymerization of AA in CS solution with the CS molecular weight 80 kDa and incubate for 48 h.

(2) Separate the NPs from the aqueous phase by ultracentrifugation (Ultra ProTM 80, Du Pont) with 50,000 rpm at 4 °C for 40 min.

(3) Wash the SP loaded CS–PAA NPs with acetone three times.

(4) Freeze in liquid nitrogen and lyophilize to obtain freeze-dried SP loaded CS–PAA NPs.

2.3.4 Micelles

Micelles are spherical amphiphilic structures that have a hydrophobic core and a hydrophilic shell.[155] The hydrophilic shell makes the micelle water soluble that allows for intravenous delivery while the hydrophobic core carries a payload of drug for therapy.[156] The nanoscale dimensions (diameter less than 50 nm)[157] and the hydrophilic shell of polymeric micelles serve as protection from elimination by the reticulo-endothelial system, thereby increasing their circulation time and ability to deliver the drug to the target.

Polymeric micelles are biocompatible, highly stable in vitro and in vivo, and can dissolve a broad variety of poorly soluble pharmaceuticals. This capability of micelles has led to the development of several types of drug-loaded micelles that are currently being tested in preclinical and clinical trials.[142,157] Among polymeric micelles, a special group is formed by lipid-core micelles, i.e., micelles formed by conjugates of soluble copolymers with lipids (such as PEG–PE conjugate). Tumor may be targeted with micelles by exploiting the enhanced permeability and retention (EPR) effect, by making micelles of stimuli-responsive amphiphilic block copolymers, or by attaching specific targeting ligand molecules to the micelle surface.[158]

2.4 CARBON NANOPLATFORMS

CNTs are among the most widely discussed NMs[159–169] and can be fabricated into biodegradable nanostructures (cylindrical buckytubes). These structures are currently being studied for use in nanomedicine and in tissue engineering as nanovectors.[169–171] The CNTs are synthesized by rolling sheets of carbon into hollow tubes that can be in the form of single-walled (0.4- to 2-nm diameter), double-walled (1- to 3.5-nm diameter), or multiwalled (2- to 100-nm diameter).[142] Although multiwalled CNTs have not resulted in proliferative or cytokine changes in vitro, CNT size and composition must be carefully controlled to promote intracellular delivery of these nanotubes and to prevent immune reaction to them.[172] Functionalization and alteration of CNT and other graphite nanoplatform surface chemistry can reduce or eliminate complement activation while making the CNTs more biocompatible.[166–168,173,174]

2.4.1 Protocol for the Synthesis of CNTs

There are numerous publications about CNTs in journals and in books. Only a simple method is described in this book using catalytic decomposition to form CNTs.[175] The following method was derived from Gao's group publication.[175]

(1) LaNi alloy is prepared by arc-melting an argon atmosphere.
(2) Alloy ingot is ground mechanically into its powder form to a particle size between 15 and 20 µm.
(3) Soak the powder with 6 N KOH solution at 70 °C for 8 h.
(4) Rinse thoroughly with running distilled water and dry in vacuum.
(5) Place the dried powder in a ceramic boat.
(6) Introduce into the flow reactor (quartz tube with an inner diameter of 3 cm and a length of 60 cm) for the CNT synthesis.
(7) Treat the alloy powder at 600 °C with flowing H_2 at 50 cm^3/min for 30 min to reduce nickel oxides at the particle surface.
(8) Introduce methane at 80 cm^3/min at atmospheric pressure, temperature of 670 °C for 30 min over the LaNi particle catalyst to synthesize the CNTs by catalytic decomposition.
(9) Collect the CNTs and characterize with SEM and TEM.

Another method was published by the group of Nasibulin who investigated CNT formation in two experimental setups as shown in their paper.[176] The two processes differ in the location of the catalyst particle generator that is outside (ex situ) or inside (in situ) the flow reactor. Both setups consisted of a hot wire generator (HWG) and a heated vertical tubular furnace and a ceramic tube, with an internal diameter of 22 mm inserted inside the furnace (Entech, Sweden; 44 or 90-cm long) was used as the reactor that was operated at ambient temperature.[176] The laminar flow conditions inside the reactor were maintained. The HWG was a resistively heated thin iron or nickel wire (0.25 mm in diameter) protected from the environment with either glass shielding (ex situ) or with a ceramic tube (in situ) through which a carrier gas was passed.[176] The particles formed by the HWG were transferred into the reactor by a carrier gas that consisted of a hydrogen/nitrogen mixture (with a mole component ratio of 7.0/93.0 or 99.999% high purity nitrogen at flow rates from 100 to 1000 cm^3/min).[176]

For the ex situ process, the catalyst particles were formed in a HWG positioned outside the furnace that were mixed with the carbon source and the promoter before entry into the reactor.[176] The in situ process involved a small ceramic tube (external and internal diameters of 13 and 9 mm, respectively, and 25-cm long) that was inserted inside the reactor.[176] The particles formed were mixed in the reactor at about 400 °C with an outer flow at 400 cm^3/min containing a carbon source. The carbon sources used were alcohols such as ethanol (Primalco Oy, 99.5%) or 1-octanol (J.T. Baker, 99%)[176] that were introduced by bubbling a carrier gas (CO or N$_2$) through the liquid carbon source at RT in the presence of a promoter such as thiophene (0.5%), to increase the yield of CNTs.[177] To lower the carbon source and promoter vapor pressures in the reactor the partial vapor pressures were calculated from the equilibrium vapor pressures of the constituents and their mole fractions in solution. The products were collected from the gas phase with an electrostatic precipitator (combination electrostatic precipitator, InTox Products) on carbon-coated copper grids (SPI Lacey Carbon Grid).

The ex situ experimental setup showed disadvantages that included the following: (1) the size of the particles cannot be controlled well due to the relatively long time between primary particle formation and their introduction into the reactor; (2) significant particle losses before introduction to the reactor; (3) the multiwalled CNTs formed via the gas-phase process do not posses well-graphitized wall structures. The presence of a promoter (thiophene) in the system increased harvest in the synthesis of multiwalled CNTs, while minimal increase was found for the single-walled CNT production.[176]

2.4.2 Fullerenes

Fullerenes, C60 being the most common form, is another class of carbon NMs that were predicted to exist in 1970 and officially publicized in 1985.[178,179] To date, fullerenes have led to the synthesis of fullerene derivatives, such as C61-butylic acid and other fullerene variations, such as C70, C20 (the smallest member), CNTs (elongated, tube-structured fullerene), carbon nano-onions, and nano-buds.[180–182] One of the most unique properties of fullerenes is the ability to assume different forms and to engage compounds.[176] Their unique physical, chemical, electrical, and optical properties allowed their application as added components of new or improved devices and materials leading to advancements in science, engineering, and industry.[183–186] Fullerenes with well-defined properties and containing polymers and amphiphilic systems that are sensitive to stimuli can be easily synthesized using the azido coupling and atom transfer radical addition process.[187] Research continues into ways to increase the solubility of fullerenes and to investigate the toxicity of fullerenes and their derived compounds.[188]

2.5 DENDRIMERS

One of the most versatile and most studied nanostructures as carriers of various molecules is dendrimers.[189] Dendrimers have complex structures consisting of an inner core surrounded with branches decorated with functional groups at the ends. Dendrimers become progressively larger with the addition of each generation (shell) of branches and can be built from the molecular level to nanoscale size (1 nm to over 10 nm). The generation (shell) number and the chemical composition of the core, branches, and surface functional groups determine the size, shape, and reactivity of dendrimers. The ability to precisely control their size, shape, and surface functionality during synthesis makes dendrimers one of the most versatile and customizable nanotechnologies. Dendrimers have myriad applications, including solubility enhancement[190,191] and gene therapy[192,193] drug delivery[194,195,196] nanocomposites[197–199]), photodynamic therapy,[200,201] and bioimaging of and the treatment of cancer.[202,203]

Dendrimers, also known as arborols, or cascade, cauliflower, or starburst polymers are attracting have unique structures and properties.[204–206] These synthetic molecules are constructed from ABn monomers (n usually 2 or 3) resulting in hyper-branched structures rather than the sAB monomers, which produce linear polymers. They are synthesized in an iterative fashion leading to stepwise synthetic growth, wherein the number of monomer units incorporated in each successive iteration roughly doubles (AB2) or triples (AB3) that in the previous cycle.[204] Using vide infra, one of the synthetic approaches to dendrimers each repetition cycle leads to the addition of additional layer of branches, *generation*, to the dendrimer framework. In this process, the generation number is equal to the number of repetition cycles performed that is determined by counting the number of branch points from the core to the periphery.[204] But, an activated ABn monomer may be polymerized in a single step resulting in a polymer with a higher polydispersity (PD) and a lower degree of branching called *hyperbranched polymers*.[204,207]

The ability to synthesize dendrimer in a controlled manner to yield very high molecular weight polymers with narrower molecular weight distributions is desired.[204] Smaller dendrimers (e.g., M_w 10–50 kDa) are often produced from short syntheses leading to single compounds (PD) and not mixtures of polymer molecular weights. Dendrimers with molecular weights over 103 kDa and molecular dimensions in the 1–100 nm range have been synthesized in a few steps which are not as homogeneous as the smaller dendrimers.[204] Since the initial report about dendrimers by Vogtle in 1978, a multitude of dendrimers of different structural classes have been reported ranging from pure hydrocarbons to peptides to coordination compounds.

The two most commonly used dendrimers, the poly(amidoamine) (PAMAM) dendrimers and poly(propylene imine) dendrimers, are commercially available.[204] There are two main synthetic strategies for synthesizing dendrimers: the divergent and convergent approaches.

The divergent strategy, which was pioneered by Newkome and Tomalia (*vide infra*), is that dendrimers are built from the central core going outward to the periphery. A number of reactive groups, n, on the dendrimer periphery react with n monomer units to add a new generation to the dendrimer in each repeat cycle. This creates $2n$ or $3n$ reactive sites in the succeeding repeat cycles depending on whether the monomer unit's branch multiplicity is 2 or 3 (i.e., AB2 vs AB3 monomer).[204] In this manner, the number of coupling reactions increases with each successive generation.[205,208–210]

In the convergent strategy,[211–213] the dendrimer is built from the periphery toward the central core.[204] The initial reaction sites are on the periphery of the dendrimer, while the reactions take place at the reactive core (called the *focal point*).[204] The number of coupling reactions to add each new generation is usually 2 or 3, depending on branch multiplicity during the synthesis that makes defective products easier to separate. Thus, the dendrimers resulting from the convergent strategy are generally more homogeneous and often monodisperse unlike those prepared by a divergent approach, where defects begin to accumulate at higher generation numbers when a large number of coupling or condensation reactions have to occur on a congested dendrimer surface. Therefore, dendrimers prepared by the divergent approach are usually monomolecular species but contain significant defects while those prepared by the convergent strategy are limited to lower generation numbers.[204]

The group of Sato reported the synthesis of dendritic chiral catalysts, which have rigid hydrocarbon backbones with no heteroatoms.[214] They also showed uses as chiral catalysts in the enantioselective addition of dialkylzincs to aldehydes (Figure 1 of Sato's paper). The chiral dendrimers were synthesized using the following protocol.

2.5.1 Protocol for Synthesis Dendrimers[214]

(1) Use the Hagihara–Sonogashira coupling reaction[215] between ethyl 4-iodobenzoate (2) and ethynyltrimethylsilane followed by subsequent reduction of the ester and removal of a trimethylsilyl group that leads to the formation of the intermediate product 4-ethynylbenzyl alcohol 3 (Scheme 2.1).

(2) Methylation of 3 and treatment with (1R,2S)-ephedrine and potassium carbonate produces the chiral amino alcohol labeled 4.

(3) Following Scheme 2.2, when 1,3,5-triiodobenzene (5) was treated with two molar equivalents of 4, a biscoupled product 6 was obtained as a major product.

(4) When compound 5 was treated with excess 4, 1a (G1) with three ephedrine moieties was synthesized at 66% yield.

(5) Compound 6 was further converted to a terminal alkyne 7 by coupling with ethynyltrimethylsilane and subsequent removal of the trimethylsilyl group.

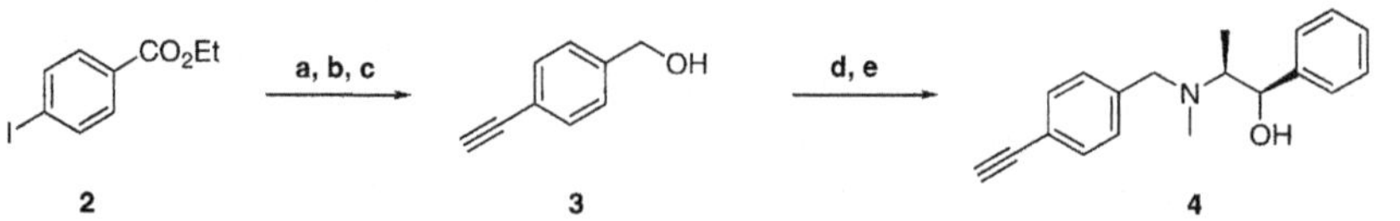

SCHEME 2.1 Reagents and conditions: (a) HC_C-SiMe3, cat. Pd(PPh3)4, cat. CuI, Et3N, THF, reflux; (b) LiAlH4, ether; (c) Bu4NF, THF, overall 83% (three steps); (d) MsCl, Et3N, CH2Cl2; (e) (1R,2S)-ephedrine_HCl, K2CO3 CH3CN, reflux, overall 76% (two steps)[214]. *Copyright permission from reference 214.*

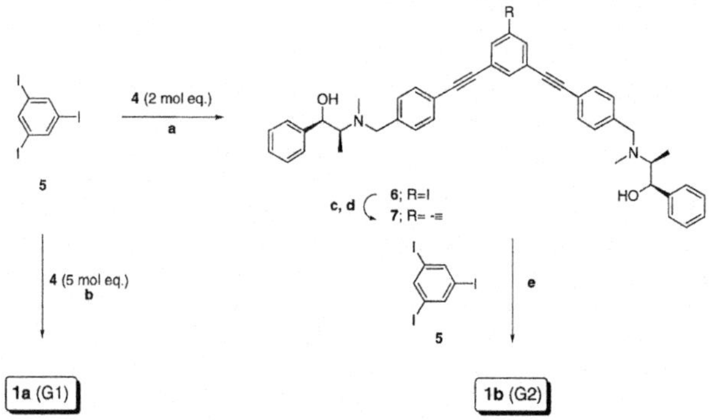

SCHEME 2.2 Reagents and conditions: (a) **4** (2 mol equiv.), cat. Pd(PPh3)4, cat. CuI, Et3N, THF, reflux, 49%; (b) **4** (5 mol equiv.), cat. Pd(PPh3)4, cat. CuI, Et3N, DMF, 66%; (c) HC_C-SiMe3, cat. Pd(PPh3)4, cat. CuI, Et3N, DMF, 69%; (d) Bu4NF, THF, 83%; (e) **7** (5 mol equiv.), cat. Pd(PPh3)4, cat. CuI, Et3N, DMF, 88% based on **5**[214]. *Copyright permission from reference 214.*

(6) On the other hand, coupling reaction of **7** with **5** result in **1b** (G2) containing six catalytic sites giving 88% yield.

Using this process developed by Sato's group, chiral dendrimers **1a** (G1) and **1b** (G2) with rigid hydrocarbon backbones are useful catalysts for the enantioselective addition of dialkylzincs. Application of these chiral dendrimers to other asymmetric syntheses is currently being studied at the same laboratory.

2.6 CHARACTERIZATION OF NMs[215]

The novel properties of materials with nanometer dimensions (and not associated chemical changes) require surface chemical characterization of paramount necessity to establish topographical properties that are important for biomedical and biological applications.[215] Thus, it is inevitable to include some techniques that have been used for NM surface chemical characterization and the determination of protein biomolecule interactions aside from those already discussed in the previous sections of this chapter. Techniques that are discussed here are attenuated total reflectance Fourier transform infrared (ATR-FTIR) spectroscopy, XPS, time-of-flight secondary ion mass spectroscopy (SIMS), colorimetric methods, and atomic force microscopy (AFM).

2.6.1 ATR-FTIR Spectroscopy

Chemical bonding interactions between structures can be studied using ATR-FTIR spectroscopy when samples are placed in contact with internal reflection elements (IREs) such as zinc selenide (ZnSe) or germanium (Ge).[215] In this process, the IR radiation is first focused in order to penetrate the end of the IRE and reflects down the length of the IRE. The IR radiation penetrates a short distance (~1 µm) from the surface of the IRE into the specimens. The absorption of radiation is related to the fundamental vibrations of chemical bonds, while internal reflection spectrometry provides information with respect to the presence or absence of specific functional groups and the chemical structures of polymer membranes. Absorption bands are assigned to functional groups (such as the C=O stretch and the C–H bend) such as in ordinary IR spectra, which can be used to identify changes in chemical structure when shifts in the frequency of absorption bands and changes in relative band intensities are observed. This can also be used to indicate changes in the chemical structure or alterations in the environment around the polymer membranes.

The ATR-FTIR analysis of vibrational spectra can be applied to characterize the organic fouling layer that may be present on a nanopolymer surface.[215] It can also be used to determine changes in surface chemistry after application of specific nanotechnology-based chemical or physical treatments or to identify unique chemical features on the polymer surface after NaOH etching of polymers to obtain nanosurface features. Information gathered with this technique has been correlated with polymer performance in biological systems as well as in understanding surface interactions with cells and proteins.[215] But, the penetration depth of ATR-FTIR has the same order of magnitude as the wavelength of IR light that ranges from several hundred nanometers to more than 1 µm. Thus, ATR-FTIR is not a very sensitive surface analysis method for NMs that are in the tens of nanometer dimensions.[215]

2.6.2 XPS

XPS is a technique for surface characterization that is used for polymeric nano-biomaterials.[215] It has a <10 nm sampling depth that makes it a more sensitive surface analysis technique than ATR-FTIR. This technique uses photoionization and energy-dispersive analysis of the emitted photoelectrons to establish the composition and electronic state of a sample. Every element has a characteristic binding energy associated with a specific atomic orbital giving a characteristic set of peaks in the photoelectron spectrum at specific kinetic energies controlled by the photon energy and their respective binding energies. Therefore, the presence of characteristic peaks at particular energies indicates the presence of a specific element on the sample. Hence, unlike ATR-FTIR, XPS provides a quantitative analysis of the surface chemical composition making it also called as electron spectroscopy for chemical analysis (ESCA).[215] The intensity of the peaks is directly related to the concentration of the element within the sampled region. Furthermore, the shape of each peak and the binding energy can be slightly altered by the chemical state of the emitting surface component atoms, thereby providing chemical bonding information as well.[216] Although XPS can be used for all other elements, it is not sensitive to hydrogen or helium. An additional advantage of XPS is its capability to provide information about the coverage and thickness of molecules adsorbed on a surface.[217–222] This has been used in comparing initial protein adsorption on NMs compared with conventional surfaces for tissue regeneration.[215]

2.6.3 Time-of-Flight SIMS

A technique with sampling depth between 1 and 2 nm that is more sensitive than XPS is time-of-flight SIMS. SIMS is used for analyzing elemental and chemical compositions of the outermost molecular or atomic layer of a solid surface.[215] With this technique, the NM surface is bombarded with a beam of energetic ions of argon or gallium, usually. As the ions hit the surface, atoms and molecules are removed from the material surface such as in sputtering process.[215] A portion of the sputtered particles is ionized to produce secondary ions that are accelerated to a constant kinetic energy. These are allowed to travel a certain distance in a field free environment and collected by a detector that measures their time-of-flight which is correlated with their individual mass. The positively charged secondary ions are characteristic fragments of chemical structures on the material surface that provide significant information about surface chemistry.

Two kinds of SIMS have been developed: static and dynamic SIMS. Static SIMS uses low-energy primary ion beam (10^{-9} A/cm^2) to scan the sample surface to obtain a "static" surface analysis.[215] Dynamic SIMS uses a high-energy primary ion beam (1 A/cm^2) at a short length of time to erode the material surface continuously while the real-time signal is recorded. A plot of the signal against the depth of the sample provides a profile of the chemical composition and/or structures from the surface into the bulk of the sample with high-resolution depth of several nanometers.

SIMS is used to study the composition, conformation, orientation, and denaturation of proteins on NM surfaces.[223] Very little is known about protein orientation and conformation after adsorption on NM surfaces because of the complexities of protein structures. Compared with XPS, SIMS provides more chemical structure information based on the fragmentation pattern. In addition, SIMS offers small sampling depths of 10–15 Å providing an amino acid level detail about the adsorbed protein on the exterior 10–15 Å portion of the protein. The relative intensities of the ion fragments detected in static SIMS are sensitive to the orientation of the protein on the surface and its degree of conformational alteration.[215] As protein adsorbs to the NM surface it may undergo changes in its conformation or orientation allowing new regions of the protein with different amino acid compositions to be more exposed to the SIMS sampling depth.[215]

2.6.4 Colorimetric Methods

Colorimetric methods are used to establish the optical characteristics of NMs as well as their concentrations. Furthermore, colorimetric methods are also used to establish the concentrations of proteins. When the wavelengths of maximum absorption for the NMs and the proteins do not overlap, these can be used to establish the identity and quantity of both the NMs and the proteins from the same sample. These properties can be used when controlling tissue regeneration on NMs that serve NMs as scaffold surfaces. The bicinchoninic acid (BCA) method is an effective approach to determine the amount of adsorbed protein on NM surface and kits are commercially available for this purpose.[215] However, the BCA method cannot be used when protein concentration is lower than its detection limit.

2.6.5 AFM

One of the earlier methods of characterizing NMs is through AFM. AFM can be used to qualitatively determine the topography of NMs. AFM technique is based on surface analysis through a precise small-scale movement of a piezo-electric scanner against a sharp tip mounted at the end of a cantilever. AFM is advantageous because of minimal sample preparation in comparison with other imaging techniques (such as SEM or TEM). Unlike SEM or TEM, AFM can produce detailed three-dimensional rather than two-dimensional images without the need for a vacuum providing a potential to image samples in ambient air or liquid.[215] Because of this, AFM is used to view and scan samples in their quasi-native environment for real-time imaging of live biological samples. AFM provides distinct topographic contrast with direct height measurements and a direct view of surface features for nonconductive materials (such as polymers and biological tissues)[215] but the depth of the field of view for AFM is limited by the travel distance of the piezoelectric tube as well as the cantilever tip size and geometry.

2.6.6 DLS for Zeta Potential

Zeta potential can be measured by dynamic light scattering (DLS) using a Zetasizer Nano ZS instrument (Malvern). One example of this process is to measure the zeta potential of Si nanocrystals. The average hydrodynamic diameter of the polymer-coated Si nanocrystals in PBS is measured by DLS using the Zetasizer instrument. The particles are placed in the disposable capillary cell at ~10^{16} nanocrystals mL^{-1} concentration for light scattering measurements. The Zetasizer detects the intensity of backscattered photons at a 173° angle from an incident 4 mW He–Ne (633 nm) laser over a time interval of 10 s, using a sample time (τ) of 0.5 µs. The hydrodynamic diameter is then extracted from the light scattering data using the method of cumulants.[224] Using the same sample, the zeta potential can be measured with the same instrument. The zetasizer applies an alternating electric field across the cell that is equipped with two electrodes. The particle mobility in the electric field is recorded as a phase shift of an incident laser beam. This particle mobility is converted to zeta potential by the Zetasizer software using the Smoluchowski theory.

2.7 CONCLUSIONS

This chapter provided an overview of the various NMs that are currently very useful in nanomedicine. A few of the sNMs were provided with protocols for synthesis, while others that are more well documented in some other references were given an overview. There are NMs at their infancy and require much more testing before their full potential in medicine can be realized. For this reason, only a selected group of NMs that are well advanced in their medical applications were given much attention. In addition, selected current NM characterization techniques were included to provide an overview of how the properties of NMs are established. Again, there are many other techniques at their infancy of development that were not included in this chapter. Instruments that are useful for NM topography, chemical composition, size, and shape analysis techniques of particular benefit to NM characterization were discussed. For clearer and better understanding of NMs and their interactions with biological systems for medical applications, novel high-resolution imaging and analysis tools, which allow for easy sample preparation and in situ monitoring, are still needed.[215]

REFERENCES

1. Brus, L. E. Electron–Electron and Electron–Hole Interaction in Small Semiconductor Crystallines–The Size Dependence of the Lowest Excited Electronic State. *J. Chem. Phys.* **1984,** *80,* 4403–4409.
2. Norris, D. J.; Sacra, A.; Murray, C. B.; Bawendi, M. G. Measurement of the Size-dependent Hole Spectrum in CdSe Quantum Dots. *Phys. Rev. Lett.* **1994,** *72.*
3. Efros, A. L.; Rosen, M. The Electronic Structure of Semiconductor Nanocrystals. *Ann. Rev. Mater. Sci.* **2000,** *30,* 475–521.
4. Castranova, V. Overview of Current Toxicological Knowledge of Engineered Nanoparticles. *J. Occup. Environ. Med.* **2011,** *53,* S14–S17.

5. Hu, J.; Li, L.; Yang, W.; Manna, L.; Wang, L.; Alivisatos, A. P. Linearly Polarized Emission from Colloidal Semiconductor Quantum Rods. *Science* **2001,** *292,* 2060–2063.
6. Martel, R.; Derycke, V.; Lavoie, C.; Appenzeller, J.; Chan, K. K.; Tersoff, J. Ambipolar Electrical Transport in Semiconducting Single-wall Carbon Nanotubes. *Phys. Rev. Lett.* **2001,** *87,* 256805.
7. Peng, X.; Manna, L.; Yang, W.; Wickham, J.; Scher, E.; Kadavanich, A.; Alivisatos, A. P. Shape Control of CdSe Nanocrystals. *Nature* **2000,** *404,* 59–61.
8. Carbó-Argibay, E.; Rodríguez-González, B.; Pastoriza-Santos, I.; Pérez-Juste, J.; Liz-Marán, L. M. Growth of Pentatwinned Gold Nanorods into Truncated Decahedra. *Nanoscale* **2010,** *2,* 2377–2383.
9. Li, M.; Li, R.; Li, C. M.; Wu, N. Electrochemical and Optical Biosensors Based on Nanomaterials and Nanostructures: A Review. *Front. Biosci.* **2011,** *S3,* 1308–1331.
10. Li, M.; Zhang, J.; Suri, S.; Sooter, L. J.; Ma, D.; Wu, N. Detection of Adenosine Triphosphate with and Aptamer Biosensor Based on the Surface-Enhanced Raman Scattering. *Anal. Chem.* **2012,** *84,* 2837–2842.
11. Hu, L.; Kim, H.; Lee, J.; Peumans, P.; Cui, Y. Scalable Coating and Properties of Transparent, Flexible, Silver Nanowire Electrodes. *ACS Nano* **2010,** *4,* 2955–2963.
12. Huang, S.; Chen, Y. Ultrasensitive Fluorescence Detection of Single Protein Molecules Manipulated Electrically on Au Nanowire. *Nano Lett.* **2008,** *8,* 2829–2833.
13. Khawaja, A. M. Review: The Legacy of Nanotechnology: Revolution and Prospects in Neurosurgery. *Int. J. Surg.* **2011,** in press
14. Xianmao, L.; Yavuz, M.; Tuan, H.; Korgel, B.; Xia, Y. Ultrathin Gold Nanowires can be obtained by Reducing Polymeric Strands of Oleylamine–AuCl Complexes Formed via Aurophilic Interaction. *J. Am. Chem. Soc.* **2008,** *130,* 8900–8901.
15. Gole, A.; Murphy, C. J. Seed-Mediated Synthesis of Gold Nanorods: Role of the Size and Nature of the Seed. *Chem. Mater.* **2004,** *16,* 3633–3640.
16. Barbosa, S.; Agrawal, A.; Rodríguez-Lorenzo, L.; Pastoriza-Santos, I.; Alvarez-Puebla, R. A.; Kornowski, A.; Weller, H.; Liz-Marzan, L. M. Tuning Size and Sensing Properties in Colloidal Gold Nanostars. *Langmuir* **2010,** *26,* 14943–14950.
17. Li, M.; Cushing, S. K.; Zhang, J.; Lankford, J.; Aguilar, Z. P.; Ma, D.; Wu, N. Shape-dependent Surface-enhanced Raman Scattering in Gold-Raman-Probe-Silica Sandwiched Nanoparticles for Biocompatible Applications. *Nanotechnology* **2012,** *23,* 115501–115511.
18. Liu, H.; Zhu, Z.; Kang, H.; Wu, Y.; Sefan, K.; Tan, W. DNA-based Micelles: Synthesis, Micellar Properties and Size-dependent Cell Permeability. *Chemistry* **2010,** *16,* 3791–3797.
19. Sekhon, B.; Kamboj, S. Inorganic Nanomedicine: Part 1. *Nanomed. Nanotechnol. Biol. Med.* **2010,** *6,* 516–522.
20. Smith, A. M.; Gao, X.; Nie, S. Quantum Dot Nanocrystals for *in vivo* Molecular and Cellular Imaging. *Photochem. Photobiol.* **2004,** *80,* 377–385.
21. Pradhan, N.; Battaglia, D. M.; Liu, Y.; Peng, X. Efficient, Stable, Small, and Water Soluble Doped ZnSe Nanocrystal Emitters as Non-cadmium Based Biomedical Labels. *Nano Lett.* **2007,** *7,* 312–317.
22. Dabbousi, B. O.; Rodríguez-Viejo, J.; Mikulec, F. V.; Heine, J. R.; Mattoussi, H.; Ober, R.; Jensen, K. J.; Bawendi, M. G. (CdSe)ZnS Core–Shell Quantum Dots: Synthesis and Characterization of a Size Series of Highly Luminescent Nanocrystallites. *J. Phys. Chem. B* **1997,** *101,* 9463–9475.
23. Manna, L.; Scher, E.; Alivisatos, A. Synthesis of Soluble and Processable Rod-, Arrow-, Teardrop-, and Tetrapod-shaped Cdse Nanocrystals. *J. Am. Chem. Soc.* **2000,** *122,* 12700–12706.

24. Murray, C.; Norris, D.; Bawendi, M. Synthesis and Characterization of Nearly Monodisperse CdE (E = sulfur, selenium, tellurium) Semiconductor Nanocrystallites. *J. Am. Chem. Soc.* **1993,** *115,* 8706–8715.

25. Su, H.; Xu, H.; Gao, S.; Dixon, J.; Aguilar, Z. P.; Wang, A.; Xu, J.; Wang, J. Microwave Synthesis of Nearly Monodisperse Core/Multishell Quantum Dots with Cell Imaging Applications. *Nanoscale Res. Lett.* **2010,** *5,* 625–630.

26. Medintz, I. L.; Uyeda, H. T.; Goldman, E. R.; Mattoussi, H. Quantum Dot Bioconjugates for Imaging, Labeling and Sensing. *Nat. Mater.* **2005,** *4,* 435–446.

27. Michalet, X.; Pinaud, F. F.; Bentolila, L. A.; Tsay, J. M.; Doose, S.; Li, J. J., et al. Quantum Dots for Live Cells, *in vivo* Imaging, and Diagnostics. *Science* **2005,** *307,* 538–544.

28. Somers, R.; Bawendi, M.; Nocera, D. CdSe Nanocrystal Based Chem-/Bio- Sensors. *Chem. Soc. Rev.* **2007,** *36,* 579–591.

29. Alivisatos, A. P.; Gu, W.; Larabell, C. Quantum Dots as Cellular Probes. *Annu. Rev. Biomed. Eng.* **2005,** *7,* 55–76.

30. Jamieson, T.; Bakhshi, R.; Petrova, D.; Pocock, R.; Seifalian, A. M. Biological Applications of Quantum Dots. *Biomaterials* **2007,** *28,* 4717–4732.

31. Iyer, G.; Weiss, S.; Pinaud, F.; Tsay, J. M. Solubilization of Quantum Dots with a Recombinant Peptide from *Escherichia coli. Small* **2007,** *3,* 793–798.

32. Liu, W.; Howarth, M.; Greytak, A. B.; Zheng, Y.; Nocera, D. G.; Ting, A. Y., et al. Compact Biocompatible Quantum Dots Functionalized for Cellular Imaging. *J. Am. Chem. Soc.* **2008,** *130,* 1274–1284.

33. Susumu, K.; Uyeda, H.; Medintz, I.; Pons, T.; Delehanty, J.; Mattoussi, H. Enhancing the Stability and Biological Functionalities of Quantum Dots via Compact Multifunctional Ligands. *J. Am. Chem. Soc.* **2007,** *129,* 13987–13996.

34. Chen, Y.; Thakar, R.; Snee, P. T. Imparting Nanoparticle Function with Size-controlled Amphiphilic Polymers. *J. Am. Chem. Soc.* **2008,** *130,* 3744–3745.

35. Carion, O.; Mahler, B.; Pons, T.; Dubertret, B. Synthesis, Encapsulation, Purification and Coupling of Single Quantum Dots in Phospholipid Micelles for their Use in Cellular and *in vivo* Imaging. *Nat. Protoc.* **2007,** *2,* 2383–2390.

36. Pinaud, F.; King, D.; Moore, H. P.; Weiss, S. Bioactivation and Cell Targeting of Semiconductor CdSe/Zns Nanocrystals with Phytochelatin-Related Peptides. *J. Am. Chem. Soc.* **2004,** *126,* 6115–6123.

37. Aguilar, Z.; Xu, H.; Jones, B.; Dixon, J.; Wang, A. Semiconductor Quantum Dots for Cell Imaging. *Mater. Res. Soc. Proc.* **2010,** *1237,* 1237-TT1206-1201.

38. Xu, H.; Aguilar, Z.; Dixon, J.; Jones, B.; Wang, A.; Wei, H. Breast Cancer Cell Imaging Using Semiconductor Quantum Dots. *Electrochem. Soc. Trans.* **2009,** *25,* 69–77.

39. Xu, H.; Aguilar, Z.; Waldron, J.; Wei, H.; Wang, Y. Application of Semiconductor Quantum Dots for Breast Cancer Cell Sensing, 2009 Biomedical Engineering and Informatics. *IEEE Computer Society BMEI* **2009,** *1,* 516–520.

40. Xu, H.; Aguilar, Z.; Wang, A. Quantum Dot-based Sensors for Proteins. *Electrochem. Soc. Trans.* **2010,** *25,* 1–10.

41. Xu, H.; Aguilar, Z.; Wei, H.; Wang, A. Development of Semiconductor Nanomaterial Whole Cell Imaging Sensor on Silanized Microscope Slides. *Front. Biosci.* **2011,** *E3,* 1013–1024.

42. Rzigalinski, B. A.; Strobl, J. S. Cadmium-containing Nanoparticles: Perspectives on Pharmacology and Toxicology of Quantum Dots in New Insights into the Mechanisms of Cadmium Toxicity—Advances in Cadmium Research. *Toxicol. Appl. Pharmacol.* **2009,** *238,* 280–288.

43. Smith, A. M.; Duan, H.; Mohs, A. M. Bioconjugated Quantum Dots for in vivo Molecular and Cellular Imaging. *Adv. Drug Deliv. Rev.* **2008**, *60*.
44. Juzenas, P.; Chen, W.; Sun, Y. P.; Coelho, M. A. N.; Genralov, R.; Genralova, N.; Christensen, I. L. Quantum Dots and Nanoparticles for Photodynamic and Radiation Therapies of Cancer. *Adv. Drug Deliv. Rev.* **2008**, *60*.
45. Akerman, M. E.; Chan, W. C.; Laakkonen, P.; Bhatia, S. N.; Ruoslahti, E. Nanocrystal Targeting in vivo. *Proc. Natl. Acad. Sci. U S A* **2002**, *99*, 12617–12621.
46. Pusic, K.; Xu, H.; Stridiron, A.; Aguilar, Z.; Wang, A. Z.; Hui, H. Blood Stage Merozoite Surface Protein Conjugated to Nanoparticles Induce Potent Parasite Inhibitory Antibodies. *Vaccine* **2011**, *29*, 8898–8908.
47. Hardman, R. A Toxicologic Review of Quantum Dots: toxicity Depends on Physicochemical and Environmental Factors. *Environ. Health Perspect* **2006**, *114*, 165–172.
48. Angell, J. J. Thesis. Type, California Polytechnic State University, San Luis Obispo, 2011.
49. Biju, V.; Itoh, T.; Anas, A.; Sujith, A.; Ishikawa, M. Semiconductor Quantum Dots and Metal Nanoparticles: Syntheses, Optical Properties, and Biological Applications. *Anal. Bioanal. Chem.* **2008**, *391*, 2469–2495.
50. Hines, M. A.; Guyot-Sionnest, P. Synthesis and Characterization of Strongly Luminescing ZnS-capped CdSe Nanocrystals. *J. Phys. Chem.* **1996**, *100*, 468–471.
51. Susumu, K.; Uyeda, H. T.; Medintz, I. L. Design of Biotin-Functionalized Luminescent Quantum Dots. *J. Biomed. Biotech.* **2007**, *2007*, 90651.
52. Peng, Z. A.; Peng, X. Formation of High-quality CdTe, CdSe, and CdS Nanocrystals Using CdO as Precursor. *J. Am. Chem. Soc.* **2001**, *123*, 183–184.
53. Mattoussi, H.; Mauro, J. M.; Goldman, E. R.; Anderson, G. P.; Sundar, V. C.; Mikulec, F. V.; Bawendi, M. G. Self-assembly of CdSe–ZnS Quantum dot Bioconjugates Using an Engineered Recombinant Protein. *J. Am. Chem. Soc.* **2000**, *122*, 12142–12150.
54. Uyeda, H. T.; Medintz, I. L.; Jaiswal, J. K.; Simon, S. M.; Mattoussi, H. Synthesis of Compact Multidentate Ligands to Prepare Stable Hydrophilic Quantum Dot Fluorophores. *J. Am. Chem. Soc.* **2005**, *127*, 3870–3878.
55. Clapp, A. R.; Goldman, E. R.; Mattoussi, H. Capping of CdSe–ZnS Quantum Dots with DHLA and Subsequent Conjugation with Proteins. *Nat. Protoc.* **2006**, *1*, 1258–1266.
56. Boatman, E. M.; Lisensky, G. C.; Nordell, K. J. A Safer Easier, Faster Synthesis for CdSe Quantum Dot Nanocrystals. *J. Chem. Educ.* **2005**, *82*, 1697–1699.
57. USDHHS. Report on carcinogens. 2011 (accessed Jan 22, 2012).
58. Gao, X.; Cui, Y.; Levenson, R. M.; Chung, L. W. K.; Nie, S. In vivo Cancer Targeting and Imaging with Semiconductor Quantum Dots. *Nat. Biotechnol.* **2004**, *22*, 969–976.
59. Dubertret, B.; Skourides, P.; Norris, D. J.; Noireaux, V.; Brivaniou, A. H.; Libchaber, A. In vivo Imaging of Quantum Dots Encapsulated in Phospholipid Micelles. *Science* **2002**, *298*, 1759–1762.
60. Pong, B.-K.; Trout, B. L.; Lee, J.-Y., 2007.
61. Invitrogen. Qdot Nanocrystal Technology. 2012 [cited Jan 22, 2012].
62. NanoTech, O. Technologies. 2012 [Jan 22, 2012].
63. Bakueva, L.; Gorelikov, I.; Musikhin, S.; Zhao, X. S.; Sargent, E. H.; Kumacheva, E. PbS Quantum Dots with Stable Efficient Luminescence in the Near-IR Spectral Range. *Adv. Mater.* **2004**, *16*.
64. Wolcott, A.; Gerion, D.; Visconte, M.; Sun, J.; Schwartzberg, A.; Chen, S.; Zhang, J. Z. Silica-coated CdTe Quantum Dots Functionalized with Thiols for Bioconjugation Fot IgG Proteins. *J. Phys. Chem. B* **2006**, *110*, 5779–5789.

Nanomaterials for Medical Applications

65. Turkevich, J.; Stevenson, P. C.; Hillier, J. A Study of the Nucleation and Growth Processes in the Synthesis of Colloidal Gold. *Discuss. Faraday Soc.* **1951,** *11,* 55–75.
66. Chaudhuri, B.; Raychaudhuri, S. Manufacturing high quality gold sol. 2001 [Feb. 1 2012].
67. Jain, P. K.; Huang, X.; El-Sayed, I. H.; El-sayed, M. A. Review of Some Interesting Surface Plasmon Resonance-enhanced Properties of Noble Metal Nanoparticles and their Applications to Biosystems. *Plasmonics* **2007,** *2.*
68. Sperling, R. A.; Gil, P. R.; Zhang, F.; Zanella, M.; Parak, W. J. Biological Applications of Gold Nanoparticles. *Chem. Soc. Rev.* **2007,** *37.*
69. Ojea-Jimenez, I.; Puntes, V. Instability of Cationic Gold Nanoparticle Bioconjugates: The Role of Citrate Ions. *J. Am. Chem. Soc.* **2009,** *131,* 13320–13327.
70. Katz, E.; Willner, I. Integrated Nanoparticle–Biomolecule Hybrid Systems: Synthesis, Properties, and Applications. *Angew. Chem. Int. Ed.* **2004,** *43,* 6042–6018.
71. Handley, D. A. Methods for Synthesis of Colloidal Gold. In *Colloidal Gold: Principles, Methods, and Applications*; Hayat, M. A., Ed.; Academic Press: New York, 1989.
72. Frens, G. Controlled Nucleation for the Regulation of the Particle Size in Monodisperse Gold Suspensions. *Nat. Phys. Sci.* **1973,** *241,* 20–22.
73. Slot, J.; Geuze, H. Cryosectioning and Immunolabeling. *Nat. Protoc.* **2007,** *2,* 2480–2491.
74. Zhang, Z.; Ross, R.; Roeder, R. Preparation of Functionalized Gold Nanoparticles as a Targeted X-ray Contrast Agent for Damaged Bone Tissue. *Nanoscale* **2010,** *2,* 582–586.
75. Shalkevich, N.; Escher, W.; Burgi, T.; Michel, B.; Si-Ahmed, L.; Poulikakos, D. On the Thermal Conductivity of Gold Nanoparticle Colloids. *Langmuir* **2010.**
76. Aqil, A.; Qiu, H.; Greish, J.; Jerome, R.; De Pauw, E.; Jerome, C. Coating of Gold Nanoparticles by Thermosensitive Poly (*N*-isopropylacrylamide) End-capped by Biotin. *Polymer* **2008,** *49,* 1145–1153.
77. Sweeney, S.; Wpehrle, G.; Hutchison, J. Rapid Purification and Size Separation of Gold Nanoparticles via Diafiltration. *J. Am. Chem. Soc.* **2006,** *128,* 3190–3197.
78. McFarland, A. D.; Haynes, C. L.; Mirkin, C. A.; Van Duyne, R. P.; Godwin, H. A. Color My Nanoworld. *J. Chem. Educ.* **2004,** *81,* 544A.
79. Basu, S.; Pande, S.; Jana, S.; Bolisetty, S.; Pal, T. Controlled Interparticle Spacing for Surface-Modified Gold Nanoparticle Aggregates. *Langmuir* **2008,** *24,* 5562–5568.
80. Huang, C. C.; Chiang, C. K.; Lin, Z. H.; Lee, K. H.; Chang, H. T. Bioconjugated Gold Nanodots and Nanoparticles for Protein Assays Based on Photoluminescence Quenching. *Anal. Chem.* **2008,** *80,* 1497–1504.
81. Balasubramanian, S. K.; Yang, L.; Yung, L. -Y. L.; Ong, C. -N.; Ong, W. -Y.; Yu, L. E. Characterization, Purification, and Stability of Gold Nanoparticles. *Biomaterials* **2010,** *31,* 9023–9030.
82. Hazarika, P.; Giorgi, T.; Reibner, M.; Ceyhan, B.; Neimeyer, C. Synthesis and Characterization of Deoxyribonucleic Acid-Conjugated Gold Nanoparticles. In *Bioconjugation Protocols: Strategies and Methods*; Niemeyer, C., Ed.; Humana Press: New Jersey, 2004.
83. Demers, L.; Mirkin, C.; Mucic, R.; Reynolds, R.; Letsinger, R.; Elghanian, R.; Viswanadham, G. A Fluorescence-based Method for Determining the Surface Coverage and Hybridization Efficiency of Thiol-capped Oligonucleotides Bound to Gold Thin Films and Nanoparticles. *Anal. Chem.* **2000,** *72,* 5535–5541.
84. Qu, F.; Xu, H.; Aguilar, Z. P.; Xu, H.; Wang, Y. A.; Wei, H. Role of Reactive Oxygen Species in the Antibacterial Mechanism of Silver Nanoparticles on *Escherichia coli* O157:H7. *Biometals* **2012,** *25,* 45–53.
85. Zhu, J. J.; Liao, X. H.; Zhao, X. N.; Hen, H. Y. *Mater. Lett.* **2001,** *48,* 91–95.
86. Chou, W. L.; Yu, D. G. *Polym. Adv. Technol.* **2005,** *16,* 600–608.

87. Loeschner, K.; Hadrup, N.; Qvotrup, K.; Larsen, A.; Gao, X.; Vogel, U.; Mortensen, A.; Lam, H. R.; Larsen, E. H. Distribution of Silver in Rats Following 28 Days of Repeated Oral Exposure to Silver Nanoparticles or Silver Acetate. *Particle Fibre Toxicol.* **2011,** *8,* 18.

88. Zhang, Z.; Zhao, B.; Hu, L. PVP Protective Mechanism of Ultrafine Silver Powder Synthesized by Chemical Reduction Processes. *J. Solid State Chem.* **1996,** *121,* 105–110.

89. Aguilar, Z.; Aguilar, Y.; Xu, H.; Jones, B.; Dixon, J.; Xu, H.; Wang, A. Nanomaterials in Medicine. *Electrochem. Soc. Trans.* **2010,** *33,* 69–74.

90. Lee, H.; Yoon, T.; Figueiredo, J.; Swirski, F. K.; Weissleder, R. Rapid Detection and Profiling of Cancer Cells in Fine-needle Aspirates. *Proc. Natl. Acad. Sci.* **2009,** *106,* 12459–12464.

91. Wagner, W.; Dullaart, A.; Bock, A. K.; Zweck, A. The Emerging Nanomedicine Landscape. *Nat. Biotechnol.* **2006,** *24,* 1211–1217.

92. Yang, L.; Cao, Z.; Sajja, H.; Mao, H.; Wang, L.; Geng, H.; Xu, H.; Jiang, T.; Wood, W.; Nie, S.; Wang, A. Development of Receptor Targeted Iron Oxide Nanoparticles for Efficient Drug Delivery and Tumor Imaging. *J. Biomed. Nanotech.* **2008,** *4,* 1–11.

93. Arruebo, M.; Fernandez-Pacheco, R.; Ricardo-Ibarra, M.; Santamaria, J. Magnetic Nanoparticles for Drug Delivery. *Nanotoday* **2007,** *2,* 22–32.

94. Varadan, V. K.; Chen, L.; Xie, J.; Abaraham, J.; e. *Nanomedicine: Design and Applications of Magnetic Nanomaterials, Nanosensors and Nanosystems*; John Wiley and Sons, 2009.

95. Shubayev, V. I.; Pisanic, T. R.; Jin, S. Magnetic Nanoparticles for Theragnostics. *Adv. Drug Deliv. Rev.* **2009,** *61,* 467–477.

96. Gupta, A. K.; Gupta, M. Synthesis and Surface Engineering of Iron Oxide Nanoparticles for Biomedical Applications. *Biomaterials* **2005,** *26,* 3995–4021.

97. Bulte, J. W.; Douglas, T.; Witwer, B.; Zhang, S. C.; Strable, E.; Lewis, B. K., et al. Magnetodendrimers Allow Endosomal Magnetic Labeling and in vivo Tracking of Stem Cells. *Nat. Biotechnol.* **2001,** *19,* 1141–1147.

98. Chen, G.; Shen, B.; Zhang, F.; Wu, J.; Xu, Y.; He, P.; Fang, Y. A New Electrochemically Active–Inactive Switching Aptamer Molecular Beacon to Detect Thrombin Directly in Solution. *Biosens. Bioelectron.* **2010,** *25,* 2265–2269.

99. Gong, J.; Liang, Y.; Huang, Y.; Chen, J.; Jiang, J.; Shen, G.; Yu, R. Ag/SiO(2) Core–Shell Nanoparticle-based Surface-enhanced Raman Probes for Immunoassay of Cancer Marker Using Silica-coated Magnetic Nanoparticles as Separation Tools. *Biosens. Bioelectron.* **2006,** *22,* 1501–1507.

100. Haun, J. B.; Yoon, T.; Lee, H. J.; Weissleder, R. Magnetic Nanoparticle Biosensors. *Wiley Interdiscip. Rev. Nanomed. Nanobiotechnol.* **2010,** *2,* 291–304.

101. Herr, J. K.; Smith, J. E.; Medley, C. D.; Shangguan, D.; Tan, W. Aptamer-Conjuagted Nanoparticles for Selective Collection and Detection of Cancer Cells. *Anal. Chem.* **2007,** *78,* 2918–2924.

102. Ishiyama, K.; Sendoh, M.; Arai, K. I. Magnetic Micromachined for Medical Applications. *Biomed. Mater. Eng.* **2002,** *15,* 367–374.

103. Mathieu, J. B.; Martel, S.; Yahia, L.; Soulez, G.; Beaudoin, G. Preliminary Investigation of the Feasibility of Magnetic Propulsion for Future Microdevices in Blood Vessels. *Biomed. Mater. Eng.* **2002,** *15,* 367–374.

104. Mejias, R.; Perez-Yague, S.; Gutierez, L.; Cabrera, L. I.; Spada, R.; Acedo, P.; Serna, C. J.; Lazaro, F. J.; Villanueva, A.; Morales, M. P.; Barber, D. F. Dimercaptosuccinic Acid-coated Magnetite Nanoparticles for Magnetically Guided in vivo Delivery of Interferon Gamma for Cancer Immunotherapy. *Biomaterials* **2011,** *32,* 2938–2952.

105. Osterfeld, S. J.; Yu, H.; Gaster, R. S.; Caramuta, S.; Xu, L.; Han, S.; Hall, D. A.; Wilson, R. J.; Sun, S.; White, R. L.; Davis, R. W.; Pourmand, N.; Wang, S. X. Multiplex Protein Assays Based on Real-time Magnetic Nanotag Sensing. *Proc. Natl. Acad. Sci.* **2008**, *105,* 20637–20640.

106. Wilhelm, C.; Gazeau, F. Universal Cell Labelling with Anionic Magnetic Nanoparticles. *Biomaterials* **2008**, *29,* 3161–3174.

107. Ge, Y.; Zhang, Y.; He, S.; Nie, F.; Teng, G.; Gu, N. Fluorescence Modified Chitosan-coated Magnetic Nanoparticles for High-efficient cellular Imaging. *Nanoscale Res. Lett.* **2009**, *4,* 287–295.

108. Morrish, A. H. *The Physical Principles of Magnetism*; John Wiley: New York, 1965, Chapter 7.

109. Unruh, K. M.; Chien, C. L. In *Nanomaterials: Synthesis, Properties, and Applications*; Institute of Physics Publishing, 1996, Chapter 14.

110. Yang, L.; Peng, X.; Wang, Y.; Wang, X.; Cao, Z.; Ni, C.; Karna, P.; Zhang, X.; Wood, W.; Gao, X.; Nie, S.; Mao, H. Receptor-targeted Nanoparticles for in vivo Imaging of Breast Cancer. *Clin. Cancer Res.* **2009**, *15,* 4722–4732.

111. Xu, H.; Aguilar, Z. P.; Yang, L.; Kuang, M.; Duan, H.; Xiong, Y.; Wei, H.; Wang, A. Y. Antibody Conjugated Magnetic iron Oxide Nanoparticles for Cancer Cell Separation in Fresh Whole Blood. *Biomaterials* **2011**, *32,* 9758–9765.

112. Xie, J.; Peng, S.; Brower, N.; Pourmand, N.; Wang, S. X.; Sun, S. One-Pot Synthesis of Monodisperse Iron Oxide Nanoparticles for Potential Biomedical Applications. *Pure Appl. Chem.* **2006**, *78,* 1003–1014.

113. Hafeli, U.; Schutt, W.; Teller, J.; Zborowski, M. *Scientific and Clinical Applications of Magnetic Carriers*; Plenum Press: New York, 1997.

114. NanoTech, O. Preparation of uniform size and size tunable iron oxide magnetic nanocrystals. [February 5, 2012]. Available from: http://www.oceannanotech.com/nav.php?qid=6.

115. Hans, M. L.; Lowman, A. M. Biodegradable Nanoparticles for Drug Delivery and Targeting. *Curr. Opin. Solid State Mater. Sci.* **2002**, *6,* 319–327.

116. Mahmoudi, M.; Sant, S.; Wang, B.; Laurent, S.; Sen, T. Superparamagnetic Iron Oxide Nanoparticles (SPIONs): Development, Surface Modification and Applications in Chemotherapy. *Adv. Drug Deliv. Rev.* **2011**, *63,* 24–46.

117. Sajja, H.; East, M.; Mao, H.; Wang, Y.; Nie, S.; Yang, L. Development of Multifunctional Nanoparticles for Targeted Drug Delivery and Noninvasive Imaging of Therapeutic Effect. *Curr. Drug Discov. Technol.* **2009**, *6,* 43–51.

118. Kodama, R. H. Magnetic Nanoparticles. *J. Magn. Magn. Mater.* **1999**, *200,* 359–372.

119. Mahmoudi, M.; Simchi, A.; Imani, M.; Shokrgozar, M. A.; Milani, A. S.; Hafeli, U.; Stroeve, P. A New Approach for the in vitro Identification of the Cytotoxicity of Superparamagnetic Iron Oxide Nanoparticles. *Colloids Surf. B* **2010**, *75,* 300–309.

120. Kim, J.; Piao, T.; Hyeon, T. Multifunctional Nanostructured Materials for Multimodal Imaging, and Simultaneous Imaging and Therapy. *Chem. Soc. Rev.* **2009**, *38,* 372–390.

121. Mahmoudi, M.; Shokrgozar, M. A.; Simchi, A.; Imani, M.; Milani, A. S.; Stroeve, P.; Vali, H.; Hafeli, U. O.; Bonakdar, S. Multiphysics Flow Modeling and in vitro Toxicity of Iron Oxide Nanoparticles Coated with poly(vinyl alcohol). *J. Phys. Chem. C* **2009**, *113,* 2322–2331.

122. Moore, A.; Weissleder, R.; Bogdanov, A., Jr. Uptake of Dextran-coated monocRystalline Iron Oxides in Tumor Cells and Macrophages. *J. Magn. Reson. Imag.* **1997**, *7,* 1140–1145.

123. Philipse, A. P.; Vanbruggen, M. P. B.; Pathmamanoharan, C. Magnetic Silica Dispersions—Preparation and Stability of Surface-modified Silica Particles with a Magnetic Core. *Langmuir* **1994**, *10,* 92–99.

124. Raynal, I.; Prigent, P.; Peyramaure, S.; Najid, A.; Rebuzzi, C.; Corot, C. Macrophage Endocytosis of Superparamagnetic Iron Oxide Nanoparticles: Mechanisms and Comparison of Ferumoxides and Ferumoxtran-10. *Invest. Radiol.* **2004**, *39*, 56–63.

125. Zhao, X.; Harris, J. M. Novel Degradable poly(ethylene glycol) Hydrogels for Controlled Release of Protein. *J. Pharm. Sci.* **1998**, *87*, 1450–1458.

126. Jiang, W.; Mardyani, S.; Fischer, H.; Chan, W. C. W. Design and Characterization of Lysine Crosslinked Mercaptoacid Biocompatible Quantum Dots. *Chem. Mater.* **2006**, *18*, 872–878.

127. Aldana, J.; Wang, Y. A.; Peng, X. G. Photochemical Instability of CdSe Nanocrystals Coated by Hydrophilic Thiols. *J. Am. Chem. Soc.* **2001**, *123*, 8844–8850.

128. Guo, W. Z.; Li, J. J.; Wang, Y. A.; Peng, X. G. Conjugation Chemistry and Bioapplications of Semiconductor Box Nanocrystals Prepared via Dendrimer Bridging. *Chem. Mater.* **2003**, *15*, 3125–3133.

129. Liz-Marzán, L. M. Tailoring Surface Plasmons through the Morphology and Assembly of Metal Nanoparticles. *Langmuir* **2006**, *22*, 32–41.

130. Larson, D. R.; Zipfel, W. R.; Williams, R. M.; Clark, S. W.; Bruchez, M. P.; Wise, F. W., et al. Watersoluble Quantum Dots for Multiphoton Fluorescence Imaging in vivo. *Science* **2003**, *300*, 1434–1436.

131. Wuister, S. F.; Swart, I.; van Driel, F.; Hickey, S. G.; Donega, C. D. Highly Luminescent Water Soluble CdTe Quantum Dots. *Nano Lett.* **2003**, *3*, 503–507.

132. Surendiran, A.; Sandhiya, S.; Pradhan, S. C.; Adithan, C. Novel Applications of Nanotechnology in Medicine. *Indian J. Med. Res.* **2009**, *130*, 689–701.

133. McCormack, B.; Gregoriadis, G. Drugs-in-Cyclodextrins-Inliposomes—A Novel concept in Drug-delivery. *Int. J. Pharm.* **1994**, *112*, 249–258.

134. Illum, L.; Davis, S. S. The Organ Uptake of Intravenously Administered Colloidal Particles can be Altered Using a nonionic Surfactant (Poloxamer 338). *FEBS Lett.* **1984**, *167*, 79–82.

135. Senior, J.; Delgado, C.; Fisher, D.; Tilcock, C.; Gregoriadis, G. Influence of Surface Hydrophilicity of Liposomes on their Interaction with Plasma–Protein and Clearance from the Circulation—Studies with poly (ethylene glycol)-coated Vesicles. *Biochim. Biophys. Acta* **1991**, *1062*, 77–82.

136. Kirby, C.; Gregoriadis, G. The effEct of Lipid Composition of Small Unilamellar Liposomes Containing Melphalan and Vincristine on Drug Clearance After Injection in Mice. *Biochem. Pharmacol.* **1983**, *32*, 609–615.

137. Torchilin, V. P.; Shtilman, M. I.; Trubetskoy, V. S.; Whiteman, K.; Milstein, A. M. Amphiphilic Vinyl Polymers Effectively Prolong Liposome Circulation Time *in vivo*. *Biochim. Biophys. Acta* **1994**, *1195*, 181–184.

138. Forssen, E. A.; Coulter, D. M.; Profitt, R. T. Selective *in vivo* Localization of Daunorubicin Small Unilamellar Vesicles in Solid Tumors. *Cancer Res.* **1992**, *52*, 3255–3261.

139. Szoka, J. F.; Papahadjopoulos, D. Procedure for Preparation of Liposomes with Large Internal Aqueous Space and High Capture by Reverse-phase Evaporation. *Proc. Natl. Acad. Sci. U S A* **1978**, *75*, 4194–4198.

140. Papahadjopoulos, D.; Jacobson, K.; Nir, S.; Isac, T. Phase Transitions in Phospholipid Vesicles. Fluorescence Polarization and Permeability Measurements Concerning the Effect of Temperature and Cholesterol. *Biochim. Biophys. Acta* **1973**, *311*, 330–348.

141. Papahadjopoulos, D.; Jacobson, K.; Poste, G.; Shepherd, G. Phase Transitions in Phospholipid Vesicles. Fluorescence Polarization and Permeability Measurements Concerning the Effect of Temperature and Cholesterol. *Biochim. Biophys. Acta* **1974**, *394*, 504–519.

Nanomaterials for Medical Applications

142. Kateb, B.; Chiu, K.; Black, K.; Yamamoto, V.; Khalsa, B.; Ljubimova, J.; Ding, H.; Patil, R.; Portilla-Arias, J.; Modo, M.; Moore, D.; Farahani, K.; Okun, M.; Prakash, N.; Neman, J.; Ahdoot, D.; Grundfest, W.; Nikzad, S.; Heiss, J. Nanoplatforms for Constructing New Approaches to Cancer Treatment, Imaging, and Drug Delivery: What Should be the Policy?. *NeuroImage* **2011**, *54*, S106–S124.

143. Peer, D.; Karp, J. M.; Hong, S.; Farokhzad, O. C.; Margalit, R.; Langer, R. Nanocarriers as an Emerging Platform for Cancer Therapy. *Nat. Nanotechnol.* **2007**, *2*, 761–770.

144. Portilla-Arias, J. P.; Garcia-Alvarez, M.; Galbis, J. A.; Munoz-Guerra, S. Biodegradable Nanoparticles of Partially Methylated Fungal poly(beta-l-malic acid) as a Novel Protein Delivery Carrier. *Macromol. Biosci.* **2008**, *8*, 551–559.

145. Portilla-Arias, J. P.; Garcia-Alvarez, M.; de Ilarduya, A. M.; Holler, E.; Galbis, J. A.; Munoz-Guerra, S. Synthesis, Hydrodegradation and Drug Releasing Properties of Methyl Esters of Fungal poly(β, l-malic acid). *Macromol. Biosci.* **2008**, *8*, 540–550.

146. Gilding, D. K.; Reed, A. M. Biodegradable Polymers for use in Surgery-polyglycolic/poly (lactic acid) Homo- and Copolymers: 1. *Polymer* **1979**, *20*, 1459–1464.

147. Duncan, R. Polymer Conjugates as Anticancer Nanomedicines. *Nat. Rev. Cancer* **2006**, *6*, 688–701.

148. Zhang, N.; Chittapuso, C.; Ampassavate, C.; Siahaan, T. J.; Berkland, C. PLGA Nanoparticle–Peptide Conjugate Effectively Targets Intercellular Cell-Adhesion Molecule-1. *Bioconjug. Chem.* **2008**, *19*, 145–152.

149. Zhang, N.; Ping, Q. N.; Huang, G. H.; Xu, W. F. Investigation of Lectin-modified Insulin Liposomes as Carriers for Oral Administration. *Int. J. Pharm.* **2005**, *294*, 247–259.

150. Tobio, M.; Sanchez, A.; Vila, A.; Soriano, I.; Evora, C.; Vila-Jato, J. L.; Alonso, M. J. Investigation of Lectin-modified Insulin Liposomes as Carriers for Oral Administration. *Colloids Surf. B* **2000**, *18*, 315–323.

151. Garcia, J. T.; Farina, J. B.; Munguia, O.; Llabres, M. Comparative Degradation Study of Biodegradable Microspheres of poly(DL-lactide-*co*-glycolide) with poly(ethyleneglycol) Derivates. *J. Microencapsul.* **1999**, *16*, 83–94.

152. Tobio, M.; Gref, R.; Sanchez, A.; Lamger, R.; Alonso, M. J. Stealth PLA–PEG Nanoparticles as Protein Carriers for Nasal Administration. *Pharm. Res.* **1998**, *15*, 270–275.

153. Hu, Y.; Jiang, X.; Ding, Y.; Ge, H.; Yuan, Y.; Yang, C. Synthesis and Characterization of Chitosan–poly(acrylic acid) Nanoparticles. *Biomaterials* **2002**, *23*, 3193–3201.

154. Qurashi, T.; Blair, H. S.; Allen, S. J. Studies on Modified Chitosan Membranes. I. Preparation and Characterization. *J. Appl. Polym. Sci.* **1992**, *46*, 255–261.

155. Oh, K. T.; Bronich, T. K.; Kabanov, A. V. Micellar Formulations for Drug Delivery Based on Mixtures of Hydrophobic and Hydrophilic Pluronic(R) Block Copolymers. *J. Control. Release* **2004**, *94*, 411–422.

156. Adams, M. L.; Lavasanifar, A.; Kwon, G. S. Amphiphilic Block Copolymers for Drug Delivery. *J. Pharm. Sci.* **2003**, *92*, 1343–1355.

157. Sahoo, S. K.; Labhasetwar, V. Nanotech Approaches to Drug Delivery and Imaging. *Drug Discov. Today* **2003**, *8*, 1112–1120.

158. Dabholkar, R. D.; Sawant, R. M.; Mongayt, D. A. Polyethylene Glycol–phosphatidylethanolamine Conjugate (PEG-PE)-Based Mixed Micelles: some Properties, Loading with Paclitaxel, and Modulation of P-glycoprotein-Mediated Efflux. *Int. J. Pharm.* **2006**, *315*, 148–157.

159. Armentano, I.; Del Gaudio, C.; Bianco, A.; Dottori, M.; Nanni, F.; Fortunati, E., et al. Processing and Properties of poly(E-Caprolactone)/Carbon Nanofibre Composite Mats and Films Obtained by Electrospinning and Solvent Casting. *J. Mater. Sci.* **2009**, *44*, 4789–4795.

160. Cherukuri, P.; Bachilo, S. M.; Litovsky, S. H.; Weisman, R. B. Weisman, Near-infrared Fluorescence Microscopy of Single-walled Carbon Nanotubes in Phagocytic Cells. *J. Am. Chem. Soc.* **2004,** *126,* 15638–15639.

161. Correa-Duarte, M. A.; Wagner, N.; Rojas-Chapana, J.; Morsczeck, C.; Thie, M.; Giersig, M. Fabrication and Biocompatibility of Carbon Nanotube-based 3d Networks as Scaffolds for Cell Seeding and Growth. *Nano Lett.* **2004,** *4,* 2233–2236.

162. Dai, H.; Shim, M.; Chen, R. J.; Li, Y.; Kam, N. W. S. Functionalization of Carbon Nanotubes for Biocompatibility and Biomolecular Recognition. *Nano Lett.* **2002,** *2,* 285–288.

163. Harrison, B. S.; Atala, A. Carbon Nanotube Applications for Tissue Engineering. *Biomaterials* **2007,** *28,* 344–353.

164. Kim, B. M.; Murray, T.; Bau, H. H. The Fabrication of Integrated Carbon Pipes with Submicron Diameters. *Nanotechnology* **2005,** *16,* 1317–1320.

165. Kim, S. N.; Rusling, J. F.; Papadimitrakopoulos, F. Carbon Nanotubes for Electronic and Electrochemical Detection of Biomolecules. *Adv. Mater.* **2007,** *19,* 3214–3228.

166. Lovat, V.; Pantarotto, D.; Lagostena, L.; Cacciari, B.; Grolfo, M.; Righi, M., et al. Nanotube Substrates Boost Neuronal Electrical Signaling. *Nano Lett.* **2005,** *5,* 1107–1110.

167. Mamedov, A. A.; Kotov, N. A.; Prato, M.; Guldi, D. M.; Wicksted, J. P.; Hirsch, A. Molecular Design of Strong Single-wall Carbon Nanotube/Polyelectrolyte Multilayer Composites. *Nat. Mater.* **2002,** *1,* 190–194.

168. Mattson, M. P.; Haddon, R. C.; Rao, A. M. Molecular Functionalization of Carbon Nanotubes and Use as Substrates for Neuronal Growth. *J. Mol. Neurosci.* **2000,** *14,* 175–182.

169. Mwenifumbo, S.; Shaffer, M. S.; Stevens, M. M. Exploring Cellular Behaviour with Multiwalled Carbon Nanotube Constructs. *J. Mater. Chem.* **2007,** *17,* 1894–1902.

170. Ma, P. X. Scaffold for Tissue Engineering. *Mater. Today* **2004,** *7,* 30–40.

171. Price, R. L.; Waid, M. C.; Haberstroh, K. M.; Webster, T. J. Selective Bone Cell Adhesion on Formulations Containing Carbon Nanofibers. *Biomaterials* **2003,** *24,* 1877–1887.

172. Kateb, B.; Van Handel, M.; Zhang, L.; Bronikowski, M. J.; Manohara, H.; Badie, B. Internalization of MWCNTs by Microglia: possible Application in Immunotherapy of Brain Tumors. *NeuroImage* **2007,** *37,* S9–S17.

173. Singh, R.; Pamtarotto, D.; McCarthy, D.; Chaloin, O.; Hoebeke, J.; Partidos, C. D.; Briand, J. P.; Prato, M.; Bianco, A.; Kostarelos, K. Binding and Condensation of Plasmid DNA onto Functionalized Carbon Nanotubes: Toward the Construction of Nanotube-based Gene Delivery Vectors. *J. Am. Chem. Soc.* **2005,** *127,* 4388–4396.

174. Singh, R.; Pantarotto, D.; Lacerdo, L.; Pastorin, G.; Klumpp, C.; Prato, M.; Bianco, A.; Kostarelos, K. Tissue Biodistribution and Blood Clearance Rates of Intravenously Administered Carbon Nanotube Radiotracers. *Proc. Natl. Acad. Sci.* **2006,** *103,* 3357–3362.

175. Gao, X. P.; Qin, X.; Wu, F.; Liu, H.; Lan, Y.; Fan, S. S.; Yuan, H. T.; Song, D. Y.; Shen, P. W. Synthesis of Carbon Nanotubes by Catalytic Decomposition Of Methane Using LaNi5 Hydrogen Storage Alloy as Catalyst. *Chem. Phys. Lett.* **2000,** *327,* 271–276.

176. Nasibulin, A. G.; Moisala, A.; Jiang, H.; Kauppinen, E. I. Carbon Nanotube Synthesis by a Novel Aerosol Method. *J. Nanopart. Res.* **2006,** *8,* 465–475.

177. Tibbets, G. G.; Bernardo, C. A.; Borkiewicz, D. W.; Alig, R. L. Role of Sulfur in the Production of Carbon Fibers in the Vapor Phase. *Carbon* **1994,** *32,* 569–576.

178. Kroto, H. W.; Heath, J. R.; O'Brien, S. C.; Curl, R. F.; Smalley, R. E. C60: Buckminsterfullerene. *Nature* **1985,** *318,* 162–163.

179. Osawa, E. C60: Buckminsterfullerene. *Kagaku* **1970,** *25,* 854.

180. Langa, F.; Nierengarten, J. *Fullerenes: Principles and Applications. RSC Nanoscience and Nanotechnology Series;* 1st ed.; Royal Society of Chemistry, 2007.

181. Nasibulin, A. G.; Pikhitsa, P. V.; Jiang, H.; Brown, D. P.; Krasheninnikov, A. V.; Anisimov, A. S.; Queipo, P.; Moisala, A.; Gonzalez, D.; Lientschnig, G.; Hassanien, A.; Shandakov, S. D.; Lolli, G.; Resasco, D. E.; Choi, M.; Tomanek, D.; Kauppinen, E. I. A Novel Hybrid Carbon Material. *Nat. Nanotechnol.* **2007,** *2,* 156–161.

182. Sano, N.; Wang, H.; Chhowalla, M.; Alexandrou, I.; Amaratunga, G. A. Synthesis of Carbon 'Onions' in Water. *Nature* **2001,** *29,* 506–507.

183. Koruga, D.; Matija, L.; Misic, N.; Rakin, P. Fullerene C60: properties and Possible Applications. *Trans. Tech. Publ. Mat. Sci. Forum* **1996,** *214,* 49–56.

184. Guldi, D. M.; Prato, M. Excited-state Properties of C (60) Fullerene derivatives. *Acc. Chem. Res.* **2000,** *33,* 695–703.

185. Bakry, R.; Vallant, R. M.; Najam-ul-hag, M.; Rainer, M.; Szabo, Z.; Huck, C. W.; Bonn, G. K. Medicinal Applications of Fullerenes. *Int. J. Nanomed.* **2007,** *2,* 639–649.

186. Zagal, J. H.; Griveau, Z.; Nyokong, T.; Bedioui, F. Carbon Nanotubes, Phthalocyanines and Porphyrins: attractive Hybrid Materials for Electrocatalysis and Electroanalysis. *J. Nanosci. Nanotech.* **2009,** *9,* 2201–2214.

187. Ravi, P.; Dai, S.; Wang, C.; Tam, K. C. Fullerene Containing Polymers: a Review on their Synthesis and Supramolecular Behavior in Solution. *J. Nanosci. Nanotech.* **2007,** *7,* 1176–1196.

188. Johnston, H. J.; Hutchison, G. R.; Christenses, F. M.; Aschberger, K.; Stone, V. The Biological Mechanisms and Physicochemical Characteristics Responsible for Driving Fullerene Toxicity. *Toxicol. Sci.* **2010,** *114,* 162–182.

189. Tekade, R.; Kumar, P.; Jain, N. Dendrimers in Oncology: An Expanding Horizon. *Chem. Rev.* **2009,** *109,* 49–87.

190. Devarakonda, B.; Otto, D.; Judefeind, A., et al. Effect of pH on the Solubility and Release of Furosemide from Polyamidoamine (PAMAM) Dendrimer Complexes. *Int. J. Pharm.* **2007,** *345.*

191. Milhem, O.; Myles, C.; Mekeown, N.; Attwood, D.; Emanuelle, A. Polyamidoamine Starburst® Dendrimers as Solubility Enhancers. *Int. J. Pharm.* **2000,** *197,* 239.

192. Dufes, C.; Uchegbu, I.; Schatzlein, A. Dendrimers in Gene Delivery. *Adv. Drug Deliv. Rev.* **2005,** *57,* 2177.

193. Hecht, S.; Frechet, J. Dendritic Encapsulation of Function: applying Nature's Site Isolation Principle from Biomimetics to Materials Science. *Angew. Chem. Int. Ed.* **2001,** *40,* 74.

194. Tomalia, D.; Reyna, L.; Svenson, S. Dendrimers as Multi-purpose Nanodevices for Oncology Drug Delivery and Diagnostic Imaging. *Biochem. Soc. Trans.* **2007,** *35,* 61.

195. Lai, P.; Lou, P.; Peng, C.; Pai, C.; Yen, W.; Huang, M.; Young, T.; Shieh, M. Doxorubicin Delivery by Polyamidoamine Dendrimer Conjugation and Photochemical Internalization for Cancer Therapy. *J. Control. Release* **2007,** *122,* 39.

196. Chauhan, A.; Sridevi, S.; Chalasani, K.; Jain, A.; Jain, S.; Jain, N.; Diwan, P. Dendrimer-mediated Transdermal Delivery: Enhanced Bioavailability of Indomethacin. *J. Control Release* **2003,** *90,* 335.

197. Curry, M.; Li, X.; Zhang, J.; Weaver, M.; Street, S. Morphological and Structural Characterizations of Dendrimer-mediated Metallic Ti and Al Thin Film Nanocomposites. *Thin Solid Films* **2007,** *515,* 3567.

198. Esumi, K.; Matsumoto, T.; Seto, Y.; Yoshimura, T. Preparation of Gold, Gold/Silver-dendrimer Nanocomposites in the Presence of Benzoin in Ethanol by UV Irradiation. *J. Colloid Interface Sci.* **2005,** *284,* 199.

199. Satoh, K.; Yoshimura, T.; Esumi, K. Effects of Various Thiol Molecules Added on Morphology of Dendrimer–Gold Nanocomposites. *J. Colloid Interface Sci.* **2002,** *255,* 312.

200. Battah, S.; Balaratnam, S.; Casas, A.; O'Neill, S.; Edwards, C.; Batlle, A.; Dobbin, P.; MacRobert, A. Macromolecular Delivery of 5-Aminolaevulinic Acid for Photodynamic Therapy Using Dendrimer Conjugates. *Mol. Cancer Ther.* **2007,** *6,* 876.

201. van Nostrum, C. Polymeric Micelles to Deliver Photosensitizers for Photodynamic Therapy. *Adv. Drug Deliv. Rev.* **2004,** *56,* 9–12.

202. Barrett, T.; Ravizzini, G.; Choyke, P.; Kobayashi, H. Dendrimers in Medical Nanotechnology. *IEEE Eng. Med. Biol. Mag.* **2009,** *28,* 12–22.

203. Bharali, D.; Khalil, M.; Gurbuz, M.; Simone, T.; Mousa, S. Nanoparticles and Cancer Therapy: A Concise Review with Emphasis on Dendrimers. *Int. J. Nanomed.* **2009,** *4,* 1–7.

204. Zeng, F.; Zimmerman, S. C. Dendrimers in Supramolecular Chemistry: From Molecular Recognition to Self-assembly. *Chem. Rev.* **1997,** *97,* 1681–1712.

205. Tomalia, D. A.; Naylor, A. M.; Goddard, W. A., III Starburst Dendrimers: Control of Size, Shape, Surface Chemistry, Topology and Flexibility in the Conversion of Atoms to Macroscopic Materials. *Angew. Chem.* **1990,** *102,* 119–157.

206. Newkome, G. R.; Moorefield, C. N.; Vogtle, F. *Dendritic Macromolecules: Concepts, Syntheses, Perspectives;* VCH Weinheim: Germany, 1996.

207. Kim, Y. H. Highly Branched Polymers. *Adv. Mater.* **1992,** *4,* 764–766.

208. Denkewalter, R. G.; Kolc, J. F.; Lukasavage, W. J. Macromolecular Highly Branched Homogeneous Compound, 1983.

209. Buhleier, E.; Wehner, W.; Vogtle, F. "Cascade"- and "Nonskid-Chain-like" Synthesis of Molecular Cavity Topologies. *Synthesis* **1978,** *155.*

210. Newkome, G. R.; Gupta, V. K.; Baker, G. R.; Yao, Z. -Q. Cascade Molecules: A New Approach to Micelle. A [27]-Arborol. *J. Org. Chem.* **1985,** *50,* 2003.

211. Hawker, C. J.; Frechet, J. M. J. Preparation of Polymers with Controlled Molecular Architecture. A New Convergent Approach to Dendritic Macromolecules. *J. Am. Chem. Soc.* **1990,** *112,* 7638–7647.

212. Miller, T. M.; Neenan, T. X. Convergent Synthesis of Monodisperse Dendrimers Based Upon 1,3,5-trisubstituted Benzenes. *Chem. Mater.* **1990,** *2,* 346–349.

213. Xu, Z. F.; Moore, J. S. Stiff Dendritic Macromolecules. 3. Rapid Construction of Large-Size Phenylacetylene Dendrimers up to 12.5 Nanometers in Molecular Diameter. *Angew. Chem. Int. Ed.* **1993,** *32,* 1354–1357.

214. Sato, I.; Shibata, T.; Ohtake, K.; Kodaka, R.; Hirokawa, Y.; Shirai, N.; Soai, K. Synthesis of Chiral Dendrimers with a Hydrocarbon Backbone and Application to the Catalytic Enantioselective Addition of Dialkylzincs to Aldehydes. *Tetrahedron Lett.* **2000,** *41,* 3123–3126.

215. Liu, H.; Webster, T. J. Review: Nanomedicine for Implants: A Review of Studies and Necessary Experimental Tools, Cellular and Molecular Biology Techniques for Biomaterials Evaluation. *Biomaterials* **2007,** *28,* 354–369.

216. Rossini, P.; Colpo, P.; Ceccone, G.; al., E. Surfaces engineering of polymeric films for biomedical applications. *Master Sci. Eng. C* **2003,** *23,* 353–358.

217. Bain, C. D.; Troughton, E. B.; Tao, Y.; Evall, J.; Whitesides, G. M.; Nuzzo, R. G. Formation of Monolayer Films by the Spontaneous Assembly of Organic Thiols from Solution onto Gold. *J. Am. Chem. Soc.* **1989,** *111,* 321–335.

218. Delamarche, E.; Sundarababu, G.; Biebuyck, H.; Michel, B.; Gerber, C.; Sigrist, H.; Wolf, H.; Ringsdorf, H.; Xanthopoulos, N.; Mathieu, H. J. Immobilization of Antibodies on a Photoactive Self-assembled Monolayer on Gold. *Langmuir* **1996,** *12,* 1997–2006.

219. Hutt, D. A.; Legget, G. J. Influence of Adsorbate Ordering on Rates of UV Photooxidation of Self-assembled Monolayers. *J. Phys. Chem.* **1996,** *100,* 6657–6662.

220. Jiang, L.; Glidle, A.; Griffith, A.; McNeil, C. J.; Cooper, J. M. Characterising the Formation of a Bioelectrochemical Interface at a Self-assembled Monolayer Using XPS. *Bioelectrochem. Bioenerg.* **1997,** 15–23.

221. Schoenfish, M. H.; Pemberton, J. E. Air Stability of Self-assembled Monolayers on Silver and Gold Surfaces. *J. Am. Chem. Soc.* **1998,** *120,* 4502–4513.

222. Zhao, Y.; Pang, D.; Hu, S.; Wang, Z.; CHeng, J.; Dai, H. DNA-Modified Electrodes: Part 4: Optimization of Covalent Immobilization of DNA on Self-assembled Monolayers. *Talanta* **1999,** *49,* 751–756.

223. Tidwell, C. D.; Castner, D. G.; Golledge, S. L., et al. Static Time-of-light Secondary Ion Mass Spectrometry and X-ray Photoelectron Spectroscopy Characterization of Adsorbed Albumin and Fibronectin Films. *Surf. Interface Anal.* **2001,** *31,* 733–745.

224. Hessel, C. M.; Rasch, M. R.; Hueso, J. L.; Goodfellow, B.; Akhavan, V. A.; Puvanakrishnan, P.; Tunnel, J. W.; Korgel, B. A. Alkyl Passivation and Amphiphilic Polymer Coating of Silicon Nanocrystals for Diagnostic Imaging. *Small* **2010,** *6,* 2026–2034.

225. Sonogashira, K.; Tohda, Y.; Hagihara, N. A convenient synthesis of acetylenes: catalytic substitutions of acetylenic hydrogen with bromoalkenes, iodoarenes and bromopyridines. *Tetrahedron Letters* **1975,** *66,* 4467–4470.

Biocompatibility and Functionalization

3.1 INTRODUCTION

One of the most important challenges in the medical applications of nano-materials (NMs) is surface modification that allows for biocompatibility and functionalization. Effective surface modifications as well as highly controlled surface conjugation strategies are needed to incorporate specific biomolecules on the surface or inside the NMs. However, success in functionalization depends on many factors that include NMs' size, shape, charge, chemistry, and surface modification. These factors are often difficult to vary independently, so the contribution of each is difficult to generalize.

The small sizes of NMs that approach the atomic level, more often than not, invalidate the governing rules at the macroscopic level involving these chemicals. At the nanometer scale, quantum mechanical effects begin to emerge leading to varied and unexpected physicochemical properties.[1–4] Hence, modeling and indirect methods are frequently employed to accurately investigate the intricate interactions and properties of materials at the nanoscale. It is important to note that these novel and unique properties enable nanotechnology, specifically for nanomedicine, to provide powerful solutions to various problems. With the introduction of the scanning tunneling microscopy (STM) in the early 1980s, the

Nanomaterials for Medical Applications. http://dx.doi.org/10.1016/B978-0-12-385089-8.00003-0

manipulation of individual atoms became possible,[5,6] significantly contributing to the rapid discovery and development of fullerenes (carbon60 molecules),[7] carbon nanotubes,[8] and semiconductor quantum dots (QDs).[9–11]

The core QDs are usually prepared in high-temperature solvents that often involve a mixture of trioctylphosphine and trioctylphosphine oxide (TOP/TOPO)[12–16] followed by a layer of wide-bandgap semiconductor materials that can be coated on the surface of the QD core/shell.[12,17,18] These QDs are either used as hydrophobic nanocrystals or are made water soluble by ligand exchange or by adsorption of heterofunctional organic coating on the QD surface.[12,17–20] A comprehensive review by Medintz et al.[12,21] summarizes the group of compounds that give functionality to the QD surface. These include thiols,[12,21–23] silanes/silanols,[24,25] bidentate thiols,[12,24] amine box dendrimers,[12,26] oligomeric phosphines,[12,27] phosphatidyl compounds,[12,28,29] amphiphilic saccharides,[12,30] proteins and peptides, etc.[12,31,32] In a similar manner, iron oxide magnetic nanoparticles (IOMNPs) and other magnetic nanoparticles can be modified like the QDs to make them biocompatible. This chapter is devoted to a discussion of various ways of modifying the NM surface to make them water soluble and ultimately biocompatible.[33–45]

3.2 NANOMATERIAL CONVERSION INTO THE WATER-SOLUBLE FORM

Most nanomaterial (NMs) including quantum dots (QDs),[46] iron oxide magnetic nanoparticles (IOMNPs), gold or silver nanoparticles (NPs) are usually synthesized in nonpolar organic solvents. In general, NM synthesis uses long-chain ligands such as oleic acid (OA) (C18) to control nucleation and particle growth. However, an OA capping introduces a 2-nm thick tunneling barrier on NMs that is detrimental for applications that rely on charge transfer. To make these useful for biological and medical applications, they have to be converted into water-soluble form by replacing the hydrophobic surface ligands with amphiphilic ligands. Different NM water solubilization processes have been developed over the past few years. These are (i) ligand exchange with simple thiol-containing molecules[20,47–49] or more sophisticated ones such as oligomeric phosphines,[27] peptides,[50] and dendrons,[26] and (ii) encapsulation by a layer of amphiphilic diblock[51] or triblock copolymers[52] or in silica shells,[25,53,54] polymer shells,[19] phospholipid micelles,[29,55] or amphiphilic polysaccharides,[30] and (iii) a combination of layers of different molecules.[56–58]

NP surface modification is often necessary for specific applications. While QDs synthesized in organic solvents tend to have higher quality due to lower density of surface trap states leading to higher photoluminescence (PL) yield, their hydrophobic surfaces are not compatible with applications that require hydrophilic surfaces such as various medical applications. In order to convert the hydrophobic into hydrophilic surfaces, a number of strategies have been developed. Three types of modifications will be discussed in this chapter, which include[59–61] ligand exchange,[48] silanization,[25,53,62] and surface coating using amphiphilic polymers

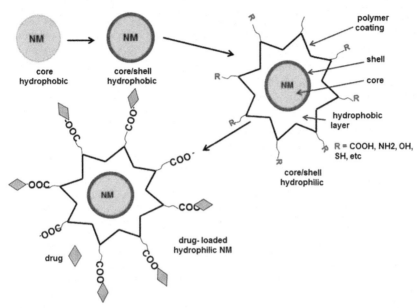

FIGURE 3.1   Schematic of converting hydrophobic NMs to hydrophilic NMs loaded with a drug. *(For color version of this figure, the reader is referred to the online version of this book)*

or surfactants such as phospholipids.[51,52,63,64] All these strategies for surface modification result in surface functionalized water-soluble nanostructures.

For fluorescent tagging or labeling of relevant molecules for medical and biological applications, it is desirable to have water-soluble QDs and other NPs with stable physical, electrical, magnetic, and/or optical properties that are not affected by environmental factors. High-quality QDs, IOMNPs, and other NMs are often synthesized under high-temperature organometallic conditions,[12,16,65] and are not compatible with biological systems. This chapter is dedicated to the discussion of various methods of surface modifications that convert NMs from hydrophobic to hydrophilic form that allows them to be biocompatible and loaded with medically relevant molecules such as drugs or antibodies (Abs) or both (Figure 3.1).

3.2.1 Ligand Exchange

Ligand exchange is one of the methods by which the surfaces of NMs are modified to make them water soluble in preparation for medical and biological applications. A ligand may be in the form of an ion, atom, molecule, or functional group that forms a complex with an NP, making up the interface between the NMs or core/shell and its surroundings (Figure 3.1). Ligands play a very important role in various applications of NMs that involve interactions between the NM and its surroundings. There is a wide range of ligands for NM ligand exchange, including hexanethiol, dodecanethiol, octadecanethiol, trioctylphosphine (TOP), triphenylphosphine, trioctylphosphine oxide (TOPO), perfluorated lauric acid, OA, didodecylamine, trioctyl aluminum, and a mixture of dodecanethiol and TOP. Of these, only thiols and OA result in increased air stability.[66] The other ligands precipitate NPs (perfluorated lauric acid and the mixture of dodecanethiol and TOP) or show identical behavior to lauric acid (TOP, triphenylphosphine, TOPO, didodecylamine, trioctyl aluminum). The latter may indicate that no exchange occurred, resulting from weaker adsorption than that of lauric acid.

Most medical and health-related applications of NMs depend on specific ligands and replacing the existing ligands with other ligands is often an essential processing step called ligand exchange. Ligand exchange is typically accomplished by exposing the particles containing the original ligands to the new ligands, which are usually present in excess. Ligand exchange can be achieved in the following ways:

- Dissolving the NPs in solid form (dried or precipitated through centrifugation or other means) in a solution containing the new ligand, which is a method used to functionalize CdSe and InP with pyridine.[20,67,68]
- A phase-transfer approach where, for example, water-soluble particles are transferred to an organic phase or vice versa by adding a suitable ligand that acts as a phase-transfer agent—for example, dodecanethiol promotes the transfer of charge-stabilized gold NPs to a toluene phase or mercapto acids have been used to transfer CdTe NMs from an organic phase to an aqueous phase.[69–71]

The outcome of ligand-exchange processes is difficult to assess except by indirect methods such as a change in solubility or even electrophoretic mobility. Verification is usually not an issue as long as the ligand exchanged NPs behave differently and that they do their job. Ligand exchange is one of the successful ways to integrate functionality that provides versatility for various applications of NMs. Ligand exchange has serious effects on the properties of NMs especially their luminescence or fluorescence properties. For instance, semiconductor NMs that have absorbed light can relax back to its ground state through luminescence and the efficiency of this process crucially depends on the NPs' surface. Surface trap states or surface defects in the nanocrystal structure act as a temporary hole for the electron preventing their radiative recombination.[60] The alternate occurrence of ion trapping and untrapping events results in intermittent fluorescence (blinking) that is visible at the single-molecule level,[72,73] which reduces the overall quantum yield (QY) which is the ratio of emitted to absorbed photons. To overcome these problems and to protect surface atoms from oxidation and other chemical reactions, a shell consisting of a few atomic layers of a material with a larger bandgap is grown on top of the nanocrystal core. This shell can be designed to enhance photostability by several orders of magnitude compared with conventional dyes[74] and at the same time obtain a QY close to 90%.[75] Binding of ligands to surface atoms that can passivate these trap states strongly affects the luminescence efficiency of the semiconductor NMs but because of stability issues, surface state passivation with ligands is not the way to create highly luminescent NMs with a robust emission. However, this change in luminescence can be used to monitor the ligand–NM interaction.[60]

The use of bifunctional ligands that contain one functional group that attaches at the NMs surface and a second group that is exposed to the surroundings is a very useful development. This is demonstrated by the use of thiols that make CdSe NMs adsorb at gold surfaces or by polymeric materials such as PEG that carry carboxyl, amine, hydroxyl, or a combination of these functional groups (Figure 3.1). An excellent application is for NM sensors that are modified with functional groups that provide affinity to a specific analyte that results in a change in the NMs' optical properties. One such NM prepared by Nath and Chilkoti[76] gave gold NMs (AuNMs) affinity for streptavidin through functionalization with biotin. Changes in the AuNMs plasmon resonance were used to indicate the binding of streptavidin to biotin. Colloidal CdSe NMs were engineered through encapsulation with an amphiphilic polymer upon which a pH-sensitive squaraine dye was conjugated.[77] In this NM structure, the CdSe/ZnS nanocrystal may either fluoresce or undergo fluorescence energy transfer (FRET) to the squaraine dye. The FRET efficiency in these nanostructures is a function of the surroundings that results from the dye's absorption profile which is controlled by pH while the ratio of the NM to dye emission is a measure of the pH of the environment. An alternative to long-chain ligands in the preparation of nanocrystal solids is short bifunctional ligands, such as hydrazine, forming a tightly packed nanocrystal solid that has sufficient conductivity to be used in different charge-transfer applications.[78]

3.2.2 Thiols for Ligand Exchange

Monothiols,[12,21,28] bidentate thiols,[12,24] silanes/silanols,[12,24,25] oligomeric phosphines,[12,27] amine box dendrimers,[12,24,26] dithiothreitol,[47] amphiphilic saccharides,[12,30] proteins and peptides, etc.[12,31,32] are used to prepare NMs for medical applications. For example, CdSe nanocrystals coated with hydrophilic deprotonated thiol (thiolate) ligands were studied systematically in a pseudo-steady-state titration, and introduced for determining the precipitation pH of nanocrystals coated with electron-donating ligands.[79] For comparison, CdTe and CdS nanocrystals coated with the same types of ligands were also examined. The results showed that the precipitation of the nanocrystals was caused by the dissociation of the nanocrystal–ligand coordinating bonds from the nanocrystal surface. The ligands were removed from the surface due to protonation in a relatively low pH range, between 2 and 7 depending on the size, approximately within the quantum confinement size regime, and chemical composition (bandgap) of the nanocrystals. In contrast, the re-dispersion of the nanocrystals was found to be solely determined by the deprotonation of the ligands. The size-dependent dissociation pH of the ligands was tentatively used as a means for determining the size-dependent free energy associated with the formation of a nanocrystal–ligand coordinating bond.

To solve the instability of NMs that are converted into water-soluble form through thiol ligand exchange, two methods have been developed. One is based on the direct adsorption of bifunctional ligands on the nanocrystal surface[20] and the other is based on surface coating with a silica layer.[25] The direct adsorption of bifunctional ligands on the nanocrystal surface is carried using ligands that have organic soluble and water-soluble functional groups. In this process, the organic soluble group orients toward the hydrophobic NMs, while the hydrophilic groups project away from the organic soluble region and toward the aqueous solution making the modified NM water soluble. Surface coating with a silica layer encapsulates multiple NMs inside a silica NP of 100 nm or greater diameter.

Mercaptoacetic acid is one of the thiols used to make QDs water soluble, because the mercapto portion has a large affinity to Zn atoms, while the carboxylic acid group is hydrophilic and reactive to biomolecules.[20] However, this process causes the fluorescence QYs to drop below 10% after water solubilization.[80] Another issue is the slow desorption of mercaptoacetic acid on the QD surface often leads to aggregation and precipitation of the QDs. A modified version of this process involves attachment of engineered proteins to QDs through electrostatic interactions,[58] and the use of dithiothreitol has been adopted for nanocrystal stabilization and bioconjugation.[47]

3.2.2.1 Protocol for Ligand Exchange[81]

The following method was used for the preparation of water-soluble CdSe/CdS/ZnS QDs for imaging and other biomedical applications.

(1) Precipitate the organic soluble CdSe/CdS/ZnS QDs with acetone two times to remove free octadecylamine (ODA) in the solution.
(2) Re-disperse in chloroform.
(3) Add 40 mg of polyethylene imine (PEI, M_w 10 kDa) to 0.5 nmol of CdSe/CdS/ZnS QDs in chloroform.
(4) Shake the mixture for 2 h at room temperature (RT).
(5) Evaporate the solvent under argon.
(6) Dissolve the dried film in ultrapure water (18 MΩ).
(7) Centrifuge at 6000g for 10 min to yield a clear supernatant with white deposits.
(8) Dialyze with M_w 50 kDa to remove the unbound PEI molecules against water or borate buffer solution (10 mM, pH 7.4).
(9) Store at 2–8 °C to avoid bacterial and mold contamination.

Characterize the water-soluble QDs with transmission electron microscopy (TEM) to establish the diameter and shape. Use a Zeta tracker to establish the zeta potential and the hydrodynamic size. Run a scan to establish the absorption and emission wavelength.

3.2.3 Encapsulation of NMs

Encapsulation with amphiphilic diblock or triblock copolymers[82] or in silica shells,[59,83] phospholipid micelles,[84] or polymer shells is another way to convert NMs into their water soluble form.[19] The encapsulation process introduces new functional groups on the surface of NMs such as carboxylic acids, amines, or hydroxides. These functional groups can be used to attach different biomolecules including drugs and vaccines on the surface of NMs (Figure 3.2).

Silanes have been used to functionalize semiconductor QDs leading to multiple advantages. The siloxane shell gives extra stability to nanostructures, and the silanized nanosystems remain stable over a wide range of pH and impede the release of undesirable heavy elements. Silanization can be carried out by Stöber-process-based approaches, in which alkoxysilanes are condensed in acidic or basic medium[62] that lead to synthesis of highly fluorescent silica-coated QDs with various surface charges by adopting a process similar to Stöber's process. One of the disadvantages of silanization is the self-condensation between the silane molecules. To overcome this, Yang and Gao[85] employed the reverse microemulsion method to coat CdTe nanocrystals with silica. Various organosilanes in toluene are used to treat nanocrystals to carry out multifunctionalization of semiconductor QDs.[86]

Silane, such as 3-mercaptopropyltrimethoxysilane, is directly adsorbed on the nanocrystals to displace the TOPO molecules and form a silica/siloxane shell on the surface by introduction of a base and hydrolysis of the silanol groups. The polymerization of the silanol groups stabilizes the nanocrystals against aggregation making the QDs soluble in intermediate polar solvents, such as methanol and dimethylsulfoxide. Reaction with bifunctional methoxy

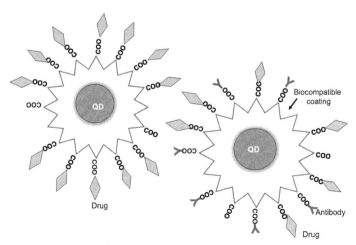

FIGURE 3.2   Schematic of hydrophilic carboxyl-functionalized NMs carrying a drug (left) or a drug and an Ab (right). *(For color version of this figure, the reader is referred to the online version of this book)*

compounds (i.e., aminopropyl trimethoxysilane or trimethoxysilyl propyl urea) converts the particles in the water-soluble form. Compared with the mercaptoacetic acid process, polymerized siloxane-coated QDs are more highly stable against aggregation. However, only milligram quantities can be prepared per batch using this process. Furthermore, this process leaves residual silanol groups on the nanocrystal surface, which can lead to precipitation and gel formation at neutral pH when not properly removed.

3.2.3.1 Protocol for NM Silica Encapsulation

One process for the synthesis of silica-coated NPs is described below.[59] The process can be scaled for making CdSe/ZnS nanocrystals with any size between 2 and 8 nm.

(1) Using anhydrous methanol, precipitate 1 mL of nanocrystals in butanol/TOPO (optical density (OD) of nanocrystals ~2).

(2) Add 50 μL of mercaptopropyltris(methyloxy)silane (MPS) and vortex to mix thoroughly.

(3) Add 5 μL of tetramethylammonium hydroxide (TMAH) and mix thoroughly into an optically clear solution.

(4) Add 120 mL of anhydrous methanol.

(5) Add 750 μL of TMAH to make it basic with a pH of 10.

(6) Place in a 500 mL three-neck-flask with a stream of N_2 with mild stirring for 1 h.

(7) Gently heat the solution to ~60 °C for 30 min.

(8) Cool down to RT.

(9) Add 90 mL of methanol, 10 mL of 18 MΩ Millipore water, 600 μL of (trihydroxysilyl)propyl methylphosphonate and 20 μL of MPS.

(10) Stir for ~2 h, heat to ~60 °C for less than 5 min, and cool down to ~30 °C.

(11) Quench the remaining silanol groups with a mixture of 20 mL of methanol and 2 mL of chlorotrimethylsilane to which ~3 g of solid TMAH pentahydrate is added to make it basic.

(12) Stir for ~2 h and then heat back to ~60 °C for ~30 min.

(13) Store at RT for 2–4 days with constant stirring in an N_2 atmosphere.

(14) Evaporate with a rotary evaporator down to 2–5× less than the original volume.

(15) Leave at RT for 24 h.

(16) Dialyze in a 10,000 molecular-weight cutoff (MWCO) dialysis tubing against methanol for 1 day.

(17) Filter through a 0.45 μm pore size nylon syringe filter.

(18) Remove the excess of free silane with centrifugal filter devices (YM-100 centriplus/centricon 100, MWCO 100,000) that leaves about 2 mL solution.

(19) Store the 2 mL solution at RT for 12 h.

(20) Pass the solution of silanized nanocrystals in methanol through a solvent exchange column (either NAP columns or a homemade 20-cm long column with a 0.7 cm diameter filled with ~5 g of Sephadex G25 medium and equilibrated with 10 mM phosphate buffer (PB), pH ~7.

(21) Only the fluorescent eluted fractions are collected and filtered with a 22-μm pore size acetate filter.

(22) Centrifuge at 20,000g for 30 min and discard the precipitate.

(23) Store the solutions in air.

(24) Establish the OD using the extinction coefficient as 10^5 M^{-1} cm^{-1}.

Characterize the water-soluble QDs with TEM to establish the diameter and shape. Use a Zeta tracker to establish the zeta potential and the hydrodynamic size. Run a scan to establish the absorption and emission wavelength.

Another process of preparing silane-coated QDs leads to organic soluble ones that are treated with ligand exchange before they become water soluble. Similar to the procedure above, the process starts with CdSe@ZnS NMs that are synthesized according to a previously published procedure.[87] The resulting QD core/shell nanocrystals are encapsulated with an SiO_2 shell using the following process.[88]

(1) Place 10 mL of cyclohexane, 1.3 mL of NM-5, 400 μL of CdSe@ZnS stock solution in chloroform, and 80 μL of tetraehtylorthosilicate (TEOS) in a flask with vigorous stirring.

(2) Thirty minutes after the microemulsion system is formed add 150 μL of ammonia aqueous solution (33 wt%) to initiate the polymerization process.

(3) Allow the process to grow silica over 24 h with vigorous stirring.

(4) Isolate the NMs from the microemulsion by adding acetone followed by centrifugation.

(5) Collect the precipitate consisting of CdSe@ZnS@SiO$_2$ composite particle.

(6) Sequentially wash with 1-butanol, 1-propanol, ethanol, and water to remove any surfactant and unreacted molecules. Completely disperse the precipitate in each solvent to remove any physically adsorbed molecules on the particle surfaces.

The resulting silica-encapsulated NMs are resuspended in the desired solvent and characterized for size, QY, concentration, and maximum wavelengths of emission and absorption. These CdSe@ZnS@SiO$_2$ are converted into their water-soluble form using ligand exchange discussed in previous section.

3.2.4 Polymer Coating

Polymer coating on various organic synthesized NMs has been used to convert these into their water-soluble form. Polymer-coated nanocrystals have been used in biological studies.[89–93] These hydrophobic nanocrystals are modified with amphiphilic polymer shell making them hydrophilic, thus water soluble. This is achieved by the reaction of the amphiphilic polymer, bis(6-aminohexyl) amine with surfactant-protected molecules that results in the cross-linking of the polymer chains around the NMs that renders them water soluble.[19] In another process, biomolecules and phospholipid micelles have been covalently linked with semiconductor QDs for application in ultrasensitive biological detection.

Polyethylene glycol (PEG) is a polymer widely used for various applications including encapsulation of NMs (Figure 3.3) due to its hydrophilicity and low antigenicity. In addition to steric stabilization of superparamagnetic iron oxide nanoparticles (SPIONs), PEG prevents plasma opsonization as well as uptake by macrophages, thereby increasing SPION circulation time in vivo. PEG-coated SPIONs are efficiently internalized by cells via fluid-phase endocytosis and through amphiphilic affinity to lipid bilayers on plasma membranes. [94]. These qualities, however, increase their potential to overload cells with iron and become toxic.[95]

Polyvinyl alcohol (PVA) is another organic polymer used as a coating for SPIONs. It has excellent film-forming, emulsifying, and adhesive properties. The use of PVA for intravenous (i.v.) delivery is limited due to poor persistence as well as agglomeration in a ferrofluid. However, when cross-linked to form a magnetic gel, PVA can be used as a vitreous eye substitute because it is a highly biocompatible material.[96] Potentially, when used with SPIONs, this biocompatibility can be utilized in targeted drug delivery, tissue engineering, and biosensor technology.[95]

Thioctic acid and PEGs have been used in simple esterification schemes, followed by reduction of the 1,2-dithiolane to synthesize a series of PEG-terminated dihydrolipoic acid (DHLA-PEG) as capping substrates.[24,97] The cap exchange reaction of TOP/TOPO-capped QDs with these substrates produced water-soluble nanocrystals that are stable over extended periods of time. These were also stable over a broad pH range, from weakly acidic to basic conditions (pH 5–12) but these ligands lacked specific functional end groups for easy implementation of simple conjugation techniques, such as avidin–biotin binding. Uyeda's

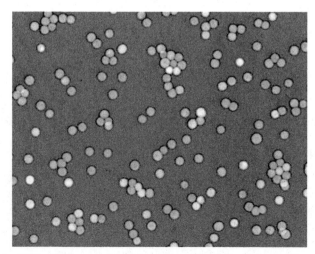

FIGURE 3.3   TEM of PEG-encapsulated 30-nm diameter IOMNPs. *Courtesy of Ocean NanoTech.*

group studied the design and synthesis of ligands functionalized with a biotin end group. The designed ligands had a central tetraethylene glycol (TEG) segment, a dithiol terminal group for anchoring on the QD surface and a lateral biotin. Attaching biotin at the end of QD surface-attached ligands provided an avidin bridge for avidin–biotin binding for attachment of proteins and other biomolecules on the QD surface. Exchange reactions were carried out with mixed ligands and binding assays of the biotin-coated water-soluble QDs to NeutrAvidin-functionalized substrates showed specific capture through avidin–biotin interactions.

Chitosan, a polysaccharide consisting of randomly distributed β-(1-4)-linked D-glucosamine (deacetylated unit) and N-acetyl-D-glucosamine (acetylated unit) provides a natural, biocompatible, cationic, and hydrophilic polymer coating that is suitable for affinity purification of proteins and magnetic bioseparation.[95] Chitosan-coated SPIONs that were used to label fibroblasts improved their invasive potential under a magnetic force, showing promise for tissue engineering.[98]

Dextran, a polysaccharide, has also been applied in coating NMs. For biological applications, SPIONs are usually coated with organic biodegradable compounds such as dextran or carbohydrate derivatives that are commonly used as plasma expanders that have very high affinity to iron oxides.[99] Several such formulations are now commercially available for human consumption such as Ferridex, Resovist, Combidex, and AMI-288/ferumoxytol that are successfully used as magnetic resonance imaging (MRI) contrast agents.[100]

Biocompatible polymers that are amphiphilic in nature have been reported for coating NPs to make them hydrophilic.[101,102] Hu's group reported the epoxidation of the surface OA ligand and further coupling with polyethylene glycol monomethyl ether (mPEG-OH) to coat the surface of nanophosphors.[102] The effective coating of the surface of the nanophosphors with mPEG-OH was confirmed by ^{1}H NMR spectrometry, Fourier-transform infrared (FTIR) spectroscopy, and dynamic light scattering (DLS) studies, but TEM and PL spectroscopy showed no obvious variations in the morphologies and luminescence before and after coating.

3.2.4.1 Protocol for Amphiphilic Polymer Coating of NMs

The following protocol was adopted from Hessel's paper.[101]

Part 1. Synthesis of the amphiphilic polymer

(1) In a capped, single neck round-bottom flask, place 100 mL anhydrous tetrahydrofuran (THF), 15 mmol dodecylamine (about 3.45 mL), and poly(isobutylene-*alt*-maleic anhydride) (20 mmol of monomer units, 3.084 g) sequentially to form a turbid white solution.

(2) Sonicate the flask for 1 min to suspend the insoluble polymer.

(3) Heat the suspension to 60 °C for 3 h under vigorous stirring. The suspension will become clear after 15 min of stirring, indicating that the polymer became soluble in THF after covalently coupling with hydrophobic dodecylamine molecules.

(4) Cool the solution down to RT.

(5) Using a rotary evaporator, reduce the volume to 20 mL.

(6) Stir the clear solution again at 60 °C for 12 h to ensure complete coupling between the polymer and dodecylamine.

(7) Cool back down to RT and evaporate the remaining solvent with a rotary evaporator that leaves a pale yellow, solid amphiphilic polymer.

(8) Transfer the polymer to a nitrogen filled glove box (< 0.1 ppm O_2) and dissolve in anhydrous $CHCl_3$ (25 mL) to give a monomer unit concentration of 0.8 M.

(9) Store the amphiphilic polymer solution in a glass vial in the glove box until use.

Part 2. Coating the Si nanocrystals with polymer[101]

(1) In a 50 mL round bottom flask mix the amphiphilic polymer stock solution (0.8 M monomer units in $CHCl_3$, 53 µL) and alkyl-Si NMs at 3.0 mg/mL in anhydrous $CHCl_3$, 0.40 mL, and anhydrous $CHCl_3$ (2.55 mL). You may use other NMs as well.

(2) Vortex the mixture and stir with magnetic stirrer for 15 min at RT.

(3) Remove the solvent by rotary evaporation to yield a yellow Si-polymer film on the inner wall of the flask.

(4) Add aqueous sodium borate buffer (SBB) (50 mM borate, 2.0 mL, pH 12) and stir for 15 min at RT to disperse the Si–polymer.

(5) Add 13.0 mL DI water to dilute the NMs.

(6) Pass the suspension through a 0.2-µm pore syringe filter (Corning, PES membrane) followed by a 0.1-µm pore syringe filter (Whatman, inorganic membrane).

(7) Place the filtered nanocrystal solution in an ultracentrifugation filter (Amicon Ultra, regenerated cellulose membrane, 50 kDa MWCO) and centrifuge at 4000g for 4 min at RT.

(8) Discard the colorless filtrate and retain the concentrated NMs solution above the membrane.

(9) Dilute the NMs solution with 15.0 mL sterile-filtered phosphate buffered saline (PBS, 150 mM, pH 7.4).

(10) Repeat the ultracentrifugation two more times using PBS to dilute the retained NMs solution.

(11) Store the final aqueous NMs solution in a glass vial under ambient conditions until use.

(12) Characterize the amphiphilic polymer coated NMs.

Hessel and coworkers used X-ray diffraction (XRD), attenuated total reflectance FTIR (ATR-FTIR) spectra (400–4000 cm^{-1}), and X-ray photoelectron spectroscopy (XPS) to characterize the surface composition and to demonstrate that the amphiphilic polymer successfully coated the NM surface. A UV–vis spectrophotometer, PL, and photoluminescence excitation (PLE) were used to establish the optical properties. Zeta potential was measured by laser Doppler anemometry using a Zetasizer Nano ZS instrument (Malvern). TEM and DLS are good nondestructive instruments to establish physical characteristics of NMs (Figure 3.4).

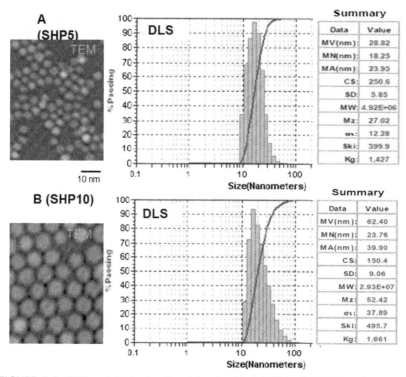

FIGURE 3.4 TEM and DLS of carboxyl-functionalized PEGylated IOMNPs. *Courtesy of Ocean NanoTech. (For color version of this figure, the reader is referred to the online version of this book)*

3.3 NM BIOCONJUGATION

In order to be useful in various specific medical applications, the hydrophilic water-soluble NMs need to be functionalized in order to load the biomolecules of interest. Water-soluble functionalized NMs have the necessary bioreceptors to carry the activity that it is intended for. The bioreceptors include proteins, DNA, lipids, carbohydrates, or parts of or whole microorganisms.[103] Various NMs such as QDs, carbon nanotubes (CNTs), metal NPs (gold, silver, and silica), metal oxides, and semiconductor and polymer nanowires attached to bioreceptors make them useful for various medical applications.[103,104] The NMs are functionalized with biocompatible materials to allow for selective and specific interactions with biomolecules that are unique to each NM application. Functionalization of NMs is also essential to facilitate self-assembly and nanopatterning on solid surfaces. Biocompatible-functionalized NMs may be used for medical diagnostics, imaging, single or multiple drug delivery, theranostics, and many more.

New developments include water-based synthesis methods for NMs[23,105] that yield particles emitting from the visible to the near-infrared (NIR) spectrum.

These particles are intrinsically water soluble and are very useful in biological environments. The surface-modified NMs require biological interfacing in order to be useful for specific applications.

3.3.1 NM Bioconjugation Techniques

The surface-functionalized NMs are conjugated to biomolecules making it useful for various biological and medical applications. Conjugation can be done using conventional conjugation techniques depending upon the surface functional group on the NM and on the biomolecule.[108] Conjugation to NMs may be done through ligand-like attachment by chemisorption to the NMs' core as in the case of sulfur-containing groups,[12,109] electrostatic adsorption (including those involving engineered proteins),[12,109] hydrophobic interactions,[12,97,110] conjugation by covalent binding of groups on both particle and the surface modifier,[12,111] or through a receptor–ligand interaction as in the case of avidin–biotin system.[12] Table 3.1 shows a list of various functional groups on the surface of NMs that can be used for the attachment of a biomolecule.

Studies have been reported on the use of thioctic acid and PEGs in simple esterification schemes, followed by reduction of the 1,2-dithiolane to synthesize a series of PEG-terminated dihydrolipoic acid (DHLA-PEG)[24,97] capping substrates. The exchange reaction of TOP/TOPO-capped QDs with these materials led to the production of water-soluble NMs that were stable over long time points over a broad pH range from weakly acidic (pH 5) to basic conditions (pH 12). However, although highly stable, these ligands did not possess

TABLE 3.1 Common NMs' Bioconjugation Techniques to load NM With Drugs, Gene, or Proteins

NMs' functional group	Molecule to be coupled with the NM	Cross-linker/mediator/reagent
Amine (–NH2)	Drug-NH$_2$	Disuccinymidyl glutarate[106]
	DNA	Succinymydyl-[4-(psoralen-8-yloxy)]-butyrate[106]
	Protein-NH$_2$	Disuccinymidyl glutarate[106]
Carboxyl (–COOH)	Drug-NH$_2$; protein-NH$_2$; DNA-NH$_2$	Carbodiimide[42,107]
Sulfhydryl (–SH)	Protein; drug	Maleimide[108]
Biotin	Streptavidin–protein	Buffer

specific functional groups and are, therefore, not useful for simple conjugation techniques, such as avidin–biotin binding. Additional studies were reported[24,97] on the design and synthesis of ligands functionalized with a biotin end group. These ligands had a central TEG segment, a dithiol terminal group for anchoring on the QD surface, and a lateral biotin. The presence of biotin at one end was expected to allow avidin–biotin binding motif to conjugate QDs to proteins and other biomolecules via the avidin surface. Their cap exchange reactions involved mixed ligands that resulted in binding assays of the biotin-coated water-soluble QDs to NeutrAvidin-functionalized substrates that exhibited specific capture of the QDs through avidin–biotin interactions.

The nanoscale dimensions of NMs bring optical, electronic, magnetic, catalytic, and other properties that are distinct from those of atoms/molecules or bulk materials. In order to exploit the special properties that arise due to the nanoscale dimensions of NMs, researchers must control and manipulate the size, shape, and surface functional groups and structure them into periodically ordered assemblies to create new products, devices, and technologies or improve existing ones.[112–119] The art of controlling/manipulating the properties and utilizing these NMs for the purpose of building microscopic machinery can be done using the "top-down" or "bottom-up" approach. In the "top-down" approach, large chunks of materials are broken down into nanostructures by lithography or any other outside force that imposes order on NMs.[120] The "bottom-up" approach follows nature's lead in making extraordinary materials and molecular machines by building nanostructures from atoms or molecules or any stable building blocks through the understanding and exploitation of order-inducing factors that are inherent in the system.[121] The mechanism of formation/fabrication of novel nanostructures from self-assembly of peptides, proteins, and lipids has been elucidated as described in a review article by Zhang[121] providing an understanding of the factors that govern growth and ordering of NMs that has led to a number of novel structures and functionalities. These nanostructures include nanofibers, bionanotubes, amphiphilic protein scaffolds, and nanowires that have potential applications in the electronic industry, biomedical field, computer information technology, etc.

The application of NMs in medicine is rapidly gaining ground in the field of medical diagnostics.[122] Driskell and Tripp[103] and Kaittanis et al.[123] discussed the different strategies for different disease diagnostics and how nanotechnology can revolutionize these strategies. Lee et al.[124] reviewed recent advances in nano/microfluidic technologies for clinical point-of-care (POC) applications at resource-limited settings in developing countries. Hauck et al.[125] described the use of NMs as labels or barcodes in conjunction with microfluidic systems for automated sample preparation and sample assays for infectious diseases diagnostics.

One of the applications of NMs that rely almost completely on the functionalization of the NM is a biosensor. A biosensor is composed of a biorecognition element that interacts with the target molecules and a transducer and detects the interaction and converts the binding event to a measurable analytical signal.

Biosensors are classified according to the bioreceptor used or biological process involved such as biocatalytic (enzyme-based)[104,126–133] immunologic (Ab–antigen based)[126,127,132–137] or DNA (nucleic acid-based)[130,134,138] sensors. Biosensors that use NMs are called nanosensors.[139–151] Nanosensors are designed in various novel ways using the enhancement of performance through the various properties of the NMs employed.[148,151,152] Recent advances in materials science and synthetic chemistry have made it possible to produce high-quality NMs in the form of NPs (nanotubes, nanorods, nanospheres, nanowires, nanoarrays, and their composites)[153,154] that have been used for the development of biosensors [140,141,148,150,155–159] because of their significant advantages over microscale and bulk materials that include (a) size-tunable properties, (b) large surface–volume ratio, (c) shape-dependent properties, (d) lower energy consumption, (e) miniaturized bisensors, and (f) low cost. These nanosensors are discussed in greater detail in Chapter 4.

3.3.2 Covalent Conjugation of Biomolecules to NPs

Covalent attachment of a biorecognition moiety to a functionalized NM is one of the more widely used strategies for converting an NM for a specific application.[139–151,160] For example, tumor cells that are circulating in the blood can be tagged and diagnosed using this approach. Aguilar et al.[161–164] exhibited specific targeting of breast cancer cell lines SK-BR3 using QDs that were functionalized with Abs against human endothelial receptors (AbHER2) forming QD–Ab. HER2 is a surface coating protein that is overexpressed in breast cancer cells. SK-BR3 breast cancer cells that were exposed to QD–Ab, appeared fluorescent under a UV illuminated microscope (Figure 3.5) making the imaging of the cells under a microscope a lot easier. Furthermore, cells that are specifically stained with biomolecule-functionalized QDs offer advantages over those that

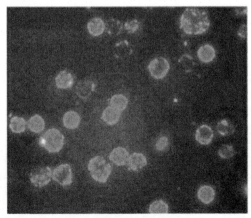

FIGURE 3.5 Digital photograph of SK-BR3 cells exposed to QD–anti-EpCAM. The QDs were ~8 nm in diameter emitting at 620 nm. *Courtesy of Ocean NanoTech (For color version of this figure, the reader is referred to the online version of this book)*

are stained with organic dyes because QDs are resistant to photobleaching, have high brightness, and are stable in cells for over six months at ambient RT.

NM bioconjugation through covalent binding is preferred to avoid desorption of the biomolecule from the surface of the NMs.[109,146,160–162,164–179] Bioconjugation of NMs with carboxyl (–COOH) functional groups on the surface often uses the carbodiimide derivative 1-ethyl-3-(3-dimethylaminopropyl) carbodiimide (EDC) for linking to the amine (–NH$_2$) groups on the biomolecules.[161,162,164,165] NMs functionalized with sulfyhydryl (–SH) groups are activated with the linker 4-(N-maleimidomethyl)-cyclohexanecarboxylic acid N-hydroxysuccinimide ester (SMCC) for linking with the –NH$_2$ groups of the biomolecule.

One example of the carbodiimide chemistry in infectious diseases diagnostics is the conjugation of the pathogen biomarkers hepatitis B surface antigen (HBsAg), HCV nonstructural protein 4 (NSP4), and HIV glycoprotein 41 (gp41) to the surface of quantum dot barcodes (QdotBs).[58] The use of the QdotBs along with advances in microfluidic and photon detection technologies, signal processing, and proteomic biomarkers of infection, have shown potential to be developed as a handheld device for POC diagnostics.[180] Agrawal et al.[181] showed how carbodiimide chemistry was also used to conjugate oligonucleotides to green and red NP probes for the determination of intact respiratory syncytial virus (RSV) and that the use of bioconjugation of two-color NPs to simultaneously recognize two binding sites in a single target allows for detection of intact viruses without the need for target amplification or the need to separate probe from target molecules.

The same carbodiimide chemistry was also used to conjugate Abs against epithelial cell adhesion molecules (EpCAM) to detect breast cancer cells[161,164,165] through QD-based specific imaging (Figure 3.6). The breast cancer cells under white light were more difficult to observe under the microscope than when these were stained specifically with the Ab-conjugated QDs. Furthermore, the

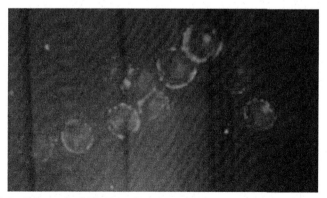

FIGURE 3.6 Photograph of SK-BR3 cells stained with green emitting QDs emitting at 530 nm attached to Ab against cell membrane proteins. The QDs–Ab are seen as dots along the cell membrane to bring fluorescence color to the cells. *Courtesy of Ocean NanoTech, LLC. (For color version of this figure, the reader is referred to the online version of this book)*

QD–Ab stained breast cancer cells remained fluorescent even after six months of storage at RT.

Carbodiimide chemistry using 1-ethyl-3-3(3-dimethylaminopropyl) carbodiimide hydrochloride (DAPC) as a cross-linker has been used to functionalize a tris(2,2′-bipyridyl) dichlororuthenium(II) hexahydrate (RuBpy)-doped silica NPs for the subsequent immobilization of Ab for *Escherichia coli*.[182] The Ab-bioconjugated NPs allowed for rapid and accurate detection of a single bacterium without the need for amplification or enrichment.[80]

Another bioconjugation scheme uses the homobifunctional coupler, 1,4-phenylenediisothiocyanate (PDITC), to bind the 38-kDa tuberculosis antigen to both the amino group of the aminopropyltriethoxysilane (APTS)-modified sensor surface and the amino groups of the antigen as well.[183] The coupling chemistry allowed for specific binding but suppressed nonspecific binding of blood serum and whole blood compounds in a serodiagnostic measurement of TB infection using three optical sensing platforms.

Common conjugation techniques such as carbodiimide or SMCC chemistries are generally used in NMs.[108] However, Mattousi's group[58] argued against EDC conjugation of QDs for a few reasons: the formation of aggregates due to instability of QDs and the various possible cross-linking reactions that lead to the formation of large and uncontrolled number of conjugates on a single nanocrystal. Nevertheless, EDC chemistry is widely used for the preparation of commercial QD-avidin/streptavidin conjugates with high QY, which in turn is used to attach different functionalities on QDs to allow for a more specific interaction with different target analytes. To solve Mattousi's concerns, Ocean NanoTech came up with QD-coupling kit that includes all the reagents and buffers necessary to prevent aggregation and maintain colloidal stability while controlling the number of biomolecules on the NM surface.[184,185] The process involves the activation of the carboxylated NPs with EDC/NHS followed by addition of the biomolecule. Conjugation efficiency is tested through gel electrophoresis or through appropriate biomolecule assay.

Applications of NMs such as QD tagging of a specific target biomolecule or a cell or microorganism involve grafting a recognition receptor to the functionalized QD surface (e.g., DNA oligonucleotide or aptamer, Ab, etc.).[186] Patolsky et al. used semiconductor QDs made from CdSe/ZnS core/shell QDs, as solid surfaces to which the nucleic acid containing the RNA primer was mobilized. These QDs exhibit photochemical centers for lighting-up the dynamics of telomerization, which occurs on the NPs by fluorescence resonance energy transfer (FRET).[187] The attachment of the nucleic acid unit, containing the G-rich sequence recognized by telomerase for the generation of telomerase activity, contained a thiolated end group, which made it possible for the attachment to the CdSe/ZnS QDs. In the presence of telomerase from HeLa cancer cells and a mixture containing dNTP and Texas-Red 14-dUTP (TR-dUTP, upon excitation of the CdSe/ZnS QDs), an emission peak at a wavelength equal to 560 nm was observed.[186] Emission of light decreases with time, since the light emitted is passed on and absorbed by the dye-modified dUTP, in the presence of the telomerase activity, showing an absorbance at a wavelength equal to 610 nm. Functionalized QD and other NMs contain either an amine or a carboxyl group that offers the possibility of cross-linking or covalent bonding molecules containing a thiol group,[188,189] carboxyl group, hydroxyl group, or an *N*-hydroxysuccinimydyl ester moiety[125,126] by means of standard bioconjugation reactions.[108]

Another approach for NM functionalization uses electrostatic interactions between NMs and adapter biomolecules, or between NMs and proteins, DNA, etc.[190] These functionalization steps can be repeated to add two or more functional moieties or to change functionality. One example is streptavidin-coated QDs (QDstrep) used in combination with biotinylated proteins or Abs (biotinAb)[191] forming QDstrep–biotinAb. This structure, QDstrep–biotinAb, depending upon the specificity of the Ab, can be used for (a) specific whole cell or tissue staining, or (b) specific medical sensing.

3.3.2.1 Protocol for Covalent Conjugation of NPs to QDs (available at Ocean NanoTech, LLC website, www.oceananotech.com)

This biomolecule conjuagtion protocol can be used for water-soluble NMs that contain carboxyl groups (–COOH) on the surface.

(1) Place 50 µL of 4 µM QD (2 nmol) aqueous solution in a low protein binding 1.5 mL centrifuge tube.
(2) Add 300 µL of QD reaction buffer (or 10 mM PBS, pH 7.4) to the QDs and mix well.
(3) Add 50 µL of EDC solution (2 mg EDC/mL reaction buffer).
(4) Add at least 5 nmol of protein to make a 1 nmol QD to 5 nmol protein. This ratio can be increased or decreased as necessary such as when the proteins are too expensive.
(5) Mix well and react for 2 h in a vortex mixer or shaker.
(6) Add 10 µL of quenching buffer and allow it to react for 10–15 min at RT.
(7) Dialyze, spin filter, or use ultracentrifugation to purify.
(8) Resuspend in storage buffer or in 10 mM PBS buffer.
(9) Refrigerate until use.

To keep the activity of the proteins and to avoid contamination, only use autoclaved buffers during the conjugation process. It is best to perform conjugation in aseptic conditions as much as possible.

3.3.2.2 Specific Staining of Cancer Cells with QDs attached to Ab against Cell Membrane Surface Proteins

This protocol can be applied to the specific attachment of NMs that are covalently conjugated with Ab on the cell membrane.

(1) Insert a cover slip in each well of a 6-well culture plate.
(2) Place 5000 cells in each well and add 1 mL culture media.

(3) Incubate the cells under manufacturer's recommended conditions (usually at 37 °C with 5% CO_2 in an incubator oven).

(4) When the growth reaches 70–80% confluence, remove the growth medium.

(5) Add 500 μL of 1× Dulbecco phosphate buffered saline (DPBS).

(6) Add 10 μL of 1–50 nM QDs–Ab and aspirate gently to mix.

(7) Incubate at 37 °C with 5% CO_2 in an incubator oven for 3–10 min.

(8) Wash three or more times with 1× DPBS with 0.02% Tween 20 and 1% BSA to remove excess QDs–Ab.

(9) Observe under a fluorescence microscope.

The SK-BR3 cells in Figure 3.6 under a fluorescent microscope show the QDs–Ab as dots along the cell surface. This is the result of the QDs–Ab targeting and attaching to specific proteins on the surface of the cell membrane. Specific targeting with NMs attached to Abs is a very useful application of NMs for sensor development as well as for targeted drug delivery.[42,44,140,141,159,192]

3.3.3 Physical Adsorption

Surface functionalization of NMs is carried out with the use of molecules that serve as stabilizers, which may be added during or after the synthesis process (in situ functionalization). These molecules are attached to the surface of the NMs by physisorption or by ligand-like interactions as in the case of sulfur containing molecules as discussed in various review articles.[193,194,109] In addition, the surface groups on NMs such as the carboxyl, amine or hydroxyl groups can lead to interaction with similarly modified biomolecules allowing physical adsorption (PA). Thus, cell tracking with water-soluble NMs dispersed in DI water very easily cling on the surfaces of proteins, DNA, lipids, carbohydrates, and cells. Although this is useful for some studies such as the easy visualization of cells under the microscope, this leads to problems of nonspecific adsorption especially during biosensor or diagnostic tool development. Some ways to minimize PA had been the subject of studies.[195] Aguilar and coworkers[195] developed buffers that minimize background signal from QDs that physically adsorb to cell surfaces. The protocol below has been designed for PA of QDs on cells followed by a process to minimize it.

3.3.3.1 Protocol for PA of QDs on Cells

The following protocol is used in the nonspecific adsorption of QDs and other NMs on human cell lines such as SK-BR3, MDA MB231, etc.

Cell cultures of human breast cancer cells (SK-BR3) that were originally obtained from ATCC (Manassas, VA).

(1) Grow the cells in a flask containing RPMI-1640 medium supplemented with 10% fetal bovine serum (FBS) and 1% of streptomycin/penicillin antibiotics.

(2) Place the flask in a cell culture incubator at a humidified atmosphere with 5% CO_2 at 37 °C.

(3) Replace the growth media at least once every three days until the cells reach about 80–90% confluence.

(4) Remove the growth medium and wash the cells two times with DPBS followed by 1 mL of trypsin to detach the cells from the flask.

(5) Add 5 mL of fresh RPMI-1640 medium neutralized trypsin in the flask.

(6) Transfer the cell suspension into a centrifuge tube and pellet the cells at 4000 rpm for 5 min.

(7) Resuspend the cells in fresh RPMI-1640 and subculture when necessary.

(8) Centrifuge at 4000 rpm for 5 min to precipitate the cells.

(9) Resuspend in 1 mL 1× DPBS.

(10) Count the cells.

(11) Take 10,000 cells and place in a centrifuge tube.

(12) Precipitate the cells at 4000 rpm for 4–5 min.

(13) Resuspend in 10–50 μL DPBS.

(14) Add 10 μL of 1–50 nM QDs and shake gently.

(15) Incubate at 37 °C with 5% CO_2 in an incubator oven for 5–15 min.

(16) Precipitate the cells at 4000 rpm for 4–5 min.

(17) Wash three or more times with 1× DPBS with 0.02% Tween 20 and 1% BSA to remove excess QDs.

(18) Resuspend in 1× DPBS.

(19) Observe under a fluorescence microscope.

Figure 3.6 shows SK-BR3 cells that were stained with red QDs (QSH620) from Ocean NanoTech. The cells were rapidly growing when harvested and exposed to 10 nM QDs for 5 min. Nonspecific staining with QDs shows almost a very even distribution of the QDs all over the cell in contrast with specific staining. Staining nonspecifically is useful for microscopic examination of cells.

Part 2. Cells grown on a cover slip inserted in a 6-well plate

Nonspecific staining of cells can also be done on adherent cells. The following protocol is for staining cells attached to glass cover slip:

(1) Insert a cover slip in each well of a 6-well cell culture plate.

(2) Place 5000 cells in each well and add 1 mL culture media.

(3) Incubate the cells under manufacturer's recommended conditions (usually at 37 °C with 5% CO_2 in an incubator oven).

(4) When the growth reaches 70–80% confluence, remove the growth medium.

(5) Add 500 μL of 1× DPBS.

(6) Add 10 μL of 1–50 nM QDs and aspirate gently to mix.

(7) Incubate at 37 °C with 5% CO_2 in an incubator oven for 3–10 min.

(8) Wash three or more times with 1× DPBS with 0.02% Tween 20 and 1% BSA to remove excess QDs.

(9) Observe under a fluorescence microscope (Figure 3.7). The cells appear fluorescent and are easier to find and to count. Sophisticated microscope can exhibit external and internal features of the cells when stained with QDs.

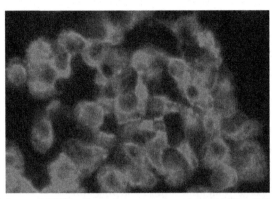

FIGURE 3.7   Adherent SK-BR3 cells on glass cover slip stained with QDs (530 nm). *Courtesy of Ocean NanoTech, LLC. (For color version of this figure, the reader is referred to the online version of this book)*

3.3.3.2 Minimizing PA of NMs on Biological Samples

To minimize nonspecific attachment of NMs on cells and other biological materials, washing and blocking buffers have been developed. These special buffers contain blocking agents such as fish gelatin, bovine serum albumin (BSA), casein, polyvinylpyrrolidone (PVP), ovalbumin, and other proteins that absorb excess NMs during the staining process. These blockers are combined with surfactants and detergents such as sodium dodecyl sulfate, Tween 20, Triton X, and others. Combined at proper ratios in buffer solutions such as 10 mM PBS, pH 7.4 or 10 mM borate buffer, pH 7.4, the blocking agents and detergents help eliminate nonspecifically adsorbed NMs.[195]

The nonspecific adsorption of NMs could lead to clinical difficulties such as failure of the medical application. Nonspecific adsorption of NMs can lead to drug delivery to the wrong cell that can lead to a cascade of cellular processes that may be triggered depending upon where the NMs are adsorbed causing alteration to biological activity. In addition PA of NMs can lead to false positives when used for diagnostics.

Elimination of PA has been the focus of one study conducted by the group of Aguilar.[195] In this study, they performed elimination of NMs' PA on cells in vitro in the immunoassay detection of breast cancer cells using the SK-BR3 cell line.[150,196] The studies involved the use of QDs that were functionalized with –COOH on the surface. The QDs were used to conjugate Abs to form secondary Abs, 2°Ab–QD against the primary Abs that were used to label the surface antigen HER2/neu, proteins found on the cell membrane that are overexpressed in cancer cells. The complete assay consisted of the SK-BR3 + anti-HER2/neu + 2°Ab–QD while the incomplete assay did not contain the specific cell membrane label, anti-HER2/neu. The process used to eliminate PA is as follows:

(1) Grow the cells in a culture flask following the manufacturer's recommendations.

(2) Incubate the cells under manufacturer's recommended conditions (usually at 37 °C with 5% CO_2 in an incubator oven).

(3) When the growth reaches 70–80% confluence, harvest the cells.

(4) Remove the growth medium and wash the cells two times with DPBS followed by 1 mL of trypsin to detach the cells from the flask.

(5) Transfer the cell suspension into a centrifuge tube and pellet the cells at 4000 rpm for 5 min.

(6) Resuspend in 1 mL 1× DPBS.

(7) Take 10,000 cells and place in separate centrifuge tubes labeled 1, 2, 3, and 4.

(8) Precipitate the cells at 4000 rpm for 4–5 min.

(9) Resuspend in 10–50 μL DPBS.

(10) Add 10 μL of 1–50 nM 2°Ab–QD to tube 1/2 and shake gently for 5 min.

(11) Add 10 μL of 1 μg/mL anti-HER2/neu to tube 3/4 and shake gently for 5 min.

(12) Precipitate the cells at 4000 rpm for 4–5 min.

(13) Remove the supernatant and wash twice with DPBS

(14) Resuspend in 10–50 μL DPBS.

(15) Add 50 μL of blocking buffer (an example of a blocking buffer may consist of a combination of 1% BSA, 5% PVP, 0.02% Tween 20, and 0.02% Triton X in PBS or tris buffer, pH 7.0–7.4) to tubes 1 and 3.

(16) Shake gently for 5–15 min.

(17) Precipitate the cells at 4000 rpm for 4–5 min.

(18) Remove the supernatant and wash twice with DPBS.

(19) Add 10 μL of 1–50 nM 2°Ab–QD to tubes 3/4 and incubate for 5–30 min.

(20) Precipitate the cells at 4000 rpm for 4–5 min.

(21) Remove the supernatant and wash twice with DPBS.

(22) Resuspend in 10–50 μL DPBS.

(23) Add 50 μL of blocking buffer (an example of a blocking buffer may consist of a combination of 1% BSA, 5% PVP, 0.02% Tween 20, and 0.02% Triton X in PBS or tris buffer, pH 7.0–7.4) to tube 3.

(24) Shake gently for 5–15 min.

(25) Precipitate the cells at 4000 rpm for 4–5 min.

(26) Remove the supernatant and wash twice with DPBS.

(27) Place 1–2 μL of the cell suspensions from each tube on a microscope slide.

(28) Observe tube under a fluorescence microscope.

Microscopic examination of cells is expected to show QDs for specific adsorption in tube 3 due to the formation of the complete assay consisting of SK-BR3 + anti-HER2/neu + 2°Ab–QD. A combination of both specific adsorption and PA is expected in tube 4 because the cells were not blocked with a blocking buffer. On the other hand, only PA is expected from tubes 1 and 2 because the cells were not exposed to anti-HER2/neu making the assay incomplete. However, because tube 1 is washed and blocked, it is expected that there will be a minimal signal from PA of 2°Ab–QD on the cell surface. PA of the 2°Ab–QD is possible because the 2°Ab is not only specific for the cell membrane surface proteins but is also specific to the anti-HER2/neu that were used to label the membrane proteins in tubes 3 and 4. This process can be used to minimize PA for in vitro diagnostics of cells, proteins, and other biomolecules using NMs.

3.3.4 Electrostatic Charge–charge Interaction

Other schemes that have been used in biosensors for infectious disease diagnostic devices include the electrostatic interactions.[12,109] For example, silver NPs in polystyrene sulfonate/polyacrylic acid capsules were coated with avidin via electrostatic interactions and used as label for electrochemical detection of *E. coli* DNA hybridization through a biotin–avidin interaction.[183]

Their use of capsules of silver NPs (AgNPs) was reported to: (1) lower the detection limit as compared to other AgNPs-based assays; (2) lower the detection limit in comparison to many hybridization assays using other NMs; and (3) approach the sensitivity of chemiluminescence, which is reported to be one of the most sensitive DNA detection methods using AgNPs.[183]

The group of Meyer has exploited the specific biotin–avidin interaction when they used commercially prepared magnetic beads coated with streptavidin for the detection of *Yersinia pestis*[197] and *Francisella tularensis*.[198] The detection principle used anti-Ft or anti-YPFI Abs for capturing the Ft or YPFI antigen. Biotinylated Abs were coupled with the streptavidin in magnetic beads. Binding resulted to a change in the induced magnetic field. These streptavidin-modified magnetic beads showed promise in the development of easy, fast, and highly sensitive biosensor for the detection and quantification of the infectious diseases mentioned.

3.4 APPLICATIONS OF BIOCOMPATIBLE NMS

Biomedical applications of NMs in the field of medicine and the life sciences research in general are growing rapidly. Nanomedicine not only aspires to develop a valuable set of research tools and devices,[199,200] but also garners a lot of attention for its possible commercial applications in the pharmaceutical industry that may include targeted drug delivery systems, new therapies, and in vivo imaging.[201] NM-based neuro-electronic interfaces, nanobiosensors, NMs-based strip immunoassays, and nanoelectronic-based sensors are among the on-going and active areas of research in nanotechnology.[202] Going into the molecular level, nanotechnology holds promise that cell repair can be carried out by molecular nanomachines that could revolutionize medicine and the medical field. Nanomedicine sales reached 6.8 billion dollars in 2004 with over 200 companies and 38 products worldwide putting a minimum of 3.8 billion dollars in nanotechnology R&D investment every year.[203] This unprecedented growth rate in nanomedicine is expected to have a significant impact that can improve worldwide economy.

Although methods for bioconjugation of NMs have been in existence for some time, it is apparent that their application to infectious diseases diagnostics is limited. At present, bioconjugation of NMs are done to make them as probes for imaging, as delivery vehicles for cancer drugs,[204] and as therapeutics for the removal of tumor cells.[205,206] NMs are currently being studied for drug delivery to improve the bioavailability of a drug, where they are most needed in the body over a time frame which will be achieved by molecular targeting using nano-engineered devices.[207,208] NMs have unusual properties that can be used to improve drug delivery.[82,209–224] Attachment of specific probes that guide the NMs to the specific cell as a specific tissue can save more than \$65 billion that is wasted each year due to poor bioavailability. Drug delivery systems using lipid- or polymer-based NMs or magnetic NPs (MNPs) can be designed to improve the pharmacological and therapeutic properties of generally nonpotent and possibly harmful drugs to nearby healthy cells. Drugs made of proteins and peptides show enormous potential for treatment of various diseases and disorders. Targeted and/or controlled delivery of these biopharmaceuticals using NMs is a rapidly growing area of research.

NMs are also actively being developed for in vitro and in vivo imaging.[18,43,44,141,150,155,156,159,225–228] MNPs are now being used as contrast agents giving improved images from ultrasound and MRI. Diagnosis of diseases such as cancer and infectious diseases at their early stages for effective treatment may be achieved with brighter, more stable, and more sensitive NMs.[18,150,228] QDs with quantum confinement properties like size-tunable light emission, when used in conjunction with MRI can produce exceptional images of tumor sites. These NPs are much brighter than organic dyes and only need one light source for excitation. This means that the use of fluorescent QDs could produce a higher contrast image and at a lower cost than today's organic dyes that are used as contrast agents. The small size of NPs (10–100 nm) allows them to preferentially accumulate at tumor sites, which lack an effective lymphatic drainage system.[229]

Biosensor development is one of the rapidly growing areas of NM applications in medicine.[140,141,143–145,147–151,156,230–232] These sensors may be in the form of lateral flow immunoassay, glass slide-type sensors, or disposable lab on a chip-type of sensors.[141,143,144,147,148,150,231,232] An approach using a solid phase involving a sandwich-type assay with an Ab against a specific target and a QD-labeled Ab allows QD-based detection of the analyte of interest.[140,141,144,150] The large number (5–200) of potential surface attachment groups on QDs allows possible incorporation of various molecules for sensing.

In one study, Xu and his collaborators[42] demonstrated the use of IOMNPs for the immunomagnetic separation of tumor cells from fresh whole blood. The process involved 30 nm IOMNPs that are amphiphilic polymer coated. These were covalent conjugated with Abs against human epithelial growth factor receptor 2 (anti-HER2 or anti-HER2/neu) forming IO-Ab. HER2 is a cell membrane protein that is overexpressed in several types of human cancer cells. Using a HER2/neu overexpressing human breast cancer cell line SK-BR3 as a model cell, the IO-Ab successfully isolated about 73.6% (with a maximum capture of 84%) of SK-BR3 cells that were spiked in 1 mL of fresh human whole blood. The IO-Ab preferentially bound to SK-BR3 cells over the 10^9 normal cells found in blood due to the high level of HER2/neu receptor on the surface of the cancer cell membrane unlike the normal cell membrane surfaces. Their studies exhibited an enrichment factor (cancer cells over normal cells) of 1:10,000,000 in a magnetic field (with gradient of 100 T/m) through the binding of IO-Ab on the cell surface that resulted in the preferential capture of the cancer cells.

In addition, as shown in the examples above, a number of studies on bioconjugated NMs for infectious diseases diagnostics have started to emerge. These studies have shown that the use of NMs as conjugates to biorecognition elements have great potential in the development of biosensing devices that are easy to use, fast, highly sensitive (lower detection limit compared to conventional assays), and capable of detecting analytes even in complex media like blood. Moreover, due to the small dimensions of the NMs, they can be incorporated into portable handheld devices for POC diagnostics.

Bioconjugation of NMs for diagnostic applications has led to more selective and even more specific sensing of target analytes. However, for the development of cost effective sensing devices that allow for multiplex sensing and at the same time, provide fast and high-resolution analysis (more sensitive), the transducer surface are often nanomanipulated. Nanomanipulation techniques include electron beam lithography (EBL), oblique angle deposition (OAD), nanoimprint lithography (NIL), nanosphere lithography (NSL), dip-pen lithography, microcontact printing (μCP), and various self-assembly approaches[233,234] This section will only present sensor fabrication/modification of the most promising sensors in the field of POC medical diagnostics—amperometric and field effect transistor (FET)-based potentiometric sensors and localized surface plasmon resonance (LSPR), and surface enhanced Raman spectroscopy (SERS).

In applications where uniformity and reproducibility of surface property is very important, the expensive top-down approaches like EBL is still the method of choice.[235] This is due to the fact that bottom-up approaches such as NIL and NSL suffer from reproducibility and reliability issues. Nevertheless, bottom-up techniques are gaining importance owing to the low cost, simplicity, and speed of the methods.[236,237,238,239]

One of the most promising applications of biocompatible NMs is drug delivery. Today, a number of nano-enabled drugs are available for various applications. A few of these are shown in Table 3.2. Aside from the use of NMs for MRI contrast agents and drug encapsulation, some are also being studied for vaccine delivery.[192] In this study, they focused on the use of the semiconductor NMs, in particular the QDs as an alternative vaccine delivery platform. They used <15 nm QDs with a crystal shell of alternating cationic and anionic layers, which consisted of

TABLE 3.2 NMs with Medical Applications

NMs	Drug/application	Reference
Polybutyl(cyanoacrylate)	Dalargin/analgesic	Kreuter et al.[241]
Polybutyl(cyanoacrylate)	Doxorubicin/antitumor	Gelperina et al.[242]
Dextran-coated iron oxide NMs	Ferridex/MRI contrast agent	Sakamoto et al.[243]
Carboxydextran-coated iron oxide NMs	Resovist/ MRI contrast agent	Sakamoto et al.[243]
Polymersomes	Paclitaxel/drug delivery	Singh et al.[244]

CdSe/ZnS.[150,196,240] The QDs were nonimmunogenic, stable, and when coated with an organic layer allowed for an array of proteins, DNA, and other biomolecules to be conjugated to their 60 surfaces. Because of their small size and surface modification, the QDs were conjugated with vaccine candidates against malaria.[192] These NMs not only served as a delivery platform for protein antigens, but also activated key immune cells to further increase the immunogenicity of the vaccine. Their in vivo tests demonstrated no immediate toxic effects but QDs that contain Cd are not compatible for human use. However, the toxicity of the CdSe/ZnS QDs was limited by coating the core with a shell layer of ZnS that is further coated with an amphiphilic polymer. Because of the possibility of eventual polymer and NMs degradation, attempts are currently being made to develop cadmium-free QD NMs as well as the use of other NMs that do not contain Cd such as IOMNPs, AuNPs, etc.

Most biosensors reported in the literature use electrochemical transduction. This is due to the low cost, high sensitivity, ease of miniaturization, low power requirements, and simple fabrication of electrochemical transducers.[245] Electrode materials are often made up of carbon, gold, platinum, or conducting polymers. Nanostructured electrode materials are gaining importance in electrochemical transduction since their greater surface area allows incorporation of more biorecognition elements thereby enabling lower detection limits and faster response times. NMs have unique optical, electrical, magnetic, and catalytic properties that facilitate label-free detection of target analytes.

CNTs have been increasingly used as substrates in electrochemical sensors due to their size and interesting physical and chemical properties. CNTs as substrates for amperometric sensors can be grown via microwave plasma vapor deposition using dendrimer-templated Fe NMs as catalyst.[246] CNT arrays have been grown via chemical vapor deposition on platinum. Multiwalled carbon nanotubes (MWNTs) have been deposited on glassy carbon electrode using the layer-by-layer technique with polyaniline as the oppositely charged polyelectrolyte.[247] CNT in a vertically aligned "forest" configuration can be grown by self-assembly of shortened CNTs and functionalized after the assembly. Despite the number of ways of assembling CNTs on electrode surfaces and the well-documented electron-transfer reactions on their surfaces, the application of CNTs in amperometric sensors remains mostly limited to small molecules. Wang et al.[248] have shown CNT-modified transducers can detect proteins and DNA down to 1.3 and 160 zmol, respectively in 25–50 μL samples indicating great promise for PCR-free DNA analysis. Yet, despite this promise, little work has been done for the application of amperometric biosensors on infectious diseases diagnostics. This has been attributed to lack of works to establish that amperometric biosensors do not suffer from biofouling.[249]

Potentiometric transducers are not as sensitive as amperometric transducers but architectures for immunosensing of pathogens involving the use of nanowires as FETs have been considered as viable candidates for ultrasensitive biosensing applications.[104] Reliable ultrasensitive biosensors using FETs are fabricated by the expensive top-down approaches such as EBL and molecular beam epitaxy, and then functionalized with biorecognition elements using bottom-up approaches as discussed by He et al.[250] They have also pointed out that bottom-up approaches of fabricating FETs offer flexibility of surface functionalization but suffer from low reproducibility and reliability. Among the mentioned bottom-up assembly of nanowires FETs are electric field and magnetic field controlled deposition, Langmuir–Blodgett method, alignment and selective growth on the device, programmed dip coating, growth substrate contact printing, blown bubble film, and electroplating in nanochannels.

Silicon nanowire FETs have been employed for the detection of influenza A and adenovirus in a study by Patolsky et al.[251] Their studies showed that single viruses can be detected directly with high selectivity and their methods allowed parallel detection of different viruses. Using virtually unpurified samples, the method exceeded the capabilities of existing methods such as PCR.

In the case of optical sensors (especially SPR-based and SERS-based), research on improving sensitivity is focused on sensor design. Conventional SPR-based or SERS-based optical sensors used planar transducer surfaces made from bulk materials or colloidal materials. Surfaces roughened with nanosized materials were found to increase the sensitivity of signal transduction. In this section, examples of nanomanipulations of the optical sensor surface to improve the sensitivity of diagnostic sensing devices are presented.

NSL involves assembly of 2D hexagonally close packed nanosphere array and then thermally depositing metals on the sphere mask. The nanospheres are removed in the LSPR applications whereas they are kept intact in the SERS application. The technique has been shown to provide a sensing platform that can detect anthrax spores well below the infectious dose and with a faster detection time.[234]

OAD involves physical vapor deposition creating NMs on tilted substrate that causes nanorods to grow on the substrate in the direction of the deposition. This process is used to make silver nanorod arrays that serve as SERS substrates for the detection and differentiation of three different virus RNAs (such as adenovirus, rhinovirus, and HIV RNA).[127] OAD has been used to fabricate a microwell-arrayed SERS chip on glass[252] that provided a uniform Raman signal enhancement from well to well with a detection limit of 10^{-8} M for the Raman active molecule—1,2-di(4-pyridyl)ethylene solution. This system has been used for biosensor development using avian influenza virus as model ananlyte. A similar method called oblique angle polymerization was used for the preparation of SERS substrates.[253] Nanostructured poly(chloro-*p*-xylelene) was used as template for the electroless deposition of Ag or Au that led to reproducible SERS signal for the detection of RSV.

Aside from containing a recognition moiety, NMs can be equipped with a coating that allows membrane transport or cell-internalization capability, and/or an enzymatic function. The natural peptide coating or the amphiphilic coating approach produces biocompatible NMs that can penetrate membrane surfaces without damaging the cells.

3.5 CONCLUSIONS

The physical, electronic, chemical, and optical properties of NMs are being exploited to benefit biomolecules that are useful in medicine. At the nanometer scale, quantum mechanical effects emerge leading to varied and unexpected physicochemical properties that make them useful for biosensor applications that provide solutions to the problems of existing methods. The novel and unique properties enable nanotechnology to provide promising solutions for nanomedicine.

The NMs that have been exploited in medicine are usually produced in organic solvents making them hydrophobic and incompatible to biological molecules. Alongside the organic synthesis of NMs, conversion methods into the water-soluble form to make them biocompatible have also emerged. Various techniques such as ligand exchange, encapsulation, and polymer coating have been developed and used in the preparation of water-soluble NMs. The water-soluble NMs that are now currently commercially available contain functional groups on their surfaces making them easy to manipulate for various medical applications. Functional groups anchored to the surface of NMs during synthesis or modification into their water-soluble forms provide reactive sites for subsequent bioconjugation reactions. These functional groups often involve sulfhydryl –SH, carboxyl –COOH, amine –NH$_2$, hydroxyl –OH, and others that allow attachment of biomolecules through various bioconjugation or cross-linking chemistry. Linkers for these NMs are carbodiimide, succinimide, maleimide, and bifunctional cross-linkers through direct attachment (hydrophobic or electrostatic interactions) and sometimes, through biodin–avidin system. These various methods have their unique qualities and applications along with inherent disadvantages such as possible low yield and loss of functionality after conjugation which researchers are actively studying to solve and improve.

NMs are now found in biosensors with high sensitivity and high stability that are easier to use, faster, and more inexpensive as compared with conventional diagnostics methods. In addition, inexpensive instrumentation that accompanies these NM-based biosensors is also currently being developed and is the focus of Chapter 4. The small dimensions of NMs allow their assembly into barcodes and high-density arrays to detect multiple analytes using miniature handheld sensing devices that may only need light emitting diodes as power source.

NMs have also now been used for drug formulations. A few of these examples were discussed in this chapter and more on targeted drug delivery will be discussed in Chapter 5. Drugs that are coated polymer NMs and iron oxide NMs coated with dextran have emerged as very sensitive contrast agents for MRI. Additionally, cancer drugs have also been loaded in NPs for ease of delivery. More studies are underway for the specific targeting of these drugs so that the effect on healthy cells can be minimized while focusing the unloading of the drugs on the sick cells such as cancer cells. Other studies have also focused on the use of NMs for eradicating viral infections, which have been one of the most difficult challenges of the human population during the last century and into the millennium. Several studies have also been focused on the use of NMs for the delivery of vaccines especially those diseases that have no existing vaccines in the market.

Thus, transforming the NMs into their water-soluble forms opened seemingly endless possibilities of their applications in medicine. Such applications go from detection to treatment of various diseases that may be molecular in nature or may be caused by infective materials. More studies toward improving success in attachment of biomolecules on the NM surfaces or for loading of molecules into the NMs are necessary to ensure successful incorporation of relevant and important molecules for medical applications. The succeeding chapters will focus more seriously on the various applications that have been introduced and partly discussed in this chapter.

REFERENCES

1. Zhang, X.; Jenekhe, S.; Perlstein, J. Nanoscale Size Effects on Photoconductivity of Semiconducting Polymer Thin Films. *Chem. Mater.* **1996,** *8,* 1571–1574.
2. Jenekhe, S.; Zhang, X.; Chen, X.; Choong, V.; Gao, Y.; Hsieh, B. Finite Size Effects on Electroluminescence of Nanoscale Semiconducting Polymer Heterojunctions. *Chem. Mater.* **1997,** *9,* 409–412.
3. Manandhar, P.; Jang, J.; Schatz, G.; Ratner, M.; Hong, S. Anomalous Surface Diffusion in Nanoscale Direct Deposition Processes. *Phys. Rev. Lett.* **2003,** *90,* 115505.
4. Clark, L.; Ye, G.; Snurr, R. Molecular Traffic Control in a Nanoscale System. *Phys. Rev. Lett.* **2000,** *84,* 2893.
5. Soler, J.; Baro, A.; Garcia, N.; Rohrer, H. Interatomic Forces in Scanning Tunneling Microscopy: Giant Corrugations of the Graphite Surface. *Phys. Rev. Lett.* **1986,** *57,* 444–447.
6. Binnig, G.; Garcia, N.; Rohrer, H. Conductivity Sensitivity of Inelastic Scanning Tunneling Microscopy. *Phys. Rev. B* **1985,** *32,* 1336–1338.

7. Curl, R.; Smalley, R. Probing C60. *Science* **1988**, *242*, 1017–1022.

8. Rao, C.; Satishkumar, B.; Govindaraj, A.; Manashi, N. Nanotubes. *Chem. Phys. Chem.* **2001**, *2*, 78–105.

9. Voura, E.; Jaiswal, J.; Mattoussi, H.; Simon, S. Tracking Metastatic Tumor Cell Extravasation with Quantum Dot Nanocrystals and Fluorescence Emission Scanning Microscopy. *Nat. Med.* **2004**, *10*, 993–998.

10. Stroh, M.; Zimmer, J.; Duda, D.; Levchenko, T.; Cohen, K.; Brown, E., et al. Quantum Dots Spectrally Distinguish Multiple Species within the Tumor Milieu *in vivo*. *Nat. Med.* **2005**, *11*, 678–682.

11. Alivisatos, A. Semiconductor Clusters, Nanocrystals, and Quantum Dots. *Science* **1992**, *271*, 933–937.

12. Murray, C.; Norris, D.; Bawendi, M. Synthesis and Characterization of Nearly Monodisperse CdE (E = Sulfur, Selenium, Tellurium) Semiconductor Nanocrystallites. *J. Am. Chem. Soc.* **1993**, *115*, 8706–8715.

13. Manna, L.; Scher, E.; Alivisatos, A. Synthesis of Soluble and Processable Rod-, Arrow-, Teardrop-, and Tetrapod-Shaped Cdse Nanocrystals. *J. Am. Chem. Soc.* **2000**, *122*, 12700–12706.

14. Peng, Z.; Peng, X. Formation of High-Quality CdTe, CdSe, and CdS Nanocrystals using CdO as Precursor. *J. Am. Chem. Soc.* **2001**, *123*, 183–184.

15. Qu, L.; Peng, X. Control of Photoluminescence Properties of CdSe Nanocrystals in Growth. *J. Am. Chem. Soc.* **2002**, , 2049–2055.

16. Hines, M.; Guyot-Sionnest, P. Synthesis of Strongly Luminescing ZnS-Capped CdSe Nanocrystals. *J. Phys. Chem. B* **1996**, *100*, 468–471.

17. Resch-Genger, U.; Grabolle, M.; Cavaliere-Jaricot, S.; Nitschke, R.; Nann, T. Quantum Dots Versus Organic Dyes as Fluorescent Labels. *Nature Methods* **2008**, *5*, 763–775.

18. Xing, Y.; Rao, J. Quantum Dot Bioconjugates for *in vitro* Diagnostics & *in vivo* Imaging. *Cancer Biomarkers* **2008**, *4*, 307–319.

19. Pellegrino, T.; Manna, L.; Kudera, S.; Liedl, T.; Koktysh, D.; Rogach, A.; Keller, S.; Raldler, J.; Natile, G.; Parak, W. Hydrophobic Nanocrystals Coated with an Amphiphilic Polymer Shell: A General Route to Water Soluble Nanocrystals. *Nano Lett.* **2004**, *4*, 703–707.

20. Chan, C.; Nie, S. Quantum Dot Bioconjugates for Ultrasensitive Nonisotopic Detection. *Science* **1998**, *281*, 2016–2018.

21. Willard, D.; Carillo, L.; Jung, J.; van Orden, A. CdSe–ZnS Quantum Dots as Resonance Energy Transfer Donors in a Model Protein–Protein Binding Assay. *Nano Lett.* **2001**, *1*.

22. Mitchell, G.; Mirkin, C.; Letsinger, R. Programmed Assembly of DNA Functionalized Quantum Dots. *JACS* **1999**, *121*, 8122–8123.

23. Rogach, A.; Harrison, M.; Kershaw, S.; Kornowski, A.; Burt, M.; Eychmuller, A.; Weller, H. Colloidally Prepared CdHgTe and HgTe Quantum Dots with Strong Near-Infrared Luminescence. *Phys. Status Solid B* **2001**, *224*, 153–158.

24. Uyeda, H.; Medintz, I.; Jaiswal, J.; Simon, S.; Mattoussi, H. Synthesis of Compact Multidentate Ligands to Prepare Stable Hydrophilic Quantum Dot Fluorophores. *J. Am. Chem. Soc.* **2005**, *127*, 3870–3878.

25. Bruchez, M., Jr.; Moronne, M.; Gin, P.; Weiss, S.; Alivisatos, A. Semiconductor Nanocrystals as Fluorescent Biological Labels. *Science* **1998**, *281*, 2013–2015.

26. Guo, W.; Li, J.; Wang, Y.; Peng, X. Conjugation Chemistry and Bioapplications of Semiconductor Box Nanocrystals Prepared via Dendrimer Bridging. *Chem. Mater.* **2003**, *15*, 3125–3133.

27. Kim, S.; Bawendi, M. Oligomeric Ligands for Luminescent and Stable Nanocrystal Quantum Dots. *J. Am. Chem. Soc.* **2003**, *125*, 14652–14653.

28. Mitchell, G.; Mirkin, C.; Letsinger, R. Programmed Assembly of DNA Functionalized Quantum Dots. *J. Am. Chem. Soc.* **1999,** *121,* 8122–8123.

29. Dubertret, B.; Skourides, P.; Norris, D.; Noireaux, V.; Brivanlou, A.; Libchaber, A. In Vivo Imaging of Quantum Dots Encapsulated in Phospholipids Micelles. *Science* **2002,** *298,* 1759–1762.

30. Osaki, F.; Kanamori, T.; Sando, S.; Sera, T.; Aoyama, Y. A Quantum Dot Conjugated Sugar Ball and its Cellular Uptake on the Size Effects of Endocytosis in the Subviral Region. *J. Am. Chem. Soc.* **2004,** *126,* 6520–6521.

31. Delehanty, J.; Medintz, I.; Pons, T.; Brunel, F.; Dawson, P.; Mattoussim, H. Self-Assembled Quantum Dot–Peptide Bioconjugates for Selective Intracellular Delivery. *Bioconjug. Chem.* **2006,** *17,* 920–927.

32. Sapsford, K.; Pons, T.; Medintz, I.; Higashiya, S.; Brunel, F.; Dawson, P.; Mattoussi, H. Kinetics of Metal-Affinity Driven Self-Assembly between Proteins or Peptides and CdSe ZnS Quantum Dots. *J. Phys. Chem.* **2007,** *111,* 11528–11538.

33. Mahmoudi, M.; Sant, S.; Wang, B.; Laurent, S.; Sen, T. Superparamagnetic Iron Oxide Nanoparticles (SPIONs): Development, Surface Modification and Applications in Chemotherapy. *Adv. Drug. Deliv. Rev.* **2011,** *63,* 24–46.

34. Hans, M. L.; Lowman, A. M. Biodegradable Nanoparticles for Drug Delivery and Targeting. *Curr. Opin. Solid St. M.* **2002,** *6,* 319–327.

35. Jaffrezic-Renault, N.; Martelet, C.; Chevolot, Y.; Cloarec, J. Biosensors and Bio-Bar Code Assays Based on Biofunctionalized Magnetic Microbeads. *Sesors* **2007,** *7,* 589–614.

36. Kim, J.; Piao, T.; Hyeon, T. Multifunctional Nanostructured Materials for Multimodal Imaging, and Simultaneous Imaging and Therapy. *Chem. Soc. Rev.* **2009,** *38,* 372–390.

37. Mahmoudi, M.; Simchi, A.; Imani, M.; Shokrgozar, M. A.; Milani, A. S.; Hafeli, U.; Stroeve, P. A New Approach for the in Vitro Identification of the Cytotoxicity of Superparamagnetic Iron Oxide Nanoparticles 3500. *Colloid. Surface. B* **2010,** *75,* 300–309.

38. Moore, A.; Weissleder, R.; Bogdanov, A., Jr. Uptake of Dextran-Coated Monocrystalline Iron Oxides in Tumor Cells and Macrophages. *J. Magn. Reson. Imaging* **1997,** *7,* 1140–1145.

39. Philipse, A. P.; Vanbruggen, M. P. B.; Pathmamanoharan, C. Magnetic Silica Dispersions— Preparation and Stability of Surface-Modified Silica Particles with a Magnetic Core. *Langmuir* **1994,** *10,* 92–99.

40. Sajja, H.; East, M.; Mao, H.; Wang, Y.; Nie, S.; Yang, L. Development of Multifunctional Nanoparticles for Targeted Drug Delivery and Noninvasive Imaging of Therapeutic Effect. *Curr. Drug Discov. Technol.* **2009,** *6,* 43–51.

41. Xie, J.; Peng, S.; Brower, N.; Pourmand, N.; Wang, S. X.; Sun, S. One-Pot Synthesis of Monodisperse Iron Oxide Nanoparticles for Potential Biomedical Applications. *Pure Appl. Chem.* **2006,** *78,* 1003–1014.

42. Xu, H.; Aguilar, Z. P.; Yang, L.; Kuang, M.; Duan, H.; Xiong, Y.; Wei, H.; Wang, A. Y. Antibody Conjugated Magnetic Iron Oxide Nanoparticles for Cancer Cell Separation in Fresh Whole Blood. *Biomaterials* **2011,** *32,* 9758–9765.

43. Yang, L.; Cao, Z.; Sajja, H.; Mao, H.; Wang, L.; Geng, H.; Xu, H.; Jiang, T.; Wood, W.; Nie, S.; Wang, A. Development of Receptor Targeted Iron Oxide Nanoparticles for Efficient Drug Delivery and Tumor Imaging. *J. Biomed. Nanotech.* **2008,** *4,* 1–11.

44. Yang, L.; Peng, X.; Wang, Y.; Wang, X.; Cao, Z.; Ni, C.; Karna, P.; Zhang, X.; Wood, W.; Gao, X.; Nie, S.; Mao, H. Receptor-Targeted Nanoparticles for in Vivo Imaging of Breast Cancer. *Clin. Cancer Res.* **2009,** *15,* 4722–4732.

45. Zhao, X.; Harris, J. M. Novel Degradable Poly(Ethylene Glycol) Hydrogels for Controlled Release of Protein. *J. Pharm. Sci.* **1998,** *87,* 1450–1458.

46. Michalet, X.; Pinaud, F.; Bentolila, L.; Tsay, J.; Doose, S.; Li, J.; Sundaresan, G.; Wu, A.; Gambhir, S.; Weiss, S. Quantum Dots for Live Cells, in Vivo Imaging, and Diagnostics. *Science* **2005**, *307*, 538–544.

47. Pathak, S.; Choi, S.; Arnheim, N.; Thompson, M. Hydroxylated Quantum Dots as Luminescent Probes for in Situ Hybridization. *J. Am. Chem. Soc.* **2001**, *123*, 4103–4104.

48. Chan, C. W. C.; Nie, S. M. Quantum Dot Bioconjugates for Ultrasensitive Nonisotopic Detection. *Science* **1998**, *281*, 2016–2018.

49. Pathak, S.; Choi, S. K.; Arnheim, N.; Thompson, M. E. Hydroxylated Quantum Dots as Luminescent Probes for in Situ Hybridization. *J. Am. Chem. Soc.* **2001**, *123*, 4103–4104.

50. Pinaud, F.; King, D.; Moore, H.; Weiss, S. Bioactivation and Cell Targeting of Semiconductor CdSe/ZnS Nanocrystals with Phytochelatin-Related Peptides. *J. Am. Chem. Soc.* **2004**, *126*, 6115–6123.

51. Wu, X.; Liu, H.; Liu, J.; Haley, K.; Treadway, J.; Larson, J.; Ge, N.; Peale, F.; Bruchez, M. Immunofluorescent Labeling of Cancer Marker Her2 and Other Cellular Targets with Semiconductor Quantum Dots. *Nat. Biotechnol* **2003**, *21*, 41–46.

52. Gao, X.; Cui, Y.; Levenson, R.; Chung, L.; Nie, S. In Vivo Cancer Targeting and Imaging with Semiconductor Quantum Dots. *Nat. Biotechnol.* **2004**, *22*, 969–976.

53. Gerion, D.; Pinaud, F.; Williams, S.; Parak, W.; Zanchet, D.; Weiss, S.; Alivisatos, A. Synthesis and Properties of Biocompatible Water-Soluble Silica-Coated CdSe/ZnS Semiconductor Quantum Dots. *J. Phys. Chem. B* **2001**, *105*, 8861–8871.

54. Gao, X.; Chan, C.; Nie, S. Quantum-Dot Nanocrystals for Ultrasensitive Biological Labeling and Multicolor Optical Encoding. *J. Biomed. Opt.* **2002**, *7*, 532–537.

55. Goldman, E.; Anderson, G.; Tran, P. T.; Mattoussi, H.; Charles, P.; Mauro, J. Conjugation of Luminescent Quantum Dots with Antibodies Using an Engineered Adaptor Protein To Provide New Reagents for Fluoroimmunoassays. *Anal. Chem.* **2002**, *74*, 841–847.

56. Sukhanova, A.; Devey, J.; Venteo, L.; Kaplan, H.; Artemyev, M.; Oleinikov, V.; Klinov, D.; Pluot, M.; Cohen, J.; Nabiev, I. Biocompatible Fluorescent Nanocrystals for Immunolabeling of Membrane Proteins and Cells. *Anal. Biochem.* **2004**, *324*, 60–67.

57. Matsuzaki, H.; Dong, S.; Loi, H.; Di, X.; Liu, G. Y.; Hubbell, E., et al. Genotyping Over 100,000 SNPs on a PAir of Oligonucleotide Arrays. *Nature Methods* **2004**, *1*, 109–111.

58. Mattoussi, H.; Mauro, J.; Goldman, E.; Anderson, G.; Sundar, V.; Bawendi, M. Self-Assembly of CdSe–ZnS Quantum Dot Bioconjugates using an Engineered Recombinant Protein. *J. Am. Chem. Soc.* **2000**, *122*, 12142–12150.

59. Gerion, D.; Pinaud, F.; Williams, S. C.; Parak, W. J.; Zanchet, D.; Weiss, S.; Alivisatos, A. P. Synthesis and Properties of Biocompatible Water-Soluble Silica-Coated CdSe/ZnS Semiconductor Quantum Dots. *J. Phys. Chem. B* **2001**, *105*, 8861–8871.

60. Michalet, X.; Pinaud, F. F.; Bentolila, L. A.; Tsay, J. M.; Doose, S.; Li, J. J., et al. Quantum Dots for Live Cells, *in vivo* Imaging, and Diagnostics. *Science* **2005**, *307*, 538–544.

61. Wuister, S. F.; Swart, I.; van Driel, F.; Hickey, S. G.; Donega, C. D. Highly Luminescent Waters-Soluble CdTe Quantum Dots. *Nano Lett.* **2003**, *3*, 503–507.

62. Parak, W.; Gerion, D.; Zanchet, D.; Woerz, A.; Pellegrino, R.; Micheel, C.; Williams, S.; Seitz, M.; Bruehl, R.; Bryant, Z.; Bustamante, C.; Bertozzi, C.; Alivisatos, A. Conjugation of DNA to Silanized Colloidal Semiconductor Nanocrystalline Quantum Dots. *Chem. Mater.* **2002**, *14*, 2113–2119.

63. Ballou, B.; Lagerholm, B.; Ernst, L.; Bruchez, M.; Waggoner, A. Noninvasive Imaging of Quantum Dots in Mice. *Bioconjug. Chem.* **2004**, *15*, 79–86.

64. Lin, C.; Li, J.; Sperling, R.; Manna, L.; Parak, W.; Chang, W., Eds. *Annual Rev. Nano Research* 2007.

65. Dabbousi, B.; Rodriguez-Viejo, J.; Mikulec, F.; Heine, J.; Mattoussi, H.; Ober, R.; Jensen, K.; Bawendi, M. CdSe/ZnS Core–Shell Quantum Dots: Synthesis and Characterization of a Size Series of Highly Luminescent Nanocrystallites. *J. Phys. Chem. B* **1997,** *101,* 9463–9475.

66. Kanninen, P.; Johans, C.; Merta, J.; Kontturi, K. Influence of Ligand Structure on the Stability and Oxidation of Copper Nanoparticles. *J. Colloid Interf. Sci.* **2008,** *318,* 88–95.

67. Lambert, K.; Wittebrood, L.; Moreels, I.; Deresmes, D.; Grandidier, B.; Hens, Z. Langmuir–Blodgett Monolayers of InP Quantum Dots with Short Chain Ligands. *J. Colloid Interf. Sci.* **2006,** *300,* 597–602.

68. Zhang, C.; O'Brien, S.; Balogh, L. Comparison and Stability of CdSe Nanocrystals Covered with Amphiphilic Poly(Amidoamine) Dendrimers. *J. Phys. Chem. B* **2002,** *106,* 10316–10321.

69. Gaponik, N.; Talapin, D. V.; Rogach, A. L.; Eychmuller, A.; Weller, H. Efficient Phase Transfer of Luminescent Thiol-Capped Nanocrystals: From Water to Nonpolar Organic Solvents. *Nano Lett.* **2002,** *2,* 803–806.

70. Sondi, I.; Siiman, O.; Koester, S.; Matijevic, E. Preparation of Aminodextran–CdS Nanoparticle Complexes and Biologically Active Antibodyaminodextran–CdS Nanoparticle Conjugates. *Langmuir* **2000,** *16.*

71. Wuister, S.; Swart, I.; van Driel, F.; Hickey, S.; Donega, C. Highly Luminescent Water-Soluble CdTe Quantum Dots. *Nano Lett.* **2003,** *3,* 503–507.

72. Nirmal, M.; Dabbousi, B. O.; Bawendi, M. G.; Macklin, J. J.; Trautman, J. K.; Harris, T. D.; Brus, L. E. Fluorescence Intermittency in Single Cadmium Selenide Nanocrystals. 1996.

73. Banin, U.; Bruchez, M.; Alivisatos, A. P.; Ha, T.; Weiss, S.; Chemla, D. S. Evidence for a Thermal Contribution to Emission Intermittency in Single CdSe/CdS Core/Shell Nanocrystals. *J. Chem. Phys.* **1998,** *110,* 1195–1201.

74. Sukhanova, A.; Devy, Y.; Venteo, L., et al. Biocompatible Fluorescent Nanocrystals for Immunolabeling of Membrane Proteins and Cells. *Anal. Biochem.* **2004,** *324,* 60–67.

75. Reiss, P.; Bleuse, J.; Pron, A. Highly Luminescent CdSe/ZnSe Core/Shell Nanocrystals of Low Size Dispersion. *Nano Lett.* **2002,** *2,* 781–784.

76. Nath, N.; Chilkoti, A. A Colorimetric Gold Nanoparticle Sensor to Interrogate Biomolecular Interactions in Real Time on a Surface. *Anal. Chem.* **2002,** *74,* 504–509.

77. Snee, P.; Somers, R.; Nair, G.; Zimmer, J.; Bawendi, M.; Nocera, D. A Ratiometric CdSe/ZnS Nanocrystal pH Sensor. *J. Am. Chem. Soc.* **2006,** *128,* 13320–133221.

78. Talapin, D.; Murray, C. PbSe Nanocrystal Solids for n- and p-channel Thin Film Field-Effect Transistors. *Science* **2005,** *310,* 86–89.

79. Aldana, J.; Lavelle, N.; Wang, Y.; Peng, X. Size-Dependent Dissociation pH of Thiolate Ligands from Cadmium Chalcogenide Nanocrystals. *J. Am. Chem. Soc.* **2005,** *127,* 2496–2504.

80. Chan, C. Thesis. Type, Indiana University, Bloomington, 2001.

81. Duan, H.; Nie, S. Cell-Penetrating Quantum Dots Based on Multivalent and Endosome-Disrupting Surface Coatings. *J. Am. Chem. Soc.* **2007.**

82. Gao, X.; Cui, Y.; Levenson, R. M.; Chung, L. W. K.; Nie, S. In Vivo Cancer Targeting and Imaging with Semiconductor Quantum Dots. *Nat. Biotechnol.* **2004,** *22,* 969–976.

83. Bruchez, M., Jr.; Moronne, M.; Gin, P.; Weiss, S.; Alivisatos, A. P. Semiconductor Nanocrystals as Fluorescent Biological Labels. *Science* **1998,** *281,* 2013–2016.

84. Dubertret, B.; Skourides, P.; Norris, D. J.; Noireaux, V.; Brivaniou, A. H.; Libchaber, A. In Vivo Imaging of Quantum Dots Encapsulated in Phospholipid Micelles. *Science* **2002,** *298,* 1759–1762.

85. Yang, Y.; Gao, M. Preparation of Fluorescent SiO$_2$ Particles with Single CdTe Nanocrystal Cores by the Reverse Microemulsion Method. *Adv. Mater.* **2005,** *17,* 2354–2357.

86. Zhu, M. -Q.; Chang, E.; Sun, J.; Drezek, R. Surface Modification and Functionalization of Semiconductor Quantum Dots through Reactive Coating of Silanes in Toluene. *J. Mater. Chem.* **2007,** *17,* 800–805.

87. Kukur, E.; Riegler, J.; Urban, G. A.; Nann, T. Determination of Quantum Confinement in CdSe Nanocrystals by Cyclic Voltammetry. *J. Chem. Phys.* **2003,** *119,* 2333–2337.

88. Darbandi, M.; Tohomann, R.; Nann, T. Single quantum dots in silica spheres by microemuslion synthesis. 2005.

89. Sun, Y.; Rollins, H. Preparation of Polymer-Protected Semiconductor. *Chem. Phys. Lett.* **1998,** *288,* 585–588.

90. Fahmi, A.; Oertel, U. V. S.; Froeck, C.; Stamm, M. Ring and Disk-Like CdSe Nanoparticles Stabilized with Copolymers. *Macromol. Rapid Comm.* **2003,** *24,* 625–629.

91. Wisher, A.; Bronstein, I.; Chechik, V. Thiolated PAMAM Dendrimer-Coated CdSe/ZnSe Nanoparticles as Protein Transfection Agents. *Chem. Commun.* **2006,** *15,* 1637–1639.

92. Xu, J.; Wang, J.; Mitchell, M.; Mukherjee, P.; Jeffries-EL, M.; Petrich, J.; Lin, Z. Organic-Inorganic Nanocomposites Prepared by Grafting Conjugated Polymers onto Quantum Dots. *J. Am. Chem. Soc.* **2007,** *129,* 12828.

93. Skaff, H.; Sill, K.; Emrick, T. Quantum Dots Tailored with Poly(Para-Phenylene Vinylene). *J. Am. Chem. Soc.* **2004,** *126* (36), 11322–11325.

94. Gupta, A.; Curtis, A. Surface Modified Superparamagnetic Nanoparticles for Drug Delivery: Interaction Studies with Human Fibroblasts in Culture. *J. Mater. Sci.: Mater. in M.* **2004,** *15,* 493–496.

95. Gupta, A.; Naregalkar, R.; Vaidya, V.; Gupta, M. Recent Advances on Surface Engineering of Magnetic Iron Oxide Nanoparticles and their Biomedical Applications. *Nanomedicine* **2007,** *2,* 23–39.

96. Maruoka, S.; Matsuura, T.; Kawasaki, K.; Okamoto, M.; Yoshiaki, H.; Kodama, M.; Sugiyama, M.; Annaka, M. Biocompatibility of Polyvinylalcohol Gel as a Vitreous Substitute. *Curr. eye res.* **2006,** *31,* 599–606.

97. Susumu, K.; Uyeda, H.; Medintz, I.; Mattoussi, H. Design of Biotin-Functionalized Luminescent Quantum Dots. *J. Biomed. Biotechnol.* **2007,** *2007,* 1–7.

98. Sasaki, T.; Iwasaki, N.; Kohno, K.; Kishimoto, M.; Majima, T.; Nishimura, S.; Minami, A. Magnetic Nanoparticles for Improving Cell Invasion in Tissue Engineering. *J. Biomed. Mater. Res. Part A* **2008,** *86,* 969–978.

99. Wilhelm, C.; Cebers, A.; Bacri, J.; Gazeau, F. Deformation of Intracellular Endosomes Under a Magnetic Field. *European Biophysics Journal* **2003,** *32,* 655–660.

100. McCarthy, J.; Kelly, K.; Sun, E.; Weissleder, R. Targeted Delivery of Multifunctional Magnetic Nanoparticles. *Nanomedicine* **2007,** *2,* 153–167.

101. Hessel, C. M.; Rasch, M. R.; Hueso, J. L.; Goodfellow, B.; Akhavan, V. A.; Puvanakrishnan, P.; Tunnel, J. W.; Korgel, B. A. Alkyl Passivation and Amphiphilic Polymer Coating of Silicon Nanocrystals for Diagnostic Imaging. *Small* **2010,** *6,* 2026–2034.

102. Hu, H.; Yu, M.; Li, F.; Chen, Z.; Gao, X.; Xiong, L.; Huang, C. Facile Epoxidation Strategy for Producing Up-Converting Rare-Earth Nanophosphors as Biological Labels. *Chem. Mater.* **2008,** *20,* 7003–7009.

103. Driskell, J.; Tripp, R. Emerging Technologies in Nanotechnology-Based Pathogen Detection. *Clin. Microbiol. Newslet.* **2009,** *31,* 137–144.

104. Mulchandani, A.; Chen, W.; Mulchandani, P.; Wang, J.; Rogers, K. R. Biosensors for Direct Determination of Organophosphate Pesticides. *Biosens. Bioelectron* **2001,** *16,* 225–230.

105. Gaponik, N.; Talapin, D.; Rogach, A.; Hoppe, K.; Shevchenko, E.; Kornowski, A.; Eychmüller, A.; Weller, H. Thiol-Capping of CdTe Nanocrystals: an Alternative to Organometallic Synthetic Routes. *J. Phys. Chem. B.* **2002,** *106,* 7177–7185.

106. Thermo. Cross Linkers at a Glance. 2012 [cited 2012 May 31].
107. Xu, H.; Aguilar, Z.; Wang, Y. Quantum Dot-Based Sensors for Proteins. *ECS Transactions* **2010,** *25.*
108. Hermanson, G. *Bioconjugate Techniques*; Academic Press, 2008.
109. Niemeyer, C. Nanoparticles, Proteins, and Nucleic Acids: Biotechnology Meets Materials Science. *Angew. Chem. Int. Ed.* **2001,** *40,* 4128–4158.
110. Chen, R.; Zhang, Y.; Wang, D.; Dai, H. Noncovalent Sidewall Functionalization of Single-Walled Carbon Nanotubes for Protein Immobilization 2360. *J. Am. Chem. Soc.* **2000,** *123,* 3838–3839.
111. Prencipe, G.; Tabakman, S.; Welsher, K.; Liu, Z.; Goodwin, A.; Zhang, L.; Henry, J.; Dai, H. PEG Branched Polymer for Functionalization of Nanomaterials with Ultralong Blood Circulation. *J. Am. Chem. Soc.* **2009,** *131,* 4783–4787.
112. Baranov, D.; Fiore, A.; van Huis, M.; Giannini, C.; Falqui, A.; Lafont, U.; Zandbergen, H.; Zanella, M.; Cingolani, R.; Manna, L. Assembly of Colloidal Semiconductor Nanorods in Solution by Depletion Attraction. *Nano Lett.* **2010,** *10,* 743–749.
113. Carbone, L.; Kudera, S.; Carlino, E.; Parak, W.; Giannini, C.; Cingolani, R.; Manna, L. Multiple Wurtzite Twinning in CdTe Nanocrystals Induced by Methylphosphonic Acid. *J. Am. Chem. Soc.* **2006,** *128,* 748–755.
114. Casavola, M.; Grillo, V.; Carlino, E.; Giannini, C.; Gozzo, F.; Pinel, E.; Garcia, M.; Manna, L.; Cingolani, R.; Cozzoli, P. Topologically Controlled Growth of Magnetic-Metal-Functionalized Semiconductor Oxide Nanorods. *Nano Lett.* **2007,** *7,* 1386–1395.
115. Deka, S.; Falqui, A.; Bertoni, G.; Sangregorio, C.; Poneti, G.; Morello, G.; De Giorgi, M.; Giannini, C.; Cingolani, R.; Manna, L.; Cozzoli, P. Fluorescent Asymmetrically Cobalt-Tipped CdSe@CdS core@shell Nanorod Heterostructures Exhibiting Room-Temperature Ferromagnetic Behavior. *J. Am. Chem. Soc.* **2009,** *131,* 12817–12828.
116. Pellegrino, T.; Fiore, A.; Carlino, E.; Giannini, C.; Cozzoli, P.; Ciccarella, G.; Respaud, M.; Palmirotta, L.; Cingolani, R.; Manna, L. Heterodimers Based on CoPt$_3$-Au Nanocrystals with Tunable Domain Size. *J. Am. Chem. Soc.* **2006,** *128,* 6690–6698.
117. Quarta, A.; Di Corato, R.; Manna, L.; Argentiere, S.; Cingolani, R.; Barbarella, G.; Pellegrino, T. Multifunctional Nanostructures Based on Inorganic Nanoparticles and Oligothiophenes and their Exploitation for Cellular Studies. *J. Am. Chem. Soc.* **2008,** *130,* 10545–10555.
118. Zeng, H. Synthetic Architecture of Interior Space for inorganic Nanostructures. *J. Mater. Chem.* **2006,** *16,* 649–662.
119. Cozzoli, P.; Manna, L.; Curri, M.; Kudera, S.; Giannini, C.; Striccoli, M.; Agostiano, A. Shape and Phase Control of Colloidal ZnSe Nanocrystals. *Chem. Mater.* **2005,** *17,* 1296–1306.
120. Kubik, T.; Bogunia-Kubik, K.; Sugisaka, M. Nanotechnology on Duty in Medical Applications. *Curr. Pharm. Biotechnol.* **2005,** *6,* 17–33.
121. Zhang, S. Fabrication of Novel Biomaterials through Molecular Self-Assembly. *Nat. Biotechnol.* **2003,** *21,* 1171–1178.
122. Jain, K. Nanotechnology in Clinical Laboratory Diagnostics. *Clin. Chim. Acta.* **2005,** *358,* 37–54.
123. Kaittanis, C.; Santra, S.; Perez, J. Emerging Nanotechnology-Based Strategies for the Identification of Microbial Pathogenesis. *Adv. Drug. Deliv. Rev.* **2010,** *62,* 408–423.
124. Lee, K.; Kim, E.; Mirkin, C.; Wolinsky, S. The Use of Nanoarrays for Highly Sensitive and Selective Detection of HIV-1 in Plasma. *Nano Lett.* **2004,** *4,* 1869–1872.
125. Hauck, T.; Giri, S.; Gao, Y.; Chan, C. Nanotechnology Diagnostics for Infectious Diseases Prevalent in Developing Countries. *Adv. Drug. Deliv. Rev.* **2010,** *62,* 438–448.
126. Habermüller, K.; Mosbach, M.; Schuhmann, W. Electron-Transfer Mechanisms in Amperometric Biosensors. *Fresen. J. Anal. Chem.* **2000,** *366,* 560–568.
127. Tripp, R.; Richard, A.; Dluhy, R.; Zhao, Y. Novel Nanostructures for SERS Biosensing. *Nano Today* **2008,** *3,* 31–37.

128. Aguilar, Z.; Sirisena, M.; Gertsch, J.; Pacsial-Ong, E.; Narasimhan, P.; Wansapura, C.; Kuzmicheva, G.; Henrichs, A.; Aday, J.; Norman, M.; Aguilar, Y.; Estorninos, L. Development of Self-Contained Microelectrochemical Array Assays for Whole Organisms. *ECS Transactions* **2008**, *16*, 165–176.

129. Aguilar, Z. P. *Thesis. Type*; University of Arkansas: Fayetteville, AR, 2002.

130. Aguilar, Z. P. Small Volume Detection of *Plasmodium Falciparum* CSP Gene Using a 50-µm Diameter Cavity with Self-contained Electrochemistry. *Anal. Chem.* **2006**, *78*, 1122–1129.

131. Aguilar, Z. P.; Fritsch, I. F. Immobilized Enzyme Linked DNA-hybridization Assay with Electrochemical Detection for *Cryptosporidium Parvum* hsp70 mRNA. *Anal. Chem.* **2003**, *75*, 3890–3897.

132. Aguilar, Z. P.; Van Nguyen, C.; Sirisena, M.; Gertsch, J.; Arumugam, P.; Spencer, D.; Wansapura, C.; Aguilar, Y.; Homesley, J. In *Chemical Sensors 7 and MEMS/NEMS 7*; Hesketh, P.; Hunter, G.; Akbar, S., et al. Eds.; *ECS Transactions*; Vol. 3, 2006; pp 125–137.

133. Ivnitski, D.; Abdel-Hamid, I.; Atanasov, P.; Wilkins, E. Biosensors for Detection of Pathogenic Bacteria. *Biosens. Bioelectron.* **1999**, *14*, 599–624.

134. Adjei, A. A.; Armah, H.; Duah, O. A.; Adiku, T.; Hesse, F. A. Evaluation of a Rapid Serological Chromatographic Immunoassay for the Diagnosis of Tuberculosis in Acra, Ghana. *Jpn. J. Infect. Dis.* **2003**, *56*.

135. Aguilar, Z. P.; Sirisena, M. Development of Automated Amperometric Detection of Antibodies against Bacillus anthracis Protective Antigen. *Anal. Bioanal. Chem.* **2007**, *389*, 507–515.

136. Luppa, P.; Sokoll, L.; Daniel, W.; Chan, D. Immunosensors-Principles and Applications to Clinical Chemistry. *Clin. Chim. Acta.* **2001**, *314*, 1–26.

137. Liu, G.; Lin, Y. Nanomaterial Labels in Electrochemical Immunosensors and Immunoassays. *Talanta* **2007**, *74*, 308–317.

138. Wang, J. Electrochemical Nucleic Acid Biosensors. *Anal. Chim. Acta.* **2002**, *469*, 63–71.

139. Grieshaber, D.; MacKenzie, R.; Voros, J.; Reimhult, E. Electrochemical Biosensors—Sensor Principles and Architectures. *Sensors* **2008**, *8*, 1400–1458.

140. Aguilar, Z.; Aguilar, Y.; Xu, H.; Jones, B.; Dixon, J.; Xu, H.; Wang, A. Nanomaterials in Medicine. *ECS Transactions* **2010**, *33*, 69–74.

141. Aguilar, Z.; Xu, H.; Jones, B.; Dixon, J.; Wang, A. Semiconductor Quantum Dots for Cell Imaging. *Mater. Res. Soc. Proc.* **2010**, *1237*, TT1206-1201.

142. Didenko, Y.; Suslick, K. Chemical Aerosol Flow Synthesis of Semiconductor Nanoparticles. *J. Am. Chem. Soc.* **2005**, *127*, 12196–12197.

143. Dyadyusha, L.; Yin, H.; Jaiswal, S.; Brown, T.; Baumberg, J.; Booye, F.; Melvin, T. Quenching of CdSe Quantum Dot Emission, a New Approach for Biosensing. *Chem. Commun.* **2005**, 3201–3203.

144. Geiber, D.; Charbonnière, L. J.; Ziessel, R. F.; Butlin, N. G.; Löhmannsröben, H.; Hildebrandt, N. Quantum Dot Biosensors for Ultrasensitive Multiplexed Diagnostics. *Angew. Chem. Int. Ed.* **2010**, *49*, 1–6.

145. Khanna, V. K. New-Generation Nano-Engineered Biosensors, Enabling Nanotechnologies and Nanomaterials. *Sens. Rev.* **2008**, *28*, 39–45.

146. Li, M.; Li, R.; Li, C. M.; Wu, N. Electrochemical and Optical Biosensors Based on Nanomaterials and Nanostructures: A review. *Front. Biosci.* **2011**, *S3*, 1308–1331.

147. Medintz, I.; Clapp, A.; Mattoussi, H.; Goldman, E.; Fisher, B.; Mauro, J. Self-Assembled Nanoscale Biosensors Based on Quantum Dot FRET Donors. *Nat. Mater.* **2003**, *2*, 630–638.

148. Wang, J. Nanomaterial-Based Electrochemical Biosensors. *Analyst* **2005**, *130*, 421–426.

149. Xiao, Y.; Patolsky, F., et al. Plugging into Enzymes: Nanowiring of Redox Enzymes by a Gold Nanoparticle. *Science* **2003**, *299*, 1877–1881.

150. Xu, H.; Aguilar, Z.; Dixon, J.; Jones, B.; Wang, A.; Wei, H. Breast Cancer Cell Imaging using Semiconductor Quantum Dots. *ECS Transactions* **2009**, *25*, 69–77.

151. Yun, Y.; Eteshola, E.; Bhattacharya, A.; Dong, Z.; Shim, J.; Conforti, L.; Kim, D.; Schulz, M.; Ahn, C.; Watts, N. Tiny Medicine: Nanomaterial-Based Biosensors. *Sensors* **2009**, *9*, 9275–9299.

152. Merkoci, A. Nanoparticles-Based Strategies for DNA, Protein and Cell Sensors. *Biosens. Bioelectron.* **2010**, *26*, 1164–1177.

153. Hu, L.; Kim, H.; Lee, J.; Peumans, P.; Cui, Y. Scalable Coating and Properties of Transparent, Flexible, Silver Nanowire Electrodes. *ACS Nano.* **2010**, *4*, 2955–2963.

154. Xianmao, L.; Yavuz, M.; Tuan, H.; Korgel, B.; Xia, Y. Ultrathin Gold Nanowires Can Be Obtained by Reducing Polymeric Strands of Oleylamine–AuCl Complexes Formed via Aurophilic Interaction. *J. Am. Chem. Soc.* **2008**, *130*, 8900–8901.

155. Byers, R.; Hitchman, E. Quantum Dots Brighten Biological Imaging. *Progr. Histochem. Cytochem.* **2011**, *45*, 201–237.

156. Jaiswal, J.; Mattoussi, H.; Mauro, J.; Simon, S. Long-Term Multiple Color Imaging of Live Cells using Quantum Dot Bioconjugates. *Nat. Biotechnol.* **2003**, *21*, 47–51.

157. Liu, J.; Lu, Y. A Colorimetric Lead Biosensor Using DNAzyme-Directed Assembly of Gold Nanoparticles. *J. Am. Chem. Soc.* **2003**, *125*, 6642–6643.

158. Vaseashta, A.; Dimova-Malinovska, D. Nanostructured and Nanoscale Devices, Sensors and Detectors. *Sci. Technol. Adv. Mat.* **2005**, *6*, 312–318.

159. Xu, H.; Aguilar, Z.; Wei, H.; Wang, A. Development of Semiconductor Nanomaterial whole Cell Imaging Sensor on Silanized Microscope Slides. *Front. Biosci.* **2011**, *E3*, 1013–1024.

160. Barbosa, S.; Agrawal, A.; Rodríguez-Lorenzo, L.; Pastoriza-Santos, I.; Alvarez-Puebla, R. A.; Kornowski, A.; Weller, H.; Liz-Marzan, L. M. Tuning Size and Sensing Properties in Colloidal Gold Nanostars. *Langmuir* **2010**, *26*, 14943–14950.

161. Xu, H.; Aguilar, Z.; Waldron, J.; Wei, H.; Wang, Y. Application of Semiconductor Quantum Dots for Breast Cancer Cell Sensing. *IEEE Computer Society BMEI* **2009**, *1*, 516–520.

162. Xu, H.; Aguilar, Z.; Su, H.; Dixon, J.; Wei, H.; Wang, Y. Breast Cancer Cell Imaging using Semiconductor Quantum Dots. *ECS Transactions* **2009**, *25*, 69–77.

163. Su, H.; Xu, H.; Gao, S.; Dixon, J.; Aguilar, Z.; Wang, A.; Xu, J.; Wang, J. Microwave Synthesis of Nearly Monodisperse Core/Multishell Quantum Dots with Cell Imaging Applications. *Nano. Res. Lett.* **2010**, *5*, 625–630.

164. Xu, H.; Aguilar, Z.; Wei, H.; Wang, A. Development of Semiconductor Nanomaterial whole Cell Imaging Sensor on Silanized Microscope Slides. *Front. Biosci.* **2011**, Accepted.

165. Aguilar, Z.; Aguilar, Y.; Xu, H.; Jones, B.; Dixon, J.; Xu, H.; Wang, A. Nanomaterials in Medicine. *ECS Transactions* **2010**, *33*, 69–74.

166. Carbó-Argibay, E.; Rodríguez-González, B.; Pastoriza-Santos, I.; Pérez-Juste, J.; Liz-Marán, L. M. Growth of Pentatwinned Gold Nanorods into Truncated Decahedra. *Nanoscale* **2010**, *2*, 2377–2383.

167. Du, P.; Li, H.; Mei, Z.; Liu, S. Electrochemical DNA Biosensor for the Detection of DNA Hybridization with the Amplification of Au Nanoparticles and CdS Nanoparticles. *Bioelectrochemistry* **2009**, *75*, 37–43.

168. Li, H.; Rothberg, L. Colorimetric Detection of DNA Sequences based on Electrostatic Interactions with Unmodified Gold Nanoparticles. *PNAS* **2004**, *101*, 14036–14039.

169. Li, M.; Zhang, J.; Suri, S.; Sooter, L. J.; Ma, D.; Wu, N. Detectionof Adenosine Triphosphate with and Aptamer Biosensor based on the Surface-Enhanced Raman Scattering. *Anal. Chem.* **2012**, *84*, 2837–2842.

170. Li-Na, M.; Dian-Jun, L.; Zhen-Xin, W. Synthesis and Applications of Gold Nanoparticle Probes. *Chin. J. Anal. Chem.* **2010**, *38*, 1–7.

171. Liu, J.; Lu, Y. Adenosine-Dependent Assembly of Aptazyme-Functionalized Gold Nanoparticles and its Application as a Colorimetric Biosensor. *Anal. Chem.* **2004,** *76,* 1627–1632.
172. Liz-Marzán, L. M. Tailoring Surface Plasmons through the Morphology and Assembly of Metal Nanoparticles. *Langmuir* **2006,** *22,* 32–41.
173. Mao, X.; Liu, G. Nanomaterial Based Electrochemical DNA Biosensors and Bioassays. *J. Biomed. Nanotechnol.* **2008,** *4,* 419–431.
174. Neely, A.; Perry, C.; Varisli, B.; Singh, A.; Arbneshi, T.; Senapati, D.; Kalluri, J.; Ray, P. Ultrasensitive and Highly Selective Detection of Alzheimer's Disease Biomarker Using Two-Photon Rayleigh Scattering Properties of Gold Nanoparticle. *ACS Nano.* **2009,** *3,* 2834–2840.
175. Paciotti, G. F.; Myer; Weinreich, D.; Goia; Pavel; McLaughlin, E.; Tamarkin, L. Colloidal Gold: A Novel Nanoparticle Vector for Tumor Directed Drug Delivery. *Drug. Deliv.* **2002,** *11,* 169–183.
176. Pellegrino, T.; Fiore, A.; Carlino, E.; Giannini, C.; Cozzoli, P. D.; Ciccarella, G.; Respaud, M.; Palmirotta, R.; Cingolani, R.; Manna, L. Heterodimers Based on CoPt₃–Au Nanocrystals with Tunable Domain Size. *J. Am. Chem. Soc.* **2006,** *128,* 6690–6698.
177. Xie, J.; Zhang, F.; Aronova, M.; Zhu, L.; Lin, X.; Quan, Q.; Liu, G.; Zhang, G.; Choi, K. Y.; Kim, K.; Sun, X.; Lee, S.; Sun, S.; Leapman, R.; Chen, X. Manipulating the Power of an Additional Phase: A Flower-Like Au–Fe₃O₄ Optical Nanosensor for Imaging Protease Expressions in Vivo. *ACS Nano.* **2011,** *5,* 3043–3051.
178. Xu, H.; Mao, X.; Zeng, Q.; Wang, S.; Kawde, A. -N.; Liu, G. Aptamer-Functionalized Gold Nanoparticles as Probes in a Dry-Reagent Strip Biosensor for Protein Analysis. *Anal. Chem.* **2008,** *81,* 669–675.
179. Yang, X.; Wang, Q.; Wang, K.; Tan, W.; Li, H. Enhanced Surface Plasmon Resonance with the modified Catalytic Growth of Au Nanoparticles. *Biosens. Bioelectron.* **2007,** *22,* 1106–1110.
180. Klostranec, M.; Xiang, Q.; Farcas, G.; Lee, J.; Rhee, A.; Lafferty, E.; Perrault, S.; Kain, K.; Chan, W. Convergence of Quantum Dot Barcodes with Microfluidics and Signal Processing for Multiplexed High-Throughput Infectious Disease Diagnostics. *Nano Lett.* **2007,** *7,* 2812–2818.
181. Aggrawal, A.; Zhang, C.; Byassee, T.; Tripp, R.; Nie, S. Counting Single Native Biomolecules and Intact Viruses with Color-Coded Nanoparticles. *Anal. Chem.* **2006,** *78,* 1061–1070.
182. Zhao, X.; Hillard, L.; Mechery, S.; Wang, Y.; Bagwe, R.; Jin, S.; Tan, W. A Rapid Bioassay for Single Bacterial Cell Quantitation using Bioconjugated Nanoparticles. *Proc. Natl. Acad. Sci.* **2004,** *101,* 15027–15032.
183. Nagel, T.; Ehrentreich-Förster, E.; Singh, M.; Schmitt, K.; Brandenburg, A.; Berk, A.; Bier, F. Direct Detection of Tuberculosis Infection in Blood Serum using Three Optical Label-Free Approaches. *Sensor. Actuator.* **2008,** *129,* 934–940.
184. Ocean. Carboxyl Magnetic Iron Oxide Nanocrystals Conjugation Kits (Catalog # ICK). 2011 [cited 2011 March 8]. Available from: http://www.oceannanotech.com/upload/090720185235954669s9vwf4.pdf.
185. Ocean. Carboxyl Quantum Dots Protein Conjugation Kits (Catalog # QCK). 2011 [cited 2011 March 8]. Available from: http://www.oceannanotech.com/upload/0908041519250478346polyw.pdf.
186. Paolsky, F.; Gill, R.; Weizmann, Y.; Mokari, T.; Banin, U.; Willner, I. Lighting-Up the Dynamics of Telomerization and DNA Replication by CdSe–ZnS Quantum Dots. *J. Am. Chem. Soc.* **2003,** *125,* 13918–13919.
187. Li, Y. CdS Nanocrystal Induced Chemiluminescence: Reaction Mechanism and Applications. *Nanotechnology* **2007,** *18,* 1–8.

188. Akerman, M.; Chan, W.; Laakkonen, P.; Bhatia, S.; Ruoslahti, E. Nanocrystal Targeting in vivo. *Proc. Natl. Acad. Sci.* **2002,** *99,* 12617–12621.

189. Mitchell, G.; Mirkin, C.; Letsinger, L. Programmed Assembly Of DNA Functionalized Quantum Dots. *J. Am. Chem. Soc.* **1999,** *121,* 8122.

190. Goldman, E.; Anderson, G.; Tran, P.; Mattoussi, H.; Charles, P.; Mauro, J. Conjugation of Luminescent Quantum Dots with Antibodies using an Engineered Adaptor Protein to Provide New Reagents for Fluoroimmunoassays. *Anal. Chem.* **2002,** *74,* 841–847.

191. Dahan, M.; Levi, S.; Luccardini, C.; Rostaing, P.; Riveau, B.; Triller, A. Diffusion Dynamics of Glycine Receptors Revealed by Single-Quantum Dot Tracking. *Science* **2003,** *302,* 442–445.

192. Pusic, K.; Xu, H.; Stridiron, A.; Aguilar, Z.; Wang, A. Z.; Hui, H. Blood Stage Merozoite Surface Protein Conjugated to Nanoparticles Induce Potent Parasite Inhibitory Antibodies. *Vaccine* **2011,** *29,* 8898–8908.

193. Daniel, M.; Astruc, D. Gold Nanoparticles: Assembly, Supramolecular Chemistry, Quantum-Size-Related Properties, and Applications Toward Biology, Catalysis, and Nanotechnology. *Chem. Rev.* **2004,** *104,* 293–346.

194. Medintz, I.; Uyeda, H.; Goldman, E.; Mattoussi, H. Quantum Dot Bioconjugates for Imaging, Labelling and Sensing. *Nat. Mater.* **2005,** *4,* 435–446.

195. Aguilar, Z.; Xu, H.; Dixon, J.; Wang, A. Blocking Non-Specific Uptake of Engineered Nanomaterials. *ECS Transactions* **2010,** *25,* 37–48.

196. Xu, H.; Aguilar, Z.; Waldron, J.; Wei, H.; Wang, Y. Application of Semiconductor Quantum Dots for Breast Cancer Cell Sensing, 2009 Biomedical Engineering and Informatics. *IEEE Computer Society BMEI* **2009,** *1,* 516–520.

197. Rijiravanich, P.; Somasundrum, M.; Surareungchai, W. Femtomolar Electrochemical Detection of DNA Hybridization using hollow Polyelectrolyte Shells Bearing Silver Nanoparticles. *Anal. Chem.* **2008,** *80,* 3904–3909.

198. Meyer, M.; Bhuju, S.; Krause, H.; Hartmann, M.; Miethe, P.; Singh, P.; Keusgen, M. Magnetic Biosensor for the Detection of *Yersinia Pestis. J. Microbiol. Meth.* **2007,** *68,* 218–224.

199. Wagner, W.; Dullaart, A.; Bock, A. K.; Zweck, A. The Emerging Nanomedicine Landscape. *Nat. Biotechnol.* **2006,** *24,* 1211–1217.

200. Freitas, R. A. Jr. What is Nanomedicine. *Nanomed.: Nanotechnol. Biol. Med.* **2005,** *1,* 2–9.

201. Coombs, R. R. H.; Robinson, D. W. *Nanotechnology in Medicine and the Biosciences,* 1996.

202. Murday, J. S.; Siegel, R. W.; Stern, J.; Wright, J. F. Translational Nanomedicine: Status Assessment and Opportunities. *Nanomed.: Nanotechnol. Biol. Med.* **2009,** *5,* 251–273.

203. Ratner, M. A.; Ratner, D. *Nanotechnology: A Gentle Introduction to the Next Big Idea* **2002.**

204. Ferrari, M. Cancer Nanotechnology: Opportunities and Challenges. *Nat. Rev. Cancer.* **2005,** *5,* 161–171.

205. Hirsch, L.; Stafford, R.; Bankson, J.; Sershen, S.; Rivera, B.; Price, R.; Hazle, J.; Halas, N.; West, J. Nanoshell-Mediated Near-Infrared Thermal Therapy of Tumors Under Magnetic Resonance Guidance. *Proc. Natl. Acad. Sci.* **2003,** *100,* 13549–13554.

206. Huang, X.; El-sayed, I.; Qian, W.; El-Sayed, M. Cancer Cell Imaging and Photothermal Therapy in the Near-Infrared Region by using Gold Nanorods. *J. Am. Chem. Soc.* **2006,** *128,* 2115–2120.

207. LaVan, D. A.; McGuire, T.; Langer, R. Small-Scale Systems for in Vivo Drug Delivery. *Nat. Biotechnol.* **2003,** *21,* 1184.

208. Cavalcanti, A.; Shirinzadeh, B.; Zhang, M.; Kretly, L. C. Nanorobot Hardware Architecture for Medical Defense. *Sensors* **2008,** *8,* 2932–2958.

209. Allen, T. M.; Mumbengegwi, D. R.; Charrois, G. J. Anti-CD19-targeted Liposomal Doxorubicin Improves the Therapeutic Efficacy in Murine B-Cell Lymphoma and Ameliorates the Toxicity of Liposomes with Varying Drug Release Rates. *Clin. Cancer. Res.* **2005,** *11,* 3567–3573.

210. Barreiro, A.; Rurali, R.; Harnandez, E. R.; Moser, J.; Pichler, T. F. L., et al. Subnanometer Motion of Cargos Driven by Thermal Gradients along Carbon Nanotubes. *Science* **2008,** *320,* 775–778.

211. Brigger, I.; Dubernet, C.; Couvreur, P. Nanoparticles in Cancer Therapy and Diagnosis. *Adv. Drug Del. Rev.* **2002,** *54,* 631–651.

212. Chauhan, A.; Sridevi, S.; Chalasani, K.; Jain, A.; Jain, S.; Jain, N.; Diwan, P. Dendrimer-Mediated Transdermal Delivery: Enhanced Bioavailability of Indomethacin. *J. Contr. Release* **2003,** *90,* 335.

213. Couvreur, P.; Barratt, G.; Fattal, E.; Legrand, P.; Vauthier, C. Nanocapsule Technology: A Review. *Crit. Rev. Ther. Drug Carrier Syst.* **2002,** *19,* 99134.

214. Dang, J. M.; Leong, K. W. Natural Polymers for Gene Delivery and Tissue Engineering. *Adv. Drug. Deliv. Rev.* **2006,** *58,* 487–499.

215. Fetterly, G. J.; Straubinger, R. M. Pharmacokinetics of Paclitaxel-Containing Liposomes in Rats. *AAPS PharmSci.* **2003,** *5,* 1–11.

216. Govender, T.; Riley, T.; Ehtezazi, T.; Garnett, M. C.; Stolnik, S.; Illum, L.; Davis, S. S. Defining the Drug Incorporation Properties of PLA-PEG Nanoparticles. *Int. J. Pharm.* **2000,** *199,* 95–110.

217. Govender, T.; Stolnik, S.; Garnett, M. C.; Illum, L.; Davis, S. S. PLGA Nanoparticles Prepared by Nanoprecipitation: Drug Loading and Release Studies of a Water Soluble Drug. *J. Contr. Release* **1999,** *57,* 171–185.

218. Kroll, R. A.; Pagel, M. A.; Muldoon, L. L.; Roman-Goldstein, S.; Fiamengo, S. A.; Neuwelt, E. A. Improving Drug Delivery to Intracerebral Tumor and Surrounding Brain in a Rodent Model: A Comparison of Osmotic Versus Bradykinin Modification of the Blood-Brain and/or Blood-Tumor Barriers. *Neurosurgery* **1998,** *43,* 879–886.

219. Labhasetwar, V. Nanotechnology for Drug and Gene Therapy: The Importance of Understanding Molecular Mechanisms of Delivery. *Curr. Opin. Biotechnol.* **2005,** *16,* 674–680.

220. Lamprecht, A.; Ubrich, N.; Yamamoto, H.; Schäfer, U.; Takeuchi, H.; Maincent, P.; Kawashima, Y.; Lehr, C. M. Biodegradable Nanoparticles for Targeted Drug Delivery in Treatment of Inflammatory Bowel Disease. *J. Pharmacol. Exp. Ther.* **2001,** *299,* 775–781.

221. Medina, O. P.; Pillarsettya, N.; Glekasa, A.; Punzalan, B.; Longo, V.; Gonen, M.; Zanzonico, P.; Smith-Jones, P.; Larson, S. M. Optimizing Tumor Targeting of the Lipophilic EGFR-Binding Radiotracer SKI 243 using a Liposomal Nanoparticle Delivery System. *J Contr. Release* **2011,** *149,* 292–298.

222. Moghimi, S. M.; Hunter, A. C.; Murray, J. C. Long-Circulating and Target-Specific Nanoparticles: Theory to Practice. *Pharmacol. Rev.* **2003,** *53,* 283–318.

223. Panyam, J.; Labhasetwar, V. Biodegradable Nanoparticles for Drug and Gene Delivery to Cells and Tissue. *Adv. Drug. Deliv. Rev.* **2003,** *12,* 329–347.

224. Sapra, P.; Allen, T. M. Ligand-Targeted Liposomal Anticancer Drugs. *Prog. Lipid. Res.* **2003,** *42,* 439–462.

225. Kateb, B.; Chiu, K.; Black, K.; Yamamoto, V.; Khalsa, B.; Ljubimova, J.; Ding, H.; Patil, R.; Portilla-Arias, J.; Modo, M.; Moore, D.; Farahani, K.; Okun, M.; Prakash, N.; Neman, J.; Ahdoot, D.; Grundfest, W.; Nikzad, S.; Heiss, J. Nanoplatforms for Constructing New Approaches to Cancer Treatment, Imaging, and Drug Delivery: What should be the Policy?. *NeuroImage* **2011,** *54,* S106–S124.

226. Koo, O. M.; Rubinstein, I.; Onyuksel, H. Role of Nanotechnology in Targeted Drug Delivery and Imaging: A Concise Review. *Nanomedicine* **2005**, *1,* 193–212.

227. Larson, D. R.; Zipfel, W. R.; Williams, R. M.; Clark, S. W.; Bruchez, M. P.; Wise, F. W., et al. Watersoluble Quantum Dots for Multiphoton Fluorescence Imaging in Vivo. *Science* **2003**, *300,* 1434–1436.

228. Su, H.; Xu, H.; Gao, S.; Dixon, J.; Aguilar, Z. P.; Wang, A.; Xu, J.; Wang, J. Microwave Synthesis of Nearly Monodisperse Core/Multishell Quantum Dots with Cell Imaging Applications. *Nano. Res. Lett.* **2010**, *5,* 625–630.

229. Allen, T. M.; Cullis, P. R. Drug Delivery Systems: Entering the Mainstream. *Science* **2005**, *303,* 1818–1822.

230. Haes, J. A.; Van Duyne, R. P. A Unified View of Propagating and Localized Surface Plasmon Resonance Biosensors. *Anal. Bioanal. Chem.* **2004**, *379,* 920–930.

231. Khanna, V. K. New-Generation Nano-Engineered Biosensors, Enabling Nanotechnologies and Nanomaterials. *Sens. Rev.* **2008**, *28,* 39–45.

232. Yang, R.; Jin, J.; Chen, Y.; Shao, N.; Kang, H.; Xiao, Z.; Tang, Z.; Wu, Y.; Zhu, Z.; Tan, W. CarbonNanotube-QuenchedFluorescentOligonucleotides:ProbesthatFluoresceuponHybridization. *J. Am. Chem. Soc.* **2008**, *130,* 8351–8358.

233. Cai, Y.; Yun, Y.; Newby, B. Generation of Contact-Printing Based Poly(Ethylene Glycol) Gradient Surfaces with Micrometer-Sized Tips. *Colloid. Surf. Biointerf.* **2010**, *75,* 115–122.

234. Zhang, X.; Yonzon, C.; Van Duyne, R. Nanosphere Lithography Fabricated Plasmonic Material and their Applications. *J. Mater. Res.* **2006**, *21,* 1083–1092.

235. Guo, L. Recent Progress in Nanoimprint Technology and its Applications. *J. Phys. D: Appl. Phys.* **2004**, *37,* R123–R141.

236. Hulteen, J.; Van Duyne, R. Nanosphere Lithography: A Materials General Fabrication Process for Periodic Particle Array Surfaces. *J. Vac. Sci. Technol. A* **1995**, *13,* 1553–1558.

237. Hulteen, J.; Treichel, D.; Smith, M.; Duval, M.; Jensen, T.; Van Duyne, R. Nanosphere Lithography: Size-Tunable Silver Nanoparticle and Surface Cluster Arrays. *J. Phys. Chem. B* **1999**, *103,* 3854–3863.

238. Riboh, J.; Haes, A.; McFarland, A.; Yonzon, C.; Van Duyne, R. A Nanoscale Optical Biosensor: Real-Time Immunoassay in Physiological Buffer Enabled by Improved Nanoparticle Adhesion. *J. Phys. Chem. B* **2003**, *107,* 1772–1780.

239. Ginger, D.; Zhang, H.; Mirkin, C. The Evolution of Dip-Pen Nanolithography. *ACIEFS* **2004**, *43,* 1–130.

240. Xu, H.; Aguilar, Z.; Wang, A. Quantum Dot-Based Sensors for Proteins. *ECS Transactions* **2010**, *25,* 1–10.

241. Kreuter, J.; Alyautdin, R. N.; Kharkevich, D. A.; Ivanov, A. A. Passage of Peptides through the Blood Brain Barrier with Colloidal Polymer Particles. *Brain Res.* **1995**, *674,* 171–174.

242. Gelperina, S. E.; Khalansky, A. S.; Skidan, I. N.; Smirnova, Z. S.; Bobruskin, A. I.; Severin, S. E.; Turowski, B.; Zanella, F. E.; Kreuter, J. Toxicological Studies of Doxorubicin Bound to Polysorbate 80-Coated Poly(Butyl Cyanoacrylate) Nanoparticles in Healthy Rats and Rats with Intracranial Glioblastoma. *Toxicol Lett.* **2002**, *126,* 131–141.

243. Sakamoto, J. H.; van de Ven, A. L.; Godin, B.; Blanco, E.; Serda, R. E.; Grattoni, A.; Ziemys, A.; Bouamrani, A.; Hu, T.; Ranganathan, S. I.; De Rosa, E.; Martinez, J. O.; Smid, C. A.; Buchanan, R.; Lee, S. Y.; Srinivasan, S.; Landry, M.; Meyn, A.; Tasciotti, E.; Li, X.; Decuzzi, P.; Ferrari, M. Review: Enabling Individualized Therapy through Nanotechnology. *Pharm. Res.* **2010**, *62,* 57–89.

244. Singh, R.; James, W.; Lillard, J. Nanoparticle-Based Targeted Drug Delivery. *Exp. Mol. Pathol.* **2009**, *86,* 215–223.

245. Thevenot, D.; Toth, K.; Durst, R.; Wilson, G. Electrochemical Biosensors: Recommended Definitions and Classification. *PureAppl. Chem.* **1999,** *71,* 2333–2348.

246. Thevenot, D. R.; Toth, K.; Durst, R. A.; Wilson, G. S. Electrochemical Biosensors: Recommended Definitions and Classification. *Biosens. Bioelectron.* **2001,** *16,* 121–131.

247. Qu, F.; Yang, M.; Jiang, J.; Shen, G.; Yu, R. Amperometric Biosensor for Choline based on Layer-by-Layer Assembled Functionalized Carbon Nanotube and Polyaniline Multilayer Film. *Anal. Biochem.* **2005,** *344,* 108–114.

248. Wang, J.; Liu, G.; Jan, M. Ultrasensitive Electrical Biosensing of Proteins and DNA: Carbon-Nanotube Derived Amplification of the Recognition and Transduction Events. *J. Am. Chem. Soc.* **2004,** *126,* 3010–3011.

249. Pejcic, B.; De Marco, R.; Parkinson, G. The Role of Biosensors in the Detection of Emerging Infectious Diseases. *Analyst* **2006,** *131,* 1079–1090.

250. He, B.; Morrow, T.; Keating, C. Nanowire Sensors for Multiplexed Detection of Biomolecules. *Curr. Opin. Chem. Biol.* **2005,** *12,* 522–528.

251. Patolsky, F.; Zheng, G.; Hayden, O.; Lakadamyali, M.; Zhuang, X.; Lieber, C. Electrical Detection of Single Viruses. *Proc. Natl. Acad. Sci.* **2004,** *101,* 14017–14022.

252. Abell, J.; Driskell, J.; Dluhy, R.; Tripp, R.; Zhao, Y. Fabrication and Characterization of a Multiwell Array SERS Chip with Biological Applications. *Biosens. and Bioelectron.* **2009,** *24,* 3663–3670.

253. Malvadkar, N.; Demirel, G.; Poss, M.; Javed, A.; Dressick, W.; Demirel, M. Fabrication and use of Electroless Plated Polymer Surface-Enhanced Raman Spectroscopy Substrates for Viral Gene Detection. *J. Phys. Chem.* **2010,** *114,* 10730–10738.

Chapter 4

Nanobiosensors

4.1 INTRODUCTION

A biosensor is a bioanalytical device that consists of a molecular recognition entity associated with a physicochemical transducer.[1] The rapid and accurate measurement of molecular entities such as protein biomarkers, genes, cells, and pathogens in biological samples is among the major challenges in medical biosensors.[2] Recently, a number of new diagnostic platforms involving dimensions in the nanometer scale

Nanomaterials for Medical Applications. http://dx.doi.org/10.1016/B978-0-12-385089-8.00004-2
    127

called nanobiosensors have been developed to detect and measure biomolecules and cells with high sensitivity. Such biosensors use nanoparticles for transduction.

A nanobiosensor can be homogeneous or heterogeneous. A homogeneous nanobiosensor occurs in solution and does not have a phase separation. A heterogeneous nanobiosensor involves a solid platform that serves to anchor the analyte being detected. The heterogeneous nanobiosensor will be the main focus of the discussions in this chapter.

Just like the biosensors in bulk, the heterogeneous nanobiosensor that will be referred to as nanobiosensor from hereon involves a solid surface called the capture platform (Figure 4.1) which is coated with a specific receptor that specifically recognizes and captures the analyte. The receptor can be a protein (antigen) when the analyte is an antibody (Figure 4.1A) or an antibody, when the analyte is a protein (Figure 4.1B). The protein analyte may be found in a cell, in which case, the whole cell will be captured on the solid surface (Figure 4.2). To detect the presence of the antigen or the antibody, a second receptor that specifically recognizes the analyte is added. This receptor may be tagged with a nanomaterial (NM) or another receptor recognizing the second receptor that is tagged with a NM is added to complete the assay. Because NMs can be detected at very low concentrations, the sensitivity of nanobiosensors is expected to be in the low picogram to attogram levels. Thus, nanobiosensors hold promise for early disease detection that can provide valuable insights into the medical biology at the systems level.

NMs exhibit unique size-tunable as well as shape-dependent physicochemical properties that do not resemble those of bulk materials. Recent advances in

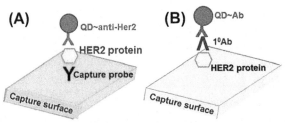

FIGURE 4.1 Schematic diagrams of QD-based nanobiosensors for analyte that is an (A) antigen and (B) antibody. *(For color version of this figure, the reader is referred to the online version of this book)*

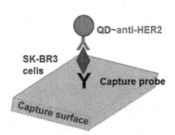

FIGURE 4.2 Schematic diagrams of a QD-based nanobiosensor for a whole cell such as breast cancer cell SK-BR3. *(For color version of this figure, the reader is referred to the online version of this book)*

NMs open new avenues to develop various novel biosensors. These NM-based biosensors, nanobiosensors, make use of electrochemical and optical properties of NMs. These nanobiosensors are expected to demonstrate improved limit of detection, sensitivity, ease of use, reproducibility, low cost, portability, and selectivity.[3–5] The size of NMs that is comparable to the dimensions of biomolecular probes and to biological analytes makes them excellent components of biosensors.[6–12]

In this chapter, nanobiosensors that involve NMs for detection of various biomolecules that are useful in the clinical diagnosis of different types of diseases will be discussed. These diseases may be genetic, metabolic, or caused by infectious disease-causing agents. Various types of NM-based nanobiosensors will be presented and a few protocols will be discussed.

4.2 NANOBIOSENSORS UNIQUE PROPERTIES

The booming nanotechnology industry has revived interest in the development of novel sensing systems as well as the enhancement of the performance of bioanalytical assays.[13–15] Recent advances in material science and synthetic chemistry have made it possible to produce high-quality nanomaterials in the form of nanoparticles (NPs; nanotubes, nanorods, nanospheres, nanowires), nanoarrays, and their composites.[16,17] These NMs have been used for the development of biosensors[6,7,10–12,14,18–20] because of their significant advantages over microscale and bulk materials that include (a) size-tunable properties, (b) large surface–volume ratio, (c) shape-dependent properties, (d) lower energy consumption, (e) miniaturized biosensors, and (f) low cost.

Bottom-up nanotechnology approaches are offering a large series of NMs with special interest for biosensing systems. Investigations of these materials are gaining interest due to the size- and shape-dependent physical, chemical, and electrochemical properties which make them extremely useful in sensing and biosensing applications.[21] The size and composition sometimes make NMs even more attractive than the corresponding bulk structure. A target binding event (i.e. DNA hybridization or immunoreaction) occurring on the NP's surface may have a significant effect on its optical (change of the light absorption/emission) or electrochemical properties (oxidation/reduction current onto a transducing platform) offering novel alternatives for bioanalysis. For example, compounds consisting of metal NPs of group II–VI which are semiconductors like CdSe, ZnSe, CdTe, etc., also called quantum dots (QDs)[22] as well as gold nanoparticles (AuNPs) are of special interest because of their properties. QDs are highly fluorescent and in comparison with organic dyes (such as rhodamine) are 20 times as bright, 100 times as stable against photobleaching, and one-third as wide in spectral line width.[23] Thus, QDs present an enormous potential for biosensors applications for fluorescence detection. The most interesting property of QDs for fluorescence detection is the very small number of QDs necessary to produce a signal. Indeed, several studies have reported flickering of some specimens, a phenomenon that is due to the blinking of a small number of QDs.[23,24]

This demonstrates that single QDs can still be observed in nanobiosensor at conditions such as those of a monolayer of molecules or atoms, with an ultimate sensitivity limit of one QD per target molecule. Additionally, QDs are available in a virtually unlimited number of well-separated colors that are all excitable by a single wavelength. Aside from simplifying image acquisition, this property could be used in confocal microscopy to perform nanometer resolution with colocalization of multiple-color individual QDs.[23–25] In addition, just like other NMs, QDs offer an increased surface area that is available for bioapplications.

The application of NMs in biosensor development is strongly related to their properties that depend on the mode of synthesis that is responsible for the quality of the resulting NPs and the postsynthesis modifications, both chemical and biological. The preparation procedures for NMs, either in colloidal solutions or grown on solid substrates, have been extensively reviewed.[26] Along with synthetic advances for varying the size, shape, and composition of nanostructured materials is the ability to tailor their binding affinities for various biomolecules through surface modification and meticulous engineering.

Thus, NM-based biosensors take advantage of the optical and electronic properties of NMs for a sensitive response to biomolecular binding events.[15,18] The sensor signal comes in the form of a change in the intensity or the peak position of optical absorption, fluorescence emission, reflection, surface plasmon resonance (SPR), surface-enhanced Raman scattering (SERS), and electrochemical potential/current under various conditions leading to the development of corresponding biosensors.[6,7,11,15,19,27,28]

The relationship between protein adsorption to particle surfaces and association of particles can be influenced by properties of the NMs, the cell surfaces, and the environment. Binding of NPs to a cell surface can involve adsorption of the proteins on the cell surface to the NM surface. For neutral chemistries such as poly(ethylene glycol) (PEG) and CH_3 on NMs surface, low protein binding is observed indicating that such groups have low affinity for both proteins and cells. For basic or acidic groups on NM surfaces, two mechanisms of protein or cell binding occur: specific or nonspecific binding could occur. Specific binding is the mechanism of choice for controlled and quantitative processes while nonspecific binding is the choice for quick and qualitative processes.

During specific interactions, NMs surfaces are modified so that proteins attached to the NMs dock within the binding sites of receptor proteins on cell surfaces. In nonspecific interactions, random binding between proteins on particles and any component of cell surfaces occurs. In both processes, the orientation of proteins on NMs surfaces plays an important role in determining the extent and stability of binding. In either case, both mechanisms hold for small to large protein molecules as wells as cells, DNA, virus, or microorganisms.

Under certain circumstances after a protein has adsorbed to a particle surface, lateral diffusion is known to occur.[29] This allows more of the NMs to attach to a bigger protein molecule or vice versa.

4.3 IMMOBILIZATION STRATEGIES

Immobilization of probes in NM-enabled biosensors requires strategies that protect the integrity of the NMs and the biomolecular probes. Proper immobilization techniques help maintain the bioactivity via control of the orientation and conformation of biomolecules. Retention of the active conformations of the biomolecules directly affects both the biosensors stability and reproducibility of signals.[7,12,32–35] Biomolecules such as proteins,[36–38] DNA,[32,33,37,39,40] and whole cells,[11,12,33,37,39,41,42] directly adsorb on various surfaces rendering the activity of the targeted biomolecules or portions of the biomolecules inactive.[39,43,44] Hence, a linker that protects the biomolecule from direct exposure to sensor surfaces is usually employed for attachment or as entrapment moiety[36,45–47] or a covalent attachment on functional groups is usually employed as the entrapment agent.[42,48] With the emergence of NMs, electrochemical biosensing with alternative ways for immobilization of biomolecule recognition probes are now being developed.[42] NMs possess a high surface-to-volume ratio and their network assemblies exhibit porous structure that is a large area of active surface that alleviates surface-fouling effects that causes the enhanced retention of bioactivity. This leads to a large amount of biological molecules (e.g. enzyme, antibody, cell, and DNA) that can be immobilized on the active surface of NMs that allows more intense response signal.[48]

4.3.1 Direct Adsorption

Direct adsorption is one of the ways by which NMs are used in biosensors development. Direct adsorption had been used in developing NM-based biosensors for the detection of DNA,[49,50] proteins,[42,51–54] whole cells,[12,39,50,55,56] and parts of cells.[39,54,57]

The group of Ehrenberg et al.[54] determined the time course of protein adsorption through the incubation of -COOH functionalized NMs in serum. Protein adsorption on the NMs surface took place in seconds and reached a plateau in less than 5 min. Steady amounts of protein were adsorbed in less than 5 min indicating rapid adsorption compared with cellular binding. This relative speed was also reported in the literature demonstrating adsorption rate constants on the order of seconds[53] compared to timescales of at least minutes for attachment to cell surfaces.

One of the materials to which many different kinds of molecules adsorb is gold. AuNPs have found various applications in medicine. Biomolecules such as single-stranded DNA (ssDNA) and double-stranded DNA (dsDNA) can be nonspecifically adsorbed on AuNPs. Double- and single-stranded oligonucleotides (ONTs) have different electrostatic properties that arise as a result of the bonding interactions among the bases in the DNA backbone. ssDNA can uncoil freely to expose the component bases while dsDNA has a stable double-helix geometry where the negatively charged phosphate backbone is exposed and the bases are shielded.[58,59] Gold citrate NMs in solution are stabilized by the adsorbed negative citrate ions with repulsive interactions preventing van der Waals attraction between AuNPs from causing them to aggregate. The phosphate backbone of dsDNA repels the citrate ions adsorbed on the AuNPs creating a distance that prevents the possibility of electrostatic interaction causing the dsDNA not to adsorb on the gold. On the other hand, the bases in ssDNA are exposed and are not repelled by the citrate ions allowing interaction with the AuNPs.[51]

Li and Rothberg[60] documented the selective adsorption of ssDNA on AuNPs. They showed that adsorption of ssDNA stabilizes the AuNPs against aggregation at salt concentrations that would ordinarily screen the repulsive interactions of the citrate ions. The color of AuNPs as determined by SPR that is dramatically affected by aggregation of the NPs was used to design a simple ssDNA and dsDNA sensor using the difference in their electrostatic properties in a simple colorimetric hybridization assay. The assay can be designed for sequence-specific detection of untagged ONTs for visual detection at the level of 100 fmol that can be used to detect single-base mismatches between probe and target.

Wang et al.[51] studied the adsorption of dye-labeled DNA on AuNP. They compared adsorption with thiol-mediated assembly and determined that DNA adsorption on AuNP is simple, fast, and convenient. However, nonspecific adsorption of DNA on AuNPs was highly inhomogeneous and the detection limit was not very sensitive. Nevertheless, it is obvious that the nonspecific adsorption of DNA on AuNPs is highly inhomogeneous, leading to broad distribution of both the equilibrium constant and rate constant in desorption.

The group of Ehrenberg et al.[54] demonstrated the capacity of NM surfaces to adsorb protein on endothelial cells. Quantification of adsorbed protein showed that high binding NMs were maximally coated in seconds to minutes which indicated that proteins on cell surfaces can mediate cell association. They removed the most abundant proteins from culture media that alters the profile of adsorbed proteins on NMs without affecting the level of cell association. They concluded that cellular association was not dependent on the identity of adsorbed proteins which indicted that there is no need for specific binding to any particular cellular receptors.

Their results indicated that NMs surface chemistry mediates their protein-adsorbing capacity during cellular binding. They showed that nonspecific interactions account for a large portion of NMs binding to endothelial cell surfaces. Carboxyl-based surface chemistry that is covalently modified reduced protein-binding capacity that resulted in decreased cell association. In terms of protein binding and cell association, Ehrenberg reported that the least effect was observed from positively charged lysine, followed by neutral groups CH_3 and cysteine, and the greatest from PEG.

Fujiwara et al. recently found that duplex DNA in phosphoric acid form (or in acidic solution) was successfully adsorbed into mesoporous silicas even in low-salt aqueous solution. The adsorption behaviors of DNA in diluted NaCl solutions into mesoporous silicas were influenced by the pore diameter between 2.80- and 3.82-nm peak pore diameters. They predicted that the adsorption resulted from the formation of the hydrogen bond between P(O)OH groups in DNA and adsorbed water, SiOH groups, or both on silica surfaces were the main factors for the adsorption.

4.3.2 Direct Adsorption Protocol

Direct adsorption of biomolecules on NMs may be done following conventional adsorption techniques.[51] The adsorption method results from hydrophobic interaction or electrostatic interaction between the biomolecules and the NP surface. A sample adsorption method used by Wang et al. is described below.

4.3.2.1 Chemicals

(1) 136 µL of 10-µM dye-labeled ssDNA.
(2) 400 µL of 5-nm AuNP hydrosol or to 200 µL of 10-nm AuNP hydrosol.
(3) 10 mM phosphate buffer, pH 7.0.
(4) TE (20 mM Tris–HCl and 20 mM EDTA, pH 7.5) with 0.1 M NaCl.

4.3.2.2 Protocol

(1) ssDNA was adsorbed on AuNPs by adding 136 µL of 10-µM dye-labeled ssDNA solution to 400 µL of 5-nm AuNP hydrosol or to 200 µL of 10-nm AuNP hydrosol.
(2) To this was added 10 mM phosphate buffer (pH 7.0) to make the final concentration of ssDNA 1.36 µM for 5-nm AuNPs or 2.72 µM for 10-nm AuNPs.
(3) The mixture was incubated for 24 h inside the refrigerator.
(4) NaCl solution was added to a final concentration of 0.1 M.
(5) The solution was incubated further for 40 h.
(6) The DNA+AuNP was purified through centrifugation for the removal of excess DNA.
(7) The red oily precipitate was washed with 0.1 M PBS and then redispersed in TE with 0.1 M NaCl.
(8) The absorption signal was measured using a spectrophotometer.

This protocol was used as described.[51] The parameters must be optimized in every situation to suit the needs of the experiment.

Detection of specific ONT sequences has important applications in medical research and diagnosis.[13,20,21,33,40,61–64] In most cases, specific sequence are identified through hybridization of an immobilized probe that is complementary to the target analyte after the latter has been modified with a covalently linked label such as a fluorescent or enzyme tag.[13,33,37,40,61,65] ONT detection schemes

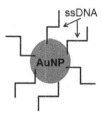

FIGURE 4.3 Schematic diagram of AuNP with ssDNA attached through charge–charge interaction through the negative phosphate backbone of the DNA. *(For color version of this figure, the reader is referred to the online version of this book)*

without analyte tagging such as SPR, imaging ellipsometry, and sandwich assays using chemically functionalized AuNPs have been invented.[13,21,60,66] These approaches involve surface modification, require expensive transduction instrument, and hybridization is separate from detection.

One of the most studied NMs for medical applications is gold. AuNPs are very versatile because biomolecules can easily adsorb through electrostatic interaction. Colloidal AuNPs prepared as gold citrate are stabilized by adsorbed negative ions (e.g. citrate) that prevent the strong van der Waals attraction between gold particles from aggregation.[59,67] These AuNPs have been used to directly adsorb ssDNA to be used to create dsDNA (Figure 4.3). ssDNA has the bases exposed whereas dsDNA has stable double-helix geometry with the negatively charged phosphate backbone exposed. Repulsion between the charged phosphate backbone of dsDNA and the adsorbed citrate ions dominates the electrostatic interaction between AuNPs and dsDNA so that dsDNA will not adsorb. Under these conditions, the negative charge on the backbone is sufficiently distant so that attractive van der Waals forces between the bases and the AuNP are sufficient to cause ssDNA to stick to the gold. The same mechanism is not operative with dsDNA because the duplex structure does not have the bases readily exposed to AuNPs. Li and Rothberg[60] used adsorption of ssDNA on colloidal AuNP solution to create a hybridization assay based on color changes associated with gold aggregation. The assay took only 5 min detecting as low as <100 fmol of target without instrumentation. It can be used to detect single-base pair mismatches.

Titanium dioxide nanoparticles are accepted to be environmentally non-threatening, chemically benign in physiological fluids, and possess good mechanical strength. The titanate surface contains functional hydroxyl groups making it hydrophilic. This titanate hydrophilic surface is expected to provide an aqueous-like environment that facilitates the stabilization of the adsorbed immobilized proteins on nanocrystalline TiO_2 which exhibited less denaturation.[52,68] Titanate nanotubes (TNTs) have been used to develop a reagentless electrochemical biosensor for lactate detection.[69] Their studies demonstrated that the nanotubes formed a porous three-dimensional (3D) network that served as the enzyme support matrix. The negatively charged groups that are present on the TNT surface in phosphate-buffered saline (PBS) solution that could favor enzyme adsorption from electrostatic interactions between the negatively charged groups on the TNT surface and the positively charged surface lysine and arginine residues of lactate oxidase. As a result of this, a large quantity of enzyme can be loaded into the electrode due to the large specific surface area of the individual TNTs and the unique porous 3D network. Furthermore, this architecture provides a friendly microenvironment for the immobilization of enzymes that retain their biocatalytic activity. In their studies, cyclic voltammetry (CV) and amperometry tests revealed that the enzyme immobilized on the TNTs maintained their substrate-specific catalytic activity. This structure formation directly resulted in the excellent performance of the biosensor giving a sensitivity of $0.24\,\mu A/cm^2/mM$, a 90% response time of 5 s, and a linear response in the range from 0.5 to 14 mM.

4.4 COVALENT BINDING

An alternative way to avoid the instability and inactivation of biomolecules is to covalently bind these to spacer or linker molecules that are attached to the NM surfaces.[6,7,11,12,41,70,71] Low-molecular weight bifunctional linkers, which have the anchor groups for their attachment to NM surfaces and the functional groups for their covalent coupling to the target biomolecules, have been extensively used in the generation of covalent-tethered conjugates of biomolecules with various NMs.[72] Anchor groups such as thiols, disulfides, or phosphine ligands are often used for the binding of the bifunctional linkers to Au, Ag, CdS, and CdSe NPs.[73] Various terminal functional groups such as amine, active ester, and maleimide groups are commonly used to covalently couple biological compounds by means of carbodiimide-mediated esterification and amidation reactions or through reactions with thiol groups.[72]

Superparamagnetic NMs as labels or as capture surfaces in biosensors has become a very important tool in research and in medicine.[74–76] These magnetic NMs are especially designed for concentration, separation, purification, and identification of molecules and specific cells. Magnetic separation technology involving NMs is a simple technique based on a two-step process:

(1) tagging or labeling of the desired biological entity with magnetic material and
(2) separating these tagged entities using a magnetic separation device.

The magnetic NMs can be used as the binding platform or linker between the analyte and the label (Figure 4.4). The strong and specific antibody–antigen interaction provides a highly accurate way to label cells.[77] These magnetic NMs coated with immunospecific agents have been successfully used to monitor lung cancer cells[78] and breast cancer cells.[69,74,75]

Hassen et al.[79] reported a new approach based on DNA hybridization for detecting hepatitis B virus (HBV) and HIV virus involving non-faradic electrochemical impedance spectroscopy using modified magnetic NMs for the solid

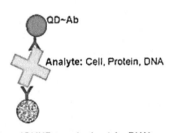

Capture: IOMNP + probe (protein, DNA)

FIGURE 4.4   Schematic diagram of IOMNP that is used as the capture platform in an assay. *(For color version of this figure, the reader is referred to the online version of this book)*

substrate. The 200-nm streptavidin-coated magnetic iron oxide nanoparticles (IOMNPs) with an iron oxide content of about 70% were used to immobilize 5′ biotinylated DNA probes using the strong biotin–streptavidin interaction. A layer of these functionalized IOMNPs was directly immobilized on bare gold electrode using a magnet. Using this technique, the values of Z real measured in the case of HIV DNA detection were lower compared to those obtained with HBV DNA. For the same concentration (12.65 nmol/mL), a value of Z real of 98.38 KΩ cm^2 was recorded for HBV DNA detection and only 15.88 KΩ cm^2 in the case of HIV DNA. This can be explained in terms of the length of the DNA target being 74 base pairs (bp) in the case of the HBV target and only 33 bp in the case of the HIV target because at the same concentration, the value of Z real is an increasing function of the DNA target length. For both biosensors, saturation was reached at the same concentration, 12.65 nmol/mL, because the same quantity of DNA probes was immobilized on the surface of the magnetic NPs. Using non-faradic impedance spectroscopy detected 50 pmol of HBV DNA and 160 pmol of HIV DNA from 20-μL sample that may be a function of the shorter HIV target sequence.

In oncology, NM-based immunoassays that detect the presence of tumor markers are important for in vitro cancer diagnosis. Gong et al.[80] used silica-coated magnetic NMs with modified amino groups for immobilization and separation of human alpha-fetoprotein (AFP), a tumor marker in hepatocellular carcinoma. The system used novel nanostructured rhodamine B isothiocyanate dye molecule Raman tags that gave high stability compared with traditional tags. The system comprising silica-coated magnetic NPs as immobilization matrix and separation tool was simpler than traditional techniques. This sensitive and specific immunoassay for human alpha-fetoprotein used Ag/SiO$_2$ core–shell NMs that resulted in detection of human AFP at concentrations as low as 11.5 pg/mL.

4.4.1 Covalent Conjugation Protocols

Covalent conjugation of biomolecules to NMs may be done following conventional bioconjugation techniques with slight modification.[81] These methods are useful for the conjugation of proteins, ONTs,[69] or other molecules to various types of functionalized NMs[6,7,13,21,66,82,83] that are used for the detection of cells,[12,39,70,74] proteins,[42] DNA,[6,7,13,82,84] and microorganisms. There are two methods to conjugate biomolecules to NMs: (1) the one-step method and the (2) two-step method. These methods are described below.

4.4.1.1 One-Step Conjugation

The following step-by-step protocol is recommended for the one-step conjugation protocol.[6,7,12,41,71] This one-step conjugation is recommended for QDs and other NMs with carboxyl groups on the surface.

Conjugating a protein or DNA or other molecules to NMs must be optimized for each type of biomolecule. An NM to biomolecule molar ratio of 1:1 to 1:50 is recommended depending upon the need of the studies as well as the stability of the NMs. Low molar ratios are recommended for expensive biomolecules.

4.4.1.1.1 Chemicals

(1) 1–1.25 nmol of NMs with carboxyl groups (NM–COOH) on the surface in 100–125 µL deionized (DI) water.
(2) Freshly prepared solution containing 1 mg of N-ethyl-N'-dimethylaminopropyl-carbodiimide (EDC) in 0.5 mL buffer A.
(3) Buffer A: 1.5 mL of 0.01 M H_3BO_3, pH 5.5.
(4) Buffer B: 0.1 mL of 1 M glycine or 1 M lysine.
(5) Buffer C: 3 mL 0.01 M of 0.01 M H_3BO_3, pH 7.2.
(6) Biomolecules (protein, DNA, etc.) in 0.01 M H_3BO_3 (or PBS), pH 7.0–7.4. If the biomolecule is in a different buffer and/or contains glycerol, these must be removed through dialysis, ultracentrifugation, or spin filtration to replace the buffer with H_3BO_3.

4.4.1.1.2 Procedure

(1) Pipet 1–1.25 nmol of the NM–COOH into a low protein-binding centrifuge tube.
(2) Add 300 µL of buffer A to the NMs and vortex to mix well.
(3) Add the appropriate amount of biomolecule from stock solution (a 10-mg/mL stock solution is advised but dilute solutions are usable except that the reagents will also be diluted so the reaction may take longer) and mix well.
(4) Add 50 µL of fresh EDC solution and vortex to mix well.
(5) React at room temperature (RT) for 1–2 h with constant gentle shaking.
(6) Add 10 µL of buffer B and react for another 15 min.
(7) Purify by dialysis, ultracentrifugation, or spin filtration to remove excess reagents.
(8) Wash three times with buffer C.
(9) Reconstitute with buffer C to 4-µM NM or as desired and label as NM–biomolecule.

(10) Run the original NM and the NM–biomolecule in 1–1.5% agarose gel at 100 V for 30–40 min to verify conjugation efficiency.

(11) Store the purified NM–biomolecule conjugates at 4 °C until use.

4.4.1.2 Two-Step Conjugation

Some NM conjugations with biomolecules require the two-step process to maintain colloidal stability in aqueous solution. The following step-by-step protocol is recommended for the two-step conjugation protocol.[85] This step is recommended for iron oxide magnetic NMs or other NMs with carboxyl groups on the surface.

Conjugating a protein or DNA or other molecules to NMs must be optimized for each type of biomolecule. An NM to biomolecule molar ratio of 1:1 to 1:50 is recommended depending upon the need of the studies. Low molar ratios are recommended for expensive biomolecules.

4.4.1.2.1 Chemicals

(1) 1–1.25 nmol NMs with carboxyl groups (QD–COOH) on the surface in 100–125 μL DI water.

(2) 2 mg of EDC in 0.5 mL buffer A.

(3) 1 mg NHS (sulfo-N-hydroxysuccinimide).

(4) Buffer A: 1.5 mL of 0.01 M H_3BO_3, pH 5.5.

(5) Buffer B: 2 mL of 0.01 M H_3BO_3, pH 8.5.

(6) Buffer C: 0.1 mL of 1 M glycine or 1 M lysine.

(7) Buffer D: 3 mL 0.01 M of 0.01 M H_3BO_3, pH 7.2.

(8) Biomolecules (protein, DNA, etc.) in 0.01 M H_3BO_3 (or PBS), pH 7.0–7.4. If the biomolecule is in a different buffer and/or contains glycerol, these must be removed through dialysis, ultracentrifugation, or spin filtration to replace the buffer with H_3BO_3.

4.4.1.2.2 Procedure

(1) Pipet 1–1.25 nmol of the NM–COOH into a low protein-binding centrifuge tube.

(2) Mix the 2 mg EDC and 1 mg NHS and add 1 mL buffer D.

(3) Add 300 μL of buffer A to the NMs and vortex to mix well.

(4) Add 80 μL of fresh EDC/NHS solution and vortex to mix well.

(5) Incubate with shaking for 5–20 min.

(6) Add 500 μL of buffer B and mix well.

(7) Add the appropriate amount of biomolecule [that may be a protein such as an antibody or bovine serum albumin (BSA)] from stock solution (a 10-mg/mL stock solution is advised but dilute solutions are usable except that the reagents will also be diluted so the reaction may take longer) and mix well.

(8) React at RT for 1–2 h with constant gentle shaking.

(9) Add 10 μL of buffer C and react for another 15 min.

(10) Purify by dialysis, ultracentrifugation, or spin filtration to remove excess reagents.

(11) Wash three times with buffer D.

(12) Reconstitute with buffer D to 4-μM NM or as desired.

(13) Run the original NM and the NM–biomolecule in 1–1.5% agarose gel at 100 V for 30–40 min to verify conjugation efficiency.

(14) Store the purified NM–biomolecule conjugates at 4 °C until use.

Although these protocols may be applied to various types of NMs with carboxyl groups on the surface, the conditions for each type of NM may vary. Thus, for each type of NM and for each type of biomolecule, the conditions for conjugation must be optimized.

Figure 4.5 shows a typical agarose gel electrophoresis of QDs with carboxyl groups on the surface, thereby allowing them to migrate toward the positive electrode. The left lane contains the unconjugated QDs and the right lane contains the QD–protein-conjugated QD. The results indicate the retardation of migration toward the positive pole after conjugation which is expected as the surface of the QD gets covered with the proteins. The QD–protein also shows tailing on the gel which is indicative of the different number of proteins that attached to the surface of each QD NP. Similarly, Figure 4.6 shows a typical agarose gel electrophoresis of 10-nm IOMNP with carboxy groups on the surface. The left lane contains the unconjugated IOMNP and the right lane contains the IOMNP–antibody. The gel electrophoresis results are similar to those of the QDs.

4.5 SELF-ASSEMBLED MONOLAYERS

Self-assembled monolayers (SAMs) refer to a single layer of molecules that assemble themselves in an orderly manner on a solid surface. Traditional formation of SAMs may be modified to manipulate NP surfaces for various applications.

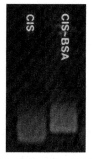

FIGURE 4.5   Agarose gel electrophoresis of QD with and without conjugated BSA. *Courtesy of Ocean NanoTech. (For color version of this figure, the reader is referred to the online version of this book)*

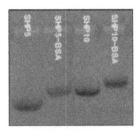

FIGURE 4.6 Agarose gel electrophoresis of IOMNP (Ocean NanoTech's catalog # SHP5 and SHP10 for 5 and 10 nm diameter with carboxyl group on the surface) with and without conjugated BSA. *Courtesy of Ocean NanoTech. (For color version of this figure, the reader is referred to the online version of this book)*

Thiol-modified biomolecules are used for the preparation of nanobiosensors. Thiols, when exposed to metallic gold, form a SAM.[47,86–89] This assembly works on metallic NMs in a similar way.

A novel method for fabrication of a diphtheria potentiometric immunosensor has been developed by means of self-assembling compound NMs to a thiol-containing sol–gel network.[90] In this study, the following protocol was used to create the NMs with self-assembled monolayers.

4.5.1 Preparation of SAMs on NMs for Protein Detection

SAMs on NMs may be prepared following ordinary protocols generally applied to formation on other substrates. SAMs may be formed from thiols or silanes. A general protocol used for AuNP and silver nanoparticle (AgNP) is described. This protocol may be adopted for other systems with optimization.

4.5.1.1 Chemicals

(1) AuNPs.
(2) AgNPs.
(3) 3-Mercaptopropyltrimethoxysilane (MPS).
(4) Aqueous NaOH.
(5) Diphtheria antigen.
(6) Antibody against diphtheria.
(7) Reference electrode.
(8) Gold electrode.
(9) 0.2 mol/L glycine–hydrochloric acid (Gly–HCl) buffer.

4.5.1.2 Protocol

(1) Immerse a clean gold electrode in an MPS sol–gel solution to assemble a silica sol–gel monolayer.
(2) Dip the silica sol–gel monolayer into aqueous NaOH to polymerize into a two-dimensional sol–gel network (2D network).

(3) Reimmerse in MPS sol–gel solution overnight to form a second silane layer.
(4) Expose this gold electrode to the AuNPs and AgNPs for chemisorption on to the thiol groups of the second silane layer.
(4) Adsorb the diphtheria antibody (anti-Diph) on the surface of the NPs.
(5) Characterize the modified gold electrode by CV.

For this particular study,[90] the detection was based on the change in the potentiometric response before and after the antigen–antibody interaction. The potentiometric response for the diphtheria antigen (Diph) was obtained as a result of capture with the immobilized diphtheria antibody. Tang's group established a potentiometric response that was rapid with a linear range from 22 to 800 ng/mL. This method established a detection limit of 3.7 ng/mL. The assay was repeated up to 19 successive assay cycles without change in sensitivity for probes that were regenerated with 0.2 mol/L Gly–HCl buffer solution. Studies using several serum samples were in agreement with those given by the enzyme-linked immunosorbent assay (ELISA) method, implying a promising alternative approach for detecting diphtheria antigen in clinical diagnosis.

4.5.2 Preparation of SAMs on Gold NMs for DNA Detection

A new method for development of a DNA sensor by means of self-assembling compound NMs to thiolated DNA was reported.[51,91] The sensor used fluorescence detection to establish the number of thiol-derivatized single-stranded ONTs bound to AuNPs as well as the extent of hybridization with complementary ONTs in solution. Their results indicated that ONT surface coverages of hexanethiol 12-mer ONTs on AuNPs (34 ± 1 pmol/cm^2) were significantly higher than on planar gold thin films (18 ± 3 pmol/cm^2), while the percentage of hybridizable strands on the AuNPs (1.3 ± 0.3 pmol/cm^2, 4%) was lower than for gold thin films (6 ± 2 pmol/cm^2, 33%). A gradual increase in electrolyte concentration during the process of ONT deposition significantly increased surface coverage that resulted in particle stability. Additionally, the ONT spacer sequences improved the hybridization efficiency of ONT-modified NPs from ~4 to 44%. The surface coverage of recognition strands that can be tailored using coadsorbed diluent ONTs provided a means of indirectly controlling the average number of hybridized strands per NP. This study presented important understanding of the interactions between modified ONTs and metal NPs, as well as optimizing the sensitivity of AuNP-based ONT detection methods. In this study, the following protocol was used to create the NMs with SAMs for DNA sensor.

4.5.2.1 Chemicals

(1) 10 nM AuNP.
(2) Fluorescein–alkanethiol ONTs, 3 µM.

(3) 10 mM phosphate buffer, pH 7, from 0.3 M stock solution of PBS.

(4) 0.3 M NaCl.

4.5.2.2 Protocol

The following protocol was used by Demers and Mirkin[91] in the preparation of AuNP-based DNA sensor.

(1) Add the 10 nM aqueous AuNPs to a 3-µM final concentration of fluorescein–alkanethiol ONTs.

(2) After 24 h, buffer the solution with 10 mM phosphate at pH 7.

(3) Add NaCl to a final concentration of 0.1 M.

(4) Incubate the solution for 40 h.

(5) Remove excess reagents by centrifugation for 30 min at 14,000 rpm.

(6) Carefully remove the supernatant.

(7) Wash the red oily precipitate with 0.3 M NaCl and 10 mM phosphate buffer (pH 7) solution.

(8) Repeat the isolation, washing, centrifugation, and redispersion of the oily precipitate.

(9) Redisperse in fresh 0.3 M PBS.

(10) Establish the AuNP–SAM concentration by a combination of Transmission electron microscopy (TEM), Inductively Coupled Plasma Atomic Emission Spectroscopy (ICP-AES), and UV–vis. The extinction coefficient of the AuNP–SAMs was earlier established at 4.2×10^8 M/cm for 15.7 ± 1.2 nm-diameter particles.

4.6 QUANTIFICATION OF BIOMOLECULES LOADED ON NMs

Surface modification of NMs is one of the preliminary steps in the preparation of nanobiosensors. Complete coverage of the NM surface with the biomolecules and the blocking agent is essential to eliminate non specific adsorption (NSA) of analytes on the exposed functional groups. Thus, it is very important to know the amount of bioreceptors on the surface of NMs before capture of the analyte of interest. The number of immobilized bioreceptors on the NM's surface is theoretically directly related to the amount of analyte that bins with the capture probe. Although, this is so, a calibration curve still needs to be established for each nanobiosensor.

4.6.1 Quantification of Protein Capture Probes on the Surface of NMs

In protein immunoassays, the capture probe that is immobilized on the NM surface can be an antibody, a hapten, or an immunogen. Taking a protein immunoassay for the detection of an antigen as a model, conjugation of the capture antibody to the functional groups on the surface of the NMs is the first step in the preparation of this type of nanobiosensors. To illustrate the quantification of immobilized capture probes on the surface of IOMNPs, an immunoassay for the well-studied mouse immunoglobulin G (IgG) will be used.

4.6.1.1 Chemicals

(1) 1–1.25 nmol NMs with carboxyl groups (IOMNP–COOH) on the surface in 100–125 μL DI water.
(2) 2 mg of EDC in 0.5 mL buffer A.
(3) 1 mg NHS.
(4) Buffer A: 1.5 mL of 0.01 M H_3BO_3, pH 5.5.
(5) Buffer B: 2 mL of 0.01 M H_3BO_3, pH 8.5.
(6) Buffer C: 0.1 mL of 1 M glycine or 1 M lysine.
(7) Buffer D: 3 mL 0.01 M of 0.01 M H_3BO_3, pH 7.2.
(8) Goat anti-mouse IgG (GAM) in 0.01 M H_3BO_3 (or PBS), pH 7.0–7.4. If the GAM is in a different buffer and/or contains glycerol, these must be removed through dialysis, ultracentrifugation, or spin filtration to replace the buffer with H_3BO_3.
(9) Donkey anti-goat IgG–horseradish peroxidase (DAG–HRP), 20 μg/mL in 0.01 M H_3BO_3 (or PBS), pH 7.0.
(10) Tetramethylbenzidene (TMB).
(11) Blocking buffer.

4.6.1.2 Procedure for Quantifying the Number of Immobilized Antibodies (Ab) on the Surface of NMs

A. Preparation of the antibody-modified NM

(1) Pipet 1 mg of the IOMNP–COOH into a low protein-binding centrifuge tube. If the IOMNP–COOH is dilute, concentrate (by magnetization or ultracentrifugation) down to 5 mg/mL.
(2) In a separate tube, mix the 2 mg EDC and 1 mg NHS and add 1 mL buffer D.
(3) Add 300 μL of buffer A to the IOMNP–COOH and vortex to mix well.
(4) Add 80 μL of fresh EDC/NHS solution and vortex to mix well.
(5) Incubate with shaking for 5–20 min.
(6) Add 500 μL of buffer B and mix well.
(7) Add 3.4 nmol of the goat anti-mouse IgG to create a 1 NM:100 Ab ratio and mix well. (Lower or higher NM to Ab ratio may also be used depending upon the stability of the resulting antibody-modified NM. This has to be optimized on a case-to-case basis depending upon the nature and the size of the NM.)
(8) React at RT for 1–2 h with constant gentle shaking.
(9) Add 10 μL of buffer C and react for another 15 min.
(10) Purify by dialysis, ultracentrifugation, or spin filtration to remove excess reagents.

(11) Wash three times with buffer D.

(12) Take 20–100 μL of the IOMNP–GAM and add to 980–900 μL buffer D.

(13) Take the absorbance at 800 and at 500 nm. Calculate the concentration of the IOMNP using the equation:

$$\frac{mg}{mL} = \frac{A500 - A800}{X}$$

where

A = absorbance and X = the factor that is a function of IOMNP diameter which is equivalent to 5 for 15–50 nm and 4 for <15-nm diameter.

(14) Reconstitute with buffer D to 1 mg/mL IOMNP–GAM or as desired.

(15) Run the original IOMNP–COOH and the IOMNP–GAM in 1–1.5% agarose gel at 100 V for 30 to 40 min to verify conjugation efficiency.

(16) Place 25 μL of the 1 mg/mL IOMNP–GAM in wells of a 96-well plate.

B. Quantification of the number of Ab on the NP surface

(17) Add 20 μg/mL of DAG–HRP at 0, 1, 5, 10, and 25 μL to the wells containing the IOMNP–GAM. Add buffer D to make a total volume of 50 μL in each of the wells. Do this in triplicate.

(18) Incubate for 30 min at RT with shaking to form the IOMNP–GAM + DAG–HRP complex.

(19) Purify the IOMNP–GAM + DAG–HRP by ultracentrifugation or by magnetic separation.

(20) Wash the IOMNP–GAM + DAG–HRP with buffer D two times.

(21) Incubate the IOMNP–GAM + DAG–HRP with blocking buffer for 10 min at RT.

(22) Wash the IOMNP–GAM + DAG–HRP with buffer D two times.

(23) Reconstitute the IOMNP–GAM + DAG–HRP with 25 μL of buffer D.

(24) Add 50 μL of TMB to each of the wells and gently shake for 5 min.

(25) Add 25 μL of 2 N HCl to quench the reaction.

(26) Magnetize and aspirate the supernatant into clean wells on the 96-well plate.

(27) Read the absorbance at 450 nm.

(28) Compare the results against a calibration standard.

C. Preparation of the calibration standard

(1) Place 50 μL of TMB in wells of a 96-well plate.

(2) Add 24.8, 24.5, 24.25, 24, 23, 21, and 25 μL of buffer D.

(3) Add 0, 0.2, 0.5, 0.75, 1, 2, 3, 4, 5, and 10 μL of DAG–HRP at 10 μg/mL.

(4) Incubate for 5 min with gentle shaking at RT.

(5) Add 25 μL of 2 N HCl to quench the reaction.

(6) Read the absorbance at 450 nm.

(7) All studies must be at least in triplicate to be statistically significant.

(8) Graph the signal versus the concentration of DAG–HRP to generate the calibration standard.

4.6.2 Quantification of DNA Capture Probes on the Surface of NMs

In DNA biosensors the capture probe that is immobilized on the NM surface is an ONT that has complementary bases to the target DNA (tDNA) or the analyte. Conjugation of the capture probe to the functional groups on the surface of the NMs is the first step in the preparation of this type of nanobiosensors. The following sample illustrates the quantification of immobilized capture probes on the surface of NPs.

4.6.2.1 Chemicals

(1) 12 mM mercaptoethanol.
(2) cy3.5-labeled oligonucleotide–AuNP (AuNP–thiolONT-cy3.5).
(3) 0.3 M PBS, pH 7.

4.6.2.2 Protocol[91]

(1) Add mercaptoethanol to a final concentration of 12 mM to AuNP–thiolONT-cy3.5 in 0.3 M PBS.
(2) Incubate for 18 h at RT with intermittent shaking.
(3) Separate the displaced ONTs from the AuNPs by centrifugation.
(4) Dilute the supernatant by twofold with 0.3 M PBS, pH 7.
(5) Measure the fluorescence maximum at 563 nm and convert this to molar concentration using the calibration curve of the cy3.5-alkanethiol-modified ONT.
(6) Prepare the standard curves with known concentrations of cy3.5-labeled ONTs using identical buffer pH, salt, and mercaptoethanol concentrations.
(7) Keep the pH and ionic strength of the sample and calibration standard solutions the same for all measurements due to the sensitivity of the optical properties of cy3.5 to these conditions.
(8) Calculate the average number of ONTs per particle by dividing the measured ONT molar concentration with the original AuNP concentration.
(9) Calculate the normalized surface coverage values by dividing with the estimated particle surface area (assuming spherical particles) in the NP solution. The assumption of roundness is based on a measured average roundness factor of 0.93. Roundness factor is computed as: $(4\pi(\text{surface area}))/(2 \times \text{perimeter})$.

4.6.2.3 AuNPs Dissolution with KCN to Establish Surface Coverage with ONT

This process is used to evaluate the surface coverage of AuNPs with thiolated ONTs. The process involves dissolution of the AuNPs to release the ONT. Absorption at specific wavelengths is used to establish the concentration using standard calibration curves.

4.6.2.3.1 Chemicals

(1) 0.2 M KCN and 2 mM $K_3Fe(CN)_6$.
(2) AuNPs.
(3) 3'-propanethiol, 5'-fluorescein 12-mer ONTs.

4.6.2.3.2 Protocol

(1) Add aqueous 0.2 M KCN and 2 mM $K_3Fe(CN)_6$ in water to 16.5 ± 1.2 nm AuNPs previously modified with 3'-propanethiol, 5'-fluorescein 12-mer ONTs in 0.3 M PBS to a final concentration of 0.08 M KCN and 0.8 mM $K_3Fe(CN)_6$ at 3.9 nM AuNPs.
(2) Mix thoroughly for a few minutes until a pale yellow solution forms.
(3) Establish the absorption of the excess ferricyanide at 420 nm and of the fluorescein-labeled ONT at 490 nm.
(4) Prepare a calibration curve by adding known amounts of 3'-propanethiol, 5'-fluorescein-12-mer ONT to AuNP solutions of known concentrations in 0.3 M PBS.
(5) Calculate the normalized surface coverage as in the previous section.

4.6.2.4 Quantification of the Hybridized Target Surface Density on AuNP Modified with the Capture ONT

The amount of ONT that is hybridized on the surface of the NMs containing the capture ONT can be established following protocols that may be used for each particular particle depending upon their respective properties. Below is a protocol for the quantification of hybridized ONT on the surface of capture ONT-modified NP, AuNP–thiolONT-dylight550.

4.6.2.4.1 Chemicals

(1) AuNP–thiolONT-dylight550.
(2) Target ONT-C6QD620 (this is the ONT that is complimentary to the ONT on the AuNP; this ONT is labeled with a QD, Ocean NanoTech catalog # QSH620, which absorbs at 610 nm and emits at 620 nm allowing for both absorbance and fluorescence detection).
(3) 0.3 M PBS, pH 7.
(4) 1 M HCl.
(5) 1 M NaOH.

4.6.2.4.1 Procedure for the AuNP-Based Detection of ONT

(1) Take AuNP–thiolONT-dylight550 and combine with equivalent amount of the complementary target ONT-QSH620 (ONT-C6QD620) at 3 μM in 0.3 M PBS, pH 7.

(2) Incubate for 2 h at hybridization temperature based on the length of the ONT-C6QD620.

(3) Wash with 0.3 M PBS, pH 7, two times to remove the unbound target ONT-C6QD620.

(4) Dehybridize by incubating in NaOH at a final concentration of 50 mM at a pH of 11–12 for 4 h.

(5) Neutralize the solution with 1 M HCl.

(6) Centrifuge to separate the AuNP–thiolONT-dylight550 which precipitates leaving the ONT-C6QD620 in the supernatant solution.

(7) Take the absorbance of the ONT-C6QD620 at 610 nm.

(8) Establish the concentration of the ONT-C6QD620 by extrapolating from the calibration curve.

(9) Prepare standard solutions of the original ONT-C6QD620. Generate the calibration curve by taking the absorbance of solutions of the original ONT-C6QD620.

4.7 TRANSDUCTION DETECTION SYSTEMS FOR NP BIOSENSORS

Different types of NMs of various sizes and compositions that are used in optical[21,92] and electrochemical[93,94] biosensors such as enzyme-based sensors, immunosensors, and DNA sensors are currently available in the market. These NMs are coated with polymer or biological coating materials that serves as bioactive and selective interface for functionalization prior to their application in biosensing systems. As discussed in the previous sections, physical adsorption, electrostatic interaction, covalent linkage, or self-assembly are the various strategies for the attachment of functional groups. Since the NMs and the functional groups are both in the nanoscale, when used in biosensors, they are appropriately termed nanobiosensors, biomolecular nanotechnology, or nanobiotechnology.[72] Aside from the physical, chemical, and biological modifications (with antibodies, DNA, RNA, peptides, cells, parts of cells, etc.), the modified NMs characterization and quantification are crucial for the biosensing application.

The size-dependent optical and electrochemical properties of NMs offer various signal transduction modes, including simultaneous approaches (optical and electrochemical) that are not available with other materials.[13,14,92,95] The range of potential applications of nanobiosensors depends on the NMs properties, the biomolecules to detect as well as the type of sample to be analyzed. Nanobiosensors can be used for the detection of DNA, protein, bacteria, virus, and cell analysis using optical and electrical biosensing systems. Aside from optical and electrochemical detection principles[13,14,21,92,95] involving nanobiosensors, NMs are also used in fluorescence quenching, magnetoelastic, and lateral flow assays.

4.7.1 Optical Detection Methods

4.7.1.1 Absorption and Emission Methods

Conventional colorimetric methods have been in existence for a long time. These have been used for DNA, proteins, bacteria, virus, cells, and other biomolecules (REFS). These have been coupled with polymerase chain reaction (PCR), high-performance liquid chromatography, ELISA, and other assays (REFS). Colorimetric assays coupled with molecular fluorophore assays offer high sensitivity of detection, but they suffer from several drawbacks that include complex handling procedures, easy contamination, high cost, and lack of portability.[6,13,66,71,82,83,96–98] In this manner, the use of NMs along with simple detection alternatives such as those based on light absorption measurement is very attractive. One of the most exploited NM for optical absorption detection is the AuNP. It has been used for various analytes including pregnancy tests, HIV, and other clinical applications.

A biosensor based upon AuNPs that were chemically modified with 5′and 3′ (alkanethiol) capped ONTs that exhibited extraordinary selectivity for DNA detection was reported.[99] This NP-based simple colorimetric detection of a target ONT in the presence of a mixture of ONTs that differed by one nucleotide in the target region. The same AuNPs were also used by the same group for a rapid, highly selective, and sensitive colorimetric assay for detecting cysteine.[100]

4.7.1.2 Fluorescence

Fluorescence-based medical biosensors involving various types of NMs have also dominated the literature. QDs are extensively used in fluorescent biosensors eventhough they are toxic. QDs, which are typically synthesized as hydrophobic molecules, are surface modified to enable hydrophilicity and biocompatibility. The strategy developed for enabling biocompatibility is to modify the surface of QDs with more biologically friendly coatings such as 3-mercaptopropanoic acid, dihydrolipoic acid, HS-poly(ethylene glycol)-carboxyl acid (HS-PEG-COOH), dextran, chitosan, or other hydrophilic and bifunctional ligands.

A QD-based fluorescence whole-cell imaging sensor that offer rapid, reproducible, accurate, and long-term cell staining system was recently reported.[12] The QD-based imaging sensor involved capture of whole cells with highly specific antibodies against the cell membrane proteins. The capture antibodies were covalently immobilized on silanized glass slides. The whole cells were exposed to a second antibody against EpCAM proteins that are found on the surface of the cells resulting in a sandwich-type assay. To complete the sensor, QD-labeled antibodies were exposed to the assay complex. QDs emitting at 620 nm giving a red color rendered the cells as bright red circular objects under UV-illuminated microscope (Figure 4.7). The results of the whole-cell sensor indicated that the QD-based imaging sensor exhibited brighter signals compared with those using the organic dye Texas red. The QD-based whole-cell imaging sensor was still brightly visible under the microscope after 1 week. The assay involved only 1 pmol of QD that was used to detect as low as 5000 cells in an unoptimized system. The whole-cell biosensor

 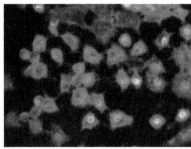

FIGURE 4.7 Breast cancer cell line SK-BR3 (under white light, left) exposed to QD emitting at 620 nm that are covalently attached to antibodies against surface proteins, EpCAM, appeared red with greenish nucleus that was stained with DAPI (4',6-diamidino-2-phenylindole) under UV light (right). *Courtesy of Ocean NanoTech. (For color version of this figure, the reader is referred to the online version of this book)*

using semiconductor NMs shows great promise for application in clinical diagnosis, environmental monitoring, food analysis, and other biological applications.

Total internal reflection fluorescence microscopy (TIRFM) was combined with fluorescent QD labeling into an ultrasensitive single-molecule detection (SMD) method for quantification of DNA.[50] In this method, the capture DNA that was immobilized on silanized coverslip was used to detect the tDNA after the QD-labeled DNA probe was hybridized to the tDNA. The images of the QD-labeled hybridized DNA were recorded with a highly sensitive CCD. The captured tDNA was quantified by counting the bright spots on the images and later compared against a with a calibration curve that gave a limit of detection (LOD) of 10 pM. Parameters that affected the signal included image acquisition, fluorescence probe, substrate preparation, noise elimination from solutions and glass coverslips, and nonspecific adsorption/binding of solution-phase detection probes. Lia's method is also applicable for quantifying messenger RNA (mRNA) in cells.

The group of Wu et al.[101] developed an optical glucose nanobiosensor with high sensitivity and selectivity at physiological pH.[101] To construct the glucose nanobiosensor, fluorescent CdS QDs, serving as the optical code, were incorporated into the glucose-sensitive poly(*N*-isopropylacrylamide-acrylamide-2-acrylamidomethyl-5-fluorophenylboronic acid) copolymer microgels, through in situ growth method and "breathing in" method. The hybrid microgels with quantum dots showed selectivity to glucose over the potential primary interferents, lactate, and human serum albumin in the physiologically important glucose concentration range. The nanobiosensors adapted to glucose concentrations and regulated the fluorescence of the embedded QDs which converted the biochemical signals into optical signals. The gradual swelling of the gel led to quenching of the fluorescence from the QDs at elevated glucose concentrations. The nanobiosensors are well tunable to the hybrid microgels through a change in the cross-linking degree of the microgels. This system is exceptional because of the easy functionalization and the potential for the combination of multiple different functions, such as glucose detection and self-regulated insulin delivery in a single nano-enabled system that can work at physiological conditions.

The size-tunable optical properties allow QDs to act as optical acceptors as well as donors for biosensing based on fluorescence resonance energy transfer (FRET).[83,97] FRET is a process that involves nonradiative energy transfer from a donor in its electronic excited state to an acceptor through dipole–dipole interactions. The acceptor will be relaxed to its ground state through emitting photons or releasing heat energy where the FRET efficiency strongly depends on the separation distance between the donors and acceptors. Generally, FRET sensors require separation of absorption profile of acceptors from the emission of donors to avoid direct excitation.[82,96]

QD-based detection of hybridization and cleavage of DNA was reported by Willner and coworkers.[66] DNA/QD conjugates were initially hybridized with the complementary Texas Red-labeled DNA. Addition of DNase I resulted in the cleavage of DNA and the partial recovery of fluorescence emission of QDs. The previous studies used organic dyes as quenchers, which have promoted the development of biosensing. AuNPs have been demonstrated to be more efficient quenchers than conventional organic dyes. The nonradiative quenching of QD's emission by AuNPs is due to long-distance dipole–metal interactions that extend significantly beyond the classical Förster distance (~6nm). The quenching efficiency strongly depends on the particle size and the quenching constant increases with increase in the AuNP size because the absorption cross-section of AuNPs is the main parameter affecting the energy transfer efficiency. The assembly with QDs as the donor and the AuNP as acceptor is extremely attractive for bioassays.

Nanotube and nanowire-based fluorescent biosensors are also attractive for optical bioassays because of their confined electron transportation along the 1D direction. Chen et al.[102] have assembled a DNA aptamer probe through attachment of thiolated thrombin-binding aptamer on gold nanowires (AuNWs). In this study, exposure of the modified AuNWs probes to the biotinylated thrombin led to specific recognition of targets that were labeled with a fluorescent reporter. Their biosensor was used to detect thrombin at a single-molecule level with a limit of detection of 100 fM.

Novel composite NMs, such as QD–carbon nanotubes and QD–graphene oxides, are among the emerging NMs that are efficient candidates for fluorescent biosensors. Applications of graphene oxide have been reported for biosensors because of its facile surface modification, high mechanical strength, good water dispersibility, and photoluminescence.[103] Aside from the advantageous planar structure that facilitates electron and energy transportation, graphene oxide is also ideal support for NP loading. Jung and coworkers reported a graphene oxide-based immunobiosensor for rotavirus pathogen detection with high sensitivity and selectivity. This sensor was based on the photoluminescence quenching of graphene oxides through the FRET process induced by the AuNPs. In this study, the antibody-modified graphene oxides could recognize the pathogen due to the specific antigen–antibody interaction showing a detection limit of 10^5 pfu/mL, which was comparable with that of the conventional ELISA technique. They used a carbon nanotubes were demonstrated to be efficient fluorescence quencher in biosensors.[69] The carbon nanotube high stability and mechanical strength allow their use in stringent detection environment. They used a hairpin-structured assembly that consisted of ONT-modified SWNTs and dye-labeled complementary ONTs, which upon the complementary recognition of oligonucleotides, quenched the fluorescence emission from the dye tags.

4.7.1.3 Light scattering

Light scattering with metal NPs that differ in size and composition can be accomplished according to their distinct SPRs. Using this property, a DNA array imaging technique using ONT functionalized NPs was reported.[90] This sensor was sensitive, ultraselective, and exhibited multicolor labeling for DNA arrays for the multiplex detection of ONT targets with AuNP probes labeled with ONTs and Raman-active dyes. The AuNPs facilitated the formation of a silver coating that acted as an SERS promoter for the dye-labeled oligonucleotides that were captured with target molecules in microarray on a chip.[104] Multiplex assay for ONT targets was performed with AuNPs labeled with ONTs and Raman-active dyes. The AuNPs facilitated the formation of a silver coating that acted as SERS promoter for the dye-labeled particles that were captured with target molecules on a chip in a microarray format. The assay strategy provided high sensitivity and high selectivity of gray-scale scanometric detection with the added attributes of multiplexing resulting from a very large number of probes that can be designed using a Raman tag as narrow-band spectroscopic fingerprint. Using his technique, six different DNA targets with six Raman-labeled NP probes were detected along with two RNA targets that had single-nucleotide polymorphisms (SNPs). The unoptimized method gave a detection limit of 20 fM. This NP-based scattering technique can be applied to various analytes.

In another study, Qian et al.[105] described the application of biocompatible and nontoxic PEGylated AuNPs for in vivo tumor targeting and detection based on SERS. In this study, signal enhancements were achieved under in vivo conditions for tumor detection in live animals. They exhibited that small-molecule Raman reporters such as organic dyes were not displaced but were stabilized by thiol-modified PEG SERS NPs that were considerably brighter than near-infrared (NIR) emitting semiconductor QDs. The AuNPs that were conjugated to tumor-targeting ligands such as single-chain variable fragment (ScFv) antibodies were able to target tumor biomarkers such as epidermal growth factor on human cancer cells and in xenograft tumor models.

A colorimetric detection method for identifying nucleic acid sequences based on the distance-dependent optical properties of AuNPs is developed by Storhoff et al.[106] In this assay, nucleic acid targets were recognized by DNA-modified AuNP probes by using a scatter-based method that enables detection of zeptomole quantities of nucleic acid targets without additional signal amplification.

In another study, a silver-plated DNA and AuNP assemblies were used for the detection of sequence-specific protein–DNA interactions.[107] In this study, a single AuNP was used for photon bursting in a highly focused laser beam due to the plasmon resonance scattering and Brownian motion of AuNPs to develop homogeneous sandwich immunoassays for cancer biomarkers, such as carcinoembryonic antigen (CEA) and alpha fetal protein (AFP), and aptamer recognition for thrombin. The detection limits were reported at 130 fM for CEA, 714 fM for AFP, and 2.72 pM for thrombin.

Resonance light scattering in a microarray format was applied for the detection of proteins and protein functionality kinase activity.[108] The sensor was based on tagging a specific antibody–protein binding or peptide phosphorylation events through attachment of AuNPs that was followed by silver deposition which lead to signal enhancement. Similarly, Sun et al.[109] reported the development of a new kinase microarray for detection of kinase inhibition. This assay also involved tagging peptide phosphorylation and biotinylation events via the attachment of AuNPs that was followed by silver deposition for signal enhancement. The α-catalytic subunit of cyclic adenosine 5'-monophosphate-dependent protein kinase (PKA) and its substrate, kemptide, were used for monitoring phosphorylation and inhibition. This sensor showed highly selective inhibition of PKA with the four inhibitors: H89, HA1077, mallotoxin, and KN62 with the inhibition assay demonstrating the ability to detect kinase inhibition as well as derive IC_{50} (half-maximal inhibitory concentration) plots.

A protein immunoassay sensor for human immunoglobulin G (h-IgG) used AuNP-based Raman label for protein detection with SERS.[110] They used 2- to 5-nm size AuNPs as labels that were attached to goat anti-h-IgG labeled with fluorescein isothiocyanate (FITC). These modified NPs were used for the detection of h-IgG using commercially available nitrocellulose strip with silver enhancement. The FITC was used as a Raman probe and its vibrational fingerprint was used for the detection of h-IgG at 1–100 ng/μl concentration.

NPs had also been used for the development of an IgE receptor (FcεRI)-targeted, pH-sensitive SERS nanosensor.[111] The nanosensor was used for spatial and temporal pH measurements. The targeting molecules on the NP were used to monitor internalization progress through the endosomal compartments in live cells. The results indicated slower progression of receptors through low-pH endocytic compartments at the lower temperature. The nanosensor was also used to directly measure changes in the pH of intracellular compartments after treatment with bafilomycin or amiloride. The sensors indicated an increase in endosome compartment pH after treatment with bafilomycin, an H(+) ATPase pump inhibitor while a decreased endosomal luminal pH was measured in cells treated with amiloride that was an inhibitor of Na(+)/H(+) exchange. The pH decline in amiloride-treated cells was transient with a recovery period of about 15–20 min to restore endosomal pH. The studies demonstrated the use of SERS to monitor local pH environment in living cells with the use of targeted nanosensors.

4.7.1.4 Surface Plasmon Resonance

A surface-sensitive analytical technique that arises from the collective oscilla-tions of conduction band electrons in resonance with the field of incident radia-tion induced by molecular adsorption at a noble metal film is called SPR.[112] Aggregation of particles results in the shift in the position of the plasmon reso-nance peak which is related to the refractive index of the surrounding medium as predicted by the Mie theory which predicts that SPR occurs when,

$$\mathrm{Re}(\epsilon(\omega)) = -2\epsilon_M$$

where $\mathrm{Re}(\epsilon(\omega))$ is the real component of the metal dielectric constant and ϵ_M is the medium dielectric constant.[113] Thus, aside from colorimetric sensing through SPR coupling in the aggregated NPs, targets of interest can also be detected through changes in the refractive index change that offers: (i) high sen-sitivity, (ii) longer sensing range through the exponential decay of the evanes-cent electromagnetic field, (iii) multiple modes of detection such as angle shift, wavelength shift, and image, (iv) real-time detection at a timescale between 0.1 and 0.001 s for measuring binding kinetics, (v) lateral spatial resolution around 10 μm, enabling multiplexing and miniaturization, and (vi) commercially avail-able instruments.[114] The SPR resonance frequency is a function of particle size, shape, dielectric constant/refractive index of the surrounding medium, the mate-rial composition, pH, and other parameters.[112,115] Noble metals such as Ag and Au have SPR bands at the visible light region.[116] However, conventional SPR sometimes fails to measure extremely small changes in refractive index limiting its application in ultrasensitive detection. This limitation is addressed with the use of NPs such as AuNP tags to increase the angle shift in SPR reflectivity.[57] This enhanced angle shift results from increased surface area, high dielectric constant of AuNPs, and the electromagnetic coupling between AuNPs and the Au film sensor surface. The detection limit of 10 pM for 24-mer ONTs at a surface density $\leq 8 \times 10^8$ molecules/cm^2 was close to that of traditional fluores-cence-based methods for DNA hybridization.

AuNPs attached to DNA was also reported to improve the sensitivity of transmission SPR spectroscopy.[117] This highly sensitive biosensor was based on the adsorption of AuNPs onto gold diffraction gratings. The sensor exhibits enhanced diffraction due to the optical coupling of the planar surface plasmons in the grating to the localized surface plasmons in the AuNPs that were used and applied to detect unmodified DNA at a concentration of 10 fM[118] that was used as a cross-linker for the immobilization of the capture antibodies.

Improvement of nanobiosensor sensitivity using the catalytic growth of AuNPs has been applied in various analytical methods or integrated with enzyme reactions for quantitative detection.[119] But, catalytic growth of AuNPs do not work in some situations, such as SPR and electrochemistry, because metal matrices used in these techniques, e.g. Au, are susceptible to metal depo-sition affecting the background seriously. To circumvent these issues, an SiO$_2$

layer was vapor deposited on the gold film that inhibited the deposition of metal on Au film. With the resulting low background achieved by SiO_2-coated Au films, sensitive detection of DNA hybridization with the catalytic growth of AuNPs was demonstrated with enhanced SPR detection.

Colloidal AuNPs was assembled on the surface of SPR gold chip through 2-aminoethanethiol (forming AuNP–gold chips) to enhance sensitivity in a label-free detection system.[120] Gold-binding polypeptides were fused to protein A resulting in the fusion protein, GBP-ProA, that was directly self-immobilized on SPR chips. h-IgG was bound on the ProA domain that targeted the Fc region of antibodies and anti-h-IgG. It was also used to immobilize antibodies against *Salmonella typhimurium* that achieved 10-fold increase in sensitivity in compared with the bare electrode. The signal enhancement in the AuNPs-gold chips demonstrated signal enhancement of biomolecular interaction. In addition, the GBP-ProA protein allowed for simple and properly oriented immobilization of antibodies onto Au chip surfaces without additional surface chemical modification.

4.7.1.5 SERS Biosensors

Raman spectroscopy is a technique that is based on inelastic scattering of monochromatic light that is usually from a laser source.[121] Inelastic scattering refers to the process where the frequency of photons in a monochromatic light changes upon interaction with a sample that are absorbed by the sample and then reemitted. The Raman effect refers to the process where the frequency of the reemitted photons is shifted up or down in comparison with the original monochromatic frequency. This shift in frequency provides information about vibrational, rotational, and other low-frequency transitions in molecules.

Raman scattering is very weak and it is difficult to separate the weak inelastically scattered light from the intense Rayleigh scattered laser light. But, this has been overcome through the discovery of SERS by Fleischmann et al.[122] in 1974 when pyridine was adsorbed onto a roughened silver electrode. The SERS signal can be enhanced by a factor proportional to the fourth power of the enhancement of the local incident near field with metals that have high optical reflectivity such as silver, gold, and copper. Transition metals such as Fe, Ni, Pd, and Pt that have low optical reflectivity do not serve for efficient SERS effect. Based on the electromagnetic (EM), theory, the size of the metal particles is required to be much smaller than the wavelength of the exciting radiation (Rayleigh approximation).

SERS-based biosensors have some advantages over fluorescent, SPR, and electrochemical biosensors including (i) label-free detection, (ii) excellent reproducibility, (iii) more reliable multiplexing capability because of fingerprinting Raman spectra, (iv) much higher sensitivity, and (v) potentially greater flexibility due to larger pools of available and nonoverlapping Raman reporters. Local electromagnetic field is significantly enhanced at the gap between two particles, the so-called "hot spot," which allows SERS enhancement factor to increase up to 10^{12}–10^{15}.[123] For this reason, nanostructures with sharp or rough junctions are preferable for SERS-based biosensors.

Citrate-coated AgNPs have been used as SERS substrate to determine the sequence of the DNA/RNA mononucleotides in the presence of $MgSO_4$.[124] The AgNPs were directly added to the solution containing mononucleotides without any modifications. Aggregation of the AgNPs was induced by the cation Mg^{2+} and mononucleotides existing at the gap between the AgNPs exhibited the enhanced Raman signal that showed a detection limit at parts per million level that resulted in in situ detection of biomacromolecules.

SERS has been used for detection of chemical and biological species at the single-molecule level.[125,126] AuNP and AgNP have optical properties that make them useful as tags in a wide variety of measurement schemes including SERS in glass-coated nanotags for a lateral flow immunoassay kit.

SERS-active platform to simultaneously detect multianalytes in a single bioassay had also been developed using Ag micropad on a silicon surface.[127] The silicon surface was functionalized with a mixture of three different aptamers that specifically bound to the three proteins: human α-thrombin, platelet-derived growth factor-BB, and immumoglobulin E. After each protein was specifically captured by the respective aptamers bound on the silicon surface, three different Raman reporter-labeled AgNPs were incubated in the aptamer-modified Ag micropad forming the aptamer–Ag micropad/protein/Raman reporter–AgNP sandwich architecture. The SERS sensor yielded a limit of detection of 100 pM.

4.7.1.6 Inductively Coupled Plasma Mass Spectrometry

Inductively coupled plasma mass spectroscopy (ICPMS) is one of the most powerful methods for qualitative and quantitative trace element detection but this technique has not been deeply explored for NMs. Merkoci explored ICPMS to detect the NM tracer for DNA analysis.[93] Not only can ICPMS be used for detecting NMs in DNA analysis, it can also be used as a transducer for protein analysis involving NM tracers.

The possibility of using the large diversity of available antibodies and their many epitope sequences makes ONT–peptide conjugates good candidates for the directed assembly of complex NMs. The DNA modification via peptide method and consecutive antigen/antibody reaction can be even used for developing multiple genosensor platforms based on the same label. Moreover, this approach can solve the problem of nonspecific adsorption coming from the limited available attachment mechanisms such as biotin–streptavidin or covalent reactions used to label the DNA strands. The proposed method is a general one with a broad range of application possibilities offered by metallic labels easily to be detected by the ICPMS technique.[128]

4.7.2 Electronic Nanobiosensors

In this section, several nanobiosensors based on electronic properties of NMs are presented. The electronic properties of NMs are based on their unique size and atomic assembly that can be harnessed for nanobiosensors applications.

4.7.2.1 Electromechanical Detection

One of the applications of NMs in nanobiosensors that are based on their electronic properties is microgravimetric quartz crystal microbalance that is used to transduce the NM-mediated biosensing reactions on the piezoelectric crystals. The amplification of DNA sensors and detection of single-base mismatches used deposition of gold on a 10-nm Au colloid/avidin conjugate label that served as a seed catalyst. The amplification of microgravimetric analysis through the catalytic deposition of Au on an Au–avidin conjugate was achieved.[129] DNA detection all the way down to a detection limit of 1×10^{-15} M was achieved.

4.7.2.2 Conductivity

Changes in conductivity resulting from NMs mediated DNA hybridization or immunosensing have been reported. A DNA detection in an array involving the binding of ONTs that were functionalized with AuNOs resulted in conductivity changes associated with the binding of the target probe that localized the AuNPs in an electrode gap. The deposition of AgNPs bridged the gap that led to measurable conductivity changes for DNA detection at concentrations as low as 500 fM.[130] Using conventional microelectrodes, this system can be used for massive multiplexing through the use of larger arrays of electrode pairs.

A nanoarray for electrical detection of hybridization events has been reported.[131] The nanoarray sensor was used for DNA sequencing with targets that were conjugated to AuNPs. During target and capture probe-binding events, a conductive bridge is formed between the two electrodes resulting in change in conductivity that enabled detection of a few (down to single) hybridization events. This system can be potentially applied to other binding events such as the specific interactions between proteins, antibodies, ligands, and receptors eliminating the need for PCR target amplification techniques.

Direct electrical detection of autometallographically enhanced Au-labeled analytes for DNA diagnostics was reported.[132–134] An online DNA diagnostics at the point-of-care uses online DC resistance monitoring during the autometallographic enhancement process. The system eliminates washing, drying, and measurement cycles by taking the direct electrical detection method. The method is applied in a simple DNA hybridization assay and the analysis of an SNP using allele-specific hybridization that resulted in unequivocal discrimination of all possible base-pairing combinations in the SNP assay. Direct electric conductivity readout resulted from secondary tagging with AuNPs and signal was enhanced with AgNPs.[179]

4.7.2.3 Stripping Analysis

A multitarget detection capability has been made possible as a result of the coupling of the amplification feature of stripping voltammetry when QDs are used as labels for DNA hybridization. This is shown to be a promising alternative for affinity bioassays. Different inorganic colloid (QDs) nanocrystals (zinc sulfide, cadmium sulfide, and lead sulfide) were used as encoding tags to differentiate the signals of three DNA targets in connection to stripping voltammetric measurements of the heavy metal dissolution products.[94] These products yield well-defined and resolved stripping peaks at -1.12 V (Zn), -0.68 V (Cd), and -0.53 V (Pb) at the mercury-coated glassy carbon electrode (vs. Ag/AgCl reference). The position and size of these peaks reflect the identity and level of the corresponding DNA target. The protocol is illustrated for the simultaneous detection of three DNA sequences related to the BCRA1 breast cancer gene in a single sample in connection to magnetic beads bearing the corresponding ONT probes. An effective and inexpensive multitarget electrochemical immunoassay based on the use of similar tags is also reported.[135] This multiprotein electrochemical stripping detection capability with femtomolar, fmol, detection limits is also combined with the efficient magnetic separation that minimizes nonspecific binding effects.

4.7.2.4 Potentiometric Analysis

Potentiometric analysis involving NP-based detection of protein and other biomolecules is another technique used with various possible medical applications. Potentiometric sensors based on polymer membrane electrodes provide electrochemical signal that are extremely useful for measurements in small volumes. Electrodes for potentiometric detection of cadmium ions with a detection limit of 6 nM utilizing a Na^+-selective electrode as pseudoreference facilitated measurements in 150-μL samples.[136] This system was applied in a potentiometric immunoassay of mouse IgG using CdSe QD labels on a secondary antibody in a sandwich immunoassay. The CdSe QDs were easily dissolved/oxidized in minutes with hydrogen peroxide maintaining a near-neutral pH. This potentiometric immunoassay exhibited a detection limit of <10 fmol in 150-μL sample wells. This system has the potential for detection of medically relevant protein biomarkers.

Another method for the sensitive sandwich assay detection of proteins through the use of NMs of gold that were silver enhanced was detected oxidatively with silver ion-selective microelectrode.[137] In this system, potentiometry was used for ultrasensitive NM-based detection of protein interactions. This approach is anticipated for bioassays with attractive detection limits for highly sensitive bioaffinity assays.

4.7.2.5 Electrocatalytic Methods

The group of Polsky et al.[138] have developed a new approach for electrochemical immunoassay sensing in which Pd NPs were loaded onto an anti-TNF-α (tumor necrosis factor-α) antibody to create an electrocatalytic antibody. Gold particles are first covalently linked to the antibody that then act as a seed for growth of a palladium shell. The Pd NPs have proven to be sensitive to the oxygen reduction reaction, thereby requiring no additional reagents except the naturally present oxygen in the solution. Electrochemical techniques like linear sweep voltammetry showed excellent catalytic activity for the Au/Pd-modified antibody toward oxygen reduction. A complete sandwich immunoassay consisting of diazonium–antibody probe immobilization, capture of the target analyte, and immobilization of the NP-antibody label has been used to detect TNF-α. Increase in the concentration of TNF-α results in a cathodic current due to the reduction of oxygen in the buffer. The assay shows detection range with very strong signals at −400 mV from 1 ppt to 100 ppb TNF-α.

In an earlier study, Lee et al.[139] reported a sensitive and selective electrochemical hybridization detection with the electrocatalytic silver-enhanced AuNP approach. The catalytic effects of various AuNPs for silver that were deposited on indium tin oxide (ITO) electrodes were successfully applied for signal amplification of a DNA hybridization assay that can be used for clinical diagnostics. The NP electrocatalytic characteristics were sensitive to surface modifications of the electrode surfaces as exhibited by coating the ITO with an electroconducting polymer, poly(2-aminobenzoic acid) (PABA), as well as avidin molecules, which are promising immobilization platforms for DNA biosensors. The catalytic silver electrodeposition of the AuNPs on the PABA-coated ITO surfaces in the presence of avidin covalently bound to the PABA showed changes in electrocatalytic performance for different types of AuNPs. Streptavidin–5-nm AuNP was used as the hybridization indicator and avidin-modified (via PABA) ITO electrode served as the immobilization platform to enable signal amplification by the silver electrodeposition process. This system led to a signal-to-noise ratio of 20 using linear sweep voltammetry.

Combining Lee's idea with magnetic collection, an electrocatalytic method induced by AuNPs to improve the sensitivity of magnetoimmunosensing technology was reported.[140] This system was designed for the detection of cancer cells through the successful integration of NPs for diagnostics. The system used AuNPs coupled with an electrotransducing platform/sensor made of screen-printed carbon electrode for in situ identification/quantification of tumor cells with a detection limit of 4000 cells per 700 μL of suspension. The cells were selectively detected through specific antibodies on AuNPs that targeted cell surface proteins. Detection required only a couple of minutes that took advantage of the catalytic properties of AuNPs on hydrogen evolution, thereby requiring no chemical agents. The system can be configured as a device that could serve as an immunosensor or DNA sensor for clinical diagnostics.

4.7.3 Other Techniques

Quite a few nanosensors using different NMs are undergoing development. These nanosensors are being developed for various medical applications. A few other NM-based sensors are discussed below.

4.7.3.1 Magnetic Sensors

Magnetic NPs are used as immobilization platforms in various protein and DNA detection systems for isolation, purification, and eventual detection process using a combination of giant magnetoresistive (GMR) sensors or magnetic sensors. These offer unique merits of portability, low cost, fast assay, and ease of integration into a disposable lab-on-a-chip. Magnetic sensors are based on physical effects that relate an electrical resistance directly to an external magnetic field, namely the GMR and the tunneling magnetoresistance effect in ultrathin multilayered film stacks.[141] These physical effects have been intensively explored within the field of magneto- and spin electronics due to their direct translation of magnetization directions into resistance changes and their scalable size that is compatible with standard complementary metal oxide semiconductor processing. Down to a concentration of about 10 pg/µL of DNA molecules, for example, the magnetoresistive technique is competitive with current standard analysis methods.

GMR biosensors utilize a quantum mechanical phenomenon wherein a change in the local magnetic field induces a change in resistance due to spin-dependent scattering in elaborately engineered magnetic multilayer or sandwich films[142] which was first demonstrated for biosensors by Baselt in 1998.[143] Nontoxic paramagnetic particles ranging from micro- to nanosized particles are linked to various biomolecules enabling highly specific biological cell separations as well as therapeutics[144] such as drug-targeting and delivery, cancer therapy, lymph node imaging, and hyperthermia. Aside from iron oxide magnetic NPs, superparamagnetic or ferromagnetic Co and FePt NPs[132,145–147] may also be used for separation and therapeutics. The magnetic sensors for detecting biomolecules are fascinating because the nanoparticles can be moved by applying a magnetic field gradient.[148]

A sensitive circuit architecture that is scalable for larger sensor arrays for multiplexing allowing real-time monitoring was reported for clinical diagnosis.[149,150] They used a custom 1 by 1.2 cm sensor with sensor-to-sensor pitch of 300 µm containing an eight by eight array of spin-valve sensorants. Each sensor has an area of 90 by 90 µm constructed by combining parallel sets of GMR stripes in series to set the coverage area independently of the resistance with the maximum voltage that can be applied limited to 0.5 V to avoid breakdown of the thin passivation layer. The sensor used paramagnetic particles ranging from micro- to nanosized particles that were linked to various biomolecules enabling highly specific protein detection. The sensor was used to detect two blinded samples of human CEA spiked into mouse serum. In a 20-min assay, the CEA in the mouse serum samples were established to contain to contain 66 fM CEA for sample A and 6.9 fM CEA for sample B. The actual mouse serum sample A was revealed to have been spiked with 75 fM CEA while mouse serum sample B contained 7.5 fM CEA showing a deviation of 12 and 8% respectively. In another study, the researchers also showed the use of MNP tags to detect CEA, lactoferrin, and vascular endothelial growth factor with BSA as negative control. The GMR assay with MNP tags were capable of exceptionally sensitive and selective multiplex protein detection in a single reaction well of only 20–50 µL.

In their study, they used cyano silane surface chemistry on magnetic particles to develop a sandwich assay for the sensitive and specific detection of proteins.[151] By using smaller particles, the magnetosandwich assay performance was enhanced with respect to dynamic range and sensitivity but the detection limit was strongly hampered by the high amount of nonspecific background, especially for the smallest 125-nm particles used, which showed the most promising results. This problem was solved by applying a more stringent blocking procedure detecting S100ββ, a diagnostic marker for stroke and minor head injury, in serum samples down to ~0.2 ng/mL over a broad dynamic range (ca. two decades). However, the smaller particles might generate smaller magnetic responses because of their lower magnetization, leading to a tradeoff between MNP size for magnetic signal generation and for assay performance.

Magnetic sensors offer rapid, sensitive, and low background methods of detecting important disease biomarkers. With proper choice of MNPs, significant degree of clustering that could lead to irreproducible magnetic sensor results could be avoided with strong blockers. Furthermore, smaller particles allow for improved sensitivity and wider dynamic range of concentration detected. However, smaller particles may generate smaller magnetic responses because of their lower magnetization showing a tradeoff between MNP size for magnetic signal generation and for assay performance. More studies are ongoing to launch this system for clinical diagnostics.

4.7.3.2 Lateral Flow Devices

NPs have been successfully integrated with lateral flow immunoassay (LFIA) devices or strip tests. The first dry-reagent strip test system using ONT-conjugated AuNPs as probes maybe the one reported by Glynou.[152] The highly specific molecular recognition properties of ONTs was combined with the unique optical properties of AuNPs for the development of a dry-reagent strip-type biosensor for visual detection of dsDNA within minutes. The assay does not require multiple incubation and washing steps in most current assays and also avoids the instrumentation through the color reaction involving the AuNPs reporters with oligo(dT) attached to their surface form an integral part of the strip. PCR products (233 or 495 bp) with biotin labels are hybridized (5 min) with a poly(dA)-tailed oligo and applied on the strip. As the buffer diffuses along the strip, it rehydrates the NPs that become linked to the tDNA through poly(dA)/(dT) hybridization. The hybrids are captured by immobilized streptavidin in the test zone of the strip that resulted in a characteristic red band. A second red band is formed in the control zone of the strip to indicate proper test performance. The sensor offered about 8 times higher sensitivity than ethidium bromide staining of agarose gels. Quantification was obtained by densitometric analysis of the bands resulting in detection of as low as 2 fmol of amplified DNA and 500 copies of prostate-specific antigen complementary DNA by combining PCR and the strip sensor. The sensor was used for 20 patient plasma samples in the detection of hepatitis C virus.

Herpes simplex virus type 2 (HSV-2) IgG-specific antibody LFIA based on colloidal AuNPs has been reported.[153] A total of 359 serum samples and 100 whole-blood samples were tested and compared to those from the HerpeSelect HSV-2

ELISA, and whole-blood sample results were compared to those of both ELISA and HerpeSelect HSV-1 and HSV-2 immunoblotting. The HSV-2 LFIA had a sensitivity of 100% compared with HerpeSelect ELISA. Although the specificity was 97.3% there was cross-reactivity with HSV-1 IgG-positive serum samples, 2.9% for rubella virus, and 6.2% for Epstein–Barr virus. There was concordance of results between capillary whole blood, Ethylenediamine tetraacetic acid-treated (EDTA-treated) venous whole blood, heparin-treated venous whole blood, and serum.

Hepatitis virus B was detected in LFIAs using antibodies that were covalently conjugated onto europium chelate-loaded silica NPs with dextran as a linker.[154] The resulting NP conjugates were used as labels in LFIA for the quantitative detection of hepatitis B surface antigen (HBsAg) with a digital camera and Adobe Photoshop software. This assay was used to detect as low as 0.03 µg/L HBsAg which was 100 times lower than the colloidal gold-based LFIAs and lower than ELISA. The assay gave a linear range at 0.05–3.13 µg/L. It was used to detect hepatitis B in 286 clinical samples the resulted in complete agreement with AuNP–LFIA and ELISA.

Tanaka et al.[155] used secondary antibodies labeled with AuNPs to enhance the signal in an immunochromatographic assay for the detection of human chorionic gonadotropin and total prostate-specific antigen in serum. The colorimetric assay resulted in lower detection limits of 1 pg/mL and 0.2 ng/mL, respectively, in less than 15 min. This research showed that AuNPs can be used for whole-blood analysis using their near-infrared emission.

Aside from excellent sensitivity and specificity, low cost, and rapid assays, LFIA using NPs allow easy diagnosis of various diseases. There are over the counter LFIA colloidal AuNPs for detection of pregnancy, ovulation, and HIV infection. These AuNPs based LFIA are commonly used worldwide resulting in a huge market for nanotechnology-based medical devices. It has been predicted that the market size for nanotechnologies will increase by 10–30% annually.[156]

4.8 APPLICATIONS

Today, there are already in vitro diagnostic products on the market, based on NPs with estimated $780 million in sales for 2004.[157] For in vitro diagnostics, NMs are used for the development of novel sensors and in vitro tests that offer several advantages: improve the sensitivity of existing tests; allow for point-of-care applications, or to develop new diagnostic test platforms. Nanotechnology applications can be broadly divided into two main approaches: (1) the use of NPs as markers for biomolecules and (2) novel sensor platforms that use NMs, such as carbon nanotubes, lateral nanostructures, or nanothin surface layers. A few examples of these NM-based in vitro diagnostic sensors are given below.

4.8.1 DNA Nanobiosensors

DNA nanobiosensors provide powerful tools for the rapid and sensitive determination of pathogens, diseases, genetic disorders, drug screening, and other in vitro diagnostics applications.[158] These provide early diagnosis even before the onset of clinical symptoms. A few nanobiosensors for DNA detection are discussed below.

The ONT-mediated AuNPs aggregation process has been extensively used for the colorimetric screening of DNA binders and triplex DNA binders. The applications of AuNP-based DNA colorimetric methods for disease diagnosis and gene expression have been reported and reviewed.[21,72,73] Because AuNPs have unique optical/electrical properties, various detection techniques have been applied in the AuNP-based DNA assay. A one-step homogeneous DNA detection method with high sensitivity was developed using AuNPs coupled with dynamic light scattering (DLS) measurement.[159] Single-base pair-mismatched DNAs can be readily discriminated from perfectly matched tDNAs using this assay. This DLS one-step homogeneous DNA detection method with high sensitivity was developed using AuNPs. Citrate–AuNPs with a diameter of 30nm were initially functionalized with two sets of ssDNA probes before these were used as optical probes for DNA detection. The hybridization between the tDNA and the two AuNP probes led to the formation of NP dimers, trimers, and oligomers. The NP aggregation increased the average diameter of the NP population that was monitored by DLS. A quantitative correlation was established between the average diameter of the resulting NPs and the tDNA concentration. The detection limit of this facile DLS-based assay that requires no additional separation and amplification steps was around 1 pM, which is four orders of magnitude better than that of light absorption-based methods.

A novel approach using ClearRead™ that utilizes total human RNA as target nucleic acid without the need for labeling or amplification steps for target preparation was reported.[160] In this study, the RNA is hybridized to an ONT microarray and the bound molecules are detected in a second hybridization step using ONT (oligo-dT20)-modified AuNP probes. The second probe hybridizes through their oligo-dT20 sequences to the poly-A tail of the captured mRNA molecules. The poly-A tail is a unique feature of eukaryotic mRNA molecules (except the animal histone mRNAs), conferring an increased stability to the mRNA in the cytoplasm.[161] Even the most abundant source of RNA in the cell which are the ribosomal transcripts, also lack the poly-A tail. The oligo-dT20 NPs used in this study specifically detect only expressed coding sequences. The light scatter ability of the AuNPs bound to the microarray is improved by autometallography which involves a short step where Ag+ ions are reduced to elementary silver that deposit around the AuNPs. The silver-coated AuNPs have an increased extinction coefficient, leading to about 1000-fold increase in the scatter signal.[106] The light scattering is captured with a photosensor of an imaging system (Verigene ID) that has been previously shown to be 1000 times more sensitive than fluorescent-based detection methodologies.[106] Using this method for gene expression analysis, Huber et al. were able to detect expressed genes as low as 0.5 μg of unamplified total human RNA in a 2-h hybridization assay.

A fluorescence QD-based ultrasensitive SMD method for quantification of DNA coupled with TIRFM was developed.[50] The capture DNA was immobilized on silanized coverslip that was blocked with ethanolamine and BSA before the capture of the tDNA. The QD-labeled DNA probe was hybridized to the tDNA and fluorescent images of the QD-based sandwich DNA hybridization assay on the coverslip were taken with a highly sensitive CCD. Quantification of the tDNA was carried out by counting the bright spots on the images using a calibration curve. The LOD of the method was 1×10^{-14} mol/L. The sensor can be used to quantify mRNA in cells.

4.8.2 Protein Nanobiosensors

NMs play very important roles in the development of the nanosensors for proteins because:

(1) NMs exhibit higher ratios of surface area to volume than their bulk counterparts, so inorganic NP-modified interfaces provide larger active capture area for higher detection sensitivity for target molecules;
(2) NMs can act as a supramolecular assembling surface with functional properties for constructing a variety of architectures on the surface;
(3) NMs can be conjugated with some important biomolecules (e.g. enzymes) for biorecognition events.

Biomolecules (e.g. enzymes, peptides, antigens, or DNA) exhibit dimensions comparable to those of NMs, suggesting that biomolecule–NM systems may provide new materials for a new generation of biosensors. These NM-based biosensors possess excellent prospects for interfacing biological recognition events with signal transduction resulting in high sensitivity. To date, there has been substantial progress in the past decade in biomolecule–NMs sensors for protein detection.

Development of highly sensitive assays for determination of enzymatic activities and kinetic parameters is important in the fabrication of novel pharmaceuticals and medical diagnostic devices. Researchers have developed various novel detection strategies that incorporate the optical and electronic properties of AuNPs.[108,109,162–164] The potential application of AuNPs as colorimetric indicators to evaluate enzymatic activity and to screen enzyme inhibitors has been reported.[109] This method can be adopted to screen libraries of inhibitors of endonucleases in a high throughput format by using either the naked eye or a simple colorimetric reader.

Semiconductor QDs had been used for the immunoassay detection of proteins in silanized glass slide.[71] The assay involved covalent immobilization of the capture antibody on the free end of the silane. The capture surface was used to immobilize mouse IgG protein. After washing and blocking open sections of the glass slide, the assay was exposed to QD-labeled antibody against the mouse IgG, QD–GAM conjugates; the QDs emitted at 620nm giving red color. Thus, when proteins were captured on the glass slide, these appeared as bright red colored dots under UV-illuminated microscope after exposure to the QD–GAM. Prior to observation under the microscope, the slides were thoroughly washed with PBS buffer and blocking buffer (Ocean catalog # BBB). The QD-based fluorescent detection of mouse IgG proteins were stable at 4 °C even after 48 h of storage. These preliminary results show great promise for application in clinical diagnosis of disease biomarkers from cancer, heart disease, and from infectious disease agents.

Rare-earth-doped β-NaYF$_4$:Yb,Er upconversion NPs were synthesized and coated with a thin layer of SiO$_2$ to form core–shell NPs that were further modified with amino groups.[55] The amino group was used to covalently attach rabbit anti-CEA8 antibodies that were used as fluorescent biolabels for the detection of CEA. CEA is a cancer biomarker expressed on the surface of HeLa cells that was detected under 980-nm NIR excitation and enabled the fluorescent imaging and detection of the HeLa cells. With proper cell-targeting or tumor-homing peptides or proteins conjugated, the NaYF$_4$:Yb,Er NPs can find potential applications in the in vivo imaging, detection, and diagnosis of cancers.

NMs consisting of aniline monomer polymerized around gamma iron(III) oxide (γ-Fe$_2$O$_3$) cores were used in a direct-charge transfer biosensor for the detection of hemagglutinin A (HA) from the Influenza A virus (FLUAV) H5N1 (A/Vietnam/1203/04).[165] The NMs were functionalized with antibodies against HA and were used for the immunomagnetic separation of HA from mouse serum matrix. CV was able to detect HA at 1.4 μM in 10% mouse serum, with high specificity for H5 as compared to H1 (H1N1 A/South Carolina/1/18).

An AuNP/multiwalled carbon nanotube (MWCNT) layer deposited on Au electrode was used for the carbodiimide covalent immobilization of uricase.[166] Uric acid was detected by oxidation of enzymically generated H2O2 at 0.4V with optimal response within 7 s at 40 °C in 50 mM Tris–HCl buffer (pH 7.5). The biosensor exhibited a linear working range of 0.01–0.8 mM with an LOD at 0.01 mM. The uric acid levels in serum of healthy individuals and persons suffering from gout were measured with the sensor giving 98.0 and 96.5% correlation with the analytical recoveries of the added uric acid, 10 and 20 mg/L, respectively. The sensor exhibited a shelf life of 120 days and was used in more than 200 assays.

4.8.3 Whole-Cell Nanobiosensors

The evolution of NMs is opening new prospects for exploring individual living cells allowing for evaluation of chemical species in specific locations. The use of these NMs could provide the basis for ultrasensitive nanoscale detection of cells. Proper interfacing of biological recognition events is necessary for signal transduction that may involve electrochemical or optical signal transduction. NMs can provide excellent solutions to meet biointerfacing requirements, owing to their tailorable physical and chemical properties by varying size, composition and shape at the nanoscale.[5,167,168] NMs are very effective in sensing of whole cells that includes human cells and bacterial cells for in vitro diagnosis. The unique properties of NMs that exhibit optical, electronic, and other unique physical properties provide effective sensing of whole cells at very low levels

AuNPs have been used as biosensors in living whole cells using SPR scattering images and SPR absorption spectra.[169] The sensor involved colloidal AuNPs and AuNPs conjugated to monoclonal anti-epidermal growth factor receptor (anti-EGFR) antibodies that were incubated with a nonmalignant epithelial cell line (HaCaT) and two malignant oral epithelial cell lines (HOC 313 clone 8 and HSC 3). The colloidal AuNPs were found in dispersed and aggregated forms within the cell cytoplasm that provided anatomic labeling information, but their uptake was nonspecific for malignant cells. On the other hand, the anti-EGFR antibody conjugated NPs specifically and homogeneously bound to the surface of cancer cells with 600% greater affinity than to the noncancerous cells. This specific and homogeneous binding to the cancerous cells produced a relatively sharper SPR absorption band with a red shifted maximum compared with the noncancerous cells. These SPR scattering imaging or SPR absorption spectroscopy can be used for molecular diagnosis and investigation of oral epithelial living cancer cells in vivo and in vitro.

A diagnostic magnetic resonance sensor that combined a miniaturized nuclear magnetic resonance (NMR), probe with targeted MNPs for detection and molecular profiling of cancer cells was reported.[170] The sensor was used to measure the transverse relaxation rate of water molecules in target cells which were labeled with magnetic NPs. The sensor achieved sensitivity improvements by synthesizing new NPs with higher transverse relaxivity at the optimized assay protocols. The nanobiosensor detected as few as two cancer cells in 1-μL sample volumes of unprocessed fine-needle aspirates of tumors and profiled the expression of several cellular markers in <15 min.

Semiconductor QDs have been used to detect whole cancer cells that overexpress HER2, a surface coating protein that is found in breast cancer cell line SK-BR3.[6,11,12,41,70] Carboxyl functionalized CdSe/ZnS emitting at 620 and/or 530 nm were covalently conjugated with antibodies against HER2 and exposed to suspended or adherent SK-BR3 cells. Suspended cells were mounted on glass slides before taking microscope images using a UV light source. The results indicated that the fluorescent cancer cells were detected more easily and over a longer time frame than cells that were stained with antibodies conjugated with organic dye.

4.8.4 Procedure for QD-Based Detection of Breast Cancer Cells

The following protocol was adopted from a paper published by Xu et al.[12] In this paper, a QD-based sensor using silanized glass slide as the capture surface successfully detected breast cancer cells.

A. Grow the cells

(1) Human breast cancer cell line (SK-BR3) that overexpress HER2.[171,172] is used as a model for the development of the QD-based whole-cell imaging sensor. The cell line SK-BR3 (American Type Culture Collection, Manassas, VA) is grown in RPMI-1640 medium supplemented with 10%

fetal bovine serum and 1% of streptomycin/penicillin antibiotics solution at 37 °C with 5% CO_2 at in a cell culture incubator.

(2) Replace the media once every 3 days.

(3) At about 80–90% confluence, harvest the cells with 1 mL of trypsin for digestion and detachment from the flask.

(4) Wash the cells with Dulbecco phosphate buffered saline (DPBS), buffer and use a hemocytometer to establish the cell concentration under an inverted microscope (Leica, Germany). Use the cells during the day of harvest.

B. Prepare the sensor slides

(1) Soak the glass slides overnight in 10% KOH, followed by soaking in 40% (3-aminopropyl) triethoxysilane for 5 h to form self-assembled silane.

(2) Wash the silanized slides thoroughly with DI water and dry under nitrogen gas.

(3) Place 0.2 M EDC (actual name) and 5 μg of anti-HER2/neu antibody on the silanized slide surface.

(4) Incubate overnight at 4 °C and washed thoroughly with autoclaved DI water to remove excess antibody and other reagents.

(5) Expose SK-BR3 cells to the anti-HER2/neu antibody-modified silanized glass slide for 30–60 min at 37 °C with 5% CO_2.

(6) Wash thoroughly with 1× DPBS, pH 7.4.

(7) Place Anti-EpCAM–QD on the slide that was exposed to the SK-BR3 cells and incubate for 30–60 min at 37 °C with 5% CO_2.

(8) Wash thoroughly with 1× DPBS, pH 7.4.

(9) Inspect under a fluorescence microscope (Figure 4.8).

(10) Generate the quantitative fluorescence signal using an Ocean Optics Fluorescence Analyzer (OOI USB 2000).

The cells captured on the glass slide will fluoresce as a result of the QD-labeled antibody against epithelial cell adhesion molecules which are abundant on the cell surface. Figure 4.8 shows a digital photograph of SK-BR3 cells captured on a silanized antibody-modified glass slide. The cells are immobilized on the glass through attachment on antibody that target the cell membrane proteins. The QDs attach to a second type of protein which are also found on the cell surface.

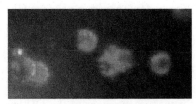

FIGURE 4.8 SK-BR3 cells captured on an antibody-modified silanized glass slide and then exposed to QD–anti-HER2. *Courtesy of Ocean NanoTech. (For color version of this figure, the reader is referred to the online version of this book)*

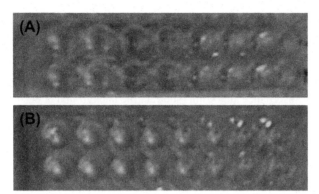

FIGURE 4.9   IOMNP-based capture of proteins from SK-BR3 breast cancer cells in an ELISA using HRP enzyme label for detection. Signal after removing IOMNP ELISA (A) without stop solution and (B) with the stop solution. *Courtesy of Ocean NanoTech. (For color version of this figure, the reader is referred to the online version of this book)*

A quantitative detection of cells or proteins captured on a solid platform and detected with fluorescence resulting from QDs attached to specific antibodies is illustrated in Figure 4.9.

4.9 AN IOMNP-BASED ELISA FOR THE DETECTION OF PROTEIN BIOMARKERS FOR CANCER

Aside from using the NMs such as AuNPs and QDs as signal generator, magnetic NMs such as the IOMNPs can also be used as the capture platform in an ELISA. Similar to the magnetic beads, spherical IOMNPs have a high surface area to volume ratio which allows for a better capture surface in heterogeneous assay. In addition, the IOMNPs do not interfere with the signal detection because these can be easily removed from the detection solution by magnetization.

4.9.1 A Protocol for IOMNP-Based ELISA Detection of Breast Cancer Protein Biomarkers

The following protocol involves the development of a heterogeneous ELISA using IOMNPs as the solid platform. The protocol involves IOMNPs that have been previously used for magnetic NP cancer cell separation.[56] The IOMNPs used in this protocol are 30 nm in diameter and larger ones can also be used for faster magnetic separation.

(1) Grow and harvest the SK-BR3 cells as in Section 4.6.1.
(2) While growing the cells, conjugate anti-HER2 antibodies to 30 nM IOMNP following the covalent conjugation protocol in Section 3.2.1.1 using IOMNP instead of the QDs.

(3) Purify the antibody-modified IOMNPs, Ab–IOMNP, through magnetic separation.

(4) Wash the Ab–IOMNP two to three times with 10 mM borate buffer, pH 7.4.

(5) Establish the concentration of the IOMNPs in the Ab–IOMNP by measuring the absorbance at 500 nm (subtract the background at 800 nm) against a standard IOMNP.

(6) To establish the concentration of the Ab in the Ab–IOMNP:

    (a) Take 1 μg of the Ab–IOMNP and add to 200 μg of anti-Ab–HRP.

    (b) Incubate for 30–60 min with gentle shaking.

    (c) Purify by magnetic separation.

    (d) Wash thoroughly (four to five times) with 10 mM borate buffer, pH 7.4.

    (e) Reconstitute with borate buffer.

    (f) Place in a 96-well plate and add 100 μL of TMB.

    (g) Cover the plate and incubate for 5 min.

    (h) Quench the reaction with 2 M H_2SO_4.

    (i) Record the absorbance at 450 nm.

    (j) Prepare a calibration standard by using various concentrations of the anti-Ab–HRP.

    (k) Calculate the concentration of the Ab in Ab–IOMNP using the slope of the anti-Ab–HRP curve.

(7) Lyse the cells (10,000–100,000 cells in 100 μL 10 mM PBS, pH 7.4) with trypsin or lysozyme for 30 min to release the cell membrane surface proteins.

(8) Add the lysed cells to 100 μL of 5 mg/mL of Ab–IOMNP.

(9) Incubate for 1–2 h with gentle shaking.

(10) Magnetize the proteins–Ab–IOMNPs for 1–2 h.

(11) Wash the proteins–Ab–IOMNPs three times with 10 mM borate buffer, pH 7.4

(12) Expose the proteins–Ab–IOMNPs to 100 μL of at least 2 μg/mL HRP–anti-proteins (the concentrations need to be optimized for optimum signals) for 1–2 h with gentle shaking.

(13) Wash the HRP–anti-proteins–Ab–IOMNPs three times with 10 mM borate buffer, pH 7.4.

(14) Place 25 μL of the proteins–Ab–IOMNPs in 96-well plate.

(15) Add 50–100 μL TMB.

(16) Incubate for 5 min.

(17) Remove the proteins–Ab–IOMNPs by magnetic separation for 10–15 min resulting in a total incubation with the TMB for 20 min.

(18) Transfer the TMB into a fresh plate.

(19) Quench the reaction with 2 M H_2SO_4.

(20) Record the absorbance at 450 nm.

(21) Calculate the concentration of HRP–anti-protein HRP using a calibration curve prepared as that of the anti-Ab–HRP.

The concentration of the anti-Ab–HRP is directly proportional to the concentration of the proteins captured by the Ab–IOMNPs. This protocol is written as a general procedure. All the parameters of the assay need to be optimized to establish an IOMNP-based assay with selectivity based on the antibody attached to the IOMNPs. The sensitivity of the assay has to be established using the optimized parameters that includes the optimum (a) concentration of the IOMNP, (b) concentration of the Ab attached to the IOMNP (or capture Ab), (c) concentration of the HRP–anti-protein, and (d) the incubation times. Figure 4.7 is a typical result of an IOMNP-based ELISA that was used to detect the protein HER2 from lysed SK-BR3 cells. The parameters used in this assay were not optimized.

4.10 CONCLUSIONS

Recent advances in nanoscience and nanotechnology have enabled a paradigm shift in biosensing technology. The use of NPs in diagnostics promises enhanced sensitivity, shorter turnaround time, and possibly cost-effectiveness. This means that NP-based assays may even come to surpass current reigning techniques such as PCR and ELISA. Despite the fact that there are pending regulatory, safety, and intellectual property issues, and the technologies themselves still need further optimization, NPs are primed to transform the field of clinical diagnostics.

When NMs are used as components of biosensors, their unique physico-chemical properties open up new possibilities for the improvement of the sensing performance. The new area of nanobiosensors involves interaction among material sciences, engineering, physics, chemistry, and biology at the nanoscale. Because the unique physicochemical properties of NM, the field of nanobiosensors is quite promising especially in areas that could not be accomplished by conventional bulk materials.

Inorganic semiconductor QDs have emerged as novel fluorescent labels in biosensing and imaging, and are substituting the conventional organic fluorophores. This is ascribed to great advantages of inorganic nanocrystals over the conventional organic dyes. Semiconducting QDs exhibit broad excitation profiles, narrow and symmetric emission spectra, high photostability and high quantum efficiency and excellent multiplexed detection capability.[96,173] For example, QDs with different emission wavelengths can be excited by single excitation source while organic dyes with different emission wavelengths must be excited by multiple excitation sources. Demand of simultaneous detection of more targets in single assay drives the development of inorganic nanocrystal-based fluorescent probes to replace organic fluorophores.[23,174–177]

It is worth noting that, different from the traditional separation between transducers and molecular recognition probes, a novel tactic is to integrate transducers with molecular recognition probes to form nanotransducers that recognize the binding events and actively transduce sensing signals simultaneously.[178]

Most of past research on the nanostructured biosensors was the proof-of-concept work that demonstrated the advantages of NMs and nanostructures. In the future, more efforts need to be made to move the proof-of-concept studies to the applications of biosensors to the real-world samples. One trend of future research is the integration of nanostructured sensors with microfluidics to form lab-on-chip devices. Furthermore, more studies need to be performed to integrate the nano-structured sensors with signal-processing instruments to build portable devices for on-site measurement of analytes to meet the need for on-time (real time) moni-toring the targets of interest and rapid assessment of risks. One of the resulting examples is the point-of-care device that has an increasing need in the commercial market.

REFERENCES

1. Tothill, I. T. Review: Biosensors for Cancer Markers Diagnostics. *Semin. Cell Dev. Biol.* **2009,** *20,* 55–62.
2. Haun, J. B.; Yoon, T.; Lee, H. J.; Weissleder, R. Magnetic Nanoparticle Biosensors. *Wiley Interdiscipl. Rev. Nanomed. Nanobiotechnol.* **2010,** *2,* 291–304.
3. Velasco, M. N. Optical Biosensors for Probing at the Cellular Level: A Review of Recent Progress and Future Prospects. *Semin. Cell Dev. Biol.* **2009,** *20,* 27–33.
4. Fan, X.; White, I. M.; Shopova, S. I.; Zhu, H.; Suter, J. D.; Sun, Y. Sensitive Optical Biosen-sors for Unlabeled Targets: A Review. *Anal. Chim. Acta* **2008,** *620,* 8–26.
5. Khanna, V. K. New-Generation Nano-engineered Biosensors, Enabling Nanotechnologies and Nanomaterials. *Sens. Rev.* **2008,** *28,* 39–45.
6. Aguilar, Z.; Aguilar, Y.; Xu, H.; Jones, B.; Dixon, J.; Xu, H.; Wang, A. Nanomaterials in Medi-cine. *Electrochem. Soc. Trans.* **2010,** *33,* 69–74.
7. Aguilar, Z.; Xu, H.; Jones, B.; Dixon, J.; Wang, A. Semiconductor Quantum Dots for Cell Imaging. *Mater. Res. Soc. Symp. Proc.* **2010,** *1237,* 1237-TT1206-1201.
8. Dyadyusha, L.; Yin, H.; Jaiswal, S.; Brown, T.; Baumberg, J.; Booye, F.; Melvin, T. Quench-ing of CdSe Quantum Dot Emission, a New Approach for Biosensing. *Chem. Commun.* **2005,** 3201–3203.
9. Neely, A.; Perry, C.; Varisli, B.; Singh, A.; Arbneshi, T.; Senapati, D.; Kalluri, J.; Ray, P. Ultrasensitive and Highly Selective Detection of Alzheimer's Disease Biomarker Using Two-Photon Rayleigh Scattering Properties of Gold Nanoparticle. *ACS Nano* **2009,** *3,* 2834–2840.
10. Vaseashta, A.; Dimova-Malinovska, D. Nanostructured and Nanoscale Devices, Sensors and Detectors. *Sci. Technol. Adv. Mat.* **2005,** *6,* 312–318.
11. Xu, H.; Aguilar, Z.; Dixon, J.; Jones, B.; Wang, A.; Wei, H. Breast Cancer Cell Imaging Using Semiconductor Quantum Dots. *Electrochem. Soc. Trans.* **2009,** *25,* 69–77.
12. Xu, H.; Aguilar, Z.; Wei, H.; Wang, A. Development of Semiconductor Nanomaterial Whole Cell Imaging Sensor on Silanized Microscope Slides. *Front. Biosci.* **2011,** *E3,* 1013–1024.
13. Merkoci, A. Nanoparticles-Based Strategies for DNA, Protein and Cell Sensors. *Biosens. Bioelectron.* **2010,** *26,* 1164–1177.
14. Wang, J. Nanomaterial-Based Electrochemical Biosensors. *Analyst* **2005,** *130,* 421–426.
15. Yun, Y.; Eteshola, E.; Bhattacharya, A.; Dong, Z.; Shim, J.; Conforti, L.; Kim, D.; Schulz, M.; Ahn, C.; Watts, N. Tiny Medicine: Nanomaterial-Based Biosensors. *Sensors* **2009,** *9,* 9275–9299.
16. Hu, L.; Kim, H.; Lee, J.; Peumans, P.; Cui, Y. Scalable Coating and Properties of Transparent, Flexible, Silver Nanowire Electrodes. *ACS Nano* **2010,** *4,* 2955–2963.
17. Xianmao, L.; Yavuz, M.; Tuan, H.; Korgel, B.; Xia, Y. Ultrathin Gold Nanowires Can Be Obtained by Reducing Polymeric Strands of Oleylamine-AuCl Complexes Formed via Auro-philic Interaction. *J. Am. Chem. Soc.* **2008,** *130,* 8900–8901.

18. Byers, R.; Hitchman, E. Quantum Dots Brighten Biological Imaging. *Prog. Histochem. Cytochem.* **2011,** *45,* 201–237.

19. Jaiswal, J.; Mattoussi, H.; Mauro, J.; Simon, S. Long-Term Multiple Color Imaging of Live Cells Using Quantum Dot Bioconjugates. *Nat. Biotechnol.* **2003,** *21,* 47–51.

20. Liu, J.; Lu, Y. A Colorimetric Lead Biosensor Using DNAzyme-Directed Assembly of Gold Nanoparticles. *J. Am. Chem. Soc.* **2003,** *125,* 6642–6643.

21. Rosi, N.; Mirkin, C. Nanostructures in Biodiagnostics. *Chem. Rev.* **2005,** *105,* 1547–1562.

22. Murphy, S. *Interpretation of Boulder Creek Phosphorous Data.* 2002, [accessed June 15, 2012] http://bcn.boulder.co.us/basin/data/NEW/bc/TP.html.

23. Chan, C.; Nie, S. Quantum Dot Bioconjugates for Ultrasensitive Nonisotopic Detection. *Science* **1998,** *281,* 2016–2018.

24. Xiao, Y.; Barker, P. Semiconductor Nanocrystal Probes for Human Metaphase Chromosomes. *Nucleic Acids Res.* **2004,** *32,* e28.

25. Lacoste, T.; Michalet, X.; Pinaud, F.; Chemla, D.; Alivisatos, A.; Weiss, S. Ultrahigh-Resolution Multicolor Colocalization of Single Fluorescent Probes. *Proc. Natl. Acad. Sci. U.S.A.* **2000,** *97,* 9461.

26. Parak, W.; Gerion, D.; Pellegrino, T.; Zanchet, D.; Micheel, C.; Williams, S.; Boudreau, R.; Le Gros, M.; Larabell, C.; Alivisatos, A. Biological Applications of Colloidal Nanocrystals. *Nanotechnology* **2003,** *14,* R15–R27.

27. Li, M.; Li, R.; Li, C. M.; Wu, N. Electrochemical and Optical Biosensors Based on Nanomaterials and Nanostructures: A Review. *Front. Biosci.* **2011,** *S3,* 1308–1331.

28. Li, M.; Zhang, J.; Suri, S.; Sooter, L. J.; Ma, D.; Wu, N. Detection of Adenosine Triphosphate with and Aptamer Biosensor Based on the Surface-Enhanced Raman Scattering. *Anal. Chem.* **2012,** *84,* 2837–2842.

29. Tilton, R.; Robertson, C.; Gast, A. Lateral Diffusion of Bovine Serum Albumin Adsorbed at the Solid-Liquid Interface. *J. Colloid Interface Sci.* **1990,** *137,* 192–203.

30. Su, T.; Lu, J.; Thomas, R.; Cui, Z.; Penfold, J. The Conformational Structure of Bovine Serum Albumin Layers Adsorbed at the Silica-Water Interface. *J. Phys. Chem. B* **1998,** *102,* 8100–8808.

31. Onoda, G.; Liniger, E. Experimental Determination of the Random-Parking Limit in Two Dimensions. *Phys. Rev. A* **1986,** *33,* 715–716.

32. Aguilar, Z. P. Dissertation for the completion of the degree of Doctor of Philosophy, University of Arkansas, Fayetteville, AR, 2002.

33. Aguilar, Z. P. Small Volume Detection of Plasmodium falciparum CSP Gene Using a 50-μm Diameter Cavity with Self-contained Electrochemistry. *Anal. Chem.* **2006,** *78,* 1122–1129.

34. Aguilar, Z. P.; Fakunle, E. S.; Fritsch, I. Immobilized Electrochemical Enzyme-Linked Immunosorbent Assay for Mouse IgG as a Model System on Low Temperature Co-fired Ceramic. In preparation, 2007.

35. Richarsdson, J. R.; Aguilar, Z. P.; Kaval, N.; Andria, S.; Shtoyko, T.; Seliskar, C. J.; Heineman, W. R. Optical and Eletrochemical Evaluation of Colloidal Au Nanoparticle-ITO Hybrid Optically Transparent Electrode and Their Applications to Attenuated Total reflections Spectroelectrochemistry. *Electrochim. Acta* **2003,** *48,* 4291–4299.

36. Aguilar, Z. P.; Sirisena, M. Development of Automated Amperometric Detection of Antibodies against Bacillus anthracis Protective Antigen. *Anal. Bioanal. Chem.* **2007,** *389,* 507–515.

37. Aguilar, Z. P.; Van Nguyen, C.; Sirisena, M.; Gertsch, J.Arumugam, P.; Spencer, D.; Wansapura, C.; Aguilar, Y.; Homesley, J. Automated Microarray Technology for Biomedical and Environmental Sensors. In Chemical Sensors 7 and MEMS/NEMS 7. Hesketh, P., Hunter, G., Akbar, S., et al. Eds.; *ECS Transactions*; 2006 Vol. 3; pp 125–137.

38. Aguilar, Z. P.; Vandaveer, W. R.; Fritsch, I. Self-contained Microelectrochemical Immunoassay for Small Volumes Using Mouse IgG as a Model System. *Anal. Chem* **2002,** *74,* 3321–3329.

39. Aguilar, Z.; Xu, H.; Dixon, J.; Wang, A. Blocking Non-specific Uptake of Engineered Nano-materials. *Electrochem. Soc. Trans.* **2010,** *25,* 37–48.
40. Aguilar, Z. P.; Fritsch, I. F. Immobilized Enzyme Linked DNA-hybridization Assay with Electrochemical Detection for *Cryptosporidium parvum* hsp70 mRNA. *Anal. Chem.* **2003,** *75,* 3890–3897.
41. Xu, H.; Aguilar, Z.; Waldron, J.; Wei, H.; Wang, Y. Application of Semiconductor Quantum Dots for Breast Cancer Cell Sensing, 2009 Biomedical Engineering and Informatics. *IEEE Comput. Soc. BMEI* **2009,** *1,* 516–520.
42. Chu, X.; Duan, D.; Shen, G.; Yu, R. Amperometric Glucose Biosensor Based on Electrodeposition of Platinum Nanoparticles onto Covalently Immobilized Carbon Nanotube Electrode. *Talanta* **2007,** *71,* 2040–2047.
43. Buijs, J.; Norde, W. Changes in the Secondary Structure of Adsorbed IgG and F(ab')2 Studied by FTIR. *Langmuir* **1996,** *12,* 1605–1613.
44. Soderquist, M. E.; Walton, A. G. Structural Changes in Proteins Adsorbed on Polymer Surfaces. *J. Colloid Interface Sci.* **1980,** *75,* 386–397.
45. Xu, H.; Aguilar, Z.; Wang, Y. Quantum Dot-Based Sensors for Proteins. *ECS Transactions.* **2010,** *25,* 1–10.
46. Aguilar, Z.; Sirisena, M.; Gertsch, J.; Pacsial-Ong, E.; Narasimhan, P.; Wansapura, C.; Kuzmicheva, G.; Henrichs, A.; Aday, J.; Norman, M.; Aguilar, Y.; Estorninos, L. Development of Self-contained Microelectrochemical Array Assays for Whole Organisms. *Electrochem. Soc. Trans.* **2008,** *16,* 165–176.
47. Zull, J. E.; Reed-Mundell, J.; Lee, Y. W.; Vezenov, D.; Ziats, N. P.; Anderson, J. M.; Sukenik, C. N. Problems and Approaches in Covalent Attachment of Peptide and Proteins to Inorganic Surfaces for Biosensor Applications. *J. Ind. Microbiol.* **1994,** *13,* 137–143.
48. Wu, N.; Li, H., Eds.; *One-Dimensional Nanostructures for Chemical Sensors and Biosensors. Handbook of Nanoceramics and Their Based Nanodevices*; American Scientific Publishers: Valencia, CA, 2009.
49. Fujiwara, M.; Yamamoto, F.; Okamoto, K.; Shiokawa, K.; Nomura, R. Adsorption of Duplex DNA on Mesoporous Silicas: Possibility of Inclusion of DNA into Their Mesopores. *Anal. Chem.* **2005,** *77,* 8138–8145.
50. Li, L.; Li, X.; Li, L.; Wang, J.; Jin, W. Ultrasensitive DNA Assay Based on Single-Molecule Detection Coupled with Fluorescent Quantum Dot-Labeling and Its Application to Determination of Messenger RNA. *Anal. Chim. Acta* **2011,** *685,* 52–57.
51. Wang, W.; Chen, C.; Qian, M.; Zhao, X. Aptamer Biosensor for Protein Detection Using Gold Nanoparticles. *Anal. Biochem.* **2008,** *373,* 213–219.
52. Topoglidis, E. A.; Cass, E., et al. Protein Adsorption on Nanocrystalline TiO_2 Films: An Immobilization Strategy for Bioanalytical Devices. *Anal. Chem.* **1998,** *70,* 5111–5113.
53. Docoslis, A.; Wu, W.; Giese, R.; van Oss, C. Measurements of the Kinetic Constants of Protein Adsorption onto Silica Particles. *Colloids Surf. B Biointerfaces* **1999,** *13,* 83–104.
54. Ehrenberg, M.; Friedman, A.; Finkelstein, J.; Oberdorster, G.; McGrath, J. The Influence of Protein Adsorption on Nanoparticle Association with Cultured Endothelial Cells. *Biomaterials* **2009,** *30,* 603–610.
55. Wang, M.; Mi, C.; Wang, W.; Liu, C.; Wu, Y.; Xu, Z.; Mao, C.; Xu, S. Immunolabeling and NIR-Excited Fluorescent Imaging of HELA Cells by Using NaYF4:Yb, Er Upconversion Nanoparticles. *ACS Nano* **2009,** *3,* 1580–1586.
56. Xu, H.; Aguilar, Z. P.; Yang, L.; Kuang, M.; Duan, H.; Xiong, Y.; Wei, H.; Wang, A. Y. Antibody Conjugated Magnetic Iron Oxide Nanoparticles for Cancer Cell Separation in Fresh Whole Blood. *Biomaterials* **2011,** *32,* 9758–9765.

57. Herr, J. K.; Smith, J. E.; Medley, C. D.; Shangguan, D.; Tan, W. Aptamer-Conjugated Nanoparticles for Selective Collection and Detection of Cancer Cells. *Anal. Chem.* **2007**, *78*, 2918–2924.
58. Stryer, L. *Biochemistry*; 3rd ed.; W. H. Freeman and Company: New York, 1988.
59. Bloomfield, V.; Crothers, D. J.; Tinoco, I., Eds.; *Nuclei Acids: Structures, Properties, and Functions*; University Science Books: Sausalito, CA, 1999.
60. Li, H.; Rothberg, L. Colorimetric Detection of DNA Sequences Based on Electrostatic Interactions with Unmodified Gold Nanoparticles. *Proc. Natl. Acad. Sci. U.S.A.* **2004**, *101*, 14036–14039.
61. Bauemner, A. J.; Humiston, M. C.; Montagna, R. A.; Durst, R. A. Detection of Viable Oocysts of Cryptosporidium parvum Following Nucleic Acid Sequence Based Amplification. *Anal. Chem* **2001**, *73*, 1176–1180.
62. He, W.; Yang, Q.; Liu, Z.; Yu, X.; Xu, D. DNA Array Biosensor Based on Electrochemical Hybridization and Detection. *Analytical Lett.* **2005**, *38*, 2567–2578.
63. Kerman, K.; Kobayashi, M.; Tamiya, E. Recent Trends in Electrochemical DNA Biosensor Technology. *Meas. Sci. Technol.* **2004**, *15*, R1–R11.
64. Wang, J.; Fernandes, J. R.; Kubota, L. T. Polishable and Renewable DNA Hybridization Biosensors. *Anal. Chem* **1998**, *70*, 3699–3702.
65. Ivnitski, D.; Abdel-Hamid, I.; Atanasov, P.; Wilkins, E. Biosensors for Detection of Pathogenic Bacteria. *Biosens. Bioelectron.* **1999**, *14*, 599–624.
66. Gill, R.; Willner, I.; Shweky, I.; Banin, U. Fluorescence Resonance Energy Transfer in CdSe/ZnS-DNA Conjugates: Probing Hybridization and DNA Cleavage. *J. Phys. Chem. B* **2005**, *109*, 23715–23719.
67. Wang, L.; Liu, X.; Hu, X.; Song, S.; Fan, C. Unmodified Gold Nanoparticles as a Colorimetric Probe for Potassium DNA Aptamers. *Chem. Commun.* **2006**, 3780–3782.
68. Tokudome, H.; Miyauchi, M. Electrochromism of Titanate-Based Nanotubes. *Angew. Chem. Int. Ed.* **2005**, *44*, 1974–1977.
69. Yang, R.; Jin, J.; Chen, Y.; Shao, N.; Kang, H.; Xiao, Z.; Tang, Z.; Wu, Y.; Zhu, Z.; Tan, W. Carbon Nanotube-Quenched Fluorescent Oligonucleotides: Probes That Fluoresce upon Hybridization. *J. Am. Chem. Soc.* **2008**, *130*, 8351–8358.
70. Su, H.; Xu, H.; Gao, S.; Dixon, J.; ZP, A.; Wang, A.; Xu, J.; Wang, J. Microwave Synthesis of Nearly Monodisperse Core/Multishell Quantum Dots with Cell Imaging Applications. *Nanoscale Res. Lett.* **2010**, *5*, 625–630.
71. Xu, H.; Aguilar, Z.; Wang, A. Quantum Dot-Based Sensors for Proteins. *ECS Trans.* **2010**, *25*, 1–10.
72. Niemeyer, C. Nanoparticles, Proteins, and Nucleic Acids: Biotechnology Meets Materials Science. *Angew. Chem. Int. Ed.* **2001**, *40*, 4128–4158.
73. Katz, E.; Willner, I. Integrated Biomolecule Hybrid Systems: Synthesis, Properties, and Applications. *Angew. Chem. Int. Ed.* **2004**, *43*, 6042–6108.
74. Yang, L.; Cao, Z.; Sajja, H.; Mao, H.; Wang, L.; Geng, H.; Xu, H.; Jiang, T.; Wood, W.; Nie, S.; Wang, A. Development of Receptor Targeted Iron Oxide Nanoparticles for Efficient Drug Delivery and Tumor Imaging. *J. Biomed. Nanotech.* **2008**, *4*, 1–11.
75. Yang, L.; Peng, X.; Wang, Y.; Wang, X.; Cao, Z.; Ni, C.; Karna, P.; Zhang, X.; Wood, W.; Gao, X.; Nie, S.; Mao, H. Receptor-Targeted Nanoparticles for In Vivo Imaging of Breast Cancer. *Clin. Cancer Res.* **2009**, *15*, 4722–4732.
76. Sajja, H.; East, M.; Mao, H.; Wang, Y.; Nie, S.; Yang, L. Development of Multifunctional Nanoparticles for Targeted Drug Delivery and Noninvasive Imaging of Therapeutic Effect. *Curr. Drug Discov. Technol.* **2009**, *6*, 43–51.
77. Jaffrezic-Renault, N.; Martelet, C.; Chevolot, Y.; Cloarec, J. Biosensors and Bio-Bar Code Assays Based on Biofunctionalized Magnetic Microbeads. *Sensors* **2007**, *7*, 589–614.

78. Kularatne, B.; Lorigan, P.; Browne, S.; Suvarna, S.; Smith, M.; Lawry, J. Monitoring Tumour Cells in the Peripheral Blood of Small Cell Lung Cancer Patients. *Cytometry* **2002**, *50*, 160–167.

79. Hassen, W.; Chaix, C.; Abdelghani, A.; Bessueille, F.; Leonard, D.; Jaffrezic-renault, N. An Impedimetric DNA Sensor Based on Functionalized Magnetic Nanoparticles for HIV and HBV Detection. *Sens. Actuators B Chem.* **2008**, *134*, 755–760.

80. Gong, J.; Liang, Y.; Huang, Y.; Chen, J.; Jiang, J.; Shen, G.; Yu, R. Ag/SiO(2) Core-Shell Nanoparticle-Based Surface-Enhanced Raman Probes for Immunoassay of Cancer Marker Using Silica-Coated Magnetic Nanoparticles as Separation Tools. *Biosens. Bioelectron.* **2006**, *22*, 1501–1507.

81. Hermanson, G. T. In *Bioconjugate Techniques*; Academic Press, Inc.: San Diego, CA, 1996; pp 169–173.

82. Clapp, A.; Medintz, I.; Mauro, J.; Fisher, B.; Bawendi, M.; Mattoussi, h Fluorescence Resonance Energy Transfer between Quantum Dot Donors and Dye-Labeled Protein Acceptors. *J. Am. Chem. Soc.* **2004**, *126*, 301–310.

83. Dennis, A.; Bao, G. Quantum Dot-Fluorescent Protein Pairs as Novel Fluorescence Resonance Energy Transfer Probes. *Nano. Lett.* **2008**, *8*, 1439–1445.

84. Du, P.; Li, H.; Mei, Z.; Liu, S. Electrochemical DNA Biosensor for the Detection of DNA Hybridization with the Amplification of Au Nanoparticles and CdS Nanoparticles. *Bioelectrochemistry* **2009**, *75*, 37–43.

85. Ehrenberg, M.; McGrath, J. Binding between Particles and Proteins in Extracts: implications for Microrheology and Toxicity. *Acta Biomater.* **2005**, *1*, 305–315.

86. Badia, A.; Singh, S.; Demers, L.; Cuccia, L.; Brown, G. R.; Lennox, R. B. Self-assembled Monolayers on Gold Nanoparticles. *Chem. Eur. J.* **1996**, *2*, 359–363.

87. Gooding, J.; Hibbert, D. B. The Application of Alkanethiol Self-assembled Monolayers to Enzyme Electrodes. *Trends Anal. Chem.* **1999**, *18*, 525–533.

88. Mrksich, M.; Whitesides, G. M. Using Self-Assembled Monolayers to Understand the Interactions of Man-Made Surfaces with Proteins and Cells. *Annu. Rev. Biophys. Biomol. Struct* **1996**, *25*, 55–78.

89. Zhang, Y.; Terrill, R. H.; Tanzer, T. A.; Bohn, P. W. Ozonolysis is the Primary Cause of UV Photooxidation of Alkanethiolate Monolayers at Low Irradiance. *J. Am. Chem. Soc.* **1998**, *120*, 2654–2655.

90. Tang, D.; Yuan, R.; Chai, Y.; Liu, Y.; Dai, J.; Zhong, X. Novel Potentiometric Immunosensor for Diphtheria Antigen Based on Compound Nanoparticles and Bilayer Two Dimensional Sol-Gel as Matrices. *Anal. Bioanal. Chem.* **2005**, *381*, 674–680.

91. Demers, L.; Mirkin, C.; Mucic, R.; Reynolds, R.; Letsinger, R.; Elghanian, R.; Viswanadham, G. A Fluorescence-Based Method for Determining the Surface Coverage and Hybridization Efficiency of Thiol-Capped Oligonucleotides Bound to Gold Thin Films and Nanoparticles. *Anal. Chem.* **2000**, *72*, 5535–5541.

92. Merkoci, A. Elecrochemical Biosensing with Nanoparticles. *FEBS J* **2007**, *274*, 310–316.

93. Merkoci, A.; Aldavert, M.; Tarrasón, G.; Eritja, R.; Alegret, S. Toward an ICPMS-Linked DNA Assay Based on Gold Nanoparticles Immunoconnected through Peptide Sequences. *Anal. Chem.* **2005**, *77*, 6500–6503.

94. Wang, J. Nanoparticle-Based Electrochemical DNA Detection. *Anal. Chim. Acta* **2003**, *500*, 247–257.

95. Ambrosi, A.; Castaneda, M.; Killard, A.; Smyth, M.; Alegret, S.; Merkoci, A. Double-Codified Gold Nanolabels for Enhanced Immunoanalysis. *Anal. Chem.* **2007**, *79*, 5232–5240.

96. Medintz, I.; Clapp, A.; Mattoussi, H.; Goldman, E.; Fisher, B.; Mauro, J. Self-assembled Nanoscale Biosensors Based on Quantum Dot FRET Donors. *Nat. Mater.* **2003**, *2*, 630–638.

97. Roy, R.; Hohng, S.; Ha, T. A Practical Guide to Single-Molecule FRET. *Nat. Methods* **2008,** *5,* 507–516.

98. Li, J.; Zhao, X.; Zhao, Y.; Gu, Z. Quantum-Dot-Coated Encoded Silica Colloidal Crystals Beads for Multiplex Coding. *Chem. Commun.* **2009,** 2329–2331.

99. Storhoff, J. J.; Elghanian, R.; Mucic, R. C.; Mirkin, C. A.; Lertsinger, R. L. One-Pot Colorimetric Differentiation of Polynucleotides with Imperfections Using Gold Nanoparticle Probes. *J. Am. Chem. Soc.* **1998,** *120,* 1959–1964.

100. Lee, J.; Ulmann, P. A.; Han, M. S.; Mirkin, C. A. A DNA-Gold Nanoparticle-Based Colorimetric Competition Assay Detection of Cysteine. *Nano Lett.* **2008,** *8,* 529–533.

101. Wu, W.; Zhou, T.; Aiello, M.; Zhou, S. Construction of Optical Glucose Nanobiosensor with High Sensitivity and Selectivity at Physiological pH on the Basis of Organic-Inorganic Hybrid Microgels. *Biosens. Bioelectron.* **2010,** *25,* 2603–2610.

102. Huang, S.; Chen, Y. Ultrasensitive Fluorescence Detection of Single Protein Molecules Manipulated Electrically on Au Nanowire. *Nano Lett.* **2008,** *8,* 2829–2833.

103. Jung, J.; Cheon, D.; Liu, F.; Lee, K.; Seo, T. A Graphene Oxide Based Immuno-biosensor for Pathogen Detection. *Angew. Chem. Int. Ed.* **2010,** *49,* 1–5.

104. Cao, Y.; Jin, R.; Mirkin, C. Nanoparticles with Raman Spectroscopic Fingerprints for DNA and RNA Detection. *Science* **2002,** *297,* 1536–1540.

105. Qian, X.; Peng, X. -H.; Ansari, D. O.; Yin-Goen, Q.; Chen, G. Z.; Shin, D. M.; Yang, L.; Young, A. N.; Wang, M. D.; Nie, S. In Vivo Tumor Targeting and Spectroscopic Detection with Surface-Enhanced Raman Nanoparticle Tags. *Nat. Biotech.* **2008,** *26,* 83–90.

106. Storhoff, J. J.; Marla, S. S.; Bao, P.; Hagenow, S.; Mehta, H.; Lucas, A.; Garimella, V.; Patno, T. J.; Buckingham, W.; Cork, W. H., et al. Gold Nanoparticle-Based Detection of Genomic DNA Targets on Microarrays Using a Novel Optical Detection System. *Biosens. Bioelectron.* **2004,** *19,* 875–883.

107. Bonham, A. J.; Braun, G.; Pavel, I.; Moskovits, M.; Reich, N. Detection of Sequence-Specific Protein-DNA Interactions via Surface Enhanced Resonance Raman Scattering. *J. Am. Chem. Soc.* **2007,** *129,* 14572–14573.

108. Wang, Z.; Levy, R.; Fernig, D.; Brust, M. Kinase-Catalyzed Modification of Gold Nanoparticles: A New Approach to Colorimetric Kinase Activity Screening. *J. Am. Chem. Soc.* **2006,** *128,* 2214–2215.

109. Sun, L.; Liu, D.; Wang, Z. Microarray-Based Kinase Inhibition Activity by Gold Nanoparticle Probes. *Anal. Chem.* **2007,** *79,* 773–777.

110. Manimaran, M.; Jana, N. R. Detection of Protein Molecules by Surface-Enhanced Raman Spectroscopy-Based Immunoassay Using 2-5 nm Gold Nanoparticle Labels. *J. Raman Spec.* **2007,** *38,* 1326–1331.

111. Nowak-Lovato, K. L.; Wilson, B. S.; Rector, K. D. SERS Nanosensors That Report the pH of Endocytic Compartments During FceRI Transit. *Anal. Bioanal. Chem.* **2010,** *398,* 2019–2029.

112. Murphy, C. J.; Gole, A. M.; Hunyadi, S. E.; Stone, J. W.; Sisco, P. N.; Alkilany, A.; Kinard, B. E.; Hankins, P. Chemical Sensing and Imaging with Metallic Nanorods. *Chem. Commun.* **2008,** 544–557.

113. Le Ru, E. C.; Etchegoin, P. G. *Principles of Surface-Enhanced Raman Spectroscopy and Related Plasmonic Effects;* Elsevier, 2009.

114. Haes, J. A.; Van Duyne, R. P. A Unified View of Propagating and Localized Surface Plasmon Resonance Biosensors. *Anal. Bioanal. Chem.* **2004,** *379,* 920–930.

115. Live, L. S.; Bolduc, O. R.; Masson, J. -F. Propagating Surface Plasmon Resonance on Micro-hole Arrays. *Anal. Chem.* **2010,** *82,* 3780–3787.

116. Liz-Marzán, L. M. Tailoring Surface Plasmons through the Morphology and Assembly of Metal Nanoparticles. *Langmuir* **2006,** *22,* 32–41.

117. Hutter, E.; Pileni, M. P. Detection of DNA Hybridization by Gold Nanoparticle Enhanced Transmission Surface Plasmon Resonance Spectroscopy. *J. Phys. Chem. B* **2003,** *107,* 6497–6499.

118. Wark, A. W.; Lee, H. J.; Qavi, A. J.; Corn, R. M. Nanoparticle-Enhanced Diffraction Gratings for Ultrasensitive Surface Plasmon Biosensing. *Anal. Chem.* **2007,** *79,* 6697–6701.

119. Yang, X.; Wang, Q.; Wang, K.; Tan, W.; Li, H. Enhanced Surface Plasmon Resonance with the Modified Catalytic Growth of Au Nanoparticles. *Biosens. Bioelectron.* **2007,** *22,* 1106–1110.

120. Ko, S.; Park, T. J. Directed Self-assembly of Gold Binding Polypeptide-Protein A Fusion for Development of Gold Nanoparticle-Based SPR Immunosensors. *Biosens. Bioelectron.* **2009,** *24,* 2592–2597.

121. Princeton. Raman Spectroscopy Basics. http://content.piacton.com/Uploads/Princeton/Documents/Library/UpdatedLibrary/Raman_Spectroscopy_Basics.pdf. (accessed May 26, 2011).

122. Fleischmann, M.; Hendra, P. J.; McQuillan, A. J. Raman Spectra of Pyridine Adsorbed at a Silver Electrode. *Chem. Phys. Lett.* **1974,** *26,* 163–166.

123. Jackson, J. B.; Halas, N. J. Surface-Enhanced Raman Scattering on Tunable Plasmonic Nanoparticle Substrates. *Proc. Natl. Acad. Sci. U.S.A.* **2004,** *101,* 17930–17935.

124. Bell, S. E. J.; NarayanaSirimuthu, N. M. S. Surface-Enhanced Raman Spectroscopy (SERS) for Sub-Micromolar Detection of DNA/RNA Mononucleotides. *J. Am. Chem. Soc.* **2006,** *128,* 15580–15581.

125. Doering, W. E.; Piotti, M. E.; Natan, M. J.; Freeman, R. G. SERS as a Foundation for Nanoscale, Optically Detected Biological Labels. *Adv. Mater.* **2007,** *19,* 3100–3108.

126. Nie, S.; Emory, S. R. Probing Single Molecules and Single Nanoparticles by Surface-Enhanced Raman Scattering. *Science* **1997,** *275,* 1102–1106.

127. Fabris, L.; Schierhorn, M.; Moskovits, M.; Bazan, G. C. Aptatag-Based Multiplexed Assay for Protein Detection by Surface-Enhanced Raman Spectroscopy. *Small* **2010,** *14,* 1550–1557.

128. Allabashi, R.; Stach, W.; de la Escosura-Muniz, A.; Liste-Calleja, L.; Merkoci, A. ICP-MS: A Powerful Technique for Quantitative Determination of Gold Nanoparticles without Previous Dissolving. *J. Nanoparticle Res.* **2008,** *11,* 2003–2011.

129. Weizmann, Y.; Patolsky, F.; Willner, I. Amplified Detection of DNA and Analysis of Single-Base Mismatches by the Catalyzed Deposition of Gold on Au-Nanoparticles. *Analyst* **2001,** *126,* 1502–1504.

130. Park, S. -J.; Taton, T. A.; Mirkin, C. A. Array-Based Electrical Detection of DNA with Nanoparticle Probes. *Science* **2002,** *295,* 1503–1506.

131. Maruccio, G.; Primiceri, E.; Marzo, P.; Arima, V.; Torre, A. D.; Rinaldi, R.; Pellegrino, T.; Krahne, R.; Cingolani, R. A Nanobiosensor to Detect Single Hybridization Events. *Analyst* **2009,** *134,* 2458–2461.

132. Puntes, V. F.; Krishnan, K. M.; Alivisatos, A. P. Colloidal Nanocrystal Shape and Size Control: The Case of Cobalt. *Science* **2001,** *291,* 2115–2117.

133. Bonham, A. J.; Braun, G.; Pavel, I.; Moskovits, M.; Reich, N. Detection of Sequence-Specific Protein-DNA Interactions via Surface Enhanced Resonance Raman Scattering. *J. Am. Chem. Soc.* **2007,** *129,* 14572–14573.

134. Diessel, E.; Grothe, K.; Siebert, H. -M.; Warner, B. D.; Burmeister, J. Online Resistance Monitoring during Autometallographic Enhancement of Colloidal Au Labels for DNA Analysis. *Biosens. Bioelectron.* **2004,** *19,* 1229–1235.

135. Liu, G.; Wang, J.; Kim, J.; Jan, M. R.; Collins, G. E. Electrochemical Coding for Multiplexed Immunoassays of Proteins. *Anal. Chem.* **2004,** *76,* 7126–7130.

136. Thuurer, R.; Vigassy, T.; Hirayaman, M.; Wang, J.; Bakker, E.; Pretsch, E. Potentiometric Immunoassay with Quantum Dots. *Anal. Chem.* **2008,** *80,* 707–712.

137. Chumbimuni-Torres, K. Y.; Dai, Z.; Rubinova, N.; Xiang, Y.; Pretsch, E.; Wang, J.; Bakker, E. Potentiometric Biosensing of Proteins with Ultrasensitive Ion-Selective Microelectrodes and Nanoparticles Labels. *J. Am. Chem. Soc.* **2006,** *128,* 13676–13677.

138. Polsky, R.; Harper, J. C.; Wheeler, D. R.; Dirk, S. M.; Rawlings, J. A.; Brozik, S. M. Reagent-Less Electrochemical Immunoassay Using Electrocatalytic Nanoparticle-Modified Antibodies. *Chem. Commun.* **2007,** 2741–2743.

139. Lee, T. M. H.; Cai, H.; Hsing, I. M. Effects of Gold Nanoparticle and Electrode Surface Properties on Electrocatalytic Silver Deposition for Electrochemical DNA Hybridization Detection. *Analyst* **2005,** *130,* 364–369.

140. de la E.scosura-Miniz, A.; Diaz-Freitas, B.; Sanchez-ESpinel, C.; Gonzalez-Fernandez, A.; Merkoci, A. Rapid Identification and Quantification of Tumour Cells Using a Novel Electrocatalytic Method Based in Gold Nanoparticles. *Anal. Chem.* **2009,** *81,* 10268–10274.

141. Reiss, G.; Brueckl, H.; Huetten, A.; Schotter, J.; Brzeska, M.; Panhorst, M.; Sudfeld, D. Magnetoresistive Sensors and Magnetic Nanoparticles for Biotechnology. *J. Mater. Res.* **2005,** *20,* 3294–3302.

142. Hall, D. A.; Gaster, R. S.; Lin, T.; Osterfeld, S. J.; Han, S.; Murmann, B.; Wang, S. X. GMR Biosensor Arrays: A System Perspective. *Biosens. Bioelectron.* **2010,** *25,* 2051–2057.

143. Baselt, D. R.; Lee, G. U.; Natesan, M.; Metzger, S. W.; Sheehan, P. E.; Colton, R. J. A Biosensor Based on Magnetoresistance Technology. *Biosens. Bioelectron.* **1998,** *13,* 731–749.

144. Hafeli, U.; Schutt, W.; Teller, J., Eds.; *Scientific and Clinical Applications of Magnetic Carriers*; Plenum: New York, 1997.

145. Murray, C. B.; Sun, S.; Gaschler, W.; Doyle, H.; Betley, T. A.; Kagan, C. R. Colloidal Synthesis of Nanocrystals and Nanocrystal Superlattices. *IBM J. Res. Dev.* **2001,** *45,* 47–56.

146. Dinega, D. P.; Bawendi, M. G. A Solution-Phase Chemical Approach to a New Crystal Structure of Cobalt. *Angew. Chem. Int. Ed.* **1999,** 1906–1909.

147. Sun, S.; Murray, C. B.; Weller, D.; Folks, L.; Moser, A. Monodisperse FePt Nanoparticles and Ferromagnetic FePt Nanocrystal Superlattices. *Science* **2000,** *287,* 1989–1992.

148. Brzeska, M.; Panhorst, M.; Kamp, P. B.; Schotter, J.; Reiss, G.; Pühler, A.; Becker, A.; Brückl, H. Detection and Manipulation of Biomolecules by Magnetic Carriers. *J. Biotechnol* **2004,** *112,* 25–33.

149. Gaster, R. S.; Hall, D. A.; Nielsen, C. H.; Osterfeld, S. J.; Yu, H.; Mach, K. E.; Wilson, R. J.; Murmann, B.; Liao, J. C.; Gambhir, S. S.; Wang, S. X. Matrix-Insensitive Protein Assays Push the Limits of Biosensors in Medicine. *Nat. Med.* **2009,** *15,* 1327–1332.

150. Osterfeld, S. J.; Yu, H.; Gaster, R. S.; Caramuta, S.; Xu, L.; Han, S.; Hall, D. A.; Wilson, R. J.; Sun, S.; White, R. L.; Davis, R. W.; Pourmand, N.; Wang, S. X. Multiplex Protein Assays Based on Real-Time Magnetic Nanotag Sensing. *Proc. Natl. Acad. Sci. U.S.A.* **2008,** *105,* 20637–20640.

151. De Palma, R.; Reekmans, G.; Laureyn, W.; Borghs, G.; Maes, G. The Optimization of Magnetosandwich Assays for the Sensitive and Specific Detection of Proteins in Serum. *Anal. Chem.* **2007,** *79,* 7540–7548.

152. Glynou, K.; Loannou, P. C.; Christopoulos, T. K.; Syriopoulou, V. Oligonucleotide-Functionalized Gold Nanoparticles as Probes in a Dry-Reagent Strip Biosensor for DNA Analysis by Hybridization. *Anal. Chem.* **2003,** *75,* 4155–4160.

153. Laderman, E. I.; Whitworth, E.; Dumaual, E.; Jones, M.; Hudak, A.; Hogerefe, W.; Carney, J.; Groen, J. Rapid, Sensitive, and Specific Lateral Flow Immunochromatographic Point of Care Detection of Herpes Simplex Virus Type 2-Specific Immunoglobulin G Antibodies in Serum and Whole Blood. *Clin. Vaccine Immunol.* **2008,** *15,* 159–163.

154. Xia, X.; Xu, Y.; Zhao, X.; Li, Q. Lateral Flow Immunoassay Using Europium Chelate-Located Silica Nanoparticles as Labels. *Clin. Chem.* **2009,** *55,* 179–182.

155. Tanaka, R.; Yuhi, T.; Nagatani, N.; Endo, T.; Kerman, K.; Takamura, Y. A Novel Enhancement Assay for Immunochromatographic Test Strips Using Gold Nanoparticles. *Anal. Bioanal. Chem.* **2006,** *385,* 1414–1420.

156. Gourley, P. L. Brief Overview of BioMicroNano Technologies. *Biotechnol. Prog.* **2005,** *21,* 2–10.

157. Wagner, W.; Dullaart, A.; Bock, A. K.; Zweck, A. The Emerging Nanomedicine Landscape. *Nat. Biotechnol.* **2006,** *24,* 1211–1217.

158. Mao, X.; Liu, G. Nanomaterial Based Electrochemical DNA Biosensors and Bioassays. *J. Biomed. Nanotech.* **2008,** *4,* 419–431.

159. Dai, Q.; Liu, X.; Coutts, J.; Austin, L.; Huo, Q. A One-Step Highly Sensitive Method for DNA Detection Using Dynamic Light Scattering. *J. Am. Chem. Soc.* **2008,** *130,* 8138–8139.

160. Huber, M.; Wei, T. F.; Muller, U. R.; Lefebvre, O. A.; Marla, S. S.; Bao, Y. P. Gold Nanoparticle Probe-Based Gene Expression Analysis with Unamplified Total Human RNA. *Nat. Biotechnol.* **2004,** *32,* e137.

161. Hentschel, C. C.; Birnstiel, M. L. The Organization and Expression of Histone Gene Families. *Cells* **1981,** *25,* 301–313.

162. Wilson, R. The Use of Gold Nanoparticles in Diagnostics and Detection. *Chem. Soc. Rev.* **2008,** *37,* 2028–2045.

163. Wang, Z.; Lee, J.; Cossins, A. R.; Brust, M. Microarray-Based Detection of Protein Binding and Functionality by Gold Nanoparticle Probes. *Anal. Chem.* **2005,** *77,* 5770–5774.

164. Li-Na, M.; Dian-Jun, L.; Zhen-Xin, W. Synthesis and Applications of Gold Nanoparticle Probes. *Chinese J. Anal. Chem.* **2010,** *38,* 1–7.

165. Kamikawa, T. L.; Mikolajczyk, M. G.; Kennedy, M.; Zhang, P.; Wang, W.; Scott, D. E.; Alocilja, E. C. Nanoparticle-Based Biosensor for the Detection of Emerging Pandemic Influenza Strain. *Biosens. Bioelectron.* **2010,** *26* (4), 1346–1352.

166. Chauhan, N.; Pundir, C. S. An Amperometric Uric Acid Biosensor Based on Multiwalled Carbon Nanotube-Gold Nanoparticle Composite. *Anal. Biochem.* **2011,** *413,* 97–103.

167. Hu, J.; Li, L.; Yang, W.; Manna, L.; Wang, L.; Alivisatos, A. P. Linearly Polarized Emission from Colloidal Semiconductor Quantum Rods. *Science* **2001,** *292,* 2060–2063.

168. Peng, X.; Manna, L.; Yang, W.; Wickham, J.; Scher, E.; Kadavanich, A.; Alivisatos, A. P. Shape Control of CdSe Nanocrystals. *Nature* **2000,** *404,* 59–61.

169. El-Sayed, I. H.; Huang, X.; El-Sayed, M. A. Surface Plasmon Resonance Scattering and Absorption of Anti-EGFR Antibody Conjugated Gold Nanoparticles in Cancer Diagnostics: Applications in Oral Cancer. *Nano Lett.* **2005,** *5,* 829–834.

170. Lee, H.; Yoon, T.; Figueiredo, J.; Swirski, F. K.; Weissleder, R. Rapid Detection and Profiling of Cancer Cells in Fine-Needle Aspirates. *Proc. Natl. Acad. Sci. U.S.A.* **2009,** *106,* 12459–12464.

171. Merlin, J.; Barberi-Heyob, M.; Bachmann, N. In Vitro Comparative Evaluation of Trastuzumab (Herceptin (R)) Combined with Paclitaxel (Taxol (R)) or Docetaxel (Taxotere (R)) in HER2-Expressing Human Breast Cancer Cell Lines. *Ann. Oncol.* **2002,** *13,* 1743.

172. Menendez, J.; Vellon, L.; Mehmi, I.; Oza, B.; Ropero, S.; Colomer, R.; Lupu, R. Inhibition of Fatty Acid Synthase (FAS) Suppresses HER2/neu (erbB-2) Oncogene Overexpression in Cancer Cells. *Proc. Natl. Acad. Sci. U.S.A.* **2004,** *101,* 10715.

173. Bruchez, M., Jr.; Moronne, M.; Gin, P.; Weiss, S.; Alivisatos, A. P. Semiconductor Nanocrystals as Fluorescent Biological Labels. *Science* **1998,** *281,* 2013–2016.

174. Lidke, D. S.; Nagy, P.; Heintzmann, R.; Arndt-Jovin, D. J.; Post, J. N.; Grecco, H. E.; Jares-Erijman, E. A.; Jovin, T. M. Quantum Dot Ligands Provide New Insights into erbB/HER Receptor-Mediated Signal Transduction. *Nat. Biotechnol.* **2004,** *22,* 198–203.

175. Freeman, R.; Tali Finder, T.; Bahshi, L.; Willner, I. β-Cyclodextrin-Modified CdSe/ZnS Quantum Dots for Sensing and Chiroselective Analysis. *Nano Lett.* **2009,** *9,* 2073–2076.
176. Cai, W.; Shin, D.; Chen, K.; Gheysens, O.; Cao, Q.; Wang, S. X.; Gambhir, S. S.; Chen, X. Peptide-Labeled Near-Infrared Quantum Dots for Imaging Tumor Vasculature in Living Subjects. *Nano Lett.* **2006,** *6,* 669–676.
177. Geiber, D.; Charbonnière, L. J.; Ziessel, R. F.; Butlin, N. G.; Löhmannsröben, H.; Hildebrandt, N. Quantum Dot Biosensors for Ultrasensitive Multiplexed Diagnostics. *Angew Chem. Int. Ed.* **2010,** *49,* 1–6.
178. Grieshaber, D.; MacKenzie, R.; Voros, J.; Reimhult, E. Electrochemical Biosensors-Sensor Principles and Architectures. *Sensors* **2008,** *8,* 1400–1458.
179. Velev, O. D.; Kaler, E. W. In Situ Assembly of Colloidal Particles into Miniaturized Biosensors. *Langmuir* **1999,** *15,* 3693–3698.

Targeted Drug Delivery

5.1 INTRODUCTION

The development of nanomaterials (NMs) has recently revolutionized the technologies for disease diagnosis, treatment, and prevention. It has been envisioned that the new nanotechnological innovations have the potential to provide extensive benefit for patients. Nanomaterials can mimic and alter biological processes owing to their size that is comparable to the size of biomolecules. Thus, to date, various NMs are being developed for targeted drug delivery.

Nanomaterials for Medical Applications. http://dx.doi.org/10.1016/B978-0-12-385089-8.00005-4

Over the past few years, NMs have been studied as drug delivery systems called NM drug carriers or simply nanocarriers. Enormous focus is being directed toward developing NMs for drug delivery for controlling the release of drugs, stabilizing labile molecules (e.g. proteins, peptides, or DNA) from degradation, and site-specific drug targeting.[1] The late 1969s and early 1979s saw the advent of polyacrylamide micelle polymerization[2] along with other polymers.[2,3,4] There are already a number of nano-enabled drugs that are sold in the market.[5] This generation of nano-enabled drugs is mainly dependent on the small size of the particles to increase the surface area to enhance the bioavailability of poorly soluble drugs and to improve the structure of the particles for delayed release. In the United States, a few of the nano-enabled drugs include Rapamune®/Pfizer, Emend®/Merck, INVEGA® SUSTENNA®/Janssen, all based on Elan's NanoCrystal® technology, Abraxane®/Abraxis Bioscience, and Triglide™/Sciele Pharma.[6] In these drugs, the NPs introduced improved functionalities that include diagnosis, targeting, drug delivery, and enhanced transport and uptake properties. This chapter is dedicated to the various aspects of different NMs for targeted drug delivery.

5.2 NANOMATERIALS AS VEHICLES FOR DRUG DELIVERY

Nanomaterials possess qualities that allow for efficient drug delivery. The nanometer size of NMs allows for extravasation through the endothelium in inflammatory sites, tumors, epithelium (e.g. intestinal tract and liver), or penetrate microcapillaries.[1] Their sizes allow for efficient uptake by various cell types which, when used for drug delivery leads to selective drug accumulation at target sites.[7,8,9] Earlier studies have demonstrated that nanoparticles (NPs) are more suited for intravenous (i.v.) delivery than microparticles (>1 μm) as a drug delivery system.[9] Because the smallest capillaries in the body are 5–6 μm in diameter, the size of particles being distributed into the bloodstream must be significantly smaller than 5 μm, without forming aggregates, to ensure that the particles do not cause an embolism.[1] Colloidal NMs that vary in size from 10 to 200 nm[2] have been extensively studied for drug delivery but particles >200 nm are not heavily pursued.

When NMs are injected into the blood stream, extensive interactions with plasma proteins, cells, and other blood components take place as reviewed by Moghimi et al.[10] Liposomes are one example of NMs as drug carriers where such interactions have been studied in detail. Phospholipids in the outer bilayer of liposomes attract some known opsonins such as immunoglobulins and complement[11] and other plasma components such as lipoproteins.[12] The reticulo-endothelial macrophages that reside in the liver and spleen have been shown to involve these events during clearance of liposomes.

As liposomes and other NMs accumulate in the liver and spleen, the mechanism could be related to the nature of proteins that adsorb onto the surface of systemically administered NMs.[13] Studies have shown that in the plasma, dextran–iron oxide and dextran–poly(isobutylcyanoacrylate) NPs are extensively coated with known opsonins such as complement, fibronectin, and fibrinogen[14,15] but the significance of these interactions in the NP clearance in vivo is not known. Others suggested that dextran–iron oxide NPs could be directly recognized through a receptor mechanism that is still unknown but without plasma opsonin involvement.[16] This claim in vivo is difficult to prove or disprove because of the presence of plasma proteins in the body.

In general, the drug is dissolved, entrapped, adsorbed, attached, and/or encapsulated into or onto an NM (Figure 5.1). The NMs can be constructed to possess different drug loading and release characteristics for the best delivery of the therapeutic agent.[3,4,17] Various forms of NMs have been used as drug delivery system. The NMs may be in the form of a nanocapsule where a drug is confined to a cavity surrounded by a polymer membrane[1] or a nanosphere in which the drug is physically and or chemically dispersed uniformly inside or outside the structure. The NMs may be in the form of liposomes, dendrimers, magnetic NPs, hydrogels, polymers, or semiconductor NMs.

The use of conventional drug carriers (adjuvants) leads to modification of the drug biodistribution profile as it is mainly delivered to the mononuclear phagocyte system (MPS),[18] also called reticuloendothelial system (RES) in the liver, spleen, lungs, and bone marrow. The NMs may be recognized by the host immune system when i.v. administered, thus, cleared by phagocytes from circulation.[19] Aside from size, the NM hydrophobicity determines the level of blood components that binds on the particle surface leading to a cascade of events that result in an immune response. The NMs hydrophobicity influences the in vivo fate of NMs[20] in such a way that once in the blood stream, nonmodified NMs are rapidly opsonized and cleared by the MPS.[21]

For successful targeted drug delivery in vivo, it is necessary to reduce the opsonization to prolong the circulation of NMs. One way to achieve this is to

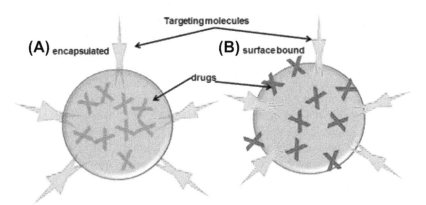

FIGURE 5.1   Schematic diagram of an NM with (A) encapsulated or (B) surface-bound drugs. The NM drug carrier is modified with a targeting molecule. *(For color version of this figure, the reader is referred to the online version of this book)*

coat the NPs with hydrophilic polymers/surfactants or by formulating NPs with biodegradable copolymers with hydrophilic characteristics such as polyethylene glycol (PEG), polyethylene oxide, polyoxamer, poloxamine, and polysorbate 80 (Tween 80).[1] Studies have shown that PEG on NP surfaces prevents opsonization by complement and other serum factors. PEG molecules reduced phagocytosis.[22]

Superparamagnetic iron oxide (SPIO) NPs that are coated with dextran are widely used as magnetic resonance imaging (MRI) contrast agents in the clinic (e.g. Ferridex™). Some SPIO NPs have been shown to exhibit prolonged circulation times that is attributed to their ultrasmall size (less than 20 nm)[23] or extensive surface cross-linking and PEGylation.[24] Larger SPIO (50–150 nm: Ferridex, Micromod SPIO, Ferumoxides) that are not dextran coated are rapidly eliminated from circulation by the liver and spleen and serve to enhance the MR contrast in these organs.[25] The mechanism of the rapid clearance of NP drug carriers must be understood in order to design long-circulating (stealth) SPIO.

In spite of the unknowns to date, NMs for drug delivery systems offer advantages that are desirable for therapeutics.[26] First, drugs and imaging agents that are associated with nanoscale carriers are distributed over smaller volumes.[27] Second, drug nanocarriers also have the ability to improve the pharmacokinetics and increase biodistribution of therapeutic agents at the target organs that result in improved efficacy.[11,28,29,30] Third, the toxicity of the drug is minimized as a result of the preferential accumulation at target diseased sites and minimized concentration in healthy tissues.[31] The nanocarriers have been engineered to target tumors and disease sites that have permeable vasculature allowing easy delivery of payload. Specific targeting and reduced clearance increases the therapeutic index that consequently lowers the dose required for efficacy.[31] Fourth, nanocarriers improve the solubility of hydrophobic therapeutics in aqueous medium allowing parenteral administration. Fifth, reports have shown that nanocarriers increase the stability of a variety of therapeutic agents such as small hydrophobic molecules, peptides, and oligonucleotides.[32,33,34] Additionally, biocompatible nanocarriers that are safe alternatives to existing drug vehicles that may cause hypersensitivity reactions and peripheral neuropathy are currently being strictly investigated.[31] Finally, nanocarriers composed of biocompatible materials[31,35,36,37,38] are investigated as safe alternatives to existing vehicles, such as Cremophor® EL (BASF, Mount Olive, NJ), that may cause hypersensitivity reactions and peripheral neuropathy.[39,40] Majority of the drugs are polycyclic making them insoluble in water.[41] Paclitaxel (TAX) and dexamethasone, for example, have low water solubility values of 0.0015[42] and 0.1 mg/mL,[43] respectively, making them unacceptable for aqueous i.v. injection.[44] A major obstacle which prevents the drug from reaching its target is its highly unspecific distribution with only 1 in 10,000 to 1 in 100,000 molecules reaching their intended site of action.[45] As a result, a much higher dose needs to be administered to obtain the desired therapeutic effect which in turn could lead closer to the toxic dose[46] as exemplified by doxorubicin (dox) which exhibits prominent cardiotoxicity.[47]

Considering these factors, it is desirable to modify the drug with features that would pharmacologically guarantee increased stability, solubility, and specific targeting to the site of action.[44] To this end, nanotechnology promises to revolutionize the area of pharmacology. Owing to their unique size and properties, NMs hold promise in improving the curative abilities of various conventional drugs which is the driving force behind the concept of nanotherapeutic drug delivery: to enhance therapeutic effects of drugs in spite of poor intrinsic pharmacological properties. NMs as drug carriers are being developed and investigated for individualized therapeutic and imaging contrast agents based on the simultaneous, anticipated advantages of targeted drug delivery at the site of the disease such as tumor growths and atherosclerotic plaque.[44] This promise is based on the ability of NMs to cross the various obstacles between the administration of the drug and the site of drug delivery.

5.3 FACTORS TO CONSIDER FOR NPS THAT WILL BE USED FOR DRUG DELIVERY

Nanotechnology is an empowering technology that holds promise in cancer therapeutics by increasing the ratio of tumor control probability to normal tissue complication probability.[31] NM drug carriers can increase the bioavailability of the drug at the target site, reduce the frequency of administration, and reach sites that are otherwise inaccessible. In order for the NM drug carriers to be useful for drug delivery, it must possess very important characteristics. Foremost among these characteristics is for the nanocarrier to be biocompatible and easy to load with the drugs.

5.3.1 Surface Charge

The surface charge of NPs plays a very important role in loading the drug for drug delivery. Furthermore, the surface charge is also important in the modification of the NMs for targeted drug delivery.

Surface charge is usually expressed and measured in terms of the NMs' zeta potential which reflects the electrical potential of particles that is influenced by its composition and the medium in which it is dispersed.[17] NMs exhibiting a zeta potential above ± 30 mV have been shown to be stable in suspension indicating that the surface charge prevents aggregation of the particles.[1]

The surface charge of an NM is important in deciding the manner by which a drug or drugs are loaded. Drugs may be loaded through covalent conjugation, hydrophobic interaction (HI), charge–charge interaction, or encapsulation. The choice of the methodology depends not only upon the surface charge but also on the nature of the drug and of the targeting molecule. Loading of the drug on the NM usually alters the surface charge. Change in the zeta potential can be used to determine whether a charged molecule has been attached or adsorbed on the NP surface. The zeta potential is measured with a zeta tracker (Chapter 2).

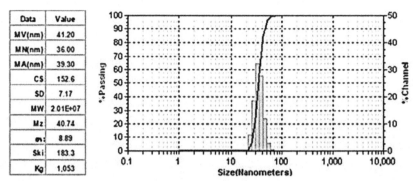

Data	Value
MV(nm)	41.20
MN(nm)	36.00
MA(nm)	39.30
CS	152.6
SD	7.17
MW	2.01E+07
Mz	40.74
σₙ:	8.89
Ski	183.3
Kg	1.053

FIGURE 5.2   DLS data for water-soluble 30-nm IOMNPs that are encapsulated with amphiphilic polymers that have carboxyl groups making them water soluble. *Courtesy of Ocean NanoTech. (For color version of this figure, the reader is referred to the online version of this book)*

A portion of the dynamic light scattering (DLS) data for 30-nm iron oxide magnetic nanoparticle (IOMNP) with carboxyl groups on the surface is shown in Figure 5.2. The DLS data sheet provides an average size based on volume, area, or diameter measurement. It also provides a particle size distribution along with the smallest size to the biggest size. Another parameter provided by the full DLS data is the average zeta potential of the NMs. The 30-nm IOMNPs (Ocean NanoTech, Catalog # SHP 30) have an average zeta potential between −30 and −50 mV.

5.3.2 Particle Size and Size Distribution

Particle size and size distribution are the most important characteristics because these determine the chemical and physical properties of NMs. Most semi-conductor and metal NMs are synthesized in organic solvent and initial size characterizations are performed on the core or core/shell particles before these are converted into the water-soluble form. The core or core/shell size and size distribution (Figure 5.3) is usually measured with transmission electron micros-copy (TEM, Chapter 2). Depending upon the sophistication of the instrument, the TEM results can provide a statistical analysis of the NMs' size distribution. In cases when the TEM does not provide size distribution, the software ImageJ has been used to calculate particle size distribution from a TEM image.

In order for the NMs to be useful for biological applications such as drug delivery, they need to be converted into water-soluble forms in order to be biocompatible. Conversion into the water-soluble form is done through amphiphilic coating (Chapter 2, Section 2.1). The size and size distribution of the water-soluble forms (Figure 5.2) of the NMs are established using DLS (Chapter 2, Section 2.4.5).

Currently, the fastest and most routine method of determining NMs' size is by photon correlation spectroscopy or DLS. Photon correlation spectroscopy

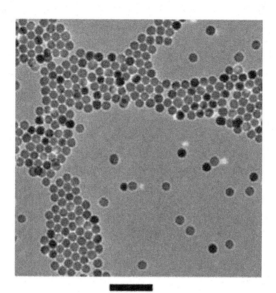

100 nm
HV=100.0kV
Direct Mag: 20000x
AMT Camera System

FIGURE 5.3 TEM image of organic soluble 20-nm IOMNP with narrow size distribution. *Courtesy of Ocean NanoTech.*

requires the viscosity of the medium to be known and determines the diameter of the particle by Brownian motion and light scattering properties.[48] The results obtained by photon correlation spectroscopy are usually verified by scanning electron microscopy (SEM) or TEM. This size of the water-soluble form called the hydrodynamic size includes the water of solvation and is, therefore, higher than the core or core/shell size. The hydrodynamic size and size distribution determine the in vivo distribution, biological fate, toxicity, and targeting ability of these NMs for drug delivery systems. In addition, they can influence drug loading, drug release, and stability of NMs. Many studies have demonstrated that NMs have a number of advantages over microparticles.[49] Generally, due to their small size and mobility, NMs have relatively higher cell uptake in comparison with microparticles making them more available to a wider range of cellular and intracellular targets. Following the opening of the endothelium tight junction (TJ), NMs can cross the blood–brain barrier (BBB) by hyperosmotic mannitol.[50] This may provide a route for sustained delivery of therapeutic agents for difficult-to-treat diseases like brain tumors.[50] Kreuter et al.[51] showed that Tween 80-coated NPs crossed the BBB as well and Zauner[52] showed that submicron NMs are taken up by the majority of cell types but not the larger microparticles. Caco-2 cells showed uptake of 100-nm NPs at 2.5-fold greater than 1-μm microparticles and a 6-fold greater uptake than 10-μm microparticles

(Desai et al., 1997)[223]. In another study, NPs were shown to penetrate throughout the submucosal layers of a rat intestinal loop model, while the microparticles were localized in the epithelial lining.[53] Thus, the particle distribution in cells can partly be tuned by controlling particle size.

5.4 DRUG LOADING

Incorporation of a drug on or in an NM is referred to as drug loading. An ideal NMs' drug delivery system should have a high drug-loading capacity without aggregation. High drug loading capacity can minimize administration or the number of doses. Dispersibility is needed for smooth and efficient delivery of the drugs.

Drug loading can be accomplished in several ways; however, drug loading and entrapment efficiency depend on drug solubility in the NMs, dispersion medium, the NMs' size and composition, drug molecular weight (MW) and solubility, drug–NM interaction, and/or the presence of surface functional groups (i.e. carboxyl, amine, ester, etc) on either the drugs or on the NMs.[54,55,56,57,58,59]

Some NM formulations use PEG because it has little or no effect on drug loading and interactions.[60] Additionally, biomolecules, drugs, or proteins encapsulated in NPs show the greatest loading efficiency when they are loaded at or near their isoelectric point (pI).[61] For small molecules, studies show that the use of ionic interaction between the drug and matrix materials can be very effective in increasing drug loading.[62,63]

Drug incorporation and loading capacity is a very important point to judge the suitability of a drug carrier system. The loading capacity is generally expressed in percent related to the NP. Westesen et al.[64] reported the incorporation of drugs using loading capacities of typically 1–5%, for ubidecarenone loading capacities of up to 50% while Iscan and coworkers[65,66] reported 10–20% for tetracaine and etomidate.

Depending upon the nature of the NM and the drug, loading may be done in several ways. The drug can be loaded on the NM surface through charge–charge interaction, covalent bonding, or through HI. It can also be loaded inside the NM core through HI or encapsulation during the NM synthesis. Examples of these methods are given below.

The protocols described below use general conditions that need to be optimized for each situation. The adsorption/absorption methods call for absorption of the drug after NP formation; this is achieved by incubating the NM with a concentrated drug solution. Furthermore, the protocols are recommended for research use only and not for clinical or human use.

It must be noted that partitioning effects of the drug between the melted lipid phase and the aqueous surfactant phase can occur during drug–NP production.[67] During the hot homogenization technique, the drug partitions from the liquid oil phase to the aqueous water phase such that the amount in the water phase increases with the solubility of the drug in the water phase which is proportional to the temperature of the aqueous phase. This is also affected by the amount of surfactant present. Thus, the higher the temperature and surfactant concentration, the greater is the saturation solubility of the drug in the water phase. In the process of cooling down the oil/water nanoemulsion temperature, the solubility of the drug in the water phase decreases as the temperature of the water phase decreases which leads to repartitioning of the drug into the lipid phase. At the lipid recrystallization temperature, a solid lipid core containing the drug forms.

In the formation of an emulsion with a lipid that is solid at room temperature (RT), the emulsion needs to be produced at a temperature above the melting point of the lipid. The lipid must be melted and its mixture with water, cosurfactants, and the surfactant (lecithin, biliary salts, and alcohols such as butanol[68]). It is heated with mild stirring until the lipid melt forms a transparent, thermodynamically stable system where the compounds are mixed in the correct ratio for the emulsion formation. The emulsion is dispersed in a cold aqueous medium (2–38 °C) with gentle mechanical mixing so that the small size of the resulting particles is caused by precipitation and not mechanically induced by the stirring process.[69,70] As high as 30% lipid solid content may be used for transfer of the dispersion to a dry product in the form of a tablet or pellet through a granulation process. To scale-up the process, the percentage composition, NP size, temperatures of the emulsion and the water, and the hydrodynamics of mixing should be maintained to keep the same product properties.[67]

In lipid NPs, the factors that determine the loading capacity of drug are: (1) solubility of drug in melted lipid, (2) miscibility of drug melt and lipid melt, (3) chemical and physical structure of solid lipid matrix, and (4) polymorphic state of lipid material. The prerequisite to obtain a substantial loading capacity in a solid lipid NP is a high solubility of the drug in the lipid melt. To be highly effective, the solubility of the drug should be higher than the dose needed because solubility decreases with the cooling down of the lipid melt and might be lowest in the solid lipid. At the same time, the drug should be miscible in the lipid. Solubilizers may be added to the lipid melt–drug mixture to enhance the drug solubility. Polydisperse lipids such those used in cosmetics showed very good drug incorporation capacities. However, crystalline structure that is related to the chemical nature of the lipid is a key factor to decide in determining whether a drug will be expelled or firmly incorporated in the long term. Therefore, for a controlled optimization of drug incorporation and drug loading, intensive characterization of the physical state of the lipid particles by NMR, X-ray, and other new techniques are highly essential.

5.4.1 Encapsulation of the Drug

Encapsulation is the general method used for solid lipid NM drug loading (Figure 5.1A). There are two basic drug encapsulation methods, the hot homogenization technique and the cold homogenization technique.[71] In both techniques, the drug is dissolved in the lipid that is melted at approximately 5–108 °C above its melting point.

Procedure for Hot homogenization technique

(1) Melt the lipid at 5 ± 108 °C above its melting point.
(2) Add the drug and stir the drug-containing melt to disperse in a hot aqueous surfactant solution.
(3) Homogenize the resulting pre-emulsion with a piston-gap homogenizer (e.g. Micron LAB40).
(4) Cool down the hot oil in water nanoemulsion to RT to allow the lipid to recrystallize into solid lipid NPs. In the case of glycerides being composed of short-chain fatty acids (e.g. Dynasan 112) and glycerides with a low melting point (too close to RT), it might be necessary to cool the nanoemulsions to even lower temperatures to initiate recrystallization. In some cases, lyophilization may be used for recrystallization.

The hot homogenization technique may be applied to drugs showing slight temperature sensitivity because the exposure to an increased temperature is relatively short. For highly temperature-sensitive compounds, the cold homogenization technique is the loading choice. This is also necessary when formulating hydrophilic drugs because during the hot homogenization process, they would partition between the lipid melt and the water phase.

Procedure for Cold homogenization technique

(1) Melt the lipid at 5 ± 108 °C above its melting point.
(2) Add the drug and stir until homogeneous.
(3) Cool the lipid melt containing the drug until it solidifies.
(4) Ground the lipid microparticles ($\sim50 \pm 100$ mm).
(5) Disperse these lipid microparticles in a cold surfactant solution to form a presuspension.
(6) Homogenize the presuspension at or below RT with a cavitation force that is strong enough to break the lipid particles directly to create solid lipid NPs. This avoids and/or minimizes the melting of the lipid and therefore minimizing the loss of hydrophilic drugs to the water phase. It is necessary that the difference between the melting point of the lipid and the homogenization temperature needs to be large enough to avoid melting the lipid in the homogenizer. Note that the homogenization process itself increases the mixture temperature (e.g. 10–20 °C per homogenization cycle), and in addition, there are temperature peaks in the homogenizer. One way to minimize the loss of hydrophilic compounds to the aqueous phase of the solid lipid NP dispersion is to replace the water with low-solubility liquids for the drug like oils or PEG 600. Encapsulation of solid lipid NPs in oil or PEG 600 is advantageous for oral drug delivery because this dispersion could be directly converted into soft gelatin capsules.

One example of a drug that had been nanocarrier encapsulated is cisplatin.[31] Cisplatin is a chemotherapeutic agent that is widely used for the treatment of malignant disorders. I.v. infusion of conventional cisplatin formulation has low bioavailability to the target organ, and in addition, it has been shown to have significant side effects, like ototoxicity and nephrotoxicity. Drug encapsulation measured by ultraviolet spectroscopy varied from 30 to 80% for different ratios of cisplatin and protein. In vitro release kinetics showed that the NP-based formulation had biphasic release kinetics and was capable of sustained release compared with the free drug (80% release in 45h). The study exhibited the feasibility of the albumin-based cisplatin NP formulation as a sustained release vehicle of cisplatin.

5.4.2 Attachment of the Drug on the NM Surface

Drug may be loaded on the surface instead of the interior of an NP. To do this, there must be functional groups on the NP surface (Figure 5.1B) that allows any of the following processes: covalent, charge–charge, or HI between the drug and the NP.

5.4.2.1 Attachment with Covalent Interaction

Common covalent coupling methods involve formation of a disulfide bond, cross-linking between two primary amines, reaction between a carboxylic acid and primary amine, reaction between maleimide and thiol, reaction between hydrazide and aldehyde, and reaction between a primary amine and free aldehyde.[72] Attachment of drugs to the NMs is discussed in the succeeding sections.

Procedure for covalent attachment of drugs on NMs

(1) Take 1 mg of carboxyl-surface-modified NM and disperse in buffer that has been optimized for the NM.

(2) Take drug that has available amine or hydroxyl group for covalent conjugation and dissolve at 0.1–2 mg/mL depending upon the loading of the drug required.

(3) Add 0.050 M borate buffer at pH 5 (or manufacturer's recommended buffer) to the NPs.

(4) Add 50 μL of 0.02 M ethyl-aminopropyl-carbodiimide hydrochloride (EDC) and 25 μL of 0.8 mM N-hydroxy succinamide (NHS) and mix well for 1–5 min (optimize the conditions depending upon the NMs and drug to be loaded).

(5) Add the drug that has been dissolved in the buffer that is appropriate for the NM.

(6) Incubate with shaking for 1–2 h at RT.

(7) Remove excess drug by centrifugation, dialysis, or magnetization for magnetic NMs. The centrifugation speed needs to be optimized depending upon the size of the NMs. The MW cutoff of the dialysis tubing also needs to be chosen based on the size of the NMs. Magnetization is recommended for ≥25 nm but not for < 25 nm because the process may take more than 24 h.

(8) Resuspend the NMs in the recommended buffer and refrigerate until use.

5.4.2.2 Attachment through Charge–Charge Interaction

One of the most studied inorganic NPs for drug delivery is IOMNP. IOM-NPs have been Food and Drug Administration approved for human use in the form of the drugs Ferridex, Resovist, Combidex, and AMI-288/feru-moxytol that are successfully utilized as MRI contrast agents.[73] Attachment of drugs to IOMNPs can be done through charge–charge interaction using carboxyl- or amine-surface modification.

Dox is one of the most commonly studied drug for NP delivery because it offers several advantages for research aside from its use as an effective anticancer drug. The hydrochloride form of dox is water soluble, it is fluorescent, and can be monitored before and after loading into the NP. Purification to eliminate excess or unloaded dox can be accomplished through centrifugation, dialysis, or magnetization.

Procedure for charge-charge loading of dox on NMs

(All the procedures in this book are for research purposes only.)

(1) Take 100 mg of carboxyl-surface-modified IOMNP and disperse in physiological saline (0.15 M NaCl, pH 7.0–7.5).

(2) Take doxorubicin hydrochloride and dissolve in physiological saline at 0.1 to 2 mg/mL depending upon the loading of the drug required.

(3) Follow the Table below for loading dox at various ratios on IOMNP.

(4) Incubate with shaking at RT for at least 60 min.

(5) Remove excess dox by centrifugation, dialysis, or magnetization. The centrifugation speed needs to be optimized depending upon the size of the IOMNPs. The MW cutoff of the dialysis tubing also needs to be chosen based on the size of the IOMNPs. Magnetization is recommended for ≥25 nm but not for <25 nm because the process may take more than 24 h.

(6) Resuspend the IOMNPs (Figure 5.4) in the physiological saline solution and refrigerate until use.

To check the efficiency of loading of the dox in IOMNPs, place the IOMNP–dox in saline at pH 2–5. Incubate at RT for 30 min with gentle shaking. Magnetize or centrifuge to precipitate the IOMNPs. Measure the absorbance or fluorescence signal from the dox. Figure 5.4 shows the 10-nm IOMNP loaded with dox (top) followed by the supernatant after release of the dox at pH 4. The bottom contains the saline used to wash the IOMNPs after the release of the dox. The supernatant contained minimal amount of dox compared with the supernatant solution.

5.4.2.3 Attachment through HI

Attachment through HI can be achieved with hydrophobic NMs and hydrophobic drugs through physical association of targeting ligands to the nanocarrier surface. HI has the advantage of eliminating the use of rigorous and potentially destructive chemicals that weaken the efficacy of the drugs. However, there are

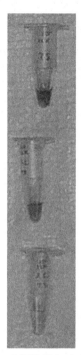

FIGURE 5.4   Ocean NanoTech Catalog # SHP 10 loaded with dox that was released at pH 2–5. *(For color version of this figure, the reader is referred to the online version of this book)*

potential problems, such as low and weak binding, poor control of the NM–drug interactions, and the ligands may not be in the desired orientation after binding.

Dagar and coworkers[74] have used vasoactive intestinal peptide (VIP), a 28-amino acid mammalian neuropeptide, as a targeting moiety to cancer and inflamed tissues because receptors for vasoactive intestinal peptide are overexpressed in human breast cancer. They established that VIPs that are HI attached to liposomes were less able to target and attach to breast cancer cells.[74] They used their sterically stabilized liposomes (SSLs) with covalently associated VIP on the surface. This was carried out by conjugating the VIP to DSPE–PEG$_{3400}$–NHS [1,2-dioleoyl-*sn*-glycero-3-phosphoethanolamine-*n*-[poly(ethylene glycol)]-*N*-hydroxy succinamide, PEG M_w 3400] under mild conditions to obtain a 1:1 conjugate of VIP and DSPE–PEG$_{3400}$ (DSPE–PEG$_{3400}$–VIP) which was confirmed by sodium dodecyl sulfate-polyacrylamide gel electrophoresis.[74] This was followed by the insertion of DSPE–PEG$_{3400}$–VIP into preformed fluorescent cholesterol (BODIPY-Chol)-labeled SSL by incubation at 37 °C. The breast cancer targeting ability in vitro was carried out by incubating these, VIP–SSL with MNU-induced rat breast cancer tissue sections. Compared with fluorescent SSL without VIP or with noncovalently attached VIP, significantly more of the covalently formed VIP–SSL were attached to rat breast cancer tissues. This indicated that SSL with covalently attached VIP can be used for targeted attachment to rat breast cancer tissues. These are currently exploring the use of covalently prepared VIP–SSL for imaging and targeted chemotherapy of breast cancer. In a different study, however, HI-attached VIP is preferred for the delivery of a therapeutic agent to inflammatory cells in animal joints with rheumatoid arthritis.[75] Thus, more investigation is necessary to establish which mode of VIP–SSL preparation is more efficient for targeted drug delivery.

Procedure for HI loading of drug on NMs[76]

To prepare the micelle NMs containing a hydrophobic drug, the dialysis method was used.[77] The protocol was as follows.

(1) Take 200 mg of the diblock copolymer and dissolve in 10 mL of DMF (dimethylformamide).
(2) Add 150 mg of drug papaverine-free base (PAP).
(3) Stir until dissolved at RT.
(4) Filter to remove dust particles.
(5) Dialyze for 24 h against 2 L of ultrapure water using cellulose dialysis membrane (MW cut off: 6000–8000). Change the water once every 5 h.
(6) Filter the NP solution to eliminate the unloaded drug and aggregated particles using a 0.45-μm pore-size Teflon filter.
(7) Freeze dry to obtain dried NMs.
(8) Use the freeze-dried NMs to calculate the concentration of the solution generated.
(9) Freeze the excess NMs solution to prevent degradation of diblock copolymer. The micelle NMs that do not contain the drug are also prepared following the same method.

5.5 NM TARGETING FOR DRUG DELIVERY

Nanotechnology provides a highly versatile platform for exploring different approaches to improving chemotherapy through specific tumor targeting of drugs that has been shown to effectively improve selective localization in human tumors in vivo of small-molecule drugs such as doxorubicin.[78] NPs as demonstrated by nanosized liposomes target tumors spontaneously because of the fenestrated blood vessels of the tumor that result in enhanced permeability and subsequent drug retention. Furthermore, liposomes offer a platform for active targeting by linking targeting agents to the liposome core.[79,80] In a study recently reported by Medina et al.,[81] they discovered that targeting on liposomal SKI 243 for tumor xenografts uptake exhibited that liposomal SKI 243 remained in the blood longer and consequently exhibited a three- to six-fold increase in uptake in the tumor among several other organs.

Targeting of NMs as drug delivery vehicles or nanocarriers for site-specific delivery has a number of advantages over targeting ligand–drug conjugates.[82] First, efficient drug loading of high concentrations of drug within the nanocarrier can be delivered specifically to the target cell or tissue when a ligand interacts with its receptor which results in the delivery of large payloads of therapeutic agent relative to number of ligand-binding sites. This is very advantageous in imaging tumor through the increase in tumor signal to background ratio. Second, the nano-carrier is attached to the ligand and the drug is loaded independent of the coupling of ligands. This avoids compromising the drug activity that may result during for-mation of the ligand–drug conjugate or inactivated by the potentially aggressive coupling reaction. Third, a large number of ligand molecules can be attached to the nanocarrier depending upon the size of the NM and the size of the drug to increase the probability of binding to target cells especially for those with low binding affinities. Fourth, active targeting enables efficient distribution of the carriers in the tumor, thereby reducing the return of drug back to the circulation that may be caused by high intratumoral pressure. Finally, when ligand is only attached to the carrier due to the small size of the conjugate, it can only extravasate at the disease site but not in normal vasculature, and as such, the ligand cannot interact with the target epitopes of normal tissues avoiding side effects. Sethi et al.[75] exhibited that VIP receptors of normal cells are not accessible after i.v. injection when VIP was associated with a nanocarrier. This showed that specific targeting in nanocarriers can play an important role in reducing toxicities of the drug.

The development of NP delivery systems for targeted drug delivery[10] can be actively or passively achieved. In active targeting, the therapeutic agent is con-jugated with the nanocarrier system that has targeting ligands to a tissue or cell-specific ligand.[83] In passive targeting, the therapeutic agent is incorporated into a macromolecule or NP that passively reaches the target organ. NP-encapsulated drugs or drugs coupled to macromolecules can passively target tumors through the enhanced permeation and retention (EPR) effect. Localized delivery of NPs bearing drugs to sites of vascular restenosis may provide sustained drug release at specific sites on the arterial wall.[84,85]

5.5.1 Antibodies

Targeting in nano-enabled drug delivery systems is accomplished by labeling the NP with receptors or biomolecules that specifically attach them to the target cells or tissues (Figure 5.4). The most common targeting molecules are antibodies (Fig-ure 5.5B) against epithelial growth factor receptors, anti-epidermal growth factor receptor (EGFR). Because EGFR is expressed in all epithelial cells, this molecule is a special target when delivering drugs to epithelial cells. Human epithelial recep-tors (HERs) are commonly overexpressed in a number of different cancer cells and, therefore, is commonly targeted in nano-enabled targeted drug delivery.[55,56]

The HER-2/neu (HER-2) oncogene is another closely related member of the EGFR family that is known to be upregulated in different types of human cancers including breast, ovarian, lung, gastric, and oral cancers. Increased malignancy and poor survival of breast cancer patients have been associated with upregulation of HER-2 that seems to impart chemoresistance upon the

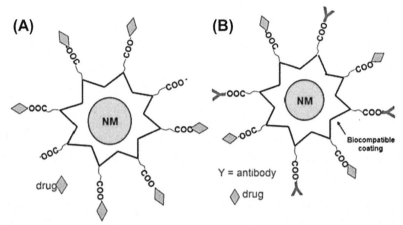

FIGURE 5.5 Schematic diagram of an NM for (A) drug delivery and (B) targeted drug delivery. *Courtesy of Ocean NanoTech. (For color version of this figure, the reader is referred to the online version of this book)*

tumors. Repression of HER-2/neu was observed in many studies indicating that HER-2 is an excellent target for developing anticancer agents specific for HER-2-upregulated cancer cells. It has been used as target with CdSe quantum dots (QDs) that had been conjugated with monoclonal anti-HER-2 antibody.[86] The following protocol was designed in preparing HER-2-targeted drug delivery.

Procedure for HER-2-targeted drug delivery

(1) Take 1 nmole of carboxyl-surface-modified iron oxide nanoparticles (IONPs) dispersed in water or appropriate buffer such as borate buffer at pH 7–7.4.

(2) Take 1–5 nmoles of monoclonal antibodies (mAbs) against HER-2 mAb and dissolve in borate buffer at pH 7–7.4.

(3) Add 50 μL of 0.02 M EDC and 26 μL of 8 mM of NHS and mix well for 1–5 min (optimize the conditions depending upon the NMs and drug to be loaded).

(4) Vortex at RT for 1 h.

(5) Remove unreacted antibody by centrifugation, dialysis, or magnetization of the magnetic NMs. The centrifugation speed needs to be optimized depending upon the size of the NMs. The MW cutoff of the dialysis tubing also needs to be chosen based on the size of the NMs. Magnetization is recommended for ≥25 nm but not for <25 nm because the process may take more than 24 h.

(6) Load the drugs based on the appropriate protocols for the drug and the NMs.

(7) Resuspend the NMs in the recommended buffer and refrigerate until use.

(8) Characterize the antibody conjugation with agarose gel electrophoresis. The NMs carrying the covalently conjugated antibody show a retarded migration compared with the NM (Figure 5.6) that does not carry a conjugated antibody. After conjugation of an antibody or a protein or any other biomolecule to an NM, the gel shows a tailing of the signal that may be attributed to the

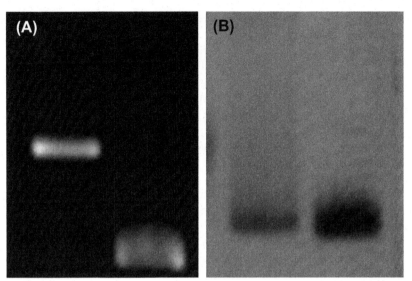

FIGURE 5.6   Agarose gel electrophoresis of (A) QD with (right) and without antibody (left) and (B) IOMNP with (left) and without antibody (right) covalent conjugated antibody. *Courtesy of Ocean NanoTech. (For color version of this figure, the reader is referred to the online version of this book)*

number of proteins or biomolecules per NM. The higher the number of biomolecules attached to the NM, the slower the rate of migration. It is usually observed that tailing occurs in all types of NMs after bioconjugation.

5.5.2 Peptides

Although antibodies have very high target selectivity and binding affinities, they are potentially immunogenic. To overcome such a drawback, antibodies may be engineered to acquire humanized or chimeric properties to avoid immune detection. In addition, antibody production and isolation are difficult and tedious. Alternative targeting molecules such as peptides, aptamers, and some small molecules have been identified.

Compared with antibodies, peptides as targeting moieties offer several advantages, such as lack of immunogenicity and lower cost of production. However, they have lower target affinities, increased chance of nonspecific binding, and an increased probability of proteolytic cleavage. A few of these issues may be improved by displaying the peptides multivalently to increase the effective binding affinity and by using D-amino acids which evade proteolysis. Peptide-based targeting ligands are identified from the binding regions of proteins for the target of interest. They can also be produced using phage display which is a technique utilized for efficient and rapid screening of peptides possessing specific binding to targets of interest.[73] This method uses bacteriophage, viruses that only infect bacteria, and are genetically modified to express multiple copies of a single peptide on their surface forming a library containing over 109 different sequences. This library can be screened against purified targets immobilized on plates, washed to remove any unbound phage, while the bound phage are isolated, expanded, and replated with the target. The screening is repeated a number of times until a consensus sequence is reached. The problem with this method is that the target molecules are not in their native state and may not truly represent the in vivo environment. For a faster identification of target peptides, PepBank, a searchable database based on sequence text mining and public peptide data sources (http://pepbank.mgh.harvard.edu) has been created and currently contains over 21,000 entries.

One peptide sequence being utilized for the targeting of diagnostic and therapeutic moieties is the tripeptide arginine–glycine–aspartate (RGD). RGD binds to anb3 integrin which is upregulated in activated endothelial cells during inflammation or angiogenesis which are both observed cancer cases.[87,88] This peptide was initially studied for treatment of cancers and later subsequently utilized for the delivery of both therapeutic and imaging agents to tumors. RGD has been conjugated with Cy5.5 to mono-, di-, and tetrameric RGD peptides and each conjugate's targeting ability had been tested on U87MG glioblastoma xenograft model. A multifunctional RGD on IONP probe for positron emission tomography (PET)/MRI imaging of human glioblastoma cancer cells has been developed.[89] The IONP were initially coated with polyaspartic acid, to which was conjugated 1,4,7,10-tetraazacyclododecane-1,4,7,10-tetraacetic acid (DOTA) to serve as a chelating agent for the ^{64}Cu radionucleotide. DOTA-labeled particles were decorated with RGD and were treated with ^{64}Cu under slightly acidic conditions to obtain ^{64}Cu-DOTA-RGD-IO NPs. These were injected into mice bearing U87MG tumors and monitored with PET/MRI imaging which revealed that the U87MG tumor was clearly visualized whereas the nontargeted ^{64}Cu-DOTA-IO particles exhibited very low nonspecific tumor uptake.

5.5.3 Aptamers

Aptamers are short oligonucleotides (15–40 bases) that are identified via selection processes called systematic evolution of ligands by exponential enrichment[90,91] that can potentially be used as both therapeutic and targeting entities.[92] Just like antibodies, aptamers are highly specific for their targets and possess high binding affinities that are largely due to the ability of the molecules complex three-dimensional structures.[93] Aptamers offer advantages over antibodies such as easy synthesis through solid-phase methodologies and minimal immunogenicity. However, nonmodified aptamers possess several deleterious properties such as rapid blood clearance that is largely due to nuclease degradation which had been circumvented by the inclusion of subunits such as 20-fluorine-substituted pyrimidines and PEG linkages.

5.5.4 Small Molecules

A popular strategy for disease detection is the use of small-molecule-modified materials as an alternative targeting strategy.[94] This is attributed to the diversity that small molecules offer through their structures and properties allowing for rapid access to libraries of diverse molecules with different functionalities.[95] When the small molecules do not demonstrate effective binding to targets, their small size allows for incorporation of a number of ligands that increase the effective target affinity via multivalency. A library of 146 various functionalized small molecules consisting of amines, alcohols, carboxylic acids, sulfhydryls, or anhydrides which were used to label magnetofluorescent iron oxide NPs had been reported.[96] This library was screened against five human cell lines such as the umbilical vein endothelial cells (HUVEC), resting primary human macrophages, granulocyte macrophage colony-stimulating factor-stimulated primary macrophages, a human macrophage-like cell line (U937), and human pancreatic ductal adenocarcinoma cells (PDAC, PaCa-2). The cell uptake (measured by fluorescence microscopy and flow cytometry) showed preferential uptake by activated resting macrophages. In vivo test with PaCa-2 tumors demonstrated significant localization of the test materials by both fluorescence reflectance imaging and histology. Surface plasmon resonance tests to study the role of multivalency using a library of structurally related small molecules for the protein FKBP12 that was conjugated to magnetofluorescent NPs[97] showed that the small molecules and their NP conjugates had the association rate k_a, dissociation rate k_d, and dissociation constant K_D (k_d/k_a) for the interaction of FKBP12 revealed significant decrease in k_d, whereas changes in k_a varied greatly, as compared to the free molecules. This indicated that the multivalent attachment of small molecules to the NM surface resulted in similar K_D for the conjugates.

A number of small molecules have been used for the delivery of therapeutic agents including folate and carbohydrates. Folic acid is a water-soluble vitamin (vitamin B6) that occurs rarely in foods while the tetrahydrofolate form is found in foods and in the human body. Diets that are rich in folate have been associated with decreased risk of cardiovascular disease. Folate is critical for the metabolism of DNA and RNA as well as for rapid cell division and growth especially during the development of embryos. The folate receptor may be upregulated in order to provide cells with the required amount of folate in cancer patients. For this reason, folic acid has been used to deliver a number of imaging and therapeutic agents to tumors.[98] Some of the clinically relevant examples include 111In-DTPA-folate, EC20 (a folate conjugate of 99mTc), EC17 (a folate-linked fluorescent hepten), and EC145 (a folate conjugate of diacetylvinylblastine hydrazide) that have been tested for clinical imaging and therapeutic purposes.

Carbohydrates is another class of small molecules that have been used as targeting ligands as a result of their biocompatibility and their ability to be selectively recognized by cell surface receptors, such as lectins.[99] Although glycoproteins are endogenously expressed in a number of tissues, certain cells such as endothelial cells have been shown to upregulate carbohydrate receptors in response to inflammation, such as selectins. The liver, particularly, the hepatocytes express asialoglycoprotein receptor (ASGP-R) which readily binds galactose that may serve as a means to ameliorate liver-specific drug delivery.[99]

5.6 BINDING AND UPTAKE

In order for the NM-mediated drug delivery to take effect, the drug-loaded NM must be bound to the target tissue and cellular uptake is a prerequisite before the drug can be delivered. Thus, movement toward the target tissue and ultimately, to the target cell, is critical. The probability of binding or adhesion in a dynamic environment, Padh, is given by the equation

$$\text{Padh} = f(d^{-x}, Q^{-y}, \delta_{rec}, f_{atr})$$

where d = particle diameter, Q = flow rate, δ_{rec} = density of the receptors, and f_{atr} = force of attraction between receptor and particle which is affected by the particle ligand coverage and the NM conformation.[100]

Conventional drug carriers lead to modification of the drug distribution profile as it is delivered to the MPS such as liver, spleen, lungs, and bone marrow. However, NMs as drug carriers can be recognized by the host immune system when i.v. administered causing them to be cleared by phagocytes from the circulation.[19] The size of the NMs, surface hydrophobicity, and surface coating functionalities determine the level of blood components (e.g. opsonins) that bind to its surface[19,20] influencing the in vivo fate of NMs. To enhance the chances of success in drug targeting, it is important to prevent the opsonization while prolonging the circulation of NMs in vivo. The NMs can achieve this by precoating with hydrophilic polymers and/or surfactants or by using NMs with biodegradable hydrophilic copolymers such as PEG, polyethylene oxide, polysorbate 80 (Tween 80), and poloxamine. Studies have shown that PEG on NM surfaces eliminates opsonization.[22,101]

NMs undergo extravasation during entry into tumor tissues which occurs by means of the EPR effect.[102,103] Thus, drugs carried by NMs for delivery or nano-enabled drugs at the lower size range are preferable to the upper submicron and micron sizes to achieve longer circulation half-lives through the reduced macrophage mononuclear uptake (Figure 5.7) and more efficient cellular uptake. Research had established that majority of solid tumors exhibit a vascular pore cutoff size between 380 and 780 nm,[104] but tumor vasculature organization may differ depending on the tumor type, its growth rate, and microenvironment.[104,105] Hence, in order for the nano-enabled drugs to reach the tumor sites, the nanocarriers must be of a size much smaller than the cutoff pore diameter. On the other hand, normal vasculature is impermeable to drug-associated nanocarriers larger than 2–4 nm compared with free, unassociated

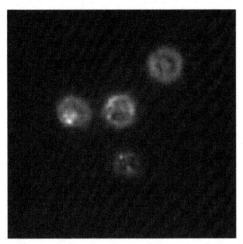

FIGURE 5.7   Macrophage uptake of QD–vaccine candidates. Macrophages were labeled with CD11 that had a green dye. The vaccine candidate was covalently conjugated with a red emitting QD that was ~12nm in diameter. *Courtesy of Dr George Hui, University of Hawaii at Manoa. (For color version of this figure, the reader is referred to the online version of this book)*

drug molecules.[27,106] This size range offers the opportunity to increase drug accumulation and local concentration in target sites by extravasation and, at the same time, significantly reduce drug distribution and toxicity to normal tissues. Researchers have also developed other approaches to increase local microvascular permeability and further enhance delivery to solid tumors and other tissues of interest through the use of: (a) physical energy such as hyperthermia[107] and (b) ultrasound.[108] To help maximize drug delivery at targeted locations, a genetic algorithm-based, area-coverage approach was developed for robot path planning to a targeted area.[109] This helps avoid obstacles (i.e. blood barriers, organs, or tissues) through a suboptimal path that will achieve near-optimal energy consumption for drug delivery. Cellular uptake of particles can occur by various mechanisms.

5.6.1 Uptake by Phagocytic Cells

The macrophage system is made up of largely phagocytic cells such as macrophages. Generally, particles >1 μm generate a phagocytic response.[110,111] In a study using immunoglobulin G-opsonized polystyrene beads of defined size ranging from 0.2 to 3 μm in murine macrophages, Koval[110] reported that phagocytosis uptake was size dependent; <30% of 0.2- to 0.75-μm particles compared to >80% of 2- and 3-μm particles were taken up. On the other hand, Moghimi reported that entrapment by hepatic and splenic endothelial fenestrations and subsequent clearance can be avoided by using nanocarriers that do not exceed 200 nm.[10] Other properties such as surface charge and chemistry can also influence nanocarrier uptake and subsequent clearance by MPS cells.[75,110,111]

5.6.2 Uptake by Nonphagocytic Cells

Uptake of NMs by nonphagocytic cells such as tumor cells can also happen if particles are <500 nm.[26,112] Nonphagocytic internalization of nano-enabled drugs into the target cells can occur macropinocytosis, clathrin-mediated endocytosis, and non-clathrin-mediated endocytosis in such a way that as particle size increased, internalization decreases. Cellular uptake was not observed for particles >500 nm.[112]

5.6.3 Uptake by Drug-Resistant Cancer Cells

Overcoming drug resistance in cancer chemotherapy by using NMs as delivery systems is a very hot area of research in this century. Various mechanisms that have been proposed include enhanced intracellular concentration of the drug by endocytosis,[113] inhibition of multidrug resistance (MDR) proteins by carrier component materials such as Pluronic block copolymers,[113,114] promotion of other uptake mechanisms such as receptor-mediated cellular internalization,[115,116] adhesion of NMs to the cell surface and increased drug concentrations at the vicinity of target cancer cells.[113] Furthermore, both drug and inhibitors of MDR proteins can be incorporated into the same carriers for simultaneous delivery to the cancer cells. For example, dox and cyclosporin A encapsulated in polyalkylcyanoacrylate NPs have been demonstrated to reverse resistance synergistically.[117]

5.7 DRUG RELEASE AND BIODEGRADATION

Drug release refers to the process by which the drug loaded in or on the NMs is released in the body through diffusion or dissolution of the NMs matrix releasing the drug in solution. Biodegradation refers to the process by which the drug delivery system is broken down inside the body.

Both drug release and biodegradation are important to consider when developing an NMs drug delivery system. Ordinarily, effectiveness of drugs is dependent not only on its active components but also on its solubility and diffusion. When the drug is delivered using an NMs delivery system, effectiveness is affected by parameters such as the particle size, release process which is in turn affected by the biodegradation of the particle matrix. The smaller the particles, the larger the surface area-to-volume ratio; therefore, most of the drug associated with small particles would be at or near the particle surface which leads to faster drug release. In contrast, larger particles have large cores, which allow more drugs to be encapsulated per particle and give slower release. Thus, control of particle size provides a means of tuning drug release rates.

5.7.1 Factors Affecting Drug Release

In general, the drug release rate depends on: (1) drug solubility, (2) desorption of the surface-bound or adsorbed drug, (3) drug diffusion out of the NM matrix into the body, (4) NM matrix erosion or degradation, and (5) the combination of erosion and diffusion processes.[118] The method of drug incorporation into the NM delivery system also affects the release profile.

Drug release when loaded by covalent attachment on the particle system is affected almost solely by drug–NM diffusion. This system has a relatively small burst effect and sustained release characteristics.[119] When the drug is encapsulated inside a NM, the release is controlled by diffusion of the drug from the NM interior.

The polymer coating acts as a drug release barrier; hence, the drug solubility and diffusion in or across the polymer membrane becomes a determining factor in drug release. The release rate can also be affected by ionic interactions between the drug and secondary ingredients. In the event that polymer-encapsulated drug interacts with auxiliary ingredients, a less water-soluble complex may form causing a slower drug release that almost has no burst release effect.[62] On the other hand, addition of auxiliary ingredients, e.g. ethylene oxide–propylene oxide block copolymer (PEO-PPO), to chitosan (CS) reduces the interaction of the drug with the matrix material via competitive electrostatic interaction of PEO-PPO with CS, and an increase in drug release could be achieved.[61]

In an encapsulated drug where the drug is uniformly distributed inside the NM matrix, drug release occurs by diffusion and/or erosion of the matrix. When the diffusion of the drug is faster than matrix erosion, diffusion largely controls the mechanism of release. The rapid, initial release, or "burst," is mainly attributed to weakly bound or adsorbed drug to the relatively large surface of NMs.[120]

There are several in vitro methods that can be used to study the release of drugs loaded in an NM. These include: (1) side-by-side diffusion in cells with artificial or biological membranes, (2) diffusion through a dialysis bag, (3) reverse dialysis bag diffusion, (4) agitation followed by ultracentrifugation or centrifugation, (5) ultrafiltration, or (6) pH change. In general, drug release study is carried out by controlled shaking to allow the drug to ooze out of the NM into a release media followed by centrifugation to separate the NM from the drug in solution. However, the difficulties in the separation of NMs from the release media favor the use of the dialysis technique. Exception to these is the use of IOMNPs where loading with drugs is performed at high pH and drug is released at low physiological pH. After the drug release, the IOMNPs can easily be separated from the media with the use of magnets (SuperMag, Ocean NanoTech) and the concentration of drug in the release media can be established depending upon the properties of the drug (unpublished paper, Ocean Nanotech).

Only a few studies have been published on drug release,[118,121] especially on the release mechanisms. The mechanisms on in vitro drug release were generated by studying the model drugs tetracaine, etomidate, and prednisolone.[66,122] However, lipid NMs exhibited burst release when incorporating tetracaine and etomidate. A prolonged drug release was obtained first with prednisolone that demonstrated the suitability of the solid lipid NMs for prolonged drug release. Drug release can be controlled as a function of the lipid matrix, surfactant concentration, and production parameters such as temperature[122] achieving as long as 5–7 weeks. The formulation can be modulated for prolonged release without any burst or with different percentages of burst followed by prolonged release.[67] The burst can be used to deliver an initial dose when desired.

5.8 NM CLEARANCE

Concerns about NM clearance after drug delivery are prevalent because the technology is still in its infancy. Thus, it is very important to understand how the human body clears NMs that are used in NP-based drug delivery.[49,123] After the body has distributed oxygen, nutrients, and systemically administered NM-mediated drugs via the vascular and lymphatic systems, it has to clear anything and everything that is introduced. I.v. introduced materials are scavenged and cleared from the circulation by Kupffer cells and macrophages.[10] Clearance is facilitated by surface deposition of blood opsonic factors and complement proteins on the injected drug–NP. Studies have recently been published on the detailed information regarding the phagocytosis and clearance of carbon nanotubes in vitro.[124,125] The size and surface properties of the injected NMs affect both clearance and opsonization. Bigger particles that are 200 nm or greater in diameter activate the complement system more efficiently and are cleared faster from the circulatory system than the smaller particles in poorly studied and less understood biological mechanisms. However, the biological mechanism of particle clearance is likely related to the basic geometry and surface characteristics (charge, functional groups, shape, etc.) of particles that mediate binding of blood proteins and opsonins.[10,11]

Theoretically, NMs may be engineered to introduce various characteristics that are designed to suit the phenotype, physiological activity, and recognition mechanisms of specific subpopulations of macrophages to enhance differential opsonization and clearance.[126] On the other hand, NMs less than 100 nm have been associated with variable levels of toxicity through different mechanisms. In a study by Nel et al.,[127] inhaled particles can elicit pulmonary inflammation and oxidative stress and disrupt distal organ function. As NMs decrease in size, their relative surface area in air is increased, causing an enhanced exposure to several proposed toxic mechanisms including HIs, redox cycling, and free radical formation. In this manner, a 20-nm particle would have roughly 100 times the inherent toxicity of a 2-μm particle in an equivalent dose based on mass, assuming a direct relationship with surface area.

The surface chemistry and design of NMs impacts the pharmacokinetic profile of a given drug it carries by altering its aggregation in the body.[49,123] Although NMs including dendrimers, QDs, and micelles are prone to aggregation, this can be circumvented by surface engineering. NMs such as QDs can be made water soluble, dispersible, and stable in serum by coating their surface with polydentate phosphine or hydrophilic polymers.[128,129,130] NMs can be coated with polymers such as PEG[10,126] that suppress macrophage recognition by reducing protein adsorption and surface opsonization. This prolongs the circulation of NMs which allows for the controlled release of the drugs in the blood. I.v. injected radiolabeled carbon nanotubes appears to be retained by the liver or spleen but are rapidly cleared (half-life of 3 h) intact from the blood by renal excretion.[125]

Control of the pharmacokinetic profile of circulating NMs allows confinement of injected particles to the vascular system by preventing leakage or avoiding splenic filtration. This control is useful cancer where the tumor-associated blood vessels are leaky and serve as a potential therapeutic target.[131] Studies revealed the molecular signatures in endothelial cells as well as the vascular and lymphatic beds[126,132] which can be used as easy targets for specific pathological sites for therapeutics and diagnostics.[128,133] Useful NMs that are sued as nanocarriers must be designed to contain the appropriate targeting ligands.[82] Long circulating nanocarriers with controlled particle stability and aggregation having appropriately engineered surface curvature and reactivity for strong receptor binding and subsequent biochemical cascades and signaling processes are among the properties of successful nanocarriers. It is possible that the preferred method of NM delivery is direct interstitial injection wherein the fate of interstitially injected NMs is dependent on the size and surface characteristics of the particles.[134,135] For the NMs to be successful, the size must be large enough (30–100 nm) to avoid leakage into blood capillaries but not too large (>100 nm) to become susceptible to macrophage-based clearance. Manipulation of the NM surface can be used to control particle aggregation at interstitial sites, controlling drainage kinetics and lymph node retention.[134] Hydrophilic but not hydrophobic NMs repulse each other and interact poorly with the interstitium, thus draining rapidly into the lymphatics. Thus, nanosize particles from 1 to 20 nm in diameter extravasate from the vasculature into the interstitial spaces during transport by lymphatic vessels to lymph nodes.[136] This phenomenon is an important aspect to consider in the design of drug nanocarriers as the extent of nodal vascularization and blood supply varies across tissues allowing differential leakage from the blood pool through the permeable endothelium in lymph nodes. Nanocarrier movement from the blood and interstitial sites to the lymph nodes provides opportunities for diagnosis where an enhancement of signal over background can be observed. The physicochemical properties of QDs,[137] superparamagnetic iron oxide nanocrystals, and other similar NMs are ideal for these purposes.

Aspects of tumor-targeted NM-based drug delivery systems that must be addressed are technical and biological concerns that influence their distribution. Challenges to these technologies are rapid opsonization in the blood and subsequent clearance by the RES. This process can be minimized by saturation since at a high enough dose of NPs, the ability of the RES to clear such particles could be exceeded.[138,139] When RES saturation was achieved, NPs not trapped in the liver or spleen could deliver drugs to solid tumors as shown by data obtained with the cAu-TNF vector. Even when a majority of the vector was cleared by RES, a fraction of the drug was delivered to the tumor.

A better and safer approach in addressing RES uptake and clearance was the modification of the NP surface to include hydrophilic blockers such as PEG as well as block copolymers in the tetronic and pluronic families of surfactants. These modifications significantly altered the biodistribution of liposomes and biopolymers since liver and splenic uptake of these hydrated particles was marginal. In addition, these preparations were shown to passively accumulate in solid tumors through extravasation of the leaky vasculature that fed them.[140,141] Unfortunately, blockers such as PEG-based stabilizers, including carbowax, or block copolymers such as poloxamine or poloxamer[53,140,141] failed to alter the biodistribution of the cAu-TNF vector when compared to the cAu-TNF vector alone which may be explained due to an inability of the tumor necrosis factor (TNF)-saturated gold particles to directly bind the hydrophilic blockers. Thus, such poorly bound blockers were unable to stop the vectors' uptake by the RES.

5.9 VARIOUS NMs FOR DRUG DELIVERY

It is a well-known fact that radiotherapy- and chemotherapy-based cancer treatments affect both tumors and healthy tissue, thereby leading to sometimes toxic side effects. Using biocompatible NPs, cancer immunotherapy attempts to specifically deliver the drugs or the treatment to the affected tissues/cells as well as to enhance the natural immune response to tumor cells. Aside from treatment of cancers, NM-based drug delivery systems can also be used to deliver vaccines and drugs for other diseases that are hard to reach.

5.9.1 Polymers

Polymeric NPs made from natural and synthetic polymers have received the majority of attention due to their stability and ease of surface modification.[113,142] These can be configured to achieve controlled drug release and tissue/cell specific localization at the site of the disease by tuning the polymer characteristics, surface chemistry, and functionalization.[8,10,49,143]

Nanopolymers carrying drugs can become concentrated preferentially to tumors, inflammatory sites, and at antigen sampling sites by virtue of the EPR effect of the vasculature.[1] Once at the target site, biodegradable polymeric NPs can act as a drug depot that provides a continuous supply of encapsulated therapeutic compounds at the disease site such as at solid tumors.

Polymeric drug delivery systems can be used to provide targeted (cellular or tissue) delivery of drugs with improved bioavailability enabling sustained release of drugs or solubilization of drugs for systemic delivery. This system can be adapted to protect therapeutic agents against enzymatic degradation (i.e. nucleases and proteases).[144] The use of biodegradable materials for NP preparation allows for sustained drug release within the target site over a period of days or even weeks. Biodegradable NPs formulated from polylactic glycolic acid

(PLGA) and PLA have been developed for drug delivery.[145] These polymeric NMs have been effective in delivering their contents to intracellular targets.

In another study, a degradable, polyamine ester polymer, polybutanediol diacrylate co amino pentanol (C32), a diptheria toxin suicide gene (DT-A) driven by a prostate-specific promoter was directly injected into normal prostate and prostate tumors in mice.[146] This C32/DT-A system resulted in notable size decrease and apoptosis in 50% of normal prostate. A single injection of C32/DT-A-triggered apoptosis in 80% of tumor cells present in the tissue; therefore, it is expected that multiple NP injection would trigger a great percentage of prostate tumor cells apoptosis.

MDR is known to develop through a variety of molecular mechanisms in tumor cells. The enzyme, glucosylceramide synthase, is responsible for the activation of ceramide, the proapoptotic mediator, to glucosylceramide, a nonfunctional moiety. This molecule is overexpressed by a number of MDR tumor types and has been implicated in cell survival during chemotherapy. Investigation of the therapeutic strategy of coadministering ceramide with TAX in an attempt to restore apoptotic signaling and overcome MDR in a human ovarian cancer cell line using modified poly(epsilon-caprolactone) (PEO-PCL) NPs to encapsulate and deliver the therapeutic agents for enhanced efficacy was carried out.[147] The studies showed that MDR cancer cells can be completely eradicated by this approach and that MDR cells can be resensitized to a dose of TAX near the IC_{50} of non-MDR cells. Molecular analysis of activity showed that the efficacy of this therapeutic approach is due to a restoration in apoptotic signaling exhibiting the potential for clinical use to overcome MDR.

5.9.1.1 Polylactic Glycolic Acid

NMs have a great risk of aggregation during storage, transport, and dispersion. Degradation of the outer polymer coating can also be affected by particle size. As an example, the rate of PLGA degradation was found to increase as the particle made from this polymer increased in size.[148] This degradation process is believed to result from PLGA degradation products that easily diffuse through shorter distances in smaller NPs, whereas the polymer matrix of larger particles increases the time of release due to the greater distance that may cause autocatalytic degradation of the polymer.[149]

PLGA has been widely studied for various medical applications. It has also been extensively reported for drug delivery for different drugs and diseases.[8,54,59,150,151,152,153,154] Seju et al.[152] focused on the use of PLGA for the delivery of olanzapine (OZ), a second-generation or atypical antipsychotic drug which selectively binds to central dopamine D_2 and serotonin (5-HT_{2c}) receptors. This drug has poor bioavailability due to hepatic first-pass metabolism and low permeability into the brain that is due to efflux by P-glycoproteins.[152] They prepared PLGA using nanoprecipitation technique and characterized by entrapment efficiency, particle size, zeta potential, modulated temperature differential scanning calorimetry, and X-ray diffraction.[152] The NP showed a mean diameter of 91.2 ± 5.2 nm with OZ entrapment efficiency of 68.91 ± 2.31%. The in vitro studies showed a biphasic drug release pattern with an initial burst release followed by sustained release (43.26 ± 0.156% after 120 h) with a Fick's diffusion-based release mechanism.[152] The ex vivo diffusion using sheep nasal mucosa showed 13.21 ± 1.59% drug diffusion from the PLGA in 210 min. Study of sheep nasal mucosa showed no significant adverse effect of the OZ-loaded PLGA. The in vivo pharmacokinetic studies showed 6.35 and 10.86 times higher uptake of intranasal (i.n.) OZ delivery with PLGA than in solution that is delivered through i.v. and i.n. route, respectively. These results hold promise for OZ delivery directly to the brain after i.n. delivery in the presence of PLGA. PLGA-enhanced delivery to the brain can increase drug concentration in the brain for improving the treatment of central nervous system (CNS) disorders.[152]

Nano-enabled formulations have also been evaluated as ocular drug delivery vehicles to enhance the absorption of therapeutic drugs, improve bioavailability, reduce systemic side effects, and sustain intraocular levels of drugs.[151] Just as in the delivery of drugs to other tissues, polymeric NMs offer unique features while preserving the ease of drug delivery in liquid form, and to improve the corneal and conjunctival penetration of therapeutic drugs and peptides, they sustain drug levels while also reducing systemic side effects.[155] Of the known polymeric NMs, PLGA is ideal for ocular therapy due to its biocompatibility, safety, regulatory approval, and wide use.[54,59,150,152,153,156,157,158,159] Jain et al.[151] designed and evaluated the use of PLGA–CS complex for ocular drug delivery. Fluorescent Rhodamine (Rd) PLGA–CS complexes were prepared by ionotropic gelation method and tested on rabbit cornea for retention, uptake, and penetration. They reported that both ex vivo and in vivo studies showed greater amounts of NMs delivered Rd in the cornea than those delivered only from solution.[151] Confocal microscopy of the corneas revealed paracellular and transcellular uptake supporting possible adsorptive-mediated endocytosis and opening of the TJs between epithelial cells.

Wang et al.[153] reported the use of combination of two or more therapeutic drugs to minimize the limitation of single-drug chemotherapy in antitumor treatment that includes development of drug resistance, high toxicity, and regimen to minimize the amount of each drug achieve the synergistic effect for cancer therapies. Other NMs had been used to deliver combination chemotherapeutic drugs using drug carriers, such as micelles, liposomes, and inorganic NPs.[153] In this paper, Wang and coworkers emulsified an amphiphilic copolymer methoxy poly(ethylene glycol)–poly(lactide-co-glycolide) (mPEG-PLGA) that were easy to produce, biocompatible, and exhibited high loading efficacy. These NPs were sued to codeliver hydrophilic dox and hydrophobic TAX. The drug release and cellular uptake of the codelivery platform showed that both drugs were effectively taken up by the cells and exhibited suppression of tumor cell growth more efficiently than the delivery of either dox or TAX at the same concentrations. This indicated that codelivery with the NMs had a synergistic effect.[153] In this study, the NMs' drug loading with a dox/TAX at a 2:1 concentration ratio showed the highest antitumor activity to three different types of tumor cells that were studied.

In another study, the length of time for PLGA circulation in the bloodstream was investigated using TAX-loaded chitosan and polyethylene glycol-coated PLGA (PLGA–CS–PEG) NMs.[160] This study also looked at efficiency of encapsulation of hydrophobic drugs and evasion of phagocytic uptake by reducing opsonization by blood proteins to increase the bioavailability of the drug by optimizing the concentration of CS and PEG.[160] The efficiency of uptake and in vitro cytotoxicity was evaluated in various cancer cell lines representing retinoblastoma, breast cancer, and pancreatic cancer. The studies showed prolonged blood circulation of the PLGA–CS–PEG NPs as well as reduced macrophage uptake with minimal sequestration in the liver. This in vitro study showed the synergistic effect of PEG–CS drug delivery NMs for prolonged blood circulation.

5.9.1.2 Liposome

Liposomes have been demonstrated to be useful for delivering pharmaceutical agents. These systems use "contact-facilitated drug delivery," which involves binding or interaction with the targeted cell membrane allowing for enhanced lipid–lipid exchange with the lipid monolayer of the NP, thereby accelerating the convective flux of lipophilic drugs (e.g. TAX) to dissolve through the outer lipid membrane of the NMs to targeted cells.[161] These types of nanosystems can serve as drug depots exhibiting prolonged release kinetics and long persistence at the target site.

Medina et al.[81] developed PET tracers which irreversibly bound to EGFR. They used a liposomal NP delivery system to alter the pharmacokinetic profile and improve tumor targeting of highly lipophilic but otherwise promising cancer imaging tracers, such as the EGFR inhibitor SKI 243. In their study, they compared the pharmacokinetics and tumor targeting of the bare EGFR kinase-targeting radiotracer SKI 212243 (SKI 243) with that of the same tracer embedded in liposomes. The results indicated that SKI 243 and liposomal SKI 243 were both taken up by tumor xenografts but liposomal SKI 243 remained in the blood longer and consequently exhibited a three- to six-fold increase in uptake in the tumor among several other organs.

NPs can be formulated to deliver drugs across several biological barriers.[162,163] Antineoplastics, antiviral drugs, and several other types of drugs are markedly hindered because of inability of these molecules to cross the BBB which can be overcome with the application of NPs to deliver across this barrier. It has been reported that NPs can cross the BBB following the opening of TJs by hyperosmotic mannitol that may provide sustained delivery of therapeutic agents for diseases that are difficult to treat like brain tumors.[164]

In another study, amorphous drug/polymer NPs were prepared from ethyl cellulose and UK-157,147 (systematic name (3S,4R)-[6-(3-hydroxyphenyl) sulfonyl]-2,2,3-trimethyl-4-(2-methyl-3-oxo-2,3-dihydropyridazin-6-yloxy)-3-chromanol), a potassium channel opener, using sodium glycocholate (NaGC) as a surface stabilizer.[165] NP suspensions were evaluated to determine if targeted drug delivery to sebaceous glands and hair follicles could be achieved. In vitro delivery of UK-157,147 to the follicles on rabbit ear tissue was demonstrated with limited distribution to the surrounding dermis. Delivery to hair follicles was demonstrated in vivo following stimulation of hair growth with 100-nm NPs with a C3H mouse model. The NPs were completely biocompatible without visible skin irritation. In vivo tests of smaller NPs with a hamster ear model indicated targeted delivery to sebaceous glands. The NPs released drug rapidly in in vitro tests and were stable in suspension for 3months. The results showed selective drug delivery to the follicles through follicular transport of NPs and rapid release of a poorly water-soluble drug showing a promising approach for targeted topical delivery of low-solubility compounds to hair follicles.

In as much as liposomes have been shown to be biocompatible, safe, and biodegradable, its potential of liposomes as a drug delivery system for use in the oral cavity has been investigated.[166] For the specific in vitro targeting of the teeth, formulations based on the adsorption of charged liposome to hydroxyapatite (HA) which is a model substance for the dental enamel, has been conducted in human parotid saliva to simulate oral-like conditions. The results showed that precipitation occurred in the presence of the lipids dipalmitoyl phosphatidylcholine (DPPC)/dipalmitoyl trimethylammoniumpropane or DPPC/dipalmitoyl phosphatidylglycerol–liposomes in parotid saliva with no HA which indicated that constituents of parotid saliva reacted with the liposomes.[166] Based on these studies, the constituents of saliva may interact with liposomes resulting in aggregation that can be circumvented by adding various ions to create ionic stability in the medium. The results of the studies by Nguyen et al. indicated that negatively charged DPPC/DPPA–liposomes showed the elast reactive to the components of parotid saliva and may be the most suitable for use in the oral cavity. Additional investigations as to how these liposomes affect the various components and physiological conditions in the oral cavity especially the cells must be conducted in vitro to evaluate the safety of the NMs for dental drug delivery.

5.9.1.3 Polymersomes

Polymersomes are hollow shell NPs that can be sued for the delivery of drugs. Biodegradable polymersomes for loading, delivery, and cytosolic uptake of drug mixtures were shown to exploit the thick membrane of these block copolymer vesicles, their aqueous lumen, and pH-triggered release within endolysosomes.[1] Target-specific and biodegradable polymersomes break down in acidic environments and release the drugs within tumor cell endosomes. Unlike cell membranes and liposomes that are created from a double layer of phospholipids, a polymersome is comprised of two layers of synthetic polymers where the individual polymers are considerably larger than individual phospholipids but have many of the same chemical features.

TAX and dox have been encapsulated in polymersomes for passive delivery to tumor-bearing mice.[167] The big molecules that compose the polymersome are used to embed the water-insoluble TAX within the NM shell. Unlike TAX, dox is water soluble and stays within the interior of the polymersome until it degrades. When the drugs are combined with the polymersome, they spontaneously self-assemble into a cocktail that lead to better tumor regression than either drugs alone. Furthermore, the polymersome drug cocktail carries both drugs efficiently to a tumor.

5.9.2 Micelles

Block copolymer micelles are spherical supermolecular assemblies of amphiphilic copolymer in which the core can accommodate hydrophobic drugs while the shell is a hydrophilic brush-like corona that makes the micelle water soluble, allowing delivery of the poorly soluble contents.[1] Camptothecin (CPT) is a topoisomerase I inhibitor that is effective against cancer but has poor solubility, instability, and toxicity limiting its clinical application. To solve these issues, biocompatible, targeted sterically stabilized micelles (SSMs) have been used as nanocarriers for CPT (CPT–SSM). SSM solubilization of CPT is expensive yet reproducible and it prevents drug aggregate formation. In addition, SSM composed of PEGylated phospholipids are attractive nanocarriers for CPT delivery because of their size (14 nm) and ability to extravasate through the leaky microvasculature of tumors and inflamed tissues. This passive targeting results in high drug concentration in tumors and reduced drug toxicity to the normal tissues.[168] Stealth micelle formulations have stabilizing PEG coronas to minimize opsonization of the micelles and maximize serum half-life. Currently, SP1049C, NK911, and Genexol-PM have been approved for clinical use.[42] SP1049C is formulated as dox-encapsulated pluronic micelles. NK911 is dox-encapsulated micelles from a copolymer of PEG-dox-conjugated poly(aspartic acid), and Genexol-PM is a TAX-encapsulated PEG–PLA micelle formulation. Polymer micelles have several advantages over other drug delivery systems, including increased drug solubility, prolonged circulation half-life, selective accumulation at tumor sites, and lower toxicity. However, this technology currently lacks tumor specificity and the ability to control the release of the entrapped agents. With these limitations, nano-enabled therapy has shifted focus from passive targeting systems (e.g. micelles) to active targeting.

5.9.3 Hydrogels

Hydrogel NPs use hydrophobic polysaccharides for encapsulation and delivery of drugs, therapeutic proteins, or vaccine antigens.[1] A system using cholesterol to form a self-aggregating hydrophobic core resulting in cholesterol NPs stabilized entrapped proteins. These particles stimulate the immune system and are readily taken up by dendritic cells. Larger hydrogel NMs can also be used to encapsulate and release monoclonal antibodies.

A naturally occurring substance found in the cooking spice turmeric, curcumin, has long been known to have anticancer properties. However, widespread clinical application of this anticancer agent has been limited due to its poor solubility and minimal systemic bioavailability. This problem has been resolved by encapsulating curcumin in a polymeric NP, creating "nanocurcumin."[169] Nanocurcumin and free curcumin have been shown to affect pancreatic cancer cells through induction of apoptosis, blockade of nuclear factor kappa B activation, and downregulation of proinflammatory cytokines [i.e. interleukin (IL)-6, IL-8, and TNF-α]. Thus, nanocurcumin provides an opportunity to expand the anticancer applications of this agent by enabling soluble dispersion.

5.9.4 Magnetic NPs

The magnetic property of a material is the atomic or subatomic response a material to an applied magnetic field wherein the electron spin and charge create a dipole moment and a magnetic field.[170] A magnetic field of measurable intensity that can be recorded results when multiple dipole moments ensue. The response of a magnetic material to an external magnetic force can be attraction (paramagnetism) or repulsion (diamagnetism) or something more complex.[170] Magnetic material structures are based on magnetic domains which are small areas that align themselves in an applied magnetic field. Spontaneous magnetization occurs in paramagnetic materials (ferromagnetic and ferromagnetic) that results in the formation of permanent magnets or gradual demagnetization. With superparamagnetic materials, such as magnetic NPs that are the size of magnetic domains, spontaneous magnetization and demagnetization occur[170] causing a much larger response to an applied magnetic field called superparamagnetic behavior.

To date, the most activity in magnetic NP-based drug delivery has focused on Fe-based NPs of the three elements (B=Ni, Co, and Fe) that are ferromagnetic under physiological conditions. This may be attributed to the to its superior magnetic susceptibility (218 and 90 emu/g for elemental Fe and Fe_3O_4, respectively), as well as the large natural reservoir of iron in the body, suggesting the comparative absence of toxicity of this element.[170] During the last few years, interest on the synthesis and drug delivery applications of Fe-based NPs has matured to in vivo studies of localization and to antitumor activity.

Magnetic NPs are ideal nanocarriers of drugs and vaccines because these NPs can also be used to diagnose the efficacy of treatment. Dimercaptosuccinic acid (DMSA)-coated monodisperse magnetic nanoparticles (MNPs) were tested as a delivery system for the antitumorigenic cytokine interferon-gamma IFN-γ in mouse models of cancer.[171] Using an external magnetic field, the IFN-γ-adsorbed DMSA-coated MNPs that were targeted to the tumor site showed a high degree of NP accumulation and of cytokine delivery at the tumor site. This caused an increased T cell and macrophage infiltration that promoted an antiangiogenic effect. This led to a notable reduction in tumor size indicating that

IFN-γ-adsorbed DMSA-coated MNPs can be used as an efficient in vivo drug delivery system for tumor immunotherapy.

To study the mechanism of cellular uptake, the lymphatic biodistribution of superparamagnetic NP ferumoxtran, AMI 227/Sinerem™/Combidex was characterized in rats.[172] Within 90 min after catheterization of the thoracic lymph duct and i.v. injection of ferumoxtran, high concentrations were found by MR relaxometry and atomic absorption spectroscopy in the thoracic lymph. There were no NMs found in the lymph cells which indicated that ferumoxtran was extracellular.[170] The highest concentration of NMs was reached 12 h later in all node groups and then plateaued thereafter.

In another study, the biodistribution of dox-loaded MNPs was assessed in mice after i.v. injection.[173] The results of electron spin resonance (ESR) showed that the dox–MNPs decreased the dox bioavailability in the heart and kidney compared with the free unconjugated dox. The dox–MNPs bioavailability at the target site was effectively increased by an applied magnetic field of 210 mT and gradient of 200 mT/cm which also reduced the hepatic clearance resulting in the increased plasma bioavailability.[173] This response was attributed to possible in vivo inhibition of phagocytic cells by the applied magnetic fields.

In a separate study using magnetic vectoring system with more complex external magnetic fields to target a tumor and enhance tumor extravasation of systemically administered magnetite-based, silica-coated MNP prodrug constructs were administred.[174] The biodistribution of magnetite MNPs were found widely distributed in tissues including the heart, liver, spleen, lungs, kidneys, brain, stomach, small intestine, and bone marrow, with the majority in the liver and spleen. Fe_3O_4 MNP levels in brain tissue were higher in the MNP-treated group than in the controls, indicating penetration of the BBB. These observed localization have already been achieved as validated by MRI and SEM in tumor tissues from human ovarian and breast carcinoma xenograft models.[175,176]

Superparamagnetic Fe_3O_4 poly e-caprolactone (PCL) NPs (~165 nm) were prepared by Gang et al.[177] with magnetizations of ~10.2 emu/g. These PCL NPs showed improved pharmacokinetic behavior. The potential for enhanced antitumor effects were examined in nude mice with subcutaneous (s.c.) xenografts of human pancreatic adenocarcinoma cells using the PCL NPs that were loaded with gemcitabine. The magnetic targeting exhibited 15-fold higher intratumoral drug levels compared with free gemcitabine administration.

The chemoadsorptive properties of activated carbon had been exploited in the form of silica-coated iron–carbon composite NPs (200–300 nm) for drug loading and for magnetic iron targeting.[178] Using dox loaded NPs, the dox content of pig hepatic tissue was ~24-fold higher in the magnetically targeted left lobe than that in the nontargeted right lobe following intra-arterial infusion.[178] From these observatios, it was suggested that the NPs penetrated through the capillary wall around the tissue interstitium and hepatic cells under the external magnetic field.

MNPs biodistribution was compared with inductively coupled plasma optical emission spectroscopy (ICP-OES) and ESR spectroscopy.[179] The biodistribution was evaluated in rats bearing 9L glioma that were administered with MNP at 12–25 mg Fe/kg under magnetic targeting. Ex vivo analysis of MNP in animal tissues was performed with both ICP-OES and ESR using a cryogenic method to overcome the technical hurdle of loading tissue samples into ESR tubes. The results from the ICP-OES and ESR measurements revealed two distinct relationships for organs accumulating *high* or *low* levels of MNP. The *high* MNP accumulation in liver and spleen showed strongly correlated data ($r =$ 0.97, 0.94 for liver and spleen, respectively), thereby validating the equivalence of the two methods at high concentrations (>1000 nmol Fe/g tissue). However, at lower levels of IOMNPs accumulations, the two methods differed significantly in organs such as brain, kidney, and the tumor. While the ESR resolved MNPs down to 10–55 nmol Fe/g tissue, ICP-OES failed due to masking by endogenous iron. These findings suggest that ESR coupled to cryogenic sample handling is more sensitive than ICP-OES.[179]

Chertok et al.[180] studied the use of 100-nm IOMNP (saturation magnetization of 94 emu/g Fe) as a drug delivery platform for MRI-monitored magnetic targeting of brain tumors. The rats bearing orthotopic 9L gliosarcomas were i.v. injected with IOMNPs (12 mg Fe/kg) under a magnetic field density of 0 T for the control and 0.4 T for the test animals for 30 min. Prior to administration, immediately after administration of the IOMNPs, and at 1-h intervals for 4 h, MR images were taken. The results revealed that magnetic targeting induced a fivefold increase in the total glioma exposure to the IOMNPs compared with nontargeted tumors ($p = 0.005$). A 3.6-fold enhancement in target selectivity index of NP accumulation in glioma over the normal brain ($p = 0.025$) was observed. This study showed that accumulation of iron oxide NPs in gliosarcomas can be significantly enhanced by magnetic targeting and successfully quantified by MR imaging, indicating that IOMNPs hold promise as platform for targeted drug delivery.

Superparamagnetic magnetite- and QD-embedded polystyrene NPs loaded with TAX were conjugated to anti-prostate-specific membrane antigen (PSMA) antibodies.[181] After i.v. injection into tumor-bearing nude mice, significant differences in fluorescent signals were demonstrated between tumor regions in animals that were treated with the PSMA-targeted nanocarrier system and the nontargeted nanocarrier system. This indicated that the targeted NMs were more efficiently delivered into the tumor regions showing that they can be used for targeted drug delivery.

The anticancer drug dox and IOMNPs were loaded into human serum albumin matrices.[182] The results indicated that the 50-nm IOMNPs translocated the dox across cell membranes (similar to the mechanism proposed for Abraxane™), followed by nuclear accumulation. Both MRI and immunostaining showed that in vivo, they retained tumor-targeting capability. In vitro studies using the 4T1 breast cancer model showed that the dox-loaded IOMNPs demonstrated marked tumor suppression that were comparable to the effect of Doxil and superior to free dox.

Super paramagnetic iron oxide particles can be used in conjunction with MRI to localize the tumor as well as for subsequent thermal ablation. This has been used, for example, to target glioblastoma multiforme (GBM), a primary malignant tumor of the brain with few effective therapeutic options. The primary difficulty in treating GBM lies in the difficulty of delivering drugs across the BBB. However, nanoscale liposomal iron oxide preparations were recently shown to improve passage across the BBB.[183]

Alexiou et al.[184] reported the successful preclinical applications of iron-based NP drug delivery systems. He and his group established the established initial parameters for targeted MNP drug delivery using intratumor arterial (i.a.) administration.[176,184,185,186] In their studies, an external magnetic field was applied to make i.a.-administered ferrofluids (100-nm diameter NPs) loaded with mitoxantrone (MTX) to accumulate at rabbit hind limb VX2 tumors fed by this artery. The ferrofluids consisted of iron oxides and hydroxides NPs that were encapsulated with a starch polymer matrix to provide biological stability with sites for chemoabsorptive/electrostatic MTX binding, forming MTX–NMs. Immediately after administration of the MTX–NMs, darkened tumor blood vessels were observed histologically with brown–black particles distributed throughout the entire tumor. At the end of a 3-month study, no tumor tissue was histologically observed in rabbits that were i.a. treated with the MTX–NMs but the i.v. administration failed. This may have been caused by the extensive clearance of NMs prior to reaching the tumor or to premature MTX release before extravasation. This approach is currently being studied for the treatment of head and neck cancer.[187]

The extensive applications of iron-based NPs for drug delivery and other medical applications that spurred extensive toxicological assessments have been conducted by various researchers. In vitro studies using human aortic endothelial cells (HAECs) were incubated with different NPs composed of Fe_2O_3, Y_2O_3, or ZnO after which the levels of messenger RNA and protein levels of intercellular adhesion molecule-1 (ICAM-1), IL-8, and monocyte chemoattractant protein-1 (MCP-1) were evaluated.[188] The interactions of the NPs with the cells were evaluated with inductively coupled plasma mass spectrometry and TEM. The results showed that all three NPs were internalized and localized to intracellular vesicles in HAECs. Out of the three NMs, Fe_2O_3 did not induce an inflammatory response unlike Y_2O_3 and ZnO NPs that did. In a separate investigation, both Fe_2O_3 and Fe_3O_4 NMs generated oxidative stress as well as increased nitric oxide (NO) production in human ECV304 umbilical endothelial cells.[189] Early signs of apoptosis such as loss of mitochondrial membrane potential and nuclear chromatin condensation were apparent.

The effect of 22- to 43-nm Fe_2O_3 NPs on HAECs and U937 resulted in cytoplasmic vacuolation, mitochondrial swelling and cell death that were accompanied by an increase in NO production and NO synthesis activity.[190] Monocytes adhesion to the HAECs was enhanced as a result of the upregulation of expressions of ICAM-1 and IL-8. The U937 phagocytosized the NMs which simultaneously provoked oxidative stress and severe endothelial cell toxicity. This study indicated that i.v.-administered IOMNPs may result in endothelial inflammation and dysfunction when NMs escape phagocytosis and directly interact with the endothelial layer, or the IOMNPs undergo phagocytosis by monocytes followed by their dissolution resulting in free iron ions, or they undergo phagocytosis and induce oxidative stress responses.[170] Cell death that were most likely due to oxidative stress were observed in polyol-produced maghemite γ-Fe$_2$O$_3$ NPs that were efficiently internalized by human endothelial cells within 24h of exposure.[191] These NMs were rapidly cleared through the urine but caused toxicity in the liver, kidneys, and lungs and did not affect the brain and the heart.[170] From these studies, it can be inferred that care must be taken with respect to surface coating, cellular targeting, and local exposure toward clinical applications.

Ferritin contains 7-nm iron (ferrous) particles and a protein shell that had failed to induce spontaneous glutamate release but induced intrasynaptosomal ROS formation that was insensitive to the inhibitor of NADPH oxidase, DPI (diphenyleneiodonium), and to carbonyl cyanide m-chloro phenyl hydrazone CCCP, a mitochondrial uncoupler.[192] As more applications of IOMNPs are studied, concerns about long-term toxicity related to the production of toxic-free iron during their biodegradation prompted an EM-based study which found that the iron oxide NPs were degraded after internalization by macrophages, leading to the core iron being incorporated into the nontoxic iron-storing protein, ferritin.[193]

5.9.5 Nanotubes

Previously, it has already been possible to attach drug molecules directly to antibodies; however, attaching a handful of drug molecules to an antibody significantly limits its targeting ability because the chemical bonds that are used for the drug attachment deactivates antibody activity. With the onset of nanotechnology, a number of NPs have been investigated to overcome this limitation. Among the NMs available commercially, carbon nanotubes have been studied quite well. Tumor targeting single-walled carbon nanotube has been developed by covalently attaching tumor-specific mAbs, radiation ion chelates, and fluorescent probes.[194] This led to a new class of anticancer compound that contains both tumor-targeting antibodies and NPs called fullerenes (C60) that can be loaded with several molecules of an anticancer drug such as Taxol®.[195] This system allows loading as many as 40 fullerenes onto a single skin cancer antibody called ZME-108 that can be used to deliver drugs directly into melanomas. Distinct sites on the antibody are hydrophobic which attract the hydrophobic fullerenes in large numbers and so multiple drugs can be loaded into a single antibody in a spontaneous manner, requiring no covalent bond, so the increased payload does not significantly change the targeting ability of the antibody. The fullerene-based therapies provide potential to carry multiple drug payloads, such as taxol plus other chemotherapeutic drugs which can solve the issue of drug resistance in cancer cells. This can avoid the possibility of their escaping treatment by attacking them with more than one kind of drug at a time.

5.9.6 Semiconductor NPs

One of the more significant advancement involves the use of semiconductor NMs for the delivery of vaccine to prevent diseases that currently do not have any cure or preventive drugs. In a proof-of-concept study, the use of <15 nm, water-soluble, inorganic NPs as a vaccine delivery system for a blood-stage malaria vaccine was recently reported.[196] The recombinant malarial antigen, merozoite surface protein 1 (rMSP1) of *Plasmodium falciparum* was used as the model vaccine.[197] Using published protocols, the rMSP1 was covalently conjugated to water-soluble amphiphilic polymer-coated QD, CdSe/ZnS NPs, using surface carboxyl groups to form rMSP1–QDs. In this study, the anti-MSP1 antibody responses induced by rMSP1–QDs were found to have 2–3 log higher titers than those obtained with rMSP1 that were administered with the conventional adjuvants, Montanide ISA51 and CFA.[196] In addition, the immune response and the induction of parasite inhibitory antibodies were significantly higher in mice that were injected with rMSP1–QDs. The results were similar whether the rMSP1–QDs were delivered via intraperitoneal, intramuscular, and s.c. routes. Very high levels of immunogenicity from injections of the rMSP1–QDs were achieved without further addition of other commercial adjuvant components. Dendritic cells that were bone marrow derived showed efficient uptake of the QDs (Figure 5.7) which were suspected to cause their activation and the expression/secretion of key cytokines, suggesting that this may be the mechanism for the enhanced immunogenicity. This study provides promising use of water-soluble, inorganic semiconductor NPs (<15 nm, Figure 5.8) as potent platforms to enhance the immunogenicity of polypeptide antigens in adjuvant-free immunizations. This

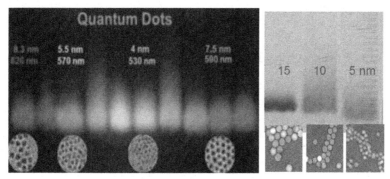

FIGURE 5.8   TEM and gel electrophoresis of QDs (left) and IOMNPs (right) that are <15 nm in diameter. *(For color version of this figure, the reader is referred to the online version of this book)*

study also shows promising applications of semiconductor NMs for efficient delivery and efficacy of vaccines for diseases that currently have no cure.

In a separate study, semiconductor QDs conjugated to tumor-targeting anti-human epidermal growth factor receptor 2 (HER-2) mAb forming QD–mAb have been used to locate tumors using high-speed confocal microscopy.[198] After injection of QD–mAb conjugates, distinct steps were identified as the particles traveled from the injection site to the tumor site. The blood-borne QD–mAb conjugates extravasated into the tumor, bound to HER-2 on cell membranes, entered the tumor cells, and migrated to the perinuclear region. The images collected provide evidence for the analysis of the delivery processes of NPs in vivo as well as valuable information on NP-based mAb-conjugated therapeutics. This is very important in the development of QDs and other semiconductor NPs for anticancer therapeutic efficacy.

5.9.7 Dendrimers

Early studies on dendrimer-based drug delivery systems focused on encapsulating drugs but it was difficult to control the release of drugs. New developments in polymer and dendrimer chemistry provided a new class of molecules, dendronized polymers which are linear polymers that bear dendrons at each repeat unit. Dendronized polymers provide drug delivery advantages because of their enhanced circulation time. The drugs can also be conjugated with the drug to the dendrimers through a degradable link that can be used to control the release of the drug. A study using dox that was conjugated to a biodegradable dendrimer with optimized blood circulation time was achieved through the meticulous design of size and molecular architecture.[199] The dox–dendrimer drug loading was controlled through multiple attachment sites and its solubility was controlled through PEGylation; the drug release was controlled through the use of pH-sensitive hydrazone dendrimer linkages. In vitro studies using colon carcinoma cells showed that the dox–dendrimers were more than 10 times less toxic than free dox. I.v. administration to tumor-bearing mice showed that the tumor uptake of dox–dendrimers was ninefold higher than i.v.-free dox and caused complete tumor regression with 100% survival of the mice after 60 days.

5.10 THE BLOOD BRAIN BARRIER (BBB)

The molecular level interaction of NMs with cells and tissues provides a distinct advantage over other substances. NMs have been recognized to pass across the BBB.[200] The BBB consists of a tightly packed layer of endothelial cells surrounding the brain that prevents high-MW molecules from passing through. The ability of NMs to pass through the BBB is an important advantage for drug delivery systems for effective treatments. However, the efficacy of NPs toward the treatment of neurological disorders, like brain tumor, stroke, and Alzheimer's disease, have been largely constrained in spite of the advances and breakthroughs in nanotechnology-based medical approaches. Thus, targeting of drugs to the CNS remains for the future success and development of nanotechnology-based diagnostics and therapeutics in neurology. The global market for drugs that target the CNS would have to grow by over 500% to come close to the global market for cardiovascular diseases.[201]

The efficient delivery of potentially therapeutic and diagnostic compounds to specific areas of the brain are hindered by the BBB, the blood cerebrospinal fluid barrier, or other specialized CNS barriers which restrict the passage of foreign particles into the brain. Thus, because of these barriers, the efficient design of noninvasive nanocarrier systems that can facilitate controlled and targeted drug delivery to the specific regions of the brain is a major challenge for neurological diseases.[101,202]

The BBB acts as a neuroprotective shield by selecting the passage of substances from the blood, supplying the brain with nutrients, and disposing harmful compounds from the brain back to the bloodstream.[203] The BBB composed of the brain endothelial cells that make up the cerebral microvascular endothelium together with astrocytes, pericytes, neurons, and the extracellular matrix constitute a "neurovascular unit" that is essential for the health and function of the CNS.[204] This maintains the transport of substances including drugs in and out of the brain, leukocyte migration, and regulates the brain microenvironment that is crucial for neuronal activity and proper functioning of CNS. The unique environment in the CNS makes the treatment of neurological diseases such as inborn metabolic errors (e.g. lysosomal storage diseases), brain tumors, infectious diseases, and aging and is a unnerving challenge.[205,206] Transport across the BBB is strictly constrained through the physical TJs and adherent junctions as well as metabolic barriers (enzymes, diverse transport systems) that excludes very small, electrically neutral, and lipid-soluble molecules.[207] The CNS also has a lack of fenestrations (perforations) and a lack of pinocytotic vesicles.[208,209,210] Combined with an intricate complex of transmembrane proteins [junctional adhesion molecule-1 (JAM-1), occludin, and claudins], it allows drugs with cytoplasmic accessory proteins, zonula drugs, or small molecules, with high lipid solubility and low molecular mass of <400–500 Daltons. On top of this intricate structure, there are other CNS barriers, such as the blood tumor barrier and the blood retina barrier shielding the brain which may play a role in drug transport.[211] Thus, conventional pharmacological drugs or chemotherapeutic agents are unable to pass through the barrier.

NMs have emerged as potential drug delivery carriers to various tissues throughout the body including the brain owing to their small size, solubility in aqueous solutions, adaptable surface, targeted drug delivery, and multifunctionality.[1] However, because entry through the almost impermeable BBB is extremely selective, the proper design of these engineered nanocarriers become extremely important to facilitate drug delivery. In addition, it is also necessary to retain the integrity and stability of the drug to prevent untimely degradation of the drugs in the NMs–drug complex. Multiple factors such as size, shape, biocompatibility, target-specific affinity, escape from the RES, stability in blood, and ability to perform in the controlled drug release must be considered during the development of the nanocarriers. Excellent candidates as nanocarriers must have the following properties[163]:

- Size: <100 nm diameter
- Nontoxic, biodegradable, and biocompatible
- No particle aggregation in blood
- No opsonization by proteins
- BBB-targeted chemistry: use of cell surface, ligands, and receptor-mediated endocytosis
- No activation of neutrophils and noninflammatory
- No platelet aggregation
- Escapes the RES
- Prolonged circulation time
- Cost-effective scaled-up manufacturing/production
- Ease of complexation with drugs that may be in the form of small molecules, peptides, proteins, or nucleic acids
- Controlled drug release or exhibit modulation of drug release profiles.

The engineering of NMs for drug delivery becomes more complicated when it comes to drug delivery to the brain because of its immunologically unique characteristics which restricts the entry of most pharmaceutical compounds. As a result, there is a severely limited research on the applicability of nanotechnology in CNS drug delivery that may be attributed to the lack of strategies that can allow localized and controlled delivery of drugs across the BBB to the site of injury or disease.

Among the few NMs that have been studied for drug delivery to the brain are the liposomes and their related lipid NPs. Lipid NMs are the alternative to traditional colloidal carriers, such as emulsions, liposomes, and polymeric particles that have been employed for brain tumor targeting.[212] The role of apolipoprotein A-I in the NP uptake and passage across the BBB was observed for different types of NPs.[213] For targeting, specific receptors on the brain capillaries such as the transferrin receptor[214] and the receptor for insulin[215] are highly expressed by the endothelial cells forming the BBB with the assumption that the endogenous ligands for these receptors as well as antibodies against them can be used for drug targeting to the CNS.[216] A collection of papers on the use of NPs or drug delivery has been included in the review by Wohlfart.[213]

The most popular alternative route for direct drug administration to the brain region that is painless and safe is i.v. administration. Some approaches such as oral route, inhalation or intratracheal instillation, i.n. drug delivery, and convection-enhanced diffusion, and intrathecal/intraventricular drug delivery systems are other conventional modes. The administration route of NMs becomes an important criterion of consideration to overcome the physiological barriers of the brain. Studies have used fluorescence-labeled bovine serum albumin loaded in biodegradable PLGA for intraspinal administration of glial cell line-derived neurotrophic factor following contusive spinal cord injury and for in vitro study.[154] Intraspinal delivery of neurotrophic factor encapsulated in biodegradable PLGA NPs following contusive spinal cord injury were well absorbed by neurons and glia showing PLGA as a useful nanocarrier delivery system for neuroprotective polypeptide into the injured spinal cord.

One important requirement for NMs' brain delivery systems is that they are rapidly biodegradable over a time frame of a few days.[213] Nonbiodegradable particles such as fullerenes, toxic systems as heavy metal containing QDs, or potentially risky drug delivery systems such as carbon nanotubes that may have hazardous effects similar to asbestos, therefore, are not useful.

5.11 CONCLUSION

Drug delivery in cancer, tumor, and other types of diseases are important for optimizing the effect of drugs and reducing toxic side effects. Several nano-technologies, mostly based on NMs, can facilitate drug delivery to tumors. However, such NMs have to be carefully and meticulously engineered before they can perform the functions they are designed for. Excellent candidates as nanocarriers must be small (less than 100 nm), nontoxic, biodegradable, biocompatible, does not aggregate, avoids the RES, and escapes opsonization, non-inflammatory, with prolonged circulation time and cost effective. Many drugs in the market that are now available for human use are already nano enabled. The ability of these drugs to minimize the side effects that are normally observed in conventional drugs open up doors for applications of NMs as safer alternatives to drug delivery.

Aside from the requirements of size, charge, shape, surface modifications, loading, and other chemical properties to effectively deliver drugs using the NM carrier systems, other challenges need further attention. These studies need to focus on the interaction of NMs and their hosts in terms of biodistribution, organ accumulation, degradation and/or toxicity, damage of cellular structures or inflammatory foreign body effects, and genetic damage. Aggregation or precipitation once in contact with biological fluids in host animals or humans must be carefully evaluated and its prevention are established to prevent adverse effects. In a preliminary study, the author conducted a stability evaluation of IOMNPs loaded with dox in fresh human whole blood (Z.P. Aguilar unpublished data). The results indicated that properly coated with amphiphilic polymer, IOMNPs loaded with dox are stable (left and middle wells) in fresh human whole blood (treated with heparin to prevent coagulation) even after 24 h of exposure (Figure 5.9). Without the proper coating, the IOMNP can be loaded with dox but aggregation occurs upon exposure to blood (two wells on the right).

It is essential to investicate the possible adverse effects or toxicity of nano-carriers.[217,218,219] But, the NM drug delivery system is still its infancy. Research protocols like absorption, distribution, metabolism, and elimination (ADME),

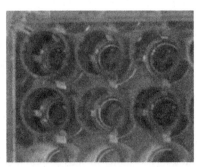

FIGURE 5.9 IOMNPs loaded with dox exposed to fresh human whole blood. *(For color version of this figure, the reader is referred to the online version of this book)*

and drug metabolism and pharmacokinetics will definitely be part of further studies on NM drug delivery systems in the future.[220,221,222]

The use of nonbiodegradable NMs such as carbon-based single- or multi-wall carbon nanotubes, metallic nanocarriers, and some inorganic oxides may not be possible in nanomedicine. Depending on their functionalization, bio-degradable drug nanocarriers can take a number of paths within tissues. The pharmacokinetics (PK) and excretion routes of the various NMs used as drug delivery systems demand exhaustive research to clear the path for their human applications. The path that the nano-enabled drugs take after entry into the living system depends on many factors which were discussed in this chapter. The NM properties that allow its in vivo imaging maybe the most useful property for elucidating the ADME and PK in nanodrug delivery systems. Further investigations on the properties of NMs that will allow in vivo imaging and other modes of detection are important as the NMs enter the realm of human consumption.

REFERENCES

1. Singh, R.; Lillard, J. W., Jr. Nanoparticle-Based Targeted Delivery. *Exp. Mol. Pathol.* **2009,** *86,* 215–223.
2. Kreuter, J. *Nanoparticles, Encyclopaedia of Pharmaceutical Technology*; Marcel Dekker Inc: New York, 1994.
3. Barratt, G. M. Therapeutic Applications of Colloidal Drug Carriers. *Pharma. Sci. Tech. Today* **2000,** *3,* 163–171.
4. Pitt, C. G.; Gratzl, M. M.; Kimmel, G. L.; Surles, J.; Schindler, A. Aliphatic Polyesters II. The Degradation of Poly(DL-lactide), Poly(epsilon-caprolactone), and Their Copolymers In Vivo. *Biomaterials* **1981,** *2,* 215–220.
5. Liversidge, G. Controlled Release and Nanotechnologies: Recent Advances and Future Opportunities. *Drug Dev. Deliv.* **2011,** *11,* 1.
6. Panagiotou, T.; Fisher, R. J. Enhanced Transport Capabilities via Nanotechnologies: Impacting Bioefficacy, Controlled Release Strategies, and Novel Chaperones. *J. Drug Deliv.* **2011**: 1–14.
7. Dekker, C. *Phys. Today* **1999,** *52,* 22–28.
8. Panyam, J.; Sahoo, S. K.; Prabha, S.; Bargar, T.; Labhasetwar, V. Fluorescence and Electron Microscopy Probes for Cellular and Tissue Uptake of Poly(D, L-lactide-co-glycolide) Nanoparticles. *Int. J. Pharm.* **2003,** *262,* 1–11.

9. Linhardt, R. J. Biodegradable polymers for controlled release of drugs. In *Controlled Release of Drugs*; Rosoff, M., Ed.; VCH Publishers: New York, 1989; pp 53–95.

10. Moghimi, S. M.; Hunter, A. C.; Murray, J. C. Long-Circulating and Target-Specific Nanoparticles: Theory to Practice. *Pharmacol. Rev.* **2001**, *53*, 283–318.

11. Moghimi, S. M.; Szebeni, J. Stealth Liposomes and Long Circulating Nanoparticles: Critical Issues in Pharmacokinetics, Opsonization and Protein-Binding Properties. *Prog. Lipid Res.* **2003**, *42*, 463–478.

12. Yan, X.; Kuipers, F.; Havekes, L. M.; Havinga, R.; Dontje, B.; Poelstra, K.; Scherpof, G. L.; Kamps, J. A. A.M. The Role of Apolipoprotein E in the Elimination of Liposomes from Blood by Hepatocytes in the Mouse. *Biochem. Biophys. Res. Commun.* **2005**, *328*, 57–62.

13. Kamps, J. A.; Scherphof, G. L. Receptor versus Non-Receptor Mediated Clearance of Liposomes. *Adv. Drug Deliv. Rev.* **1998**, *32*, 81–97.

14. Bertholon, I.; Ponchel, G.; Labarre, D.; Couvreur, P.; Vauthier, C. Bioadhesive Properties of Poly(alkylcyanoacrylate) Nanoparticles Coated with Polysaccharide. *J. Nanosci. Nanotechnol.* **2006**, *6*, 3102–3109.

15. Moore, A.; Weissleder, R.; Bogdanov, A., Jr. Uptake of Dextran-Coated Monocrystalline Iron Oxides in Tumor Cells and Macrophages. *J. Magn. Reson. Imaging* **1997**, *7*, 1140–1145.

16. Raynal, I.; Prigent, P.; Peyramaure, S.; Najid, A.; Rebuzzi, C.; Corot, C. Macrophage Endocytosis of Superparamagnetic Iron Oxide Nanoparticles: Mechanisms and Comparison of Ferumoxides and Ferumoxtran-10. *Invest. Radiol.* **2004**, *39*, 56–63.

17. Couvreur, P.; Barratt, G.; Fattal, E.; Legrand, P.; Vauthier, C. Nanocapsule Technology: A Review. *Crit. Rev. Ther. Drug Carrier Syst.* **2002**, *19*, 99–134.

18. Hume, D. A. The Mononuclear Phagocyte System. *Curr. Opin. Immunol.* **2006**, *18*, 48–53.

19. Muller, R. H.; Maassen, S.; Weyhers, H.; Mehnert, W. Phagocytic Uptake and Cytotoxicity of Solid Lipid Nanoparticles (Sln) Sterically Stabilized with Poloxamine 908 and Poloxamer 407. *J. Drug Target.* **1996**, *4*, 161–170.

20. Brigger, I.; Dubernet, C.; Couvreur, P. Nanoparticles in Cancer Therapy and Diagnosis. *Adv. Drug Deliv. Rev.* **2002**, *54*, 631–651.

21. Grislain, L.; Couvreur, P.; Lenaerts, V.; Roland, M.; D-Decampeneere, D.; Speiser, P. Pharmacokinetics and Biodistribution of a Biodegradable Drug-Carrier. *Int. J. Pharm.* **1983**, *15*, 335–345.

22. Bhadra, D.; Bhadra, S.; Jain, P.; Jain, N. K. Pegnology: A Review of PEG-ylated Systems. *Pharmazie* **2002**, *57*, 5–29.

23. Weissleder, R.; Bogdanov, A. J.; Neuwelt, E. A.; Papisov, M. Long-Circulating Iron Oxides for MR Imaging. *Adv. Drug Deliv. Rev.* **1995**, *16*, 321–334.

24. Park, J. H.; von Maltzhan, G.; Zhang, L.; Schwartz, M. P.; Ruoslahti, E.; Bhatia, S. Magnetic Iron Oxide Nanoworms for Tumor Targeting and Imaging. *Adv. Mater.* **2008**, *20*, 1630–1635.

25. Bulte, J. W.; Kraitchman, D. L. Iron Oxide MR Contrast Agents for Molecular and Cellular Imaging. *NMR Biomed.* **2004**, *17*, 484–499.

26. Koo, O. M.; Rubinstein, I.; Onyuksel, H. Role of Nanotechnology in Targeted Drug Delivery and Imaging: A Concise Review. *Nanomedicine* **2005**, *1*, 193–212.

27. Drummond, D. C.; Meyer, O.; Hong, K.; Kirpotin, D. B.; Papahadjopoulos, D. Optimizing Liposomes for Delivery of Chemotherapeutic Agents to Solid Tumors. *Pharmacol. Rev.* **1999**, *51*, 691–743.

28. Au, J. L.; Jang, S. H.; Zheng, J.; Chen, C. T.; Song, S.; Hu, L.; Wientjes, M. G.; Determinants of Drug Delivery and Transport to Solid Tumors. *J. Contr. Release* **2001**, *74*, 31–46.

29. Fetterly, G. J.; Straubinger, R. M. Pharmacokinetics of Paclitaxel-Containing Liposomes in Rats. *AAPS PharmSci.* **2003**, *5*, 1–11.

30. Hoarau, D.; Delmas, P.; David, S.; Roux, E.; Leroux, J. C. Novel Long Circulating Lipid Nanocapsules. *Pharm. Res.* **2004,** *21,* 1783–1789.

31. Das, S.; Jagan, L.; Isiah, R.; Rajech, B.; Backianathan, S.; Subhashini, J. Nanotechnology in Oncology: Characterization and In Vitro Release Kinetics of Cisplatin-Loaded Albumin Nanoparticles: Implications in Anticancer Drug Delivery. *Indian J. Pharmacol.* **2011,** *43,* 409–413.

32. Koo, O.; Rubinstein, I.; Onyuksel, H. Camptothecin in Sterically Stabilized Phospholipid Micelles: A Novel Nanomedicine. *Nanomedicine* **2005,** *1,* 77–84.

33. Kristl, J.; Volk, B.; Gasperlin, M.; Sentjurc, M.; Jurkovic, P. Effect of Colloidal Carriers on Ascorbyl Palmitate Stability. *Eur. J. Pharm. Sci.* **2003,** *19,* 181–189.

34. Arnedo, A.; Irache, J. M.; Merodio, M.; Espuelas, M.; Millan, S. Albumin Nanoparticles Improved the Stability, Nuclear Accumulation and Anticytomegaloviral Activity of a Phosphodiester Oligonucleotide. *J. Contr. Release* **2004,** *94,* 217–227.

35. Zhang, J. A.; Anyarambhatla, G.; Ma, L.; Ugwu, S.; Xuan, T.; Sardone, T.; Ahmad, I. Development and Characterization of a Novel Cremophor® EL Free Liposome-Based Paclitaxel (Lep-Etu) Formulation. *Eur. J. Pharm. Biopharm.* **2005,** *59,* 177–187.

36. Gradishar, W. J.; Tjulandin, S.; Davidson, N.; Shaw, H.; Desai, N.; Bhar, P.; Hawkins, M.; O'Shaughnessy, J. Phase III Trial of Nanoparticle Albumin-Bound Paclitaxel Compared with Polyethylated Castor Oil-Based Paclitaxel in Women with Breast Cancer. *J. Clin. Oncol.* **2005,** *23,* 7794–7803.

37. Blum, J. L.; Savin, M. A.; Edelman, G.; Pippen, J. E.; Robert, N. J.; Geister, B. V.; Kirby, R. L.; Clawson, A.; O'shaughnessy, J. A. Phase II Study of Weekly Albumin-Bound Paclitaxel for Patients with Metastatic Breast Cancer Heavily Pretreated with Taxanes. *Clin. Breast Cancer* **2007,** *7,* 850–856.

38. Krishnadas, A.; Rubinstein, I.; Onyuksel, H. Sterically Stabilized Phospholipid Mixed Micelles: In Vitro Evaluation as a Novel Carrier for Water-Insoluble Drugs. *Pharm. Res.* **2003,** *20,* 297–302.

39. Gelderblom, H.; Verweij, J.; Nooter, K.; Sparreboom, A. Cremophor EL: The Drawbacks and Advantages of Vehicle Selection for Drug Formulation. *Eur. J. Cancer* **2001,** *37,* 1590–1598.

40. tenTije, A. J.; Verweij, J.; Loos, W. J.; Sparreboom, A. Pharmacological Effects of Formulation Vehicles: Implications for Cancer Chemotherapy. *Clin. Pharmacokinet.* **2003,** *42,* 665–685.

41. Hatefi, A.; Amsden, B. Camptothecin Delivery Methods. *Pharm. Res.* **2002,** *19,* 1389–1399.

42. Sutton, D.; Nasongkla, N.; Blanco, E.; Gao, J. Functionalized Micellar Systems for Cancer Targeted Drug Delivery. *Pharm. Res.* **2007,** *24,* 1029–1046.

43. Huuskonen, J.; Salo, M.; Taskinen, J. Neural Network Modeling for Estimation of the Aqueous Solubility of Structurally Related Drugs. *J. Pharm. Sci.* **1997,** *86,* 450–454.

44. Sakamoto, J. H.; van de Ven, A. L.; Godin, B.; Blanco, E.; Serda, R. E.; Grattoni, A.; Ziemys, A.; Bouamrani, A.; Hu, T.; Ranganathan, S. I.; De Rosa, E.; Martinez, J. O.; Smid, C. A.; Buchanan, R.; Lee, S. Y.; Srinivasan, S.; Landry, M.; Meyn, A.; Tasciotti, E.; Li, X.; Decuzzi, P.; Ferrari, M. Review: Enabling Individualized Therapy through Nanotechnology. *Pharm. Res.* **2010,** *62,* 57–89.

45. Ferrari, M. Nanovector Therapeutics. *Curr. Opin. Chem. Biol.* **2005,** *9,* 343–346.

46. Canal, P.; Gamelin, E.; Vassal, G.; Robert, J. Benefits of Pharmacological Knowledge in the Design and Monitoring of Cancer Chemotherapy. *Pathol. Oncol. Res.* **1998,** *4,* 171–178.

47. Tallaj, J. A.; Franco, V.; Rayburn, B. K.; Pinderski, L.; Benza, R. L.; Pamboukian, S., et al. Response of Doxorubicin Induced Cardiomyopathy to the Current Management Strategy of Heart Failure. *J. Heart Lung Transplant.* **2005,** *24,* 196–201.

48. Swarbrick, J.; Boylan, J. *Encyclopedia of Pharmaceutical Technology*; 2nd ed.; MArcel Dekker: New York, 2002.

49. Panyam, J.; Labhasetwar, V. Biodegradable Nanoparticles for Drug and Gene Delivery to Cells and Tissue. *Adv. Drug Deliv. Rev.* **2003**, *55,* 329–347.

50. Kroll, R. A.; Pagel, M. A.; Muldoon, L. L.; Roman-Goldstein, S.; Fiamengo, S. A.; Neuwelt, E. A. Improving Drug Delivery to Intracerebral Tumor and Surrounding Brain in a Rodent Model: A Comparison of Osmotic versus Bradykinin Modification of the Blood-Brain and/or Blood-Tumor Barriers. *Neurosurgery* **1998**, *43,* 879–886.

51. Kreuter, J.; Ramge, P.; Petrov, V.; Hamm, S.; Gelperina, S. E.; Engelhardt, B.; Alyautdin, R.; von Briesen, H.; Begley, D. J. Direct Evidence That Polysorbate-80-Coated Poly(Butylcyanoacrylate) Nanoparticles Deliver Drugs to the CNS via Specific Mechanisms Requiring Prior Binding of Drug to the Nanoparticles. *Pharm. Res.* **2003**, *20,* 409–416.

52. Zauner, W.; Farrow, N. A.; Haines, A. M. In Vitro Uptake of Polystyrene Microspheres: Effect of Particle Size, Cell Line and Cell Density. *J. Contr. Release* **2001**, *71,* 39–51.

53. Redhead, H. M.; Davis, S. S.; Illum, L. Drug Delivery in Poly(lactide-co-glycolide) Nanoparticles Surface Modified with Poloxamer 407 and Poloxamine 908: In Vitro Characterisation and In Vivo Evaluation. *J. Contr. Release* **2001**, *70,* 353–363.

54. Govender, T.; Stolnik, S.; Garnett, M. C.; Illum, L.; Davis, S. S. PLGA Nanoparticles Prepared by Nanoprecipitation: Drug Loading and Release Studies of a Water Soluble Drug. *J. Contr. Release* **1999**, *57,* 171–185.

55. Yang, L.; Cao, Z.; Sajja, H.; Mao, H.; Wang, L.; Geng, H.; Xu, H.; Jiang, T.; Wood, W.; Nie, S.; Wang, A. Development of Receptor Targeted Iron Oxide Nanoparticles for Efficient Drug Delivery and Tumor Imaging. *J. Biomed. Nanotech.* **2008**, *4,* 1–11.

56. Yang, L.; Peng, X.; Wang, Y.; Wang, X.; Cao, Z.; Ni, C.; Karna, P.; Zhang, X.; Wood, W.; Gao, X.; Nie, S.; Mao, H. Receptor-Targeted Nanoparticles for In Vivo Imaging of Breast Cancer. *Clin. Cancer Res.* **2009**, *15,* 4722–4732.

57. Aguilar, Z.; Aguilar, Y.; Xu, H.; Jones, B.; Dixon, J.; Xu, H.; Wang, A. Nanomaterials in Medicine. *Electrochem. Soc. Trans.* **2010**, *33,* 69–74.

58. Govender, T.; Riley, T.; Ehtezazi, T.; Garnett, M. C.; Stolnik, S.; Illum, L.; Davis, S. S. Defining the Drug Incorporation Properties of PLA-PEG Nanoparticles. *Int. J. Pharm.* **2000**, *199,* 95–110.

59. Panyam, J.; Williams, D.; Dash, A.; Leslie-Pelecky, D.; Labhasetwar, V. Solid-State Solubility Influences Encapsulation and Release of Hydrophobic Drugs from PLGA/PLA Nanoparticles. *J. Pharm. Sci.* **2004**, *93,* 1804–1814.

60. Peracchia, M. T.; Gref, R.; Minamitae, Y.; Domb, A.; Lotan, N.; Langer, R. PEG-Coated Nanospheres from Amphiphilic Diblock and Multiblock Copolymers: Investigation of Their Drug Encapsulation and Release Characteristics. *J. Contr. Release* **1997**, *46,* 223–231.

61. Calvo, P.; Remuñan-López, C.; Vila-Jato, J. L.; Alonso, M. J. Chitosan and Chitosan/Ethylene Oxide-Propylene Oxide Block Copolymer Nanoparticles as Novel Carriers for Proteins and Vaccines. *Pharm. Res.* **1997**, *14,* 1431–1436.

62. Chen, Y.; McCulloch, R. K.; Gray, B. N. Synthesis of Albumin-Dextran Sulfate Microspheres Possessing Favourable Loading and Release Characteristics for the Anticancer Drug Doxorubicin. *J. Contr. Release* **1994**, *31,* 49–54.

63. Chen, Y.; Mohanraj, V.; Parkin, J. Chitosan-Dextran Sulfate Nanoparticles for Delivery of an Anti-angiogenesis Peptide. *Int. J. Pept. Res. Ther.* **2003**, *10,* 621–629.

64. Westesen, K.; Bunjes, H.; Koch, M. H. J. Physicochemical Characterization of Lipid Nanoparticles and Evaluation of Their Drug Loading Capacity and Sustained Release Potential. *J. Controlled Release* **1997**, *48,* 223–236.

65. Iscan, Y. Y.; Hekimoglu, S.; Kas, S.; Hinca, A. A. *Formulation and Characterization of Solid Lipid Nanoparticles for Skin Delivery, Conference Lipid and Surfactant Dispersed Systems*; Proceedings Book: Moscow, Russia, 1999, 163–166.

66. Schwarz, C.; Freitas, C.; Mehnert, W.; MuÈller, R. H. Sterilisation and Physical Stability of Drug-Free and Etomidate-Loaded Solid Lipid Nano-particles. *Proc. Int. Symp. Control. Release Bioact. Mater.* **1995**, *22*, 766–767.

67. Muller, R. H.; Mader, K.; Gohla, S. Solid Lipid Nanoparticles (SLN) for Controlled Drug Delivery ± A Review of the State of the Art. *Eur. J. Pharm. Biopharm.* **2000**, *50*, 161–177.

68. Morel, S.; Terreno, E.; Ugazio, E.; Aime, S.; Gasco, M. R. NMR Relaxometric Investigations of Solid Lipid Nanoparticles (SLN) Containing Gadolinium (III) Complexes. *Eur. J. Pharm. Biopharm.* **1998**, *45*, 157–163.

69. Gasco, M. R. Solid Lipid Nanospheres from Warm Micro-emulsions. *Pharm. Technol. Eur.* **1997**, *9*, 52–58.

70. Boltri, L.; Canal, T.; Esposito, P. A.; Carli, F. Lipid Nanoparticles: Evaluation of Some Critical Formulation Parameters. *Proc. Int. Symp. Control Release Bioact. Mater.* **1993**, *20*, 346–347.

71. Mueller, R. H.; Schwarz, C.; Mehnert, W.; Lucks, J. S. Production of Solid Lipid Nanoparticles (SLN) for Controlled Drug Delivery. *Proc. Int. Symp. Control Release Bioact. Mater.* **1993**, *20*, 480–481.

72. Nobs, L.; Buchegger, F.; Gurny, R.; Allemann, E. Current Methods for Attaching Targeting Ligands to Liposomes and Nanoparticles. *J. Pharm. Sci.* **2004**, *93*, 1980–1992.

73. McCarthy, J. R.; Kelly, K. A.; Sun, E. Y.; Weissleder, R. Targeted Delivery of Multifunctional Magnetic Nanoparticles. *Nanomedicine* **2007**, *2*, 153–167.

74. Dagar, S.; Sekosan, M.; Lee, B. S.; Rubinstein, I.; Onyuksel, H. VIP Receptors as Molecular Targets of Breast Cancer: Implications for Targeted Imaging and Drug Delivery. *J. Contr. Release* **2001**, *74*, 129–134.

75. Sethi, V.; Onyuksel, H.; Rubinstein, I. A novel therapy for rheumatoid arthritis using a-helix VIP, FASEB 2003 conference proceedings. *FASEB* **2003**, 660.

76. Lee, J.; Cho, E. C.; Cho, K. Incorporation and Release Behavior of Hydrophobic Drug in Functionalized Poly(D, L-lactide)-Block-Poly(ethylene oxide) Micelles. *J. Contr. Release* **2004**, *94*, 323–335.

77. La, S. B.; Okano, T.; Kataoka, K. Preparation and Characterization of Micelle-Forming Polymeric Drug Indomethacin-Incorporated Poly(ethylene oxide)–Poly(β-benzyl L-aspartate) Block Copolymer Micelles. *J. Pharm. Sci.* **1996**, *85*, 85–90.

78. Torchilin, V. P. Targeted Pharmaceutical Nanocarriers for Cancer Therapy and Imaging. *AAPS J.* **2007**, *9*, E128–E147.

79. Pastorino, F.; Brignole, C.; Marimpietri, D.; Sapra, P.; Moase, E. H.; Allen, T. M.; Ponzoni, M. Doxorubicin-Loaded Fab' Fragments of Anti-disialoganglioside Immunoliposomes Selectively Inhibit the Growth and Dissemination of Human Neuroblastoma in Nude Mice. *Cancer Res.* **2003**, *63*, 86–92.

80. Allen, T. M.; Mumbengegwi, D. R.; Charrois, G. J. Anti-CD19-Targeted Liposomal Doxorubicin Improves the Therapeutic Efficacy in Murine B-cell Lymphoma and Ameliorates the Toxicity of Liposomes with Varying Drug Release Rates. *Clin. Cancer Res.* **2005**, *11*, 3567–3573.

81. Medina, O. P.; Pillarsettya, N.; Glekasa, A.; Punzalan, B.; Longo, V.; Gönen, M.; Zanzonico, P.; Smith-Jones, P.; Larson, S. M. Optimizing Tumor Targeting of the Lipophilic EGFR-Binding Radiotracer SKI 243 Using a Liposomal Nanoparticle Delivery System. *J. Contr. Release* **2011**, *149*, 292–298.

82. Emerich, D. F.; Thanos, C. G. The Pinpoint Promise of Nanoparticle-Based Drug Delivery and Molecular Diagnosis. *Biomol. Eng.* **2006**, *23*, 171–184.

83. Lamprecht, A.; Ubrich, N.; Yamamoto, H.; Schäfer, U.; Takeuchi, H.; Maincent, P.; Kawashima, Y.; Lehr, C. M. Biodegradable Nanoparticles for Targeted Drug Delivery in Treatment of Inflammatory Bowel Disease. *J. Pharmacol. Exp. Ther.* **2001,** *299,* 775–781.

84. Maeda, H. The Enhanced Permeability and Retention (EPR) Effect in Tumor Vasculature: The Key Role of Tumor-Selective Macromolecular Drug Targeting. *Adv. Enzym. Regul.* **2001,** *41,* 189–207.

85. Sahoo, S. K.; Sawa, T.; Fang, J.; Tanaka, S.; Miyamoto, Y.; Akaike, T.; Maeda, H. PEGylated Zinc Protoporphyrin: A Water-Soluble Heme Oxygenase Inhibitor with Tumor-Targeting Capacity. *Bioconjugate Chem.* **2002,** *13,* 1031–1038.

86. Takeda, M.; Tada, H.; Higuchi, H., et al. In Vivo Single Molecular Imaging and Sentinel Node Navigation by Nanotechnology for Molecular Targeting Drug-Delivery Systems and Tailor-Made Medicine. *Breast Cancer* **2008,** *15,* 145–152.

87. Cairns, R. A.; Khokha, R.; Hill, R. P. Molecular Mechanisms of Tumor Invasion and Metastasis: An Integrated View. *Curr. Mol. Med.* **2003,** *3,* 659–671.

88. Felding-Habermann, B. Integrin Adhesion Receptors in Tumor Metastasis. *Clin. Exp. Metastasis* **2003,** *20,* 203–213.

89. Lee, H. Y.; Li, Z.; Chen, K.; Hsu, A. R.; Xu, C.; Xie, J.; Sun, S.; Chen, X. ET/MRI Dual-Modality Tumor Imaging Using Arginine Glycine-Aspartic (RGD)-Conjugated Radiolabeled Iron Oxide Nanoparticles. *J. Nucl. Med.* **2008,** *49,* 1371–1379.

90. Ellington, A. D.; Szostak, J. W. In Vitro Selection of RNA Molecules That Bind Specific Ligands. *Nature* **1990,** *346,* 818–822.

91. Tuerk, C.; Gold, L. Systematic Evolution of Ligands by Exponential Enrichment: RNA Ligands to Bacteriophage T4 DNA Polymerase. *Science* **1990,** *249,* 505–510.

92. Farokhzad, O. C.; Karp, J. M.; Langer, R. Nanoparticle-Aptamer Bioconjugates for Cancer Targeting. *Exp. Opin. Drug. Del.* **2006,** *3,* 311–324.

93. Levy-Nissenbaum, E.; Radovic-Moreno, A. F.; Wang, A. Z.; Langer, R.; Farokhzad, O. C. Nanotechnology and Aptamers: Applications in Drug Delivery. *Trends Biotechnol.* **2008,** *26,* 442–449.

94. McCarthy, J. R.; Bhaumik, J.; Karver, M. R.; Erdem, S. S.; Weissleder, R. Review: Targeted Nanoagents for the Detection of Cancers. *Mol. Oncol.* **2010,** *4,* 511–528.

95. McCarthy, J. R.; Weissleder, R. Multifunctional Magnetic Nanoparticles for Targeted Imaging and Therapy. *Adv. Drug Deliv. Rev.* **2008,** *60,* 1241–1251.

96. Weissleder, R.; Kelly, K.; Sun, E. Y.; Shtatland, T.; Josephson, L. Cell-Specific Targeting of Nanoparticles by Multivalent Attachment of Small Molecules. *Nat. Biotechnol.* **2005,** *23,* 1418–1423.

97. Tassa, C.; Duffner, J. L.; Lewis, T. A.; Weissleder, R.; Schreiber, S. L.; Koehler, A. N.; Shaw, S. Y. Binding Affinity and Kinetic Analysis of Targeted Small Molecule-Modified Nanoparticles. *Bioconjug. Chem.* **2010,** *21,* 14–19.

98. Low, P. S.; Kularatne, S. A. Folate-Targeted Therapeutic and Imaging Agents for Cancer. *Curr. Opin. Chem. Biol.* **2009,** *13,* 256–262.

99. Zhang, H. Y.; Ma, Y.; Sun, X. L. Recent Developments in Carbohydrate-Decorated Targeted Drug/Gene Delivery. *Med. Res. Rev.* **2010,** *30,* 270–289.

100. Ruenraroengsak, P.; Cook, J. M.; Florence, A. T. Nanosystem Drug Targeting: Facing up to Complex Realities. *J. Contr. Release* **2010,** *141,* 265–276.

101. Olivier, J. -C. Drug Transport to Brain with Targeted Nanoparticles. *NeuroRX* **2005,** *2,* 108–119.

102. Fang, T.; Sawa, X.; Maeda, H., Eds.; *Factors and Mechanism of "EPR" Effect and the Enhanced Antitumor Effects of Macromolecular Drugs Including SMANCS Book Series Advances in Experimental Medicine and Biology,* SpringerLink Netherlands: Dordrecht, Netherlands, 2004; pp 29–49.

103. Geish, K. Enhanced Permeability and Retention Effect of Macromolecular Drugs in Solid Tumors: A Royal Gate for Targeted Anticancer Medicines. *J. Drug Target.* **2007,** *15,* 457–464.

104. Hobbs, S. K.; Monsky, W. L.; Yuan, F.; Roberts, W. G.; Griffith, L.; Torchilin, V. P.; Jain, R. K. Regulation of Transport Pathways in Tumor Vessels: Role of Tumor Type and Microenvironment. *Proc. Natl. Acad. Sci. U.S.A.* **1998,** *95,* 4607–4612.

105. Jain, R. K. Delivery of Molecular and Cellular Medicine to Solid Tumors. *J. Contr. Release* **1998,** *53,* 49–67.

106. Fu, B. M.; Adamson, R. H.; Curry, F. E. Test of a Two-Pathway Model for Small-Solute Exchange across the Capillary Wall. *Am. J. Physiol.* **1998,** *274,* H2062–H2073.

107. Meyer, D. E.; Shin, B. C.; Kong, G. A.; Dewhirst, M. W.; Chilkoti, A. Drug Targeting Using Thermally Responsive Polymers and Local Hyperthermia. *J. Contr. Release* **2001,** *74,* 213–224.

108. Nelson, J. L.; Roeder, B. L.; Carmen, J. C.; Roloff, F.; Pitt, W. G. Ultrasonically Activated Chemotherapeutic Drug Delivery in a Rat Model. *Cancer Res.* **2002,** 62(24), 7280–7283.

109. Tao, W. M.; Zhang, M. A Genetic Algorithm-Based Area Coverage Approach for Controlled Drug Delivery Using Microrobots. *Nanomedicine* **2005,** *1,* 91–100.

110. Koval, M.; Preiter, K.; Adles, C.; Stahl, P. D.; Steinberg, T. H. Size of IgG Opsonized Particles Determines Macrophage Response During Internalization. *Exp. Cell Res.* **1998,** *242,* 265–273.

111. Harashima, H.; Sakata, K.; Funato, K.; Kiwada, H. Enhanced Hepatic Uptake of Liposomes Through Complement Activation Depending on the Size of Liposomes. *Pharm. Res.* **1994,** *11,* 402–406.

112. Rejman, J.; Oberle, V.; Zuhorn, I. S.; Hoekstra, D. Size-Dependent Internalization of Particles via the Pathways of Clathrin- and Caveolae-Mediated Endocytosis. *Biochem. J.* **2004,** *377,* 159–169.

113. Vauthier, C.; Dubernet, C.; Chauvierre, C.; Brigger, I.; Couvreur, P. Drug Delivery to Resistant Tumors: The Potential of Poly(alkyl cyanoacrylate) Nanoparticles. *J. Controlled Release* **2003,** *93,* 151–160.

114. Miller, D. W.; Batrakova, E. V.; Kabanov, A. V. Inhibition of Multidrug Resistance-Associated Protein (MRP) Functional Activity with Pluronic Block Copolymers. *Pharm. Res.* **1999,** *16,* 396–401.

115. Sapra, P.; Allen, T. M. Ligand-Targeted Liposomal Anticancer Drugs. *Prog. Lipid Res.* **2003,** *42,* 439–462.

116. Mamot, C.; Drummond, D. C.; Hong, K.; Kirpotin, D. B.; Park, J. W. Liposome-Based Approaches to Overcome Anticancer Drug Resistance. *Drug Resist. Update* **2003,** *6,* 271–279.

117. Soma, C. E.; Dubernet, C.; Bentolila, D.; Benita, S.; Couvreur, P. Reversion of Multidrug Resistance by Co-encapsulation of Doxorubicin and Cyclosporin A in Polyalkylcyanoacrylate Nanoparticles. *Biomaterials* **2000,** *21,* 1–7.

118. Yang, S.; Zhu, J.; Lu, Y.; Liang, B.; Yang, C. Body Distribution of Camptothecin Solid Lipid Nanoparticles after Oral Administration. *Pharm. Res.* **1999,** *16,* 751–757.

119. Fresta, M.; Puglisi, G.; Giammona, G.; Cavallaro, G.; Micali, N.; Furneri, P. M. Pefloxacine Mesilate- and Ofloxacin-Loaded Polyethylcyanoacrylate Nanoparticles: Characterization of the Colloidal Drug Carrier Formulation. *J. Pharm. Sci.* **1995,** *84,* 895–902.

120. Magenheim, B.; Levy, M. Y.; Benita, S. A New In Vitro Technique for the Evaluation of Drug Release Profile from Colloidal Carriers-Ultrafiltration Technique at Low Pressure. *Int. J. Pharm.* **1993,** *94,* 115–123.

121. zur MuËhlen, A.; Mehnert, W. Drug Release and Release Mechanism of Prednisolone Loaded Solid Lipid Nanoparticles. *Pharmazie* **1998,** *53,* 552.

122. zur MuÈhlen, A.; Schwarz, C.; Mehnert, W. Solid Lipid Nanoparticles (SLN) for Controlled Drug Delivery ± Drug Release and Release Mechanism. *Eur. J. Pharm. Biopharm.* **1998,** *45,* 149–155.

123. Labhasetwar, V. Nanotechnology for Drug and Gene Therapy: The Importance of Understanding Molecular Mechanisms of Delivery. *Curr. Opin. Biotechnol.* **2005,** *16,* 674–680.

124. Cherukuri, P.; Bachilo, S. M.; Litovsky, S. H.; Weisman, R. B. Near-Infrared Fluorescence Microscopy of Single-Walled Carbon Nanotunes in Phagocytic Cells. *J. Am. Chem. Soc.* **2004,** *126,* 15638–15639.

125. Singh, R.; Pantarotto, D.; Lacerdo, L.; Pastorin, G.; Klumpp, C.; Prato, M.; Bianco, A.; Kostarelos, K. Tissue Biodistribution and Blood Clearance Rates of Intravenously Administered Carbon Nanotube Radiotracers. *Proc. Natl. Acad. Sci. U.S.A.* **2006,** *103,* 3357–3362.

126. Moghimi, S. M.; Hunter, A. C.; Murray, J. C. Nanomedicine: Current Status and Future Prospects. *FASEB J.* **2005,** *19,* 311–330.

127. Nel, A.; Xia, T.; Madler, L.; Li, N. Tox Potential of Materials at the Nanolevel. *Science* **2006,** *311,* 622–627.

128. Akerman, M. E.; Chan, W. C.; Laakkonen, P.; Bhatia, S. N.; Ruoslahti, E. Nanocrystal Targeting In Vivo. *Proc. Natl. Acad. Sci. U.S.A.* **2002,** *99,* 12617–12621.

129. Ballou, B.; Lagerholm, B. C.; Ernst, L. A.; Bruchez, M. P.; Waggoner, A. S. Noninvasive Imaging of Quantum Dots in Mice. *Bioconjug. Chem.* **2004,** *15,* 79–86.

130. Gao, X.; Cui, Y.; Levenson, R. M.; Chung, L. W. K.; Nie, S. In Vivo Cancer Targeting and Imaging with Semiconductor Quantum Dots. *Nat. Biotechnol.* **2004,** *22,* 969–976.

131. Vasir, J.; Labhasetwar, V. Targeted Drug Delivery in Cancer Therapy. *Technol. Cancer Res. Treat.* **2005,** *4,* 363–374.

132. Oh, P.; Li, Y.; Yu, J.; Durr, E.; Krasinka, K. M.; Carver, L. A.; Testa, J. E.; Schnitzer, J. E. Subtractive Proteomic Mapping of the Endothelial Surface in Lung and Solid Tumours for Tissue-Specific Therapy. *Nature* **2004,** *429,* 629–635.

133. Murray, J. C.; Moghimi, S. M. Endothelial Cells as Therapeutic Targets in Cancer: New Biology and Novel Delivery Systems. *Crit. Rev. Ther. Drug Carrier Syst.* **2003,** *20,* 139–152.

134. Moghimi, S. M. Modulation of Lymphatic Distribution of Subcutaneously Injected Poloxamer 407-Coated Nanospheres: The Effect of the Ethylene Oxide Chain Configuration. *FEBS Lett.* **2003,** *540,* 241–244.

135. Moghimi, S. M.; Bonnemain, B. Subcutaneous and Intravenous Delivery of Diagnostic Agents to the Lymphatic System: Applications in Lymphoscintigraphy and Indirect Lymphography. *Adv. Drug Deliv. Rev.* **1999,** *37,* 295–312.

136. Winter, P.; Caruthers, S. D.; Kassner, A.; Harris, T. D.; Chinen, L. K.; Allen, J. S.; Lacy, E. K.; Zhang, H. Y.; Robertson, J. D.; Wickline, S. A. Molecular Imaging of Angiogenesis in Nascent vx-2 Rabbit Tumours using a Novel Alpha(v) Beta(3)-Targeted Nanoparticle and 1.5 Tesla Magnetic Resonance Imaging. *Cancer Res.* **2003,** *63,* 5838–5843.

137. Kim, S.; Lim, Y. T.; Soltesz, E. G.; De Grand, A. M.; Lee, J.; Nakayama, A.; Parker, J. A.; Mihaljevic, T.; Laurence, R. G.; Dor, D. M. Near-Infrared Fluorescent Type II Quantum Dots for Sentinel Lymph Node Mapping. *Nat. Biotechnol.* **2004,** *22,* 93–97.

138. Bergqvist, L.; Sundberg, R.; Ryden, S.; Strand, S. E. The "Critical Colloid Dose" in Studies of Reticuloendothelial Function. *J. Nucl. Med.* **1987,** *28,* 1424–1429.

139. Bradfield, J. W. A New Look at Reticuloendothelial Blockade. *Br. J. Exp. Pathol.* **1980,** *61,* 617–623.

140. Cleland, J. L., Ed.; *Protein Delivery from Biodegradable Microspheres*; Plenum Press: New York, 1997.

141. Molema, G.; de Leij, L. F. M. H .; Meijer, D. K. F. Tumor Vascular Endothelium: Barrier or Target in Tumor Directed Drug Delivery and Immunotherapy. *Pharm. Res.* **1999,** *14,* 2–38.

142. Herrero-Vanrell, R.; Rincón, A. C.; Alonso, M.; Reboto, V.; Molina-Martinez, I. T.; Rodríguez-Cabello, J. C. Self-assembled Particles of an Elastin-Like Polymer as Vehicles for Controlled Drug Release. *J. Contr. Release* **2005,** *102,* 113–122.

143. Kreuter, J., Ed.; *Nanoparticles*; M. Dekker: New York, 1994.

144. Ge, H.; Hu, Y.; Jiang, X.; Cheng, D.; Yuan, Y.; Bi, H.; Yang, C. Preparation, Characterization, and Drug Release Behaviors of Drug Nimodipine-Loaded Poly(epsilon-caprolactone)-Poly(ethylene oxide)-Poly(epsilon-caprolactone) Amphiphilic Triblock Copolymer Micelles. *J. Pharm. Sci.* **2002,** *91,* 1463–1473.

145. Barrera, D. A.; Zylstra, E.; Lansbury, P. T.; Langer, R. Synthesis and RGD Peptide Modification of a Newbiodegradable Copolymer: Poly(lactic acid-co-lysine). *J. Am. Chem. Soc.* **1993,** *115,* 11010–11011.

146. Peng, W.; Anderson, D. G.; Bao, Y.; Padera, R. F., Jr.; Langer, R.; Sawicki, J. A. Nanoparticulate Delivery of Suicide DNA to Murine Prostate and Prostate Tumors. *Prostate* **2007,** *7,* 855–862.

147. van Vlerken, L. E.; Amiji, M. M. Multi-functional Polymeric Nanoparticles for Tumour-Targeted Drug Delivery. *Exp. Opin. Drug Del.* **2006,** *3,* 205–216.

148. Dunne, M.; Corrigan, I.; Ramtoola, Z. Influence of Particle Size and Dissolution Conditions on the Degradation Properties of Polylactide-co-glycolide Particles. *Biomaterials* **2000,** *21,* 1659–1668.

149. Panyam, J.; Dali, M. M.; Sahoo, S. K.; Ma, W.; Chakravarthi, S. S.; Amidon, G. L.; Levy, R. J.; Labhasetwar, V. Polymer Degradation and In Vitro Release of a Model Protein from Poly(D, L-lactide-co-glycolide) Nano- and Microparticles. *J. Contr. Release* **2003,** *92,* 173–187.

150. Hu, C.; Feng, H.; Zhu, C. Preparation and Characterization of Rifampicin-PLGA Microspheres/Sodium Alginate In Situ Gel Combination Delivery System. *Colloids Surf. B* **2012,** *96,* 162–169.

151. Jain, G. K.; Pathan, S. A.; Akhter, S.; Jayabalan, N.; Talegaonkar, S.; Khar, R. K.; Ahmad, F. J. Microscopic and Spectroscopic Evaluation of Novel PLGA-Chitosan Nanoplexes as an Ocular Delivery System. *Colloids Surf. B* **2011,** *82,* 397–403.

152. Seju, U.; Kumar, A.; Sawani, K. K. Development and Evaluation of Olanzapine-Loaded PLGA Nanoparticles for Nose-to-Brain Delivery: In Vitro and In Vivo Studies. *Acta Biomater.* **2011,** *7,* 4169–4176.

153. Wang, H.; Zhao, Y.; Wu, Y.; Hu, Y.; Nan, K.; Nie, G.; Chen, H. Enhanced Anti-Tumor Efficacy by Co-delivery of Doxorubicin and Paclitaxel with Amphiphilic PEG-PLGA Copolymer Nanoparticles. *Biomaterials* **2011,** *32,* 8281–8290.

154. Wang, Y. -C.; Wu, Y. -T.; Huang, H. -Y.; Lin, H. -I.; Lo, L. -W.; Tzeng, S. -F.; Yang, C. -S. Sustained Intraspinal Delivery of Neurotrophic Factor Encapsulated in Biodegradable Nanoparticles Following Contusive Spinal Cord Injury. *Biomaterials* **2008,** *29,* 4546–4553.

155. Bu, H. Z.; Gukasyan, H. J.; Goulet, L.; Lou, X. -J.; Xiang, C.; Koudnakova, T. Ocular Disposition, Pharmacokinetics, Efficacy and Safety of Nanoparticle-Formulated Ophthalmic Drugs. *Curr. Drug Metab.* **2007,** *8,* 91–107.

156. Cohen, H.; Levy, R. J.; Gao, J.; Fishbein, I.; Kousaev, V.; Sosnowski, S.; Slomkowski, S.; Golomb, G. Sustained Delivery and Expression of DNA Encapsulated in Polymeric Nanoparticles. *Gene Ther.* **2000,** *7,* 1896–1905.

157. Miller, D. C.; Thapa, A.; Haberstroh, K. M.; Webster, T. J. Endothelial and Vascular Smooth Muscle Cell Function on Poly(lactic-co-glycolic acid) with Nano Surface Features. *Biomaterials* **2004,** *25,* 53–61.

158. Panyam, J.; Zhou, W. Z.; Prabha, S.; Sahoo, S. K.; Labhasetwar, V. Rapid Endo-lysosomal Escape of Poly(DL-lactide-co-glycolide) Nanoparticles: Implications for Drug and Gene Delivery. *FASEB J.* **2002,** *16,* 1217–1226.

159. Prabha, S.; Labhasetwar, V. Critical Determinants in PLGA/PLA Nanoparticle-Mediated Gene Expression. *Pharm. Res.* **2004,** *21,* 3354–3363.

160. Parveen, S.; Sahoo, S. K. Long Circulating Chitosan/PEG Blended PLGA Nanoparticle for Tumor Drug Delivery. *Eur. J. Pharm.* **2011,** *670,* 372–383.

161. Guzman, L. A.; Labhasetwar, V.; Song, C.; Jang, Y.; Lincoff, A. M.; Levy, R.; Topol, E. J. Local Intraluminal Infusion of Biodegradable Polymeric Nanoparticles. A Novel Approach for Prolonged Drug Delivery after Balloon Angioplasty. *Circulation* **1996,** *94,* 1441–1448.

162. Fisher, R. S.; Ho, J. Potential New Methods for Antiepileptic Drug Delivery. *CNS Drugs* **2002,** *16,* 579–593.

163. Lockman, P. R.; Mumper, R. J.; Khan, M. A.; Allen, D. D. Nanoparticle Technology for Drug Delivery across the Blood-Brain Barrier. *Drug Dev. Ind. Pharm.* **2002,** *28,* 1–13.

164. Avgoustakis, K.; Beletsi, A.; Panagi, Z.; Klepetsanis, P.; Karydas, A. G.; Ithakissios, D. S. PLGA-mPEG Nanoparticles of Cisplatin: In Vitro Nanoparticle Degradation, In Vitro Drug Release and In Vivo Drug Residence in Blood Properties. *J. Contr. Release* **2002,** *79,* 123–135.

165. Morgen, M.; Lu, G. W.; Dub, D.; Stehle, R.; Lembke, F.; Cervantes, J.; Ciotti, S.; Haskell, R.; Smithey, D.; Haley, K.; Fan, C. Targeted Delivery of a Poorly Water-Soluble Compound to Hair Follicles Using Polymeric Nanoparticle Suspensions. *Int. J. Pharm.* **2011,** 416:314–332.

166. Nguyen, S.; Hiorth, M.; Rykke, M.; Smistad, G. The Potential of Liposomes as Dental Drug Delivery Systems. *Eur. J. Pharm. Biopharm.* **2011,** *77,* 75–83.

167. Ahmed, F.; Pakunlu, R. I.; Srinivas, G.; Brannan, A.; Bates, F.; Klein, M. L.; Minko, T.; Discher, D. E. Shrinkage of a Rapidly Growing Tumor by Drug-Loaded Polymersomes: pH-Triggered Release through Copolymer Degradation. *Mol. Pharm.* **2006,** *3,* 340–350.

168. Koo, O. M. Y.; Rubinstein, I.; Onyuksel, H. Camptothecin in Sterically Stabilized Phospholipid Nano-micelles: A Novel Solvent pH Change Solubilization Method. *J. Nanosci. Nanotech.* **2006,** *6,* 2996–3000.

169. Bisht, S.; Feldmann, G.; Soni, S.; Ravi, R.; Karikar, C.; Maitra, A.; Maitra, A. Polymeric Nanoparticle-Encapsulated Curcumin ("nanocurcumin"): A Novel Strategy for Human Cancer Therapy. *J. Nanobiotechnol.* **2007,** *5,* 3.

170. Klostergaard, J.; Seeney, C. E. Magnetic Nanovectors for Drug Delivery. *Nanomed. Nanotechnol. Biol. Med.* **2012,** 73(1):33–44.

171. Mejias, R.; Perez-Yague, S.; Gutierez, L.; Cabrera, L. I.; Spada, R.; Acedo, P.; Serna, C. J.; Lazaro, F. J.; Villanueva, A.; Morales, M. P.; Barber, D. F. Dimercaptosuccinic Acid-Coated Magnetite Nanoparticles for Magnetically Guided In Vivo Delivery of Interferon Gamma for Cancer Immunotherapy. *Biomaterials* **2011,** *32,* 2938–2952.

172. Rey, F.; Clement, O.; Siauve, N.; et al. MR Lymphography Using Iron Oxide Nanoparticles in Rats: Pharmacokinetics in the Lymphatic System after Intravenous Injection. *J. Magn. Reson. Imaging* **2000,** *12,* 80–92.

173. Mykhaylyk, O. M.; Dudchenko, N. O.; Dudchenko, A. K. Pharmacokinetics of the Doxorubicin Magnetic Nanoconjugate in Mice Effects of the Nonuniform Stationary Magnetic Field. *Ukr. Biokhim. Zh.* **2005,** *77,* 80–92.

174. Lian, G.; Lewelling, K.; Johnson, M.; Dormer, K.; Gibson, D.; Seeney, C. Nanoparticles for Biomedical Applications. *Microsc. Microanal.* **2004,** *10,* 2.

175. Klostergaard, J.; Bankson, J.; Auzenne, E.; Gibson, D.; Yuill, W.; Seeney, C. Magnetic Vectoring of Magnetically Responsive Nanoparticles within the Murine Peritoneum. *J. Magn. Magn. Mater.* **2007,** *311,* 330–335.

176. Klostergaard, J.; Bankson, J.; Woodward, W.; Gibson, D.; Seeney, C. Magnetically Responsive Nanoparticles for Vectored Delivery of Cancer Therapeutics. *AIP Conf. Proc.* **2011,** *1311,* 382–387.

177. Gang, J.; Park, S. B.; Hyung, W.; Choi, E. H.; Wen, J.; Kim, H. S.; Shul, Y. G.; Haam, S.; Song, S. Y. Magnetic Poly Epsilon-Caprolactone Nanoparticles Containing Fe_3O_4 and Gemcitabine Enhance Anti-tumor Effect in Pancreatic Cancer Xenograft Mouse Model. *J. Drug Target.* **2007,** *15,* 445–453.

178. Cao, H.; Gan, J.; Wang, S., et al. Novel Silica-Coated Iron–Carbon Composite Particles and Their Targeting Effect as a Drug Carrier. *J. Biomed. Mater. Res.* **2008,** *86,* 671–677.

179. Chertok, B.; Cole, A. J.; David, A. E.; Yang, V. C. Comparison of Electron Spin Resonance Spectroscopy and Inductively-Coupled Plasma Optical Emission Spectroscopy for Biodistribution Analysis of Iron-Oxide Nanoparticles. *Mol. Pharm.* **2010,** *7,* 375–385.

180. Chertok, B.; Moffat, B. A.; David, A. E.; Yu, F.; Bergemann, C.; Ross, B. D.; Yang, V. C. Iron Oxide Nanoparticles as a Drug Delivery Vehicle for MRI Monitored Magnetic Targeting of Brain Tumors. *Biomaterials* **2008,** *29,* 486–496.

181. Cho, H. S.; Dong, Z.; Pauletti, G. M., et al. Fluorescent, Superparamagnetic Nanospheres for Drug Storage, Targeting, and Imaging: A Multifunctional Nanocarrier System for Cancer Diagnosis and Treatment. *ACS Nano* **2010,** *4,* 5398–5404.

182. Quan, Q.; Xie, J.; Gao, H., et al. HSA Coated Iron Oxide Nanoparticles as Drug Delivery Vehicles for Cancer Therapy. *Mol. Pharm.* **2011,** *8,* 1669–1676.

183. Jain, K. K. Use of Nanoparticles for Drug Delivery in Glioblastome Multiforme. *Exp. Rev. Neurother.* **2007,** *7,* 363–372.

184. Alexiou, C.; Arnold, W.; Klein, R. J., et al. Locoregional Cancer Treatment with Magnetic Drug Targeting. *Cancer Res.* **2006,** *60,* 6641–6648.

185. Lübbe, A. S.; Alexiou, C.; Bergemann, C. Clinical Applications of Magnetic Drug Targeting. *J. Surg. Res.* **2001,** *95,* 200–206.

186. Tietze, R.; Schreiber, E.; Lyer, S.; Alexiou, C. Mitoxantrone Loaded Superparamagnetic Nanoparticles for Drug Targeting: A Versatile and Sensitive Method for Quantification of Drug Enrichment in Rabbit Tissues Using HPLC–UV. *J. Biomed. Biotech.* **2010.**

187. El-Sayed, I. H. Nanotechnology in Head and Neck Cancer: The Race Is On. *Curr. Oncol. Rep.* **2010,** *12,* 121–128.

188. Gojova, A.; Guo, B.; Kota, R. S.; Rutledge, J. C.; Kennedy, I. M.; Barakat, A. I. Induction of Inflammation in Vascular Endothelial Cells by Metal Oxide Nanoparticles: Effect of Particle Composition. *Environ. Health Perspect.* **2007,** *3,* 403–409.

189. Zhu, M. T.; Wang, Y.; Feng, Y. W., et al. Oxidative Stress and Apoptosis Induced by Iron Oxide Nanoparticles in Cultured Human Umbilical Endothelial Cells. *J. Nanosci. Nanotech.* **2010,** *10,* 8584–8590.

190. Zhu, M. T.; Wang, B.; Wang, Y., et al. Endothelial Dysfunction and Inflammation Induced by Iron Oxide Nanoparticle Exposure: Risk Factors for Early Atherosclerosis. *Toxicol. Lett.* **2011,** *203,* 162–171.

191. Hanini, A.; Schmitt, A.; Kacem, K.; Chau, F.; Ammar, S.; Gavard, J. Evaluation of Iron Oxide Nanoparticle Biocompatibility. *Int. J. Nanomed.* **2011,** *6,* 787–794.

192. Alekseenko, A. V.; Waseem, T. V.; Fedorovich, S. V. Ferritin, a Protein Containing Iron Nanoparticles, Induces Reactive Oxygen Species Formation and Inhibits Glutamate Uptake in Rat Brain Synaptosomes. *Brain Res.* **2008,** *1241,* 193–200.

193. López-Castro, J. D.; Maraloiu, A. V.; Delgado, J. J., et al. From Synthetic to Natural Nanoparticles: Monitoring the Biodegradation of SPIO (P904) into Ferritin by Electron Microscopy. *Nanoscale* **2011,** *3,* 4597–4599.

194. McDevitt, M. R.; Chattopadhyay, D.; Kappel, B. J.; Jaggi, J. S.; Schiffman, S. R.; A. C.; Njardarson, J. T.; Brentjens, R.; Scheinberg, D. A. Tumor Targeting with Antibody-Functionalized, Radiolabeled Carbon Nanotubes. *J. Nucl. Med.* **2007,** *48,* 1180–1189.

195. Ashcroft, J. M.; Tsyboulski, D. A.; Hartman, K. B.; Zakharian, T. Y.; Marks, J. W.; Weisman, R. B.; Rosenblum, M. G.; Wilson, L. J. Fullerene (C60) Immunoconjugates: Interaction of Water-Soluble C60 Derivatives with the Murine Anti-gp240 Melanoma Antibody. *Chem. Commun.* **2006,** 3004–3006.

196. Pusic, K.; Xu, H.; Stridiron, A.; Aguilar, Z.; Wang, A. Z.; Hui, H. Blood Stage Merozoite Surface Protein Conjugated to Nanoparticles Induce Potent Parasite Inhibitory Antibodies. *Vaccine* **2011,** *29,* 8898–8908.

197. Aguilar, Z. P.; Xu, H.; Dixon, J. D.; Wang, A. W. *Nanomaterials for Enhanced Antibody Production*; Small Business Innovations Research for the National Science Foundation, 2012 (Ocean NanoTech, unpublished report).

198. Tada, H.; Higuchi, H.; Wanatabe, T. M.; Ohuchi, N. In Vivo Real-Time Tracking of Single Quantum Dots Conjugated with Monoclonal Anti-HER2 Antibody in Tumors of Mice. *Cancer Res.* **2007,** *67,* 1138–1144.

199. Lee, C. C.; Gillies, E. R.; Fox, M. E.; Guillaudeu, S. J.; Fréchet, J. M.; Dy, E. E.; Szoka, F. C. A Single Dose of Doxorubicin-Functionalized Bow-Tie Dendrimer Cures Mice Bearing C-26 Colon Carcinomas. *Proc. Natl. Acad. Sci. U.S.A.* **2006,** *103,* 16649–16654.

200. Czerniawska, A. Experimental Investigations on the Penetration of 198Au from Nasal Mucous Membrane into Cerebrospinal Fluid. *Acta Otolaryngol.* **1970,** *70,* 58–61.

201. Pardridge, W. M. Why Is the Global CNS Pharmaceutical Market So Underpenetrated? *Drug Discov. Today* **2002,** *7,* 5–7.

202. Juillerat-Jeanneret, L. The Targeted Delivery of Cancer Drugs across the Blood-Brain Barrier: Chemical Modifications of Drugs or Drug Nanoparticles? *Drug Discov. Today* **2008,** *13,* 1099–1106.

203. Persidsky, Y.; Ramirez, S.; Haorah, J.; Kanmogne, G. Blood-Brain Barrier: Structural Components and Function under Physiologic and Pathologic Conditions. *J. Neuroimmune Pharmacol.* **2006,** *1,* 223–236.

204. Hawkins, B. T.; Davis, T. P. The Blood-Brain Barrier/Neurovascular Unit in Health and Disease. *Pharmacol. Rev.* **2005,** *57,* 173–185.

205. Begley, D. J. Delivery of Therapeutic Agents to the Central Nervous System: The Problems and the Possibilities. *Pharmacol. Ther.* **2004,** *104,* 29–47.

206. Chen, Y.; Dalwadi, G.; Benson, H. A. E. Drug Delivery across the Blood-Brain Barrier. *Curr. Drug Del.* **2004,** *1,* 361–367.

207. Brightman, M. W.; Reese, T. S. Junctions between Intimately Apposed Cell Membranes in the Vertebrate Brain. *J. Cell Biol.* **1969,** *40,* 648–677.

208. Saunders, N.; Knott, G.; Dziegielewska, K. Barriers in the Immature Brain. *Neurobiology* **2000,** *20,* 29–40.

209. Saunders, N.; Ek, C. J.; Habgood, M. D.; Dziegielewska, K. M. Barriers in the Brain: A Renaissance? *Trends Neurosci.* **2008,** *31,* 279–286.

210. Stewart, P. A. Endothelial Vesicles in the Blood-Brain Barrier: Are They Related to Permeability? *Cell Mol. Neurobiol.* **2000,** *20,* 149–163.

211. Decleves, X.; Amiel, A.; Delattre, J. -Y.; Scherrmann, J. -M. Role of ABC Transporters in the Chemoresistance of Human Gliomas. *Curr. Cancer Drug Targets* **2006,** *6,* 433–445.

212. Tiwari, S. B.; Amiji, M. M. A Review of Nanocarrier-Based CNS Delivery Systems. *Curr. Drug Del.* **2006,** *3,* 219–232.

213. Wohlfart, S.; Gelperina, S. E.; Kreuter, J. Transport of Drugs across the Blood–Brain Barrier by Nanoparticles. *J. Contr. Release* **2012,** 161(2), 264–273.

214. Jeffries, W. A.; Brandon, M. R.; Hunt, S. V.; Williams, A. F.; Gatter, K. C.; Mason, D. Y. Transferrin Receptor on Endothelium of Brain Capillaries. *Nature* **1984,** *312,* 162–163.

215. Boado, R. J.; Zhang, Y.; Pardridge, W. M. Humanization of Anti-human Insulin Receptor Antibody for Drug Targeting across the Human Blood–Brain Barrier. *Biotechnol. Bioeng.* **2007,** *96,* 381–391.

216. Ulbrich, K.; Hekmatara, T.; Herbert, E.; Kreuter, J. Transferrin- and Transferrin Receptor-Antibody-Modified Nanoparticles Enable Drug Delivery across the Blood–Brain Barrier (BBB). *Eur. J. Pharm. Biopharm.* **2009,** *71,* 251–256.

217. Chen, X.; Schluesener, H. J. Nanosilver: A Nanoproduct in Medical Application. *Toxicol. Lett.* **2008,** *176,* 1–12.

218. Tian, F.; Cui, D.; Schwarz, H.; Estrada, G.; Kobayashic, H. Cytotoxicity of Single Wall Carbon Nanotubes on Human Fibroblasts. *Toxicol. In Vitro* **2006,** *20,* 1202–1212.

219. Beyerle, A.; Merkel, O.; Stoeger, T.; Kissel, T. PEGylation Affects Cytotoxicity and Cell-Compatibility of Poly(ethylene imine) for Lung Application: Structure Function Relationships. *Toxicol. Appl. Pharmacol.* **2010,** *242,* 146–154.

220. Hagens, W. I.; Oomen, A. G.; de Jong, W. H.; Cassee, F. R.; Sips, A. What Do We (need to) Know about the Kinetic Properties of Nanoparticles in the Body? *Regul. Toxicol. Pharmacol.* **2007,** *49,* 217–229.

221. Kreyling, W. G.; Möller, W.; Semmler-Behnke, M.; Oberdörster, G. Particle Toxicology. In Born, D. K., Ed.; CRC Press: Boca Raton, FL, 2007.

222. Kreyling, W. G.; Geiser, M. Dosimetry of Inhaled Nanoparticles. In: *Inhalation and Health Effects*; Marijnissen, J. C., Ed.; Springer: Berlin, 2009.

223. Desai, M. P.; Labhasetwar, V.; Walter, E.; Levy, R. J.; Amidon, G. L. The mechanism of uptake of biodegradable microparticles in Caco-2 cells is size dependent. *Pharm. Res.* **1997,** *14,* 1568–1573.

Nanomedical Devices

6.1 INTRODUCTION

Nanomaterials have been used in combination with biomolecules to create novel tissue substitutes, biological electronics such as biosensors, sensitive diagnostic systems, and controlled drug delivery systems with significantly improved performances. NMs are being used in a wide spectrum of nanomedical device applications. The nanomedical devices are used for nanorobots, nanochips and nanoimplants, prostheses, tissue engineering, and cell repair. The nanomaterials used as components or as additives in creating nanomedical devices have led to improved biocompatibility and functionality making them superior for tissue substitutes, tissue regeneration, prostheses, tissue engineering, and cell repair[1-7]. Nanosurgery is expected to bring a revolutionary change in terms of neighboring tissue/cell damage during surgery. [4,5,8-18]Nanorobots bring hope to early diagnosis and targeted drug delivery for early disease treatment such as cancer [1-5,7,8,11,15,19-27]. Improvements in implants can reduce cost and provide

Nanomaterials for Medical Applications. http://dx.doi.org/10.1016/B978-0-12-385089-8.00006-6

ease of use to patients while minimizing swelling, toxicity and other side effects. Various kinds of nanomaterials are currently being developed for various nanochips, nanoimplants, and even for stem cell regeneration [119,28-47]. These various applications of nanomedical devices are being developed for more accurate diagnosis and more efficient therapeutics that will benefit the human quality of life.[3,5-7,14,20,23,25,48-51] To date, majority of the NMs applications in medicine are still in the research stage, and only a a few are already in full blast clinical use. This chapter is dedicated to the various applications of nanomaterials for the creation of various nanomedical devices.[33,52-62]

6.2 NANOROBOTS

The technology of creating nanosized machines is called nanorobotics. This term, nanorobotics, refers to the section of nanotechnology that involves engineering, designing, and building of nanorobots. Nanorobots are devices ranging in size from 0.1 to 10 μm that are composed of nanoscale or molecular components. These devices can be injected into the patient to perform diagnosis or treatment on a cellular level. Such diagnosis or treatments involve the nanoscale, molecular, or atomic level. Treatments with nanorobots may involve alterations in structure and composition in the molecular or submolecular level.

The various applications for nanorobots in medicine include early diagnosis and targeted drug delivery for cancer therapeutics, nanosized biomedical instrument for surgery, pharmacokinetics, disease monitoring, and improving the affectivity and efficiency of health care.[4,11,63] These various areas of applications of nanorobots leverage the unique properties of materials and devices in the nanoscale dimensions.

6.2.1 Nanosurgery

Nanosurgery is the term that refers to surgery that uses fast laser beams which are focused by an objective microscope lens to exert a controlled force to manipulate organelles and other subcellular structures.[12] This precise technique allows for the destruction of a single cell without damaging adjacent healthy cells. It allows precise ablation of cellular and subcellular structures without compromising cell viability and with minimal damage to nearby cells.[64]

Conventional nanosurgery uses optical tweezers that consists of beams of laser light.[12] The narrowest point of the laser beam contains a strong electric field gradient at the center that attracts dielectric particles such that they move along the gradient toward the enabling the particles to be moved from one location to another, without ever touching them. The optical tweezers can be applied to biological substructures such as cell nuclei and chromosomes. In combination with a scalpel, the optical tweezers allow for even greater precision during surgery.

Ultrafast laser nanosurgery provides a high flux of photons that can be absorbed nonlinearly by the electrons.[64] The short duration of the absorption process leads to rapid and efficient plasma generation at the focal point of the beam, thereby providing only a few nanojoules for subcellular structure ablation. Damage from this technique depends on the pulse intensity, total number of pulses, and repetition rate of the laser but the wavelength has very minimal effect (see Table 6.1).[64] Disection effect on the tissue depends upon the density of free electrons.[65]

One of the applications of nanosurgery is for analysis of cell regulation.[16] At this molecular-level ablation process, there is a need to use low-repetition rate, low-energy femtosecond laser pulses. Using tightly focused pulses beneath the cell membrane, cellular material inside the cell is ablated through nonlinear processes. Using this technique, Mazur's group[16] selectively removed sub-micrometer regions of the cytoskeleton and individual mitochondria without altering neighboring structures or compromising cell viability. This nanoscissor technique enables a noninvasive manipulation of the living cells with several-hundred-nanometer resolution. This technique was used to demonstrate that the mitochondria are structurally independent functional units.

The distribution of contractile stresses across the extracellular matrix (ECM) in a cell in a spatially heterogeneous fashion underlies many cellular behaviors such as motility and tissue assembly.[17] Tanner et al.[17] investigated the biophysical basis of this process using femtosecond laser nanosurgery. They used nanosurgery to measure the viscoelastic recoil and the contributions of cell shape of contractile stress fibers (SFs, Figure 6.1). Right after laser nanosurgery and recoil, myosin light-chain kinase-dependent SFs along the cell periphery displayed less effective elasticities with severing of peripheral

TABLE 6.1 Sources of Damage during Ultrafast Laser Surgery[64]

Parameter	Photochemical damage	Thermoelastic stress confinement	Plasma-mediated ablation
Intensity threshold	$0.26 \times 10^{12}\,W/cm^2$	$5.1 \times 10^{12}\,W/cm^2$	$6.54 \times 10^{12}\,W/cm^2$
Electron density at threshold	$2.1 \times 10^{23}/cm^3$ One free electron in the focal volume	$0.24 \times 10^{21}/cm^3$ Induced thermal stress overcomes tensile	$1.0 \times 10^{21}/cm^3$ Critical electron density for optical breakdown
Description of damage	Free electrons cause formation of reactive oxygen species that break chemical bonds	Thermalization of the plasma occurs faster than accoustic relaxation time; hence, confinement of thermal stress leads to nanoscale transient bubbles	Damage caused by high-pressure and high temperature plasma plus the accompanying wave and cavitation bubble

fibers triggering a dramatic contraction of the entire cell within minutes of fiber irradiation.[17] When a population of SFs is pharmacologically dissipated, actin density flowed toward the other population as shown by image correlation spectroscopy.

Nanosurgery can be very useful to researchers investigating the development of the nervous system. During certain stages of neural development, trail-blazing "pioneer" neurons migrate and provide chemical signals which are subsequently used by migrating cells to extend their processes in the right direction. Nanosurgery could be used to eliminate pioneer neurons in order to determine exactly how they influence cells in the nervous system.

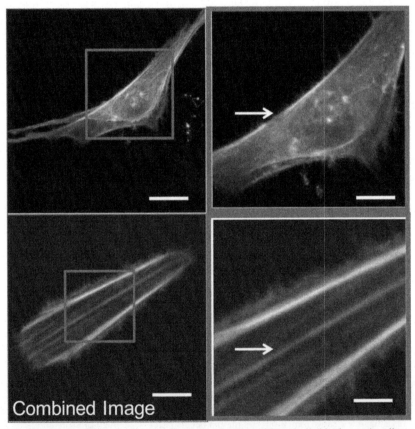

FIGURE 6.1 Femtolaser nanosurgery of central and peripheral SFs. Negligible changes in cell area occur after femtolaser disruption of a single central fiber (*top*); dramatic changes in cell area after ablation of a single peripheral fiber (*bottom*). Left: low-magnification snapshots showing the outline of the entire cell. Right: high-magnification zooms of the boxed regions that more clearly show the severed SF. All images are overlays of mCherry-LifeAct fluorescence before ablation (*red*) and 30-min postablation (*green*). Scale bar for left and right panels = 10 and 20μm, respectively. *From Tanner.[8] (For color version of this figure, the reader is referred to the online version of this book)*

One nanomaterial that has been used in the development of nanoneedles is carbon nanotubes (CNTs). These are attached to the tips of nanoneedles, and with the aid of atomic force microscopy (AFM), the needles are fabricated from pyramidal silicon AFM tips using focused ion beam etching. The nanoneedles can be potentially used by a nanosurgeon to perform an operation on a single cell without harming the cell.[66]

Today, cellular nanosurgery are already being explored using a rapidly vibrating (100Hz) micropipette with a <1-mm-tip diameter. This device is used to completely cut dendrites from single neurons without damaging cell viability.[67] It was reported that femtosecond surgery was performed on roundworm neurons and were functionally regenerated.[18] The femtolaser functions like a pair of "nanoscissors" by vaporizing local tissue without affecting adjacent tissue through the localized nanosurgical ablation of focal adhesions adjoining live mammalian epithelial cells.[68] It has also been used for microtubule dissection inside yeast cells,[69] noninvasive intratissue nanodissection of plant cell walls, and selective destruction of intracellular single plastids or selected parts of them.[70] In addition, femtolaser had also been reported for the nanosurgery of individual chromosomes to selectively knock out genomic nanometer-sized regions in the nucleus of living Chinese hamster ovary cells.[71] After these nanosurgeries, the cells survived. Bacterial cell dissection in aqueous medium has also been performed in situ using atomic force microscopes that revealed 26-nm-thick twisted strands inside the cell wall after mechanically peeling back large patches of the outer cell wall.[72]

6.2.2 Nanocameras

Unlike conventional clinical laboratory setup, medical robots like medical micro machines that are implanted or ingested can continuously gather diagnostic information and fine-tune the mode of treatments continuously over an extended period of time.[8] Some current examples are pill-sized cameras to view the digestive tract as well as implanted glucose and bone growth monitors to aid in the treatment of diabetes and joint replacements. The capabilities of micro machines are significantly extended to stand-alone millimeter-scale microrobots for possible in vivo surgical use. For example, external magnetic fields from a clinical magnetic resonance imaging (MRI) system can move microrobots containing ferromagnetic particles through blood vessels.[73–76]

In the field of nanotechnology, continuing development of in vivo machines has the potential to revolutionize health care[27,77–79] with devices small enough to reach and interact with individual cells of the body.[80,81] Current efforts focus on the development and functionalization of nanomaterials[86] that will allow their applications to enhance diagnostic imaging,[87–94] targeted drug delivery,[87–94] as well as a combination of both diagnosis and treatment which has been given the term called nanotheranostics.[95–101] Various studies have focused on the development and applications of nanomaterials that target specific cell types for imaging and/or drug delivery.[102–106]

6.2.3 Nanoradiofrequency antennas

Studies are also being focused on more complex devices that include multicomponent nanodevices called tectodendrimers that have a single-core dendrimer to which additional dendrimer modules of different types are affixed that are designed to perform specific function necessary for smart therapeutic nanodevices.[6,48,107] These nanomaterials can also be designed to provide some external control of chemistry within cells through the use of devices such as tiny nano radiofrequency antennas attached to DNA to control hybridization. Combining the excellent precision of nanomaterials with nanorobots allows a revolutionary approach to surgery in the subcellular level. These nanorobots are comparable with the size of cells that could provide significant medical benefits[2,3,27,108] but this requires that the nanorobots be fabricated at low cost in large numbers. To carry this out, the nanorobots may be created by engineering of biological systems such as attaching nanoparticles to bacteria, by using the programs within bacterial genetic machinery,[19,22,26] and creating computers out of DNA that respond to logical combinations of chemicals.[21] Nanoscale devices made of synthetic inorganic machines[8] could result from studies on nanoscale electronics, sensors, and motors.[1,7,20,24,25,109]

6.2.4 Applications of Nanorobots

One of the key benefits of nanorobots is that they can pass through the smallest vessels of the circulatory system and can, thereby, approach the individual cells of tissues to reach the desired locations and attach on these target cells through engineering processes.[8,85] Nanorobots can be used for nanomanipulations during "surgery at the nanoscale level."[9,14] Nanorobots can be introduced into the vascular system or body cavities, programmed, and controlled remotely by the surgeon in order to be able to perform various diagnostic and therapeutic precisely with minimal invasion that leads to faster recovery, while allowing communications with the on-site surgeon through signals.[9]

One nanorobot that has been investigated is a rapidly vibrating (100 Hz) micropipette with <1-micron tip that has been used to dissect the apical dendrites of rat hippocampal CA1 pyramidal cells that resulted in complete disconnection of dendrites while maintaining cell viability.[67] Femtosecond laser surgery was used in axotomy performed in roundword neurons that resulted in complete regeneration.[18] A similar femtosecond laser axotomy was performed on D-type axons of *Caenorhabditis elegans*.[15] They used confocal microscopy and laser scanning bright-field microscopy for real-time imaging of femtosecond laser nanosurgery and its dynamics in *C. elegans*. In this nanosurgery, muscular contraction and single-muscle cell stimulation were imaged. Confocal fluorescence imaging and laser scanning bright-field microscopy for real-time imaging were used to study the development of incision and observation of possible presence of any possible collateral damage and improvement of the technique. Other surgical nanorobots outfitted with operating instruments and capable of precise

Rabbit heart	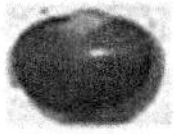	2 cm x 3 cm
Human breast cancer cell	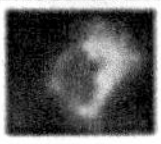	8-60 um
Bacteria	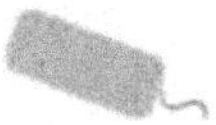	0.5 -20 um
Virus	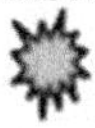	10-300 nm
Nanomaterials	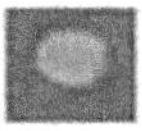	2-100 nm
Protein	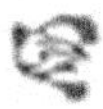	2-10 nm
Atom	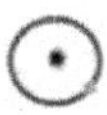	0.1 nm

FIGURE 6.2 Comparative sizes of nanomaterials with proteins, cells, tissues, etc. *(For color version of this figure, the reader is referred to the online version of this book)*

mobility for microvascular surgery, organ transplants, molecular repairs on cells, and eliminating cancerous cells have also been envisioned.[5,15]

In another context, nanorobots can come in the form of tiny engineered nanomaterials that are best suited for early diagnosis and targeted delivery for diseases such as cancer.[11,97,98,101,110] Disease-specific receptors on the surface of cells provide useful targets for nanoparticles because nanoparticles can be engineered from components that (1) recognize disease at the cellular level, (2) are visible on imaging studies, and (3) deliver therapeutic compounds.[104] Advances in nanotechnology are in the process of discovering new methods for delivery of therapeutic compounds, including genes and proteins, to diseased tissue. A variety of nano-enabled and nanostructured drugs with effective site targeting are being developed by combining a diverse selection of targeting, diagnostic, and therapeutic components. The use of immune target specificity with nanomaterials introduces a new type of treatment modality, nano-immunochemotherapy.[111]

6.3 NANOCHIPS AND NANOIMPLANTS

Understanding the structures of natural tissues is important in designing nanomaterials for nanochips and nanoimplants.[112] The size and structure of nanomaterials are very important in understanding the relationship between such structures and natural tissues at various levels. In Figure 6.2, the relative scales of proteins, cells, tissues, etc., in biological systems that nanomaterials attempt to mimic and penetrate are shown[112] (http://www.sciencedirect.com/science/article/pii/S0142961206007630 - ref_bib35). Only a few studies are dedicated to understand the degree to which nanomaterials interact with various cells to describe why nanomaterials demonstrate unique biological properties. One possible explanation lies in the nanostructures of the natural tissues and associated extracellular matrices. A more plausible explanation is that nanomaterials mimic dimensions of components of tissues for tissue engineering applications that relies on their unique surface energetics. Prior to adherence of cells, proteins are adsorbed to a material surface to potentially interact with selected cell membrane receptors.[112] Specific amino acid sequences of adsorbed vitronectin, fibronectin, and laminin may either enhance or inhibit cellular adhesion and growth. The surface chemistry, hydrophilicity or hydrophobicity, charge, topography, roughness, and energy affect the type, concentration, conformation, and bioactivity of plasma proteins adsorbed.[112,113]

The unique properties of nanomaterials include higher surface areas, higher surface roughness, higher amounts of surface defects (including grain boundaries), altered electron distributions, improved topography, and biocompatibility.[112] These affect interactions with proteins and other biomolecules which are nanoscale entities. The nanoscale surface features on nanomaterials can provide for more available sites for protein adsorption affecting the amount of cellular interactions.[112]

The cellular interactions with artificial surfaces are complex and still current unresolved.[114,115] Ideally, cell adhesion to surfaces and neighboring cells involves formation of specific short-range attractive forces that are formed through molecular ligand–receptor recognition steps to overcome specific long-range repulsive forces between hydrophilic surfaces and glycocalyx macromolecules.[114,116] After the occurrence of a short-term cell adhesion, further adhesion and spreading are governed by a subtle combination of molecular recognition and mechanosensing, which depends on surface topography, nature of functional groups, surface energy (wettability), stiffness, and the contact area between cell and substrate.[117,118] The surface parameters modulate the start of adhesion when cells are cultured without serum or when adsorbed cell-adhesive glycoproteins such as fibronectin or vitronectin are present.[119] However, cell adhesion to polystyrene surfaces can be triggered by hydroxyl groups even in the absence of serum or cell-produced fibronectin[120] (Figure 6.3).[77]

6.3.1 Nanomaterials for Bones

Natural bone is a nanostructured composite material.[112] It has three levels of structures namely: (1) the nanostructure (a few nanometers to a few hundred nanometers) that includes noncollageneous organic proteins, fibrillar collagen, and embedded mineral hydroxyapatite (HA) crystals; (2) the microstructure (from 1 to 500 μm) that includes lamellae, osteons, and Haversian systems; and (3) the macrostructure that includes cancellous and cortical bone.[121] These three levels of oriented structures assemble into heterogeneous and anisotropic bone[112] using natural porcine femur bone as seen by scanning electron microscopy (SEM) and AFM.[112]

6.3.1.1 HA in Polymers

Until recently, the effects of the nanosize hydroxyapatite (nHA) scaffold surface on protein adsorption and in vivo biocompatibility and vascularization have been analyzed. Nanoparticles strongly influence various inflammatory processes, depending on their physical and chemical properties (e.g. size, shape, surface

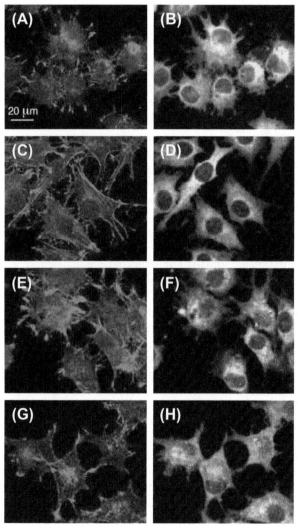

FIGURE 6.3   Confocal microscopy imaging of MG-63 grown without serum for 4h on ammonium persulfate APS-treated CNPs, bare (A and B) or with adsorbed fibronectin (C and D), RGD-pep (E and F), and RGE-pep (G and H). Actin appears red (left column) and vinculin green (right column). *From Vidal.[77] (For interpretation of the references to colour in this figure legend, the reader is referred to the online version of this book)*

chemistry)[122,123,124] while inflammation is linked to the process of angiogenesis,[125] which is necessary for the adequate vascularization of scaffolds after implantation into the host tissue.[122] Bone tissue engineering scaffolds must provide an osteoconductive surface to promote new bone ingrowth after implantation into bone defects that may be achieved by HA loading of distinct scaffold biomaterials. Lashke et al. reported the in vitro and in vivo properties of a novel nanosize hydroxyapatite particles/poly(ester-urethane) (nHA/PU) composite scaffold which was prepared by a salt leaching–phase inverse process.[122] Analysis of results with microtomography, SEM, and X-ray spectroscopy demonstrated the capability of the material processing to create a three-dimensional (3D) porous PU scaffold with nHA on the surface. The modified scaffold induced a significant increase in in vitro adsorption of model proteins compared to nHA-free PU scaffolds (control).[122] In vivo analysis of inflammatory and angiogenic host tissue response to implanted nHA/PU scaffolds indicated that the nHA particles incorporation into the scaffold material did not affect biocompatibility and vascularization.[122]

Biodegradable nHA/PU composite scaffold that was fabricated by a salt leaching–phase inverse process had been developed for bone regeneration.[122,126] The addition of 10–20%$_w$ of nHA improved the scaffold stiffness with an increase of 50% in the Young modulus, which may result in better scaffold stability after implantation into a bone defect.[122] In addition, the osteoconductive properties of the calcium phosphate-containing scaffold surface may accelerate and improve the formation of new bone tissue within the biodegradable PU foam.[122]

Nanohydroxyapatite (n-HAP) reinforced ceramic/polymer nanocomposites have gained recognition as bone scaffolds due to their composition and structural similarity with natural bones.[127] In addition, their unique functional properties such as larger surface area and superior mechanical strength make them better than those of their single-phase constituents. Rod-shaped n-HAP nanocomposite scaffold has been developed to mimic natural bone apatite morphology.[128] Incorporation of synthesized nHA in place of microparticles of HA brings higher mechanical strength and more regular microarchitecture that result from the nanoparticles' interfacial area, surface reactivity, and ultrafine structure. A variety of scaffolds using thermally have also been reported for thermally induced phase separation.[129,130]

In one study, n-HAP bone scaffolds were prepared by a homemade selective laser sintering (SLS) system based on rapid prototyping technology.[131] The SLS system developed consisted of a precise three-axis motion platform and a laser with optical focusing device which implements arbitrary complex movements based on the nonuniform rational B-spline theory is realized in this system. The effects of the processing parameters on n-HAP were tested with X-ray diffraction, Fourier transform infrared spectroscopy, and SEM. The particles of n-HAP grew into spherical like from the initial needle-like shape with a nanoscale structure at scanning speeds between 200- and 300-mm/min when the laser power was 50W, the light spot diameter 4mm, and the layer thickness

(A)

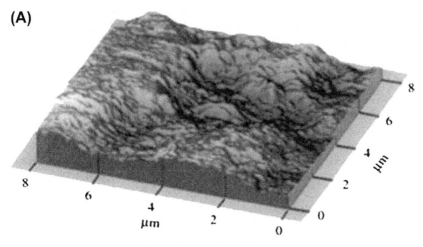

32 nm grain size titania

(B)

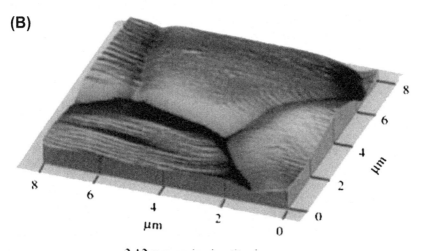

2.12 μm grain size titania

FIGURE 6.4 Atomic force micrographs of (A) nanophase and (B) conventional titania. The nanophase materials have unique surface properties that are conducive to enhanced bone cell. *Adapted and reprinted from Webster.*[99]

0.3 mm. These changes did not result in decomposition of the n-HAP during the sintering process. The newly developed n-HAP scaffolds have the potential to serve as an excellent substrate in bone tissue engineering.

6.3.1.2 Titanium Nanomaterials

Contemporary dental implants regard titanium as the "gold standard" material.[40] The high success and survival rates of titanium implants have been demonstrated in many different applications.[36,132] The spontaneous formation of a dense oxide film on the surface of titanium provides high biocompatibility, but it also poses as a disadvantage because its spontaneity can result in poor aesthetics. The grayish color results from exposure caused by soft tissue recession or thin gingival biotype especially in anterior sites in the mouth. Zirconia implants have been introduced that might offer a better alternative to titanium. Unlike titanium implants that can give the gingiva an unnatural bluish/gray appearance, zirconia has an opacity that resembles natural teeth and its bright white color may provide satisfactory aesthetics.[31]

The increased adhesion of bone-forming cells, osteoblast, on nanostructured materials was reported in 1999[133] using alumina with grain sizes between 49 and 67 nm and titania with grain sizes between 32 and 56 nm. These nanomaterials were reported to promote osteoblast adhesion compared with their respective micrograined materials. Additional studies of these nanostructured ceramics (such as alumina, titania, and HA) exhibited in vitro osteoblast proliferation. Their long-term functions as measured by intracellular and ECM protein synthesis such as collagen and alkaline phosphatase, as well as calcium-containing mineral deposition, were superior on ceramics with less than 100-nm grain or fiber sizes.[134,135] Two, three, and four times the amount of calcium deposition was observed on nanostructured materials compared with the conventional HA, titania, and alumina when osteoblasts were cultured for up to 28 days. In addition, osteoblast functions such as viable cell adhesion, proliferation, and calcium deposition were further increased on nanofiber materials compared with nanospherical structures of alumina. This was believed to result from the nanofibers having more closely approximate the shape of HA crystals and collagen fibers in bone compared with nanospherical geometries.[135] The surface chemistry and/or crystal structures of the conventional ceramics tested in these reports were similar to their respective nanophase materials except the degree of nanometer surface features that was altered.

Stadlinger[40] performed animal studies to investigate and compare the osseointegration of 14 zirconia and 7 titanium dental implants in minipigs. At the end of a healing period of 4 weeks, a histological analysis of the soft and hard tissue and a histomorphometric analysis of the bone–implant contact (BIC) and relative peri-implant bone-volume density (rBVD) was performed. Submerged zirconia and titanium implants surface showed an intimate connection to the neighboring bone, both achieving a BIC of 53%. The nonsubmerged zirconia implants showed some crestal epithelial downgrowth with a BIC of 48%. Zirconia exhibited the highest rBVD values (80%), followed by titanium (74%) and nonsubmerged zirconia (63%). These in vivo studies suggest that unloaded zirconia and titanium implants osseointegrate similarly within the 4-week healing period studied. Figure 6.4 shows a comparison between nanoscale and conventional microscale titania[133] which is the oxide that forms on the widely implanted titanium (Ti).

TABLE 6.2 Various Methods to Create Nanofeatures on cpTitanium Implants[138]

Methods	Characteristics
Self-assembly	The available functional group could serve multiple functions such as an osteoinductive or cell-adhesive molecule.
Ion beam deposition	Creates nanofeatures on the surface of the material used.
Acid etching	Creates surface nanofeatures and destroy contaminants when combined with sandblasting and/or peroxidation.

The topography of titanium implant surfaces may be affected by nanoscale modification as well as the chemistry of the surface. Implant surface quality has been divided into three categories[136]:

(1) mechanical properties
(2) topographic properties, and
(3) physicochemical properties.

These characteristics are indicated to be relative and changing any of these groups also affected the others. One limitation that is usually encountered in studies comparing nano- and micron-level surface topography is the extreme difficulty to isolate chemistry or charge effects induced by the nanotopography. However, atomic-level control of surface topography during material assembly is influenced by quantum phenomena that do not govern traditional bulk material behavior.[137] It is very extremely important to distinguish topography-specific effects from allied changes in surface energy or chemical reactivity. Nanotechnology provides novel ways of atomic-scale manipulation of matter. Some approaches are currently prevalent in the experimental application to endosseous implants (Table 6.2).[138] Physical method of compaction of nanoparticles of TiO_2 versus micron-level particles that yield surfaces with nanoscale grain boundaries is one such approach.[139] This offers conservation of the chemistry of the surface among different topographies.

Molecular self-assembly is one other factor that affects surface topography. Spontaneous chemisorption and vertical close-packed positioning of molecules onto substrates allowing the exposure of functional or active end-chain groups at the interface leads to self-assembled monolayers (SAMs).[140] The exposed functional group serves as active site for osteoinductive or cell-adhesive molecule. One such example is the use of cell-adhesive peptides (RGD domains or arginine–lysine–aspartic acid) attached to SAMs composed of polyethylene glycol (PEG) and applied to the titanium surfaces.[141] The chemical treatment of different surfaces to expose reactive groups on the material surface also creates nanoscale topography that is popular among current dental implant investigators. Treatment with NaOH catalyzes the production of titanium nanostructures outward from the titanium surface[142] producing a sodium titanate gel layer on the Ti surface while treatment with H_2O_2 produces a titania gel layer. The gel-like layer over the titanium material allows HA deposition which had been observed with other metals such as zirconium and aluminum.[143–145]

Nanotopography had been created by chemical treatments (peroxidation with H_2O_2, heat, or acid oxidation, such as hydrofluoric acid).[144,145] It has been observed that novel nanostructures of amorphous titanium oxide formed on the implant surface with the use of H_2O_2 with acid etching.[146] Increased adsorption of RGD peptides were observed after treatment of the implant surface with H_2O_2/HCl, followed by passivation (30% HNO_3) and heat treatment of the surfaces.[147] These treatment processes also increased the mineralization in the same order while hydrofluoric acid treatments created discrete nanostructures on TiO_2 grit-blasted surfaces.[148] Different reports including cell culture studies,[149,150] preclinical investigations,[151,33] and clinical studies[41] indicated that hydrofluoric acid treatment of TiO_2 grit-blasted titanium implants is associated with rapid bone accrual at the implants surface. However, further investigation must be performed to study the complex chemical changes induced by these methods.

Deposition of nanoparticles onto the titanium surface is another approach to impart nanofeatures to a titanium dental implant.[32] Deposition of nanometer-scale calcium phosphate to the implants surface can be achieved through sol–gel transformation techniques.[152,153] Materials such as alumina, titania, zirconia, and others can also be applied.[39] As a result of their resultant atomic-scale interactions, the nanomaterial buildup display strong physical interactions.[32,154,30,155] Nishimura and colleagues[156] recently demonstrated a revised directed approach to the assembly of $CaPO_4$ nanofeatures on dual acid-etched cpTitanium implant surfaces. Using a rat model, the deposition of discrete 20- to 40-nm nanoparticles on an acid-etched titanium surface led to increased mechanical interlocking with bone and the early healing of bone at the endosseous implant surface.

Nanotopography has been shown to influence cell adhesion, proliferation, differentiation, and cell-specific adhesion. Related changes in chemistry and nanostructure impart important chemical changes and permit biomimetic relationships between alloplastic surfaces and tissues. It is speculated that alloplastic nanosurfaces possess topographic elements scaled to naturally occurring substrates.

Ueno introduced nanopolymorphic features of alkali- and heat-treated titanium surfaces, comprising of tuft-like, plate-like, and nodular structures that are smaller than 100 nm and determined whether and how the addition of these nanofeatures to a microroughened titanium surface affect bone–implant integration.[157] Comprehensive assessment of biomechanical, interfacial, and histological analyses in a rat model was performed using machined surfaces without microroughness, sandblasted-microroughened surfaces, and micro–nano hybrid created by sandblasting and alkali and heat treatment. Compared with the non-microroughened surface, the microroughened surface accelerated the establishment of implant biomechanical fixation at the early healing stage but did not increase the implant fixation at the late healing stage.[157] The use of nanopolymorphic features on the microroughened surface further increased implant fixation throughout the healing time. The percentage of BIC increased four- to fivefold using microroughened surfaces that was further increased by more than twofold throughout the healing period. Using alkali- and heat-treated nanopolymorphic surface, critical parameters that were necessary to process bone–implant integration for which nanofeatures have specific and substantial roles were identified. Nanofeature-enhanced osteoconductivity, which resulted in both the acceleration and elevation of bone–implant integration was demonstrated.

The in vivo response of nanoscale titanium implants in terms of nitric oxide scavenging and fibrotic capsule formation was studied.[158] Titanium dioxide (TiO_2) nanotubes with 100-nm diameters fabricated by electrochemical anodization with TiO_2 control surfaces showed significantly lower nitric oxide, suggesting that nanotubes break down nitric oxide. The soft tissue response in vivo TiO_2 nanotube and TiO_2 control implants were placed in rat abdominal wall for 1 and 6 weeks showed a reduced fibrotic capsule thickness for the nanotube surfaces for both time points. In addition, lower nitric oxide activity, measured as the presence of nitrotyrosine ($P < 0.05$), was observed on the nanotube surface after 1 week. The differences observed may be attributed to the catalytic properties of TiO_2 that are increased by the nanotube structure. These results give insight for the interaction between titanium implants in soft tissue as well as bone tissue that provide a mechanism for the improvement of future clinical implants.

6.3.1.3 Ceramic Nanomaterials

Another interesting material that can serve as implant is ceramic that are known for their excellent biocompatibility and high resistance to wear. Ceramics find use in a wide variety of clinical applications such as in orthopedics for femoral head and hip replacements.[159] Compared with titanium, its high degree of brittleness that is due to the molecular covalent–ionic binding structure in ceramics prevents plastic deformation before failure. However, ceramics suffer from microstructural flaws that cause poor resistance to stress.[160] For applications as dental implants, ceramic implants that are yttrium-stabilized tetragonal zirconia polycrystal ceramics (PSZ) has rekindled interest in its application as implant materials. Compared with aluminum oxide ceramics, PSZ has a higher fracture resistance and flexural strength making it less sensitive to stress concentrations. This property is mostly due to the toughening transformation changing a metastable tetragonal grain structure into a monoclinic structure at room temperature.[161] This simultaneous 3% expansion in volume prevents the progression of a crack or flaw in the ceramic.[160]

Webster et al.[162,163] have focused on the mechanisms of enhanced cellular activity (such as osteoblast, chondrocyte, etc.) on nanophase materials. Mechanism-based studies exhibited that the concentration, conformation, and bioactivity of vitronectin (a protein in serum that mediates osteoblast adhesion) were responsible for the enhanced adhesion of osteoblasts (an important prerequisite for anchorage-dependent cell functions) on nanophase ceramic formulations. Vitronectin preferentially adsorbed to the small pores in nanophase ceramics (such as 0.98-nm pore diameters in nanophase titania compacts). Adsorption of vitronectin was 10% greater on nanophase compared to conventional alumina.[162,163] Increased unfolding of vitronectin was observed when this was adsorbed on nanophase ceramics compared to conventional ceramics. Unfolding of vitronectin promoted the availability of specific cell-adhesive epitopes (such as the arginine–glycine–aspartic acid or RGD sequence) that led to enhanced osteoblast adhesion.

The increased adhesion of bone-forming cells, osteoblast, on nanostructured materials was reported in 1999[133] using alumina with grain sizes between 49 and 67 nm and titania with grain sizes between 32 and 56 nm. These nanomaterials were reported to promote osteoblast adhesion compared with their respective micrograined materials. Additional studies of these nanstructured ceramics (such as alumina, titania, and HA) exhibited in vitro osteoblast proliferation. Their long-term functions as measured by intracellular and ECM protein synthesis such as collagen and alkaline phosphatase, as well as calcium-containing mineral deposition, were superior on ceramics with less than 100-nm grain or fiber sizes.[134,135] Two, three, and four times the amount of calcium deposition was observed on nanostructured materials compared with the conventional HA, titania, and alumina when osteoblasts were cultured for up to 28 days. In addition, osteoblast functions such as viable cell adhesion, proliferation, and calcium deposition were further increased on nanofiber materials compared with nanospherical structures of alumina. This was believed to result from the nanofibers having more closely approximate the shape of HA crystals and collagen fibers in bone compared with nanospherical geometries. The surface chemistry and/ or crystal structures of the conventional ceramics tested in these reports were similar to their respective nanophase materials except the degree of nanometer surface features that was altered.

Nanostructured ceramics also exhibited enhanced bone-resorbing (osteoclast) functions. Compared with conventional HA, osteoclast synthesis of tartrate-resistant acid phosphatase with subsequent formation of resorption pits on the nanoparticles showed up to two times greater.[164] Osteoblast- and osteoclast-coordinated functions are important for the formation and maintenance of healthy new bone placed adjacent to an orthopedic implant. Thus, promoted functions of osteoblasts combined with enhanced functions of osteoclasts could lead to transformation of bones formed at implant surfaces composed of nanosized ceramics.[112] A few in vivo studies have demonstrated enhanced new bone formation on metals surfaces with nanomaterials compared with conventional HA implanted in rats.[165] Enhanced new bone formation was shown on nanosized HA-coated tantalum compared with microsized HA-coated tantalum and the noncoated tantalum as seen on Figure 6.5.[112] These results are very promising for the translation of data showing greater bone growth on nanomaterials from in vitro to in vivo.

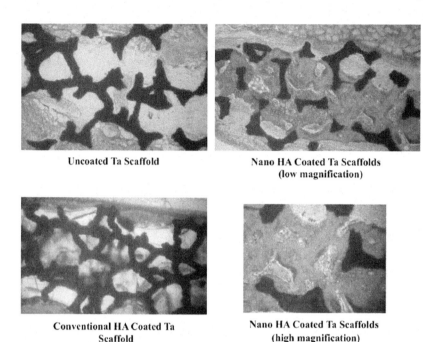

| Uncoated Ta Scaffold | Nano HA Coated Ta Scaffolds (low magnification) |
| Conventional HA Coated Ta Scaffold | Nano HA Coated Ta Scaffolds (high magnification) |

FIGURE 6.5   Histology of rat calvaria 2 weeks after the implantation of tantalum (Ta) scaffolds coated with either nanophase or conventional HA. New bone infiltration occurred in greater amounts on nano-HA-coated Ta than on either conventional HA-coated Ta or uncoated Ta (Red). *Adapted and reprinted with permission from Liu and Webster.[75] (For interpretation of the references to colour in this figure legend, the reader is referred to the online version of this book)*

For implant applications, nanoceramics and nanometals have been created by decreasing the size of component such as particles, grains, or fibers. Different techniques to create nanometer surface features on polymers such as chemical etching, mold casting, e-beam lithography, and polymer demixing[166,167] all show promise for orthopedic applications. The versatility of biodegradable polymer nanomaterials such as PLGA[168,169] in spite of increased osteoblast functions and decreased fibroblast functions on nano compared to conventional materials is that polymers may help rehabilitate damaged bone tissue due to their controllable biodegradability.[168] In this manner, while the natural tissue regenerates, these polymers degrade in vivo into nontoxic, natural metabolites (such as lactic acid and glycolic acid) which enter the metabolic pathways of the tricarboxylic acid cycle and are eventually eliminated from the body as carbon dioxide and water.[170]

6.3.1.4 Carbon Nanofiber/Polymer Composites

The bone is the hardest tissue providing mechanical support to our body, protecting other internal organs, and producing and storing blood cells in the bone marrow.[50] Thus, mechanical property is the first criteria taken into consideration when designing a material to be used as a bone scaffold. For this, the mechanical strength of CNTs and carbon nanofibers (CNFs) is excellent making them largely studied nanostructures as reinforcing agents in composite materials[171-173] and for bone scaffolds.[50,174,175] In addition, unlike other metallic or ceramic-based bone scaffolds used in orthopedics single CNTs are less dense making lighter scaffolds with very high strength.[50] Single-wall carbon nanotubes (SWCNTs) offer additional properties such as high flexibility and a very high Young's modulus (stiffness) in the range of terapascals (TPa).[175,176]

The tailorable electrical and mechanical properties of CNF/polymer composites have attracted attention for orthopedic applications. CNFs–polyurethane (PU) nanocomposites promoted osteoblast adhesion[177] in comparison with conventional carbon fibers and Ti (ASTM F-67, Medical Grade 2). These show the ability of nanophase composites to increase functions of bone cells whether used alone or in polymer composite form but which is not yet fully explored for orthopedic applications. The improved mechanical and biocompatibility properties of CNF/polymer composites hold promise for alternative orthopedic implant.

Like other nanomaterials, CNTs/CNFs can be functionalized with groups that can improve their biocompatibility[178,179] and/or mechanical strength[180] of the scaffolds.[50] Furthermore, the material surface free energies influenced cell adhesion that eventually affected subsequent functions of different types of cells causing enhanced tissue regeneration.[181-184] Hence, scaffolds containing various amounts of CNFs lead to a composite that can be used to selectively enhance functions of one type of cell but decrease functions of others.[50] These versatile nanocomposites lead to numerous applications in biological scaffolds particularly for orthopedic applications.

In an in vitro study, Price et al.[177] dispersed CNFs in polycarbonate urethane (PCU) to create composites (a PCU/CNF composite) and tested the adhesion of osteoblasts (bone-forming cells), fibroblasts (soft tissue-forming cells), chondrocytes (cartilage-synthesizing cells), and smooth muscle cells on the composite scaffolds. The results indicated that the composites with nanometer dimension carbon fibers promoted osteoblast adhesion without promoting the adhesion of other cells. Furthermore, when carbon nanofiber surface energy was increased, the adhesion of smooth muscle cell, fibroblast, and chondrocyte decreased, indicating that surface energy is an important parameter that influences cell adhesion and therefore subsequent cell functions. In this study, they reported that greater weight percentages of high surface energy carbon nanofibers in the PCU/CNF composite increased osteoblast adhesion while decreasing fibroblast adhesion. Such a material is desirable because it can promote osteoblast adhesion and decrease competitive cell adhesion that leads to faster integration of the bone to the implant surface in vivo.[177] Their study showed the versatility of CNFs to tailor the surface structure, surface chemistry, and/or surface energy of a scaffold for the selective promotion of the adhesion of one type of cell while inhibiting other types of cells.[50]

6.3.1.5 Zirconia

Zirconia implants that might offer a useful alternative to titanium have recently been introduced into dental implantology.[40,50] Zirconia has an opacity that resembles natural teeth while titanium implants can give an unnatural bluish/gray appearance.[31] Unlike titanium, the bright white color of zirconia may provide satisfactory aesthetics.[50]

The development of yttria-stabilized tetragonal PSZ has rekindled interest in ceramic implant materials for dental implants.[50] Unlike aluminum oxide ceramics used in dental implants, PSZ has a higher fracture resistance and flexural strength making it less sensitive to stress concentrations. This is due to the metastable tetragonal grain structure that is transformed into a monoclinic structure at room temperature.[161] Several studies showed the capability of zirconia implants to withstand long-term loading.[185,186]

The use of zirconia implants have shown fewer inflammatory infiltrates in soft tissue than for titanium.[34] Unlike titanium, minimal ion release is detected[187]; hence, zirconia is considered to be highly biocompatible. Zirconia implants have been reported to integrate well in the jaw bone[28,29,38] and can be produced as one-piece implants that heal nonsubmerged (i.e. transmucosal) following implantation.[50]

Andreiotelli et al.[52] concluded that zirconia may have the potential as a successful implant material but recommended that clinical application be supported by clinical studies. Implant loading can influence osseointegration.[50] Based on studies by Akagawa et al. who compared submerged and nonsubmerged zirconia implants, collagen fibers in the apical regions of submerged implants in dogs were observed after 3 months.[28] This effect was explained as the result of mastication of food. A loss of crestal bone was described after 3 months in loaded implants.[188] In a study performed in monkeys, Kohal et al. compared loaded sandblasted zirconia and sandblasted, acid-etched titanium implants in the anterior bone.[38] After 9 months of healing and 5 months of loading, the soft and hard tissue dimensions were evaluated. The results indicated that the BIC reached 67% for zirconia implants and 73% for titanium implants without statistically significant difference.

6.3.2 Nanomaterials for Cartilage Applications

Cartilage replacement is one of the necessities in medical treatments. This is because, once cartilage is damaged, it does not normally regenerate. Repeated injury plus the low cellularity and isolation from the vascular supply of bioactive molecules limit intrinsic cartilage repair. As a result, mature articular cartilage cannot heal spontaneously because of its low mitotic activity in contrast with the rapid rate of chondrocytic (cartilage-synthesizing cell) mitosis during normal cartilage growth.[189] Thus, surgical strategies for cartilage repair have focused on accessing the regenerative signaling molecules and cells within the subchondral bone marrow[112] but this requires invasive drilling or abrasion through the overlying articular cartilage into the bone marrow. This causes even further cartilage tissue damage before achieving any therapeutic effect. Besides that, the properties of the resulting tissue are inferior to that of the uninjured cartilage due to the growth of fibrocartilage.

Biomaterials are very important in engineering tissue regeneration and repair.[190] To grow an entire organ or a tissue for transplantation, it requires a pre-designed scaffold with the patient-specific anatomy.[191] In some cases, irregular shaped defects and wounds need to be filled and repaired in clinics.[192] In such situations, injectable materials are useful because they are easily manipulated and can be sued in minimally invasive procedures to reduce complications and to improve patient comfort and satisfaction.[193] One of the flexible and manipulable materials that have been explored for such purpose is hydrogel which has limitations that are being tackled by various approaches.[194–198] However, these materials are not yet in clinical use.

One material that is being studied as scaffold for cartilage tissue engineering is that electrospun polymeric nanofibers have emerged as potential scaffolds for cartilage tissue engineering[199,200] because these mimic the natural ECM making them suitable candidates for cartilage tissue engineering.[201,202] Poly-ε-caprolactone (PCL) nanofiber sheets are flexible and can be rolled or folded and contoured to cover the surface of a joint making them excellent candidates for cartilage tissue engineering. The study by Liu[192] demonstrated that it is possible to seed PCL nanofiber scaffolds with periosteal cells in vivo and subsequently produce engineered cartilage in vitro.

Other nanomaterials including polymeric nanomaterials, nanocomposites, and natural nanomaterials have also been studied for cartilage regeneration.[112] Human cartilage cells attached and proliferated well on HA nanocrystals that were homogeneously dispersed in poly(lactic acid) (PLA) nanocomposites.[35] Increased chondrocyte adhesion and migration were observed in anodized nanomaterial metals (such as Ti) with nanometer-sized pores.[203]

6.3.3 Nanomaterials for Vascular Applications

Polymeric nanomaterials have also promoted the responses of vascular cells (such as endothelial and smooth muscle cells).[112] PLGA that were treated with various concentrations of NaOH for selected period of time generated nano-structured PLGA with altered surface chemistry while retaining nanostructured topographies by using silastic mold-casting techniques. Their results demonstrated that endothelial and smooth muscle cell densities increased on nanostructured PLGA as a result of the nanometer surface features.[204] Additionally, nanometals prepared by powder metallurgy techniques also demonstrated increased endothelialization compared with conventional metals[205] showing that the use of nanometals in vascular stent applications can solve problems that were associated with endothelial monolayer formation.

Poly(butylenes succinate) (PBSU) have good biocompatibility and biodegradability but is unexplored for tissue engineering.[206] Thus, Zhao et al., compared PBSU and PLGA scaffolds prepared by electrospinning technique as vascular tissue engineering materials. Their studies showed that fiber diameter of the electrospun scaffolds ranged from 300 to 800 nm and their porosities were higher than 90%. The electrospun PLGA scaffolds gave a maximum tensile strength of 14.31 ± 5.24 MPa while the electrospun PBSU scaffolds showed a tensile strength of 2.06 ± 0.11 MPa. There was no significant difference in cell adhesion efficacy between PBSU and PLGA scaffolds, but cell proliferation rate on PLGA scaffolds was significantly higher than that on PBSU scaffolds after 7 days of culture. These in vitro studies revealed that the electrospun PBSU scaffolds showed lower tensile strength and slower proliferation rate than PLGA. On the other hand, the biocompatibility and pore structure of the electrospun PBSU scaffolds showed promising application vascular tissue engineering.

6.3.4 Nanomaterials for Bladder Implants

Nanomaterials are also being studied for bladder applications.[169] More than 90% of bladder cancers begin in the urothelium transitional epithelial layer. These are categorized as superficial and require bladder tissue replacements[166] because these often require the removal of large portions of the bladder or the entire bladder wall. As a result of biocompatibility and ability to stretch and relax, polymers are promising replacement materials. Since implant surface properties undoubtedly impact cellular responses, an important parameter for achieving maximal cell responses is the material topography.[112] Just like any natural soft tissue, the bladder has constituent ECM proteins having nanometer lengths and widths. Thus, the next generation of polymeric bladder construct materials should incorporate nanodimensional surface characteristics.

The design of synthetic bladder wall substitutes has involved polymers with microdimensional structures. Nanostructured polymers for use as synthetic bladder constructs that mimic the topography of natural bladder tissue has been studied in vitro.[166] In this study, novel nanostructured biodegradable polymeric films of PLGA (Figure 6.6), poly-ether-urethane (PU, Figure 6.7), and poly-caprolactone (PCL) were fabricated and separately treated with various concentrations of NaOH (for PLGA and PCL) and HNO_3 (for PU) for select time periods. The results provided the first evidence that adhesion of bladder smooth muscle cells was enhanced as polymer surface feature dimensions were reduced into the nanometer range. Surface analysis revealed that the polymer nanometer surface roughness was the primary design parameter that increased bladder smooth muscle cell adhesion. Results from their studies provided the first evidence that bladder smooth muscle cell adhesion and proliferation were enhanced on polymeric surfaces with nanodimensional, compared

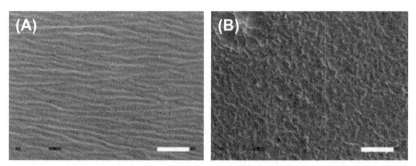

FIGURE 6.6   Scanning electron micrographs of chemically treated PLGA surfaces. Representative scanning electron micrograph images of (A) untreated (conventional) PLGA (feature dimensions 10–15 μm) and (B) chemically treated nanostructured PLGA (feature dimensions 50–100 nm). Scale bar = 10 microns (A) and 1000 nm (B). *From Thapa et al.*[140]

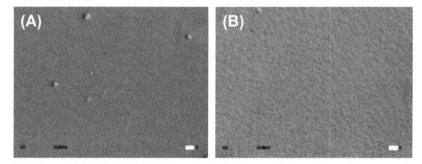

FIGURE 6.7   Scanning electron micrographs of chemically treated PU surfaces. Representative scanning electron micrograph images of (A) untreated (conventional) PU (feature dimensions > 15 μm) and (B) chemically treated nanostructured PU (feature dimensions 50–100 nm). Scale bar = 1000 nm. *From Thapa et al.*[140]

to microdimensional features.[166] In these studies, bladder smooth muscle cell adhesion and proliferation were greater on 2D nanometer surfaces of polymers such as PLGA and PU. Similar trends have recently been reported on 3D PLGA scaffolds.[207] Although most of the bladder regeneration with nanomaterials is at the in vitro level, significant promise exists for the continued exploration of these materials.

6.3.5 Nanomaterials for Neural Applications

Silicon materials are usually used for chronic neural implants but are subject to scar tissue formation at the tissue/implant interface, which interferes with their functionality.[37] CNFs that show cytocompatibility, mechanical, and electrical properties are an example of a material that may improve neural implant interactions with native cell populations. In vitro studies have shown that PCU and CNF composites have induced neurite extension. These materials have promising tunable properties for neural implants such as electrical, nanoscale structure and organization, and surface energy characteristics.

Neural prostheses are used for monitoring and applying electrical signals to neural tissue.[112] Nanomaterials with exceptional electrical properties are good candidates to transmit and receive electrical signals. In addition, nanomaterials that support and enhance nerve cell neurite/axon extension due to their excellent conductivity and biocompatibility properties are promising candidates. During neural implantation, a cellular process called gliotic response separates the implant from surrounding tissue through scar formation which is caused by the activity of astrocytes and meningeal cells. This scar formation is believed to interfere with the long-term efficacy of neural prostheses. Thus, the design of materials that will enhance nerve cell interactions while deterring astrocyte formation of scar tissue is crucial for neural implants.

Implantable probes are required for the continuous monitoring, diagnosis, and treatment of neural tissue.[208] However, such neural probes that are usually composed of silicon become encapsulated with nonconductive glial scar tissue. The same encapsulation with soft fibrous tissue usually happens to orthopedic implants such as titanium and/or titanium alloys as well instead of hard bony tissue. They have shown that functions of cells that contribute to glial scar tissue formation for neural prostheses (astrocytes) and fibrous tissue encapsulation events for bone implants (fibroblasts) decreased on PU composites containing CNFs.[208]

Studies on the use of biomaterials to improve the function of injured nervous system tissue have provided promising results[209] but not without significant hurdles, such as delayed or incomplete tissue regeneration. Because of the need for better nervous system biomaterials, recent approaches for the next generation of tissue engineering scaffolds have incorporated nanoscale surface feature dimensions that mimic natural neural tissue. Nanomaterials have enhanced desirable neural cell activity while suppressing unwanted cell activity like reactive astrocyte activity in the central nervous system. To create an environment for tissue regeneration that is superior to inert scaffolds, a combination of stimulatory cues may be used to incorporate nanoscale topographical and chemical and/or electrical cues in the same scaffold.[209] Electrically active nanomaterials are currently being used in the fabrication of composite materials with nanoscale, piezoelectric zinc oxide particles embedded into a polymer matrix. Zinc oxide can theoretically provide an electrical stimulus that is a known stimulatory cue for neural tissue regeneration. Further studies involving the combination of nanoscale surface dimensions and electrical activity that may provide enhanced neural tissue regeneration environment deserve further attention.

6.4 PROSTHESIS

Prosthesis is an artificial device that replaces a missing body part. It is typically used to replace parts of the body that are lost by injury (traumatic) or missing from birth (congenital) or to supplement defective body parts. Inside the body, artificial heart valve are in common use but artificial heart and lungs are under active technology development. Other prosthetics include hearing aids, artificial eyes, dentures, and gastric bands.

Prostheses are the medical devices that are completely finished and are technically connected to the body. One such example is the artificial limb that is made up of the C-leg, the socket, and the attachment hardware parts including the foot. New plastics and nanomaterials, such as carbon fiber, have allowed artificial limbs to be stronger and lighter, limiting the amount of energy necessary to operate the limb especially in transfemoral amputees. New materials have allowed artificial limbs to look realistic making transradial and transhumeral amputees more likely to have the artificial limb exposed.[210]

Existing body-powered arms contain sockets made of hard epoxy or carbon fiber while the wrist units are either screw-on connectors featuring the UNF 1/2–20 thread (USA) or quick release connector.[210] At the end of these arms are hooks, hands, or other devices. Hands rare usually uncomfortable because they require a large activation force unlike hooks that require a much lower force.[211]

Tang et al. studied whether the design of a transmetatarsal amputation prosthesis with a carbon-fiber plate would improve gait pattern in patients with transmetatarsal amputations.[212] In this study at a tertiary medical center, eight male patients with transmetatarsal amputations were recruited. Nine healthy male volunteers were recruited as the control group. A full-length standard shoe and a transmetatarsal amputation prosthesis with a carbon-fiber plate with a custom-molded insole, a mounted toe filler, and a thin, lightweight, carbon-fiber plate was used. The results of the kinetic and kinematic studies showed that the transmetatarsal amputation prosthesis with a carbon-fiber plate improved gait pattern significantly in patients with transmetatarsal amputations. In addition, drastic shoe modifications were not necessary to have the prosthesis inserted. The transmetatarsal amputation prosthesis with a carbon-fiber plate indicated that it was a good alternative footwear in patients with transmetatarsal amputations.

Nanomaterial-based prostheses have also been used for spine prostheses.[213] In this study, a group of 42 patients were submitted to excision of one or more vertebral bodies for the treatment of neoplastic pathology, with reconstruction by prosthetic carbon fiber modular implant to obtain immediate stability, and to stimulate solid intervertebral fusion by bone grafts introduced inside the prosthesis. At the end of 26 months after the surgery, a clinical and instrumental follow-up for all the patients showed that the use of a carbon prosthesis did not cause short- or long-term mechanical complications. The results showed that carbon fiber modular implant may have filled loss of bone substance of the vertebral column, allowed for immediate weight bearing, and favored bone fusion. Features of the carbon prosthesis favorably adapted to the surgical method of vertebrectomy, wherein (1) various components of the prosthesis adapted to bone resection of the vertebral body even in unexpected situations and (2) connection to posterior instrumentation in total vertebrectomy eliminated the use of an anterior plate, thereby reducing the time required for reconstruction of the anterior column and eliminating surgical procedures in the segmental vascular structures. Furthermore, the prosthesis allowed for easy evaluation of bone formation within and around the implant plus early diagnosis of any local recurrence.[213]

To safely and efficiently monitor, diagnose, and stimulate tissue repair neural prosthesis for damaged brain or spinal cord, neural tissue repair requires an implanted electrode of small size and excellent electrical conductivity.[50] But, dense glial scar tissue formation on conventional metal silicon and metal alloy neural implants frequently occurs that reduces the efficiency of electrical stimulation and makes the probe useless during therapy. Nguyen-Vu and colleagues fabricated a vertically aligned carbon nanofiber (VACNF) electrode array coated with a thin film of electronic conductive polypyrrole polymers for neural implants.[214] The nanoelectrode array had more open and strong 3D structures with better electrical conductivity that helped to form an intimate neural–electrical interface between cells and nanofibers crucial for neural prosthesis. Two types of VACNF electrode arrays with high aspect ratios and tested on neuronal cell (rat phenochromocytoma, PC12 cells) differentiation showed that at discrete electrodes after long-term cell cultures, the CNF arrays were responsive for the detection of oxidized species generated by the cultured cells.[215] Initial studies suggested the potential of resident CNFs for electroanalytical studies of neuronal cells indicating potential superiority over conventional metal electrodes. Thus, CNFs can be used to design a neural probe with different conductivities at different parts of the probe by controlling CNF weight percentages in polymer composites.[50]

Transradial and transtibial prostheses can cost between US $6000 and $8000 while the transfemoral and transhumeral prosthetics cost between $10,000 and $15,000 and as high as $35,000. The cost of an artificial limb does recur because wear and tear require replacement every 3–4years. The socket must be replaced within several months if it has issues and height may be an issue as well (http://en.wikipedia.org/wiki/Prosthesis - cite_note-eight-36 and http://en.wikipedia.org/wiki/Prosthesis - cite_note-eight-36).

6.5 TISSUE ENGINEERING[127]

Conventionally, tissue engineering is the process where living cells and biomolecules are incorporated into a scaffold that is placed into a bioreactor.[42] In vitro growth in the bioreactor allows engineered tissues to mature before they are implanted. Ideally, cells grow and begin to form a tissue construct within the scaffold. When the tissue construct is implanted into the body, the scaffold continues to support further cell function, proliferation, and/or differentiation.[42] Furthermore, the scaffold allows blood vessels to infiltrate while it biodegrades. Thus, tissue engineering requires three components: (1) a source of the cells, (2) a suitable scaffold to engineer the specific type of tissue, and (3) a bioreactor that resembles the body environment.[42]

Tissue engineering can be approached in three ways.[42,190] First, freshly isolated or cultured cells are implanted to treat diseased or injured tissues. The cells can be manipulated before implantation to suit the needs of the patient. Implantation eliminates possible complications and morbidity associated with surgical procedures[42] but is limited by the cells being washed out from the site of injection and the inability of the implanted cells to maintain proper function. The second approach involves in situ tissue regeneration by implanting the scaffolds or injecting tissue-inducing substance at the injured site. In this approach, the tissue-inducing materials need to be purified and a selection of appropriate delivery methods needs to be applied (i.e. controlled delivery, soluble factors).[42] The last approach is in vitro implantation of functional tissues engineered from cells and scaffolds. For this approach to work out, the mechanical and biochemical properties of the scaffolds must be optimized as well as the cell ratio and density[42] because tissue engineering requires attention to the type of materials to allow a healthy growth of the cells for the tissue.

Tissue engineering is an area of medicine where biocompatible nanomaterials finds excellent applications. It is a multidisciplinary field that uses knowledge in chemistry, physics, engineering, life, and clinical sciences toward the development of solutions to critical medical problems such as tissue loss, organ damage, and organ failure.[127,190] It requires the understanding of structure and function relationships in tissues in order to carry out the development of biological substitutes that restore, maintain, or improve tissue function.[216] During in vitro engineering of living tissues, cultured cells are grown on bioactive degradable substrates called scaffolds that serve as guide as well as provide the physical and chemical cues to the cell differentiation and assembly into 3D structures. Healthy cellular growth, proliferation, and support for new tissue formation require specific physical, mechanical, and biological properties of the scaffolds. These required properties of biomaterials that can be achieved through fabrication technologies are very important in the design of the scaffolds to stimulate specific cell response at the molecular level. The scaffolds must elicit specific interactions with the cell to allow direct cell attachment, proliferation, differentiation, and ECM production and organization. Thus, the selection of appropriate biomaterials is the major factor for the success of tissue engineering.[217] For successful tissue regeneration, the scaffold must consist of biocompatible surfaces with appropriate mechanical properties that mimic the cells environment for healthy proliferation.

Scaffolds are artificial structures that support 3D tissue formation allowing cell attachment and migration and deliver and retain cells, and biochemical factors enable diffusion of vital cell nutrients and expressed products.[127] Scaffolds must possess sufficient porosity and pore connectivity to facilitate cell seeding and diffusion of cells and nutrients and increase the specific surface area available for cell attachment and tissue ingrowth for a uniform distribution of cells and the adequate transport of nutrients and cellular waste products.[218,13,219]

To date, although existing polymeric materials have been investigated for tissue engineering, there is no single biodegradable polymer that meets all the requirements for biomedical scaffolds. Thus, the design and preparation of multicomponent polymer systems is necessary in order to develop innovative multifunctional biomaterials. One of the newest ways to do this is to introduce nanostructures in biodegradable polymer matrices to obtain nanocomposites that have specific and improved properties that can be used in tissue engineering. The basic components of cells and tissues are at the nanoscale, and therefore, the knowledge of nanobiology and application of nanotechnology in tissue engineering (TE) may be the best approach in bringing the needed improvements.[220] Nanomaterials hold promise in the development of new systems that mimic the complex, hierarchical structure of the native tissue. The combination of nanotechnology, nanobiology, and molecular biology may be used to address some biomedical problems that may revolutionize the field of health care and medicine.[221] Just like nanotechnology which involves materials that possess at least one physical dimension in the nanometer range, many biological components, such as DNA and proteins, involve nanodimensionality making nanotechnology and nanomaterials of great interest for tissue engineering.

The success of bone tissue engineering for the development of viable substitutes that can restore and maintain the function of human bone tissues depends on the design of the scaffolds.[222] The materials for such scaffolds are polymer-based composite scaffolds containing micro- and nanostructures that could provide a platform influencing osteoblastic cell adhesion, spreading, proliferation, and differentiation. Due to large surface area, better osteointegrative property, and mechanical reliability, osteoblasts may adhere strongly to the nanostructures than microstructures. Other factors such as pore size, surface topography and roughness, protein adsorption and wettability of nanostructures, and their interaction with cell-surface integrin molecules are additional factors that may influence tissue engineering success. A better understanding of the interactions of nanostructures with osteoblastic cells are important to understand potential applications in the regeneration of bone. Recently, a variety of nanocomposites based on polyester and carbon nanostructures have been explored for potential use as scaffold materials.[127,223,224]

A few studies have been reported on the impact of NMs on TE. Iron oxide superparamagnetic nanoparticles and quantum dots have been used to track the biodistribution of cells.[225] Carbon nanomaterials, in particular, have the potential for multiple uses in tissue engineering[225] as well as polymer nanocomposites.[127] Polymer nanocomposites are the result of the combination of polymers and inorganic/organic fillers at the nanometer scale.[227,228] The enhanced mechanical and functional properties of the nanocomposites results from the interaction between the nanostructures and the polymer matrix. A continuous increase in studies for the improvement of nanocomposite material properties using nanosized engineered structures make use of the inherent high surface area to volume ratio of nanomaterials.[229] Nanocomposites show an excellent balance between strength and toughness with improved characteristics compared with their individual components.[230] For example, bone is a natural organic/inorganic composite material consisting of collagen and apatites[127] making composite materials excellent choices to make bone tissue engineering scaffolds.[231]

A multitude of current opportunities for polymer nanocomposites in the biomedical field arise from the diverse applications with different functional requirements[232] but the mechanical properties of available polymeric porous scaffolds offer insufficient stiffness and compressive strength compared with human bone. This leads to the use of inorganic/organic nanostructures as components of biodegradable polymers to increase and modulate mechanical, electrical, and degradation properties.[127] Since the interface adhesion between nanoparticles and polymer matrix is the major factor affecting the nanocomposite properties, it is important to consider the mechanical properties of nanocomposites that are controlled by several microstructural parameters such as the properties of the matrix, properties and distribution of the fillers, as well as interfacial bonding and by the synthesis/processing methods.[127,233,234] To promote improved dispersion of fillers that will enhance the interfacial adhesion between the matrix and the nanostructures, surface modification of nanostructures is necessary.[127,233,235]

Scaffolds for tissue engineering that are either synthetic or natural must be biocompatible and must have properties including optimal fluid transport, delivery of bioactive molecules, material degradation, cell-recognizable surface chemistries, mechanical integrity, and the ability to induce signal transduction.[43] These properties are important in the overall success of tissue organization and development since these can ultimately dictate cell adherence, nutrient/waste transport, matrix synthesis, matrix organization, and cell differentiation. The scaffolding materials should be chemically and physically modified to allow manipulation of critical parameters for tissue engineering applications.[236,44]

6.5.1 Current Polymer Matrices for Bionanocomposites

In tissue engineering, polymers are the primary scaffold fabrication materials using many types of biodegradable polymeric materials. These materials can be classified as: (1) natural-based materials, including polysaccharides (starch, alginate, chitin/chitosan, hyaluronic acid derivatives) or proteins (soy, collagen, fibrin gels, silk) and (2) synthetic polymers, such as PLA, poly(glycolic acid) (PGA), poly(3-caprolactone) (PCL), and poly(hydroxyl butyrate) (PHB).[127,236–238] Each of these groups of materials offers many advantages and disadvantages. Generally, synthetic polymers offer good mechanical strength with easily modifiable shape and degradation rate, but their surfaces are hydrophobic and lack cell recognition signals. On the other hand, naturally derived polymers have the advantage of biological recognition that support cell adhesion and function but they have poor mechanical properties and many are limited in supply and can be costly. Thus, synthetic biodegradable polymers, which can be produced in large scale under controlled conditions and with predictable and reproducible mechanical properties, degradation rate, and microstructure, are the most viable alternatives to the naturally occurring materials.

Both PGA, PLA, and their copolymer PLGA belong to a family of linear aliphatic polyesters, which are most frequently used in tissue engineering.[127,239,240] These have been shown as biocompatible materials that degrade into nontoxic components with a controllable degradation rate in vivo that have been FDA (US Food and Drug Administration) approved as degradable surgical sutures for clinical use.[127] Degradation of these polymers through hydrolysis of the ester bonds[241] leads to degradation products that are eventually eliminated from the body in the form of carbon dioxide and water. The rates of degradation can be tailored from several weeks to several years by modifying the chemical composition, crystallinity, molecular weight value, and distribution.[127] As a result of the hydrophilic nature of PGA, rapid degradation in aqueous solution or in vivo, and ability to lose mechanical integrity in 2–4 weeks, it is widely used as polymer for scaffold.[242,243] PGA in the form of nonwoven fibrous fabrics is one of the most widely used scaffolds in tissue engineering.[127]

Compared with PGA, the extra methyl group in the PLA repeating unit makes it more hydrophobic with less affinity to water that causes a slower rate of hydrolytic de-esterification into lactic acid. The morphology and crystallinity of PLA strongly influence the rate of biodegradation and mechanical properties[244–246] making the scaffolds degrade slowly both in vitro and in vivo. Such stability leads to mechanical integrity over several months.[247] Various lactic and glycolic acid ratios are used to synthesize PLGA to achieve intermediate degradation rates between PGA and PLA.[248–250] Currently, PLGA copolymers with different PGA/PLA ratio (50:50, 65:35,75:25, 85:15, 90:10) are applied in skin tissue regeneration and for suture applications.[251]

Among the few synthetic polymers, PLA, PGA, and PLGA are approved by the FDA for certain human clinical applications.[127] Other linear aliphatic polyesters that are also used for tissue engineering research include PCL[62,252] and PHB.[253] Because PCL degrades at a significantly slower rate than PLA, PGA, and PLGA,[254] it is less attractive for biomedical applications and more attractive for long term as implants as well as controlled release applications.

One good candidate for bone tissue engineering is PCL which showed sufficient mechanical properties to serve as scaffold in bone substitution that requires physical properties to be maintained for at least 6 months.[255–258] Scaffolds involved in a bone regeneration process can be enhanced by the addition of a carbonated apatite that is the main constituent of the inorganic phase of bone.[217,218,259]

6.5.2 Examples of Bionanocomposites

Different nanocomposites have been studied for tissue engineering applications. A few of these materials are discussed below.

6.5.2.1 HA Nanomaterials

One example of a bionanocomposite that has been widely used as a biocompatible ceramic material in many areas of medicine, particularly for contact with bone tissue owing to its resemblance to mineral bone is HA ($Ca_{10}(PO_4)_6$ $(OH)_2$))[260] which is the major mineral component(69% weight) of human hard tissues. HA in natural or synthetic form possesses excellent biocompatibility with bones, teeth, skin, and muscles, both in vitro and in vivo. It is biocompatible, promotes bone growth, and hardens in situ with Ca/P ratio at 1.5–1.67 that is within the range known to promote bone regeneration.[127] These properties of HA make it widely used for hard tissue repair in orthopedic surgery and dentistry.[13,10] Inorganic and organic composites mimic the composite nature of real bone that combines the toughness of the polymer phase with the compressive strength of the inorganic component to generate bioactive materials that has improved mechanical properties and degradation profiles.[127] In these composites, the alkalinity of the inorganic particle (such as HA) neutralizes acidic autocatalytic degradation of polymers such as PLA, exploiting a bioactive function.[261] To date, calcium phosphate biomaterials have been widely used in the form of powders, granules, dense porous blocks, and various composites.[127]

Studies showed that better osteoconductivity would be achieved if synthetic HA could resemble bone minerals in composition, size, and morphology.[262] Furthermore, nanosized HA may have other special properties due to its small size and huge specific surface area resulting in significant increase in protein adsorption and osteoblast adhesion on the nanosized ceramic materials compared with traditional microsized ceramic materials.[262,263] Studies have shown that n-HAP particles influenced the conformation of adsorbed vitronectin (a linear protein 15 nm in length that mediates osteoblast adhesion).[162,264] Polysaccharide and polypeptide matrices have been used with HA nanoparticles in hybrid composites[265] that are conducive to the attachment, growth, and proliferation of human osteoblast cells. For example, collagen-based polypeptidic gelatin is currently being used in wound dressings and pharmaceutical adhesives in clinics.[266] This can be combined with the bioactivity and osteoconductivity of HA to generate potential engineering biomaterials.

6.5.2.2 Carbon Nanostructures

Carbon nanostructures such as fullerenes, CNTs, CNFs, graphene, and a wide variety of related forms[267] are attractive nanomaterials for the development of innovative devices in the form of composites, sensors, and nanoscale electronic devices.[268,269] Polymers that incorporate carbon nanostructures have been studied for different of biomedical uses.[180,270,226,223] CNTs can provide the needed structural reinforcement for biomedical scaffolds.[127] Combining a small fraction of CNTs with a polymer provides significant improvements in the composite mechanical strength (owing to the CNTs mechanical strength) making them suitable candidates for novel polymer composites.[271,272] The physical properties and performance of polymer matrix in nanocomposites can be improved by adding small percentages of CNTs less than 1% weight.[273]

Transfer of the outstanding properties of carbon nanostructures from nano- to microscale involves assembling and processing with polymers that is hindered by their intrinsic poor solubility and processability.[127] This is solved by sidewall carboxylic functionalization to improve their dispersion in polymer matrix and their compatibility in biological fluids.[180] CNTs influenced the mineralization process that was also affected by the surface functionalization. The nanotubes supported osteoblast matrix deposition, allowed mineralization, cell differentiation, and bone-like tissue formation providing an effective nucleation surface that induced the formation of a biomimetic apatite coating.[127,274] Widespread attention has been focused on the use of CNTs with living entities and biomedical application.[275,276,277]

There has been extensive interest in applying the properties of CNTs to various biological applications[278] including their use to reinforce scaffolds for tissue engineering.[45] However, the toxicity and biocompatibility of CNT nanocomposites need to be thoroughly investigated.[279] In vitro studies have successfully grown different cell types on CNTs or CNT-based nanocomposites. In unmodified nanotubes, neurons extend only one or two neurites while neurons grown on nanotube coated with bioactive molecules lead to elaborate multiple neurites, which exhibited extensive branching that established the feasibility of using nanotubes as substrates for nerve cell growth and as probes of neuronal function at the nanometer scale.[280] Because CNTs are similar in shape and size to nerve cells, they could help to structurally and functionally reconnect injured neurons.[127] Hippocampal neurons grown on nanotubes displayed a sixfold increase in the frequency of spontaneous postsynaptic currents showing functional synapse formation.[281] These results showed the performance of CNTs as support devices for bridging and integrating functional neuronal networks in vitro without causing significant neural damage.[281] Honeycomb-like matrices of multiwalled CNTs were fabricated as potential scaffolds for tissue engineering.[282] These nanotube networks were used to culture mouse fibroblast cells that formed a confluent layer that did not exhibit cytotoxicity.

Although there have been a large number of researches on the potential biomedical applications of carbon nanostructures, information on toxicity and biocompatibility has only come up recently.[283] In order to exploit the potential clinical applications of CNTs, toxicological and pharmacological studies must continue in parallel to provide clear acceptable frameworks to regulatory authorities and the public that may suggest guidelines for the safe use of CNTs in medicine.[56]

6.5.2.3 Nanocomposite Films

In order for a scaffold to be considered for use as cell culture substrate, its properties must first be properly characterized and optimized. A variety of processing methodologies to create dense nanocomposite films have been studies.

These involved the incorporation of nanostructures with polymer through one of four ways.[127] Solvent casting involves dissolution of polymers inadequate solvent with nanoscale particles and evaporation of solvent or precipitation. In the melt-mixing process, the melted polymer is directly mixed with the nanoparticle. In situ polymerization is performed in the presence of the nanoparticles that are first dispersed in the liquid monomer or monomer solution. In template synthesis, the nanoparticles are synthesized from precursor solution using polymers as template.

In solvent casting, a solvent in which the polymer is soluble is used for flexible low-cost and short-term fabrication process of the polymeric nanocomposite film.[127] This is widely used for the fabrication process where the different solvents used represent a key point in the film production that needs to be elucidated. In this methodology, the choice of solvent influences the film properties, heterogeneity of the surface structure, reorientation or mobility of the surface crystal segment, swelling, and deformation.[284–286] The polymer solubility correlated with the surface structure of the nanocomposite film; however, more studies needs to focus on the specific properties of solvent (i.e. electron-pair donation, solvochromic parameter, hydrogen bond formation, and dielectric constant) that can support an effective dispersion of nanostructures in the solvent and in the resulting polymer matrix.

Composites made from HA particles and biodegradable polymers in various forms have been used clinically due to the good osteoconductivity and osteoinductivity of HA with the biodegradability of polymer matrix in the composites. In PLA/HA blending system, only physical adsorption is achieved between HA particles and the PLA matrix leading to poor mechanical properties that result in limited load-bearing applications. Thus, it appears that the interface adhesion of HA particles and polymer matrix plays a major factor affecting the properties of the PLA/HA composites. To increase the PLA/HA interfacial strength, various methods have been applied.[233,234,235,287] Improvements in the bonding between HA particles and poly(L-lactide) (PLLA) that increases the mechanical properties of the PLLA/HA composite were accomplished by using surface-grafted hydroxyapatite (g-HA) nanoparticles with the polymer that further blended with the PLLA.[288] This process produced uniform nanocomposites with improved tensile strength, bending strength, bending modulus, and impact energy at 4% particle by weight (compared with PLLA/HA composites). Improved cell compatibility of the PLLA/g-HA composites that is attributed to the good biocompatibility of the HA nanoparticles and a more uniform distribution of the g-HA nanoparticles on the film surface were demonstrated.[233–235,287,288]

Carbon nanostructures and biodegradable polymer-based nanocomposite films showed enhanced mechanical, thermal, and electrical properties. These were shown in nanocomposite based on PLLA and SWCNTs and carboxylated SWCNTs at 1% weight.[127,289] Different PLLA crystallites were formed and an interface polymer was organized around the nanotube sidewalls with good interfacial adhesion and a good homogeneous dispersion that can be leveraged to achieve the full potential of SWCNT reinforcing material.[271,290–292]

Silver nanoparticles have been extensively used in nanocomposite films to avoid attack from a broad spectrum of microorganisms and to reduce infections.[293] Silver nanoparticles evenly dissipated in biodegradable polymers would allow timed release of the silver species in a controlled manner allowing for antibacterial action over an extended period. There are recent reports on the use of silver nanoparticles as antimicrobials in PLGA matrix nanocomposites.[294,295] These studies indicated antibacterial effect of electrospun biodegradable fibers containing silver nanoparticles over more than 20 days.[296] Presence of dispersed metal nanoparticles enhanced the thermal conductivity of the nanocomposites that can speed up the degradation of the polymeric matrix.[297] Additionally, low concentrations of silver nanoparticles induced surface morphological changes in the polymer matrix that altered surface nanocomposite wettability and roughness which influenced bacterial adhesion on the nanocomposite surface.[298,299] The contact angle increases with >5% silver content that causes hydrophobic behavior that is associated with increase in surface roughness that is induced by the presence of silver nanoparticles. Various factors such as surface preparation, texture, chemical, and physical configuration that can influence biomaterial bacteria adherence affect the contact angle.[300,301]

6.6 CELL REPAIR

Cell repair involves manipulations of cell organelles and molecules that are similar to the same tasks that living systems already prove possible.[302] Cells are accessed by inserting needles without killing them or by using molecular machines.[303] Specific biochemical reactions show that molecular systems interact with other molecules as they come in contact, thereby building and rebuilding every molecule in a cell or expelling disassembled damaged molecules. Actively growing viable cells utilize built-in molecular systems to manufacture and assemble the various components of a cell. Following these built-in mechanisms to repair a cell, nanomachine-based systems that are able to enter cells, sense differences from healthy or sick ones, can be built to make modifications to restore sick cells into their healthy state. These nanomachines will have to be biocompatible and nonforeign to the cell or to the organism in order that these will not be sequestered before those are able to perform their designated task.

The applications of nanomachines for cell repair are enormous. Smaller than the sizes of the various cell organelles, nanomachines can be engineered and designed to carry out various functions inside a cell. They can be designed for specific functions or they can be modified for multiple functions. As they go in and out of the cell membranes, travel through tissue and organs, they can correct molecular damages, deliver specific chemicals, or augment and cure deficiencies. In order to be able to wade their way into the cells, tissues, and organs of interest, the nanomachines need nanocomputers for guidance. These nanocomputers will direct and detect the nanomachines as they examine, repair, rebuild, or disassemble damaged molecular structures inside the cells. The nanomachines will work on cells and move into tissues, organs, and finally the whole organism can be restored to good health.

6.6.1 Nanomachines for Delivery in Cells

To date, nanomaterials are in use as cell delivery vehicles either to facilitate the presentation of microenvironmental cues to aid in the process of tissue regeneration [42,43,127,220,228,232,235,239,248,259,277,282,287,292] or to physically deliver molecules that repair cells or kill harmful cells such as cancer cells.[20,85,87,90,93–98,101–103,106,304–310] A cell delivery vehicle can be engineered such that it is provided with proteins or genes that serve as cues that allow cascade of biochemical events to occur such as the release of cytokines and growth factors or apoptosis. The release of cytokine or growth factor can lead to the production of antibodies that can sequester damaging unnatural materials such as cancer proteins, virus, bacteria, or toxins. It can also lead to healing of cells in a wound at physiological levels for a sustained period of time.

Various biomaterials have been used for delivery in cells including viruses. Although viruses are highly efficient for transfection, they are recognized as foreign materials causing an inherent risk of immunogenicity and pathogenicity.[311] This prompted the development of nonviral alternatives including nanoparticulate DNA–polycation complexes and other polymers that facilitate the entry of DNA into the cell and its release therein that results in higher transfection efficiencies than the DNA alone.[312,313] The polycations are typically polymers such as PEI and chitosan, but functionalized CNTs have also been employed recently.[314]

A gene-activated matrix which consists of a matrix carrier that holds DNA until endogenous wound-healing cells arrive that invade the matrix.[315,316] The recruited host cells serve as bioreactors in order for the DNA to produce the proteins needed for tissue regeneration. Gene delivery vectors within the same matrix could transfect cells with appropriate growth factor so that these can be produced in a sustained manner. Schillinger et al. transfected chondrocytes cultured in clotted fibrin glue.[317] The optimized glue is based on the fibrinogen component of TISSUCOL, a fibrin glue that is widely used in clinics, colyophilized with copolymer-protected PEI-DNA vectors (COPROGs) was used to mediate growth factor gene delivery to admixed primary keratinocytes and primary chondrocytes before clotting. The chondrocyte colonized COPROG clots showed endocytotic vector uptake. Bone morphogenetic protein (BMP-2) gene transfection in situ and subsequent expression in chondrocytes grown in COPROG clots showed in vitro upregulation of alkaline phosphatase expression and increased ECM formation. COPROG–fibrinogen chondrocytes delivered to rabbit osteochondral defects led to reporter gene expression for 2weeks.[317]

The gene-activated matrix concept for cell repair has yielded some promising results and it is being further improved and refined.[317] Various combinations of matrix materials and gene vectors have been studied.[318,319] Attachment of protein ligands (e.g. transferrin) could increase endocytic uptake and, thus, the transfection efficiency of the polycation–DNA complexes.[320] The location of genes in nanostructures within a scaffold would provide spatial control of growth factors to guide the behavior of specific cell populations.[321] The incorporation of gene delivery vectors within structured delivery vehicles, such as fibrous scaffolds, would also allow for the spatial delivery of genes to cells seeded or recruited from the host.[322]

6.6.2 Nerve Cell Repair

Another area where nanomaterials can be very useful are in peripheral nerve injuries which are a major financial burden for the public.[323] The frequency of these injuries have increased steadily over the past few decades reaching several hundred thousand cases across the world.[324] Frequently, these injuries cause disability for life because there are no efficient therapeutic repair measures, especially in severe nerve damages. Usually, end-to-end suturing and autologous nerve grafting are the most common means of treatment[325] with unsatisfactory outcomes such as reduced stretching capacity of up to 24% with end-to-end sutured nerves.[326] Nerve gaps that are not amenable to suturing are repaired using autologous nerve grafting which is the current gold standard but it is associated with morbidity, loss of sensation, painful neuroma formation, and scarring at the donor site.[327] Initial success of substitute tissues for bridging small-sized nerve gaps are dampened by the observation that the foreign tissue grafts are unsuitable to support nerve regeneration over critical size nerve injuries because they lack the appropriate biochemical and topographical elements.[323]

The peripheral nerves link the brain and spinal cord to various parts of the body. A peripheral nerve injury refers to destruction, damage, or crushing of the peripheral nerve which is a serious health problem that affects 2.8% of trauma patients annually.[328] Peripheral neuropathy is a common disease that affects about 8% of the US population.[329,331] Peripheral nerves exhibit the capacity of self-regeneration for less severe injury but serious cases can potentially lead to lifelong disabilities. Various strategies for better recovery of nerve functions have been developed including end-to-end suturing which is one effective method for short nerve gaps whereas tubular structures are necessary for bridging longer gaps.[332,333] Many kinds of bioengineered nerve grafts have been developed from polymeric materials that have conducive properties and dimensions to meet the requirements for peripheral nerve regeneration. Such materials include naturally derived polymers to conventional nondegradable and biodegradable synthetic polymers that are noncytotoxic, highly permeable, and sufficiently flexible with appropriate degradation rate and degradation products that cater to regenerative axons that minimize swelling and inflammation.[333]

Chitosan is one of the natural polymers that is utilized for fabricating nerve conduits (NCs).[334,335] Other natural polymers include collagen,[336,337] hyaluronic acid (HyA),[338] gelatin,[339] and silk fibroin.[340] Because these are natural

TABLE 6.3 Polymers that are Used in the Fabrication of Nerve Conduits for Human Use

Polymer	Brand	Maker
Cross-linked collagen	NeuraGen®	Integra
	NeuroMatrix®/Neuroflex®	Stryker
Poly(glycolic acid)	Neurotube®	Synovis
Cross-linked poly(vinyl alcohol)[330] or Salubria® hydrogel	SaluBridge®	SaluMedica
	SaluTunnel®	SaluMedica
Poly(D,L-lactide-co-caprolactone)[304]	Neurolac®	Ascension

polymers, they are biocompatible and offer excellent support for cell attachment and functions, prevents serious immune response, supports appropriate signaling to cells without the need of growth factors, and most importantly, degrade by naturally occurring enzymes.[341,342] These natural polymers have disadvantages such as batch-to-batch variance, need extensive purification and characterization, and lack adequate mechanical strength and degrade relatively fast in vivo[341,343] requiring the need to be chemically modified and cross-linked or blended with synthetic polymers to meet the mechanical requirements.

Chitosan is a biodegradable polysaccharide obtained from N-deacetylation of chitin to form a copolymer of D-glucosamine and N-acetyl-D-glucosamine which can be extracted from the shells of crabs and shrimps.[341,343] It has been used for the fabrication of nerve tubes and scaffolds because of its excellent biocompatibility and antibacterial activity.[341–343] However, chitosan has a high glass transition temperature and low thermal stability, and pure chitosan cannot be melted; therefore, it has to be used in solutions. Wang et al.[344] dissolved chitosan in trifluoroacetic acid (TFA) and added methylene chloride (MC) to prepare a chitosan/TFA/MC solution that was electrospun onto a rotating steel use stainless (SUS) bar to form macro/nanofibrous scaffolds as the inner layer while chitosan–acetic acid solution is dip coated on the SUS bar to form the outer layer. This system was successfully used to immobilize laminin peptides. More complex NCs were achieved by molding through soft lithography from chitosan/acetic acid solution in polydimethylsiloxane molds.[334]

Collagen is another natural polymer that consists of groups of 28 proteins with the same triple helical structure as an extended rod that is stabilized by hydrogen bonding.[341,345] Both type I and III collagen can be derived from animal tissues such as porcine skin[336] and bovine deep flexor (Achilles) tendon.[346] It provides excellent biocompatibility and insignificant antigenic properties [341,343] and had been utilized to form outer tubular structures and central lumen for nerve regeneration.[345] The low mechanical properties of collagen are circumvented by cross-linking collagen between amine groups to create structural stability of fabricated NCs. Some of the cross-linking reagents for collagen are glutaraldehyde, formaldehyde, and 1-ethyl-3-(3-dimethylaminopropyl)-1-carbodiimide/N-hydroxysuccinimide (NHS).[345] An FDA-approved NC was made from cross-linked bovine collagen (type I) known as NeuraGen (Integra) tube.[336]

Gelatin is derived from collagen by thermal denaturation and chemical and physical degradation[345] into a simpler natural polymer. Gelatin is water soluble, biocompatible, and has excellent plasticity and adhesiveness[341,343] but is lacking in mechanical properties and handling characteristics. To circumvent these issues, proper cross-linking agents are used to improve the chemical and physical characteristics of gelatin to prevent toxicity and to fabricate suitable tubular structures for nerve regeneration.[341,343] The degree of cross-linking has been shown to be crucial in controlling the degradation rate in order to influence nerve regenerative responses because a too low cross-linking density results in more degradation products to evoke more severe foreign body reaction while a too high cross-linking density impedes the degradation and causes nerve compression with thickened perineurium and epineurium.[345,347]

To solve some of the issues with natural polymers that are used as biological grafts, NCs made of biomaterials are currently used as flexible alternative.[323] The biomaterials significantly influence attachment, proliferation, and migration of endogenously regenerating cells[348] making the selection and processing of the biomaterial critical.[349] A suitable biomaterial should possess good biocompatibility, appropriate degradation properties, and be amenable for controlling secondary NC properties such as pore size, porosity, mechanical strength, and biological functionalization.[323] Natural and synthetic polymers have been explored for the fabrication of NCs and some have been approved for use in human[349] and are given on Table 6.3.

Nevertheless, these existing artificial NCs have limited functional capacity to repair nerve gaps[351] sometimes resulting in complete failure of nerve regeneration. Improvements in the performance of NCs involve integration of neurotrophic factors, Schwann cells or stem cells, and luminal structures such as gels, multiple channels, or longitudinally aligned nanofibers.[323]

6.6.3 Stem Cells

One of the promising areas of research for curing various diseases especially cancer are stem cells. Stem cells are unspecialized cells that can divide through mitosis and can differentiate into various specialized cell types.[352] They are capable of replenishing themselves over and over again. Stem cells are found in all multicellular organisms and can self-renew to produce more stem cells. Under certain physiologic or experimental conditions, they can be induced to become tissue- or organ-specific cells with special functions. In some organs such as the gut and bone marrow, stem cells divide to repair and replace damaged tissues perpetually as long as the person or animal is still alive. Each new cell from a stem cell has the potential either to remain a stem cell or become another type of cell with a more specialized function, such as a muscle cell, a red blood cell, or a brain cell. In some other organs like the pancreas and the heart, stem cells only divide under special conditions.

Mammalian and humans have two known kinds of stem cells: embryonic stem cells and somatic or adult stem cells. These cells are important for living organisms for many reasons. In the 3- to 5-day-old embryo called blastocyst, the inner cells give rise to the organism and many of the specialized cell types and organs such as the heart, lung, skin, sperm, eggs, and other tissues. In some adult tissues including the bone marrow, brain, and muscle discrete populations of adult stem cells generate replacements for cells that are lost through normal wear and tear, disease, or injury.

Having unsurpassed regenerative abilities, stem cells are promising alternatives for treating diseases such as diabetes and heart disease. Studies of stem cells enable scientists to learn about the cells' essential properties making them different from specialized cell types. Stem cells are now in use in the laboratory for new drug screening and to develop model systems for the study of normal growth and to identify possible causes of birth defects. At the same time, stem cell research continues to advance knowledge about how an organism develops from a single cell and how healthy cells replace damaged cells in adult organisms.

Stem cells and progenitor cells act as a repair system for the body and replenish adult tissues. On the other hand, developing embryo consists of stem cells that can differentiate into all the specialized cells called pluripotent cells and at the same time maintain the normal turnover of regenerative organs such as blood, intestinal tissues, and skin. Stem cells are young cells that can differentiate into multiple cell types making them advantageous for cellular therapy[46] and are advantageous in that they can potentially be used for cellular therapies due to the fact that they can differentiate into multiple cell types[353] including cardiovascular cells.[354,355] Studies involving nanoparticles and stem cells have recently been published.[42,44,46] Previous work demonstrated that PEGylated fibrin gels[356] promote mesenchymal stem cell (MSC) tubulogenesis and differentiation toward a vascular cell type[355,46] which suggests that MSCs could be delivered to an injury site after an ischemic event that will assist in neovascularization and tissue repair.[357,358]

MSC migration were tracked in vivo using PEGylated fibrin gels to assess the role of MSCs in the process of neovascularization and tissue repair that can potentially lead to the development of better therapies and therapeutics involving MSCs, for tissue repair.[46] The gold nanoparticle-loaded MSCs demonstrated that nanoparticle loading decreased exponentially over time[46] which previous investigators have cited as dilution of nanoparticle concentration per cell as a result of cell proliferation and division.[359] In other studies, exocytosis of cells loaded with gold nanoparticles has been shown to be dependent on nanoparticle size and shape, cell type, and extracellular environment.[360,361] In summary, these studies demonstrate that decreased nanoparticle loading over time could be attributed to cell division or exocytosis of the nanoparticles by the cells. A better understanding of the process of neovascularization, and the extent to which MSCs participate in this process, can potentially lead to the development of better therapies and therapeutics, and specifically therapies involving MSCs, for cell and ultimately for tissue repair.

6.7 CONCLUSION

The applications of nanomaterials as components or as additives for various medical devices have led to improved biocompatibility and functionality as nanorobots, novel nanochips, and nanoimplants serving as tissue substitutes, tissue regeneration, prostheses, tissue engineering, and cell repair. Nanosurgery is expected to bring a revolutionary change in terms of neighboring tissue/cell damage during surgery. Nanorobots bring hope to early diagnosis and targeted drug delivery for early cancer treatment. Improvements in implants can reduce cost and provide ease of use to patients while minimizing swelling, toxicity, and other side effects. Many different kinds of nanomaterials are currently being developed for various nanochips, nanoimplants, and even for stem cell regeneration. These various applications of nanomedical devices hold promise for better diagnosis and improved therapeutics that ultimately benefit the quality of life for humans. Although majority of these applications of nanomaterials in medicine are still in the laboratory, a few are already in full blast clinical use. Many more prototypes and more research are necessary to harness the full potential of NMs as medical devices.

REFERENCES

1. Fritz, J.; Baller, M. K.; Lang, H. P.; Rothuizen, H.; Vettiger, P.; Meyer, E., et al. Translating Biomolecular Recognition into Nanomechanics. *Science* **2000,** *288,* 316–318.
2. Hill, C.; Amodeo, A.; Joseph, J. V.; Patel, H. R. H. Nano- and Microrobotics: How Far is the Reality?. *Expert. Rev. Anticancer. Ther.* **2008,** *8,* 1891–1897.
3. Martel, S. The Coming Invasion of the Medical Nanorobots. *Nanotechnol. Percept.* **2007,** *3,* 165–173.
4. Martel, S.; Mohammadi, M.; Felfoul, O., et al. Flagellated Magnetotactic Bacteria as Controlled MRI-Trackable Propulsion and Steering Systems for Medical Nanorobots Operating in the Human Microvasculature. *Int. J. Robot. Res.* **2009,** *28,* 571–582.
5. Robert, A. F. Nanotechnology, Nanomedicine, and Nanosurgery. *Int. J. Surg.* **2005,** *34,* 243–246.
6. Baker, J. R.; Quintana, A.; Piehler, L.; Banazak-Holl, M.; Tomalia, D.; Raczka, E. The Synthesis and Testing of Anti-Cancer Therapeutic Nanodevices. *Biomed. Microdevices* **2001,** *3,* 61–69.
7. Berna, J.; Leigh, D. A.; Lubomska, M.; Mendoza, S. M.; Perez, E. M.; Rudolf, P., et al. Macroscopic transport by synthetic molecular machines. *Nat. Mater.* **2005,** *4,* 704–710.

8. Hogg, T.; Freitas, R. A., Jr. Chemical Power for Microscopic Robots in Capillaries Nanomedicine: Nanotechnology. *Biol. Med.* **2010,** *6,* 298–317.

9. Khawaja, A. M. Review: The Legacy of Nanotechnology: Revolution and Prospects in Neurosurgery. *Int. J. Surg.* **2011,** *9,* 608–614.

10. Klein, C. P. A.T.; Driessen, A. A.; de Groot, K.; van den Hooff, A. Biodegradation Behaviour of Varoius Calcium Phosphate Materials in Bone Tissue. *J. Biomed. Mater. Res.* **2004,** *17,* 769–784.

11. LaVan, D. A.; McGuire, T.; Langer, R. Small-Scale Systems for in vivo Drug Delivery. *Nat. Biotechnol.* **2003,** *21,* 1184.

12. *Neurophilosophy.* Single-cell nanosurgery. 2007 Dec 26, 2011]. Available from: http://neurophilosophy.wordpress.com/2007/01/16/single-cell-nanosurgery/

13. Rezwan, K.; Chen, Q. Z.; Blaker, J. J.; Boccaccini, A. R. Biodegradable and Bioactive Porous Polymer/Inorganic Composite Scaffolds for Bone Tissue Engineering. *Biomaterials* **2006,** *27.*

14. Saini, R.; Saini, S. Nanotechnology and Surgical Neurology. *Surg. Neurol. Int.* **2010,** *1,* 57.

15. Santos, S.; Mathew, M. Real Time Imaging of Femtosecond Laser Induced Nano-Neurosurgery Dynamics in C. elegans. *Opt. Express* **2010,** *18,* 364–377.

16. Shen, N.; Datta, D.; Schaffer, C. B.; LeDuc, P.; Ingber, D. E.; Mazur, E. Ablation of Cytoskeletal Filaments and Mitochondria in Cells using a Femtosecond Laser Nanoscissor. *Mech. Chem. of Biosyst.* **2005,** *2,* 17–26.

17. Tanner, K. E.; Boudreau, A.; Bissell, M. J.; Kumar, S. Dissecting Regional Variations in Stress Fiber Mechanics in Living Cells with Laser Surgery. *Biophys. J.* **2010,** *99,* 2775–2783.

18. Yanik, M. F.; Cinar, H.; Cinar, H. N.; Chisolm, A. D.; Jin, Y.; Ben-Yakar, A. Neurosurgery: Functional Regeneration after Laser Axotomy. *Nature* **2004,** *432,* 822.

19. Andrianantoandro, E.; Basu, S.; Karig, D. K.; Weiss, R. Synthetic Biology: New Engineering Rules for an Emerging Discipline. *Mol. Syst. Biol.* **2006,** *2,* E1–E14, msb4100073.

20. Barreiro, A.; Rurali, R.; Harnandez, E. R.; Moser, J.; Pichler, T.; Forro, L., et al. Subnanometer Motion of Cargos Driven by Thermal Gradients Along Carbon Nanotubes. *Science* **2008,** *320,* 775–778.

21. Benenson, Y.; Gil, B.; Ben-Dor, U.; Adar, R.; Shapiro, E. An Autonomous Molecular Computer for Logical Control of Gene Expression. *Nature* **2004,** *429,* 423–429.

22. Ferber, D. Microbes made to Order. *Science* **2004,** *303*(5655), 158–161.

23. Freitas, R. A. Pharmacytes: An Ideal Vehicle for Targeted Drug Delivery. *J. Nanosci. Nanotechnol.* **2006,** *6.*

24. Kufer, S. K.; Puchner, E. M.; Gumpp, H.; Liedl, T.; Gaub, H. E. Single-Molecule Cut-and-Paste Surface Assembly. *Science* **2008,** *319,* 594–596.

25. Marden, J. H.; Allen, L. R. Molecules, Muscles, and Machines: Universal Performance Characteristics of Motors. *PNAS* **2002,** *99,* 4161–4166.

26. Martel, S.; Felfoul, O.; Mohammadi, M. Flagellated Bacterial Nanorobots for Medical Interventions in the Human Body. 2nd IEEE, **2008,** p. 264–269.

27. Morris, K. Macrodoctor, Come meet the Nanodoctors. *Lancet* **2001,** *357,* 778.

28. Akagawa, Y.; Hashimoto, M.; Kondo, N.; Satomi, K.; Takata, T.; Tsuru, H. Initial Bone-Implant Interfaces of Submergible and Supramergibleendosseous Single-Crystal Sapphire Implants. *J. Prosthet. Dent.* **1986,** *55,* 96–100.

29. Akagawa, Y.; Hosokawa, R.; Sato, Y.; Kamayama, K. Comparison between Freestanding and Tooth-Connected Partially Stabilized Zirconia Implants after Two Years' Function in Monkeys: A Clinical and Histologic Study. *J. Prosthet. Dent.* **1998,** *80,* 551–558.

30. Arias, J. L.; Mayor, M. B.; Pou, J.; Leng, Y.; Leon, B.; Perez-Amor, M. Micro- and Nano-Testing of Calcium Phosphate Coatings Produced by Pulsed Laser Deposition. *Biomaterials* **2003,** *24,* 3403–3408.

31. Att, W.; Kurun, S.; Gerds, T.; Strub, J. R. Fracture Resistance of Single-Tooth Implant-Supported All-Ceramic Restorations: An In Vitro Study. *J. Prosthet. Dent.* **2006,** *95,* 111–116.

32. Ben-Nissan, B.; Choi, A. H. Sol-Gel Production of Bioactive Nanocoatings for Medical Applications. Part 1: An Introduction. *Nanomedicine* **2006,** *1,* 311–319.

33. Berglundh, T.; Abrahamsson, I.; Albouy, J. P.; Lindhe, J. Bone Healing at Implants with a Fluoride-Modified Surface: An Experimental Study in Dogs. *Clin. Oral. Implants Res.* **2007,** *18,* 147–152.

34. Carinci, F.; Pezzetti, F.; Volinia, S.; Francioso, F.; Arcelli, D.; Farina, E.; Piattelli, A. Zirconium Oxide: Analysis of MG63 Osteoblast-Like Cell Response by means of a Microarray Technology. *Biomaterials* **2004,** *25,* 215–228.

35. Cheng, L.; Zhang, S. M.; Chen, P. P. Fabrication and Characterization of Nano-Hydroxyapatite/Poly (d, l-lactide) Composite Porous Scaffolds for Human Cartilage Tissue Engineering. *Bioceramics* **2006,** *18,* 943–946.

36. Cochran, D.; Oates, T.; Morton, D.; Jones, A.; Buser, D.; Peters, F. Clinical Field Trial Examining an Implant with a Sand-Blasted, Acid-Etched Surface. *J. Periodontol.* **2007,** *78,* 974–982.

37. Khang, D.; McKenzie, J. L.; Webster, T. J. Carbon nanofibers:polycarbonate urethane composites as a neural biomaterial, IEEE 30th Annual Northeast Proceedings, April 17–18, **2004,** IN, USA, 241–242.

38. Kohal, R. J.; Weng, D.; Bachle, M.; Strub, J. R. Loaded Custom-Made Zirconia and Titanium Implants show Similar Osseointegration: An Animal Experiment. *J. Periodontol.* **2004,** *75,* 1262–1268.

39. Lee, S. H.; Kim, H. W.; Lee, E. J.; Li, L. H.; Kim, H. E. Hydroxyapatite-TiO$_2$ hybrid coating on Ti implants. *J. Biomater. Appl.* **2006,** *20,* 195–208.

40. Stadlinger, B.; Hennig, M.; Eckelt, U.; Kuhlisch, E.; Mai, R. Comparison of Zirconia and Titanium Implants after a Short Healing Period. A Pilot Study in Minipigs. *Int. J. Oral Maxillofac. Surg.* **2010,** *39,* 585–592.

41. Stanford, C. M.; Johnson, G. K.; Fakhry, A.; Gratton, D.; Mellonig, J. T.; Wanger, W. Outcomes of a Fluoride Modified Implants One Year after Loading in the Posterior-Maxilla when Placed with the Osteotome Surgical Technique. *Appl. Osseointegration Res.* **2006,** *5,* 50–55.

42. Chiu, L. L. Y.; Chu, Z.; Radisic, M. Tissue Engineering. *Compr. Nanosci. Tech.* **2010,** *2,* 175–211.

43. Dawson, E.; Mapili, G.; Ericson, K.; Taqvi, S.; Roy, K. Biomaterials for Stem Cell Differentiation. *Adv. Drug Deliv. Revi.* **2008,** *60,* 215–228, http://www.sciencedirect.com/science/journal/0169409X.

44. Drury, J. L.; Mooney, D. J. Hydrogels for Tissue Engineering: Scaffold Design Variables and Applications. *Biomaterials* **2003,** *24,* 4337–4351.

45. Jan, E.; Kotov, N. A. Successful Differentiation of Mouse Neural Stem Cells on Layer-by-Layer Assembled Single-Walled Carbon Nanotube Composite. *Nano Lett.* **2007,** *7,* 1123–1128.

46. Ricles, L. M.; Nam, S. Y.; Sokolov, K.; Emelianov, S. Y.; Suggs, L. J. Function of Mesenchymal Stem Cells Following Loading of Gold Nanotracers. *Int. J. Nanomed.* **2011,** *6,* 407–416.

47. Slotkin, J. R.; Chakrabarti, L.; Dai, H. N.; Carney, R. S.; Hirata, T.; Bregman, B. S.; Gallicano, G. I.; Corbin, J. G.; Haydar, T. F. In Vivo Quantum Dot Labeling of Mammalian Stem and Progenitor Cells. *Dev. Dyn.* **2007,** *236,* 3393–3401.

48. Quintana, A.; Raczka, E.; Piehler, L.; Lee, I.; Myc, A.; Majoros, I., et al. Design and Function of a Dendrimer-based Therapeutic Cells through the Folate Receptor. *Pharm. Res.* **2000,** *19,* 1310–1360.

49. Topoglidis, E. A.; Cass, E., et al. Protein Adsorption on Nanocrystalline TiO2 Films: An Immobilization Strategy for Bioanalytical Devices. *Anal. Chem.* **1998,** *70,* 5111–5113.

50. Tran, P. A.; Zhang, L.; Webster, T. J. Carbon Nanofibers and Carbon Nanotubes in Regenerative Medicine. *Adv. Drug. Deliv. Rev.* **2009,** *61,* 1097–1114.

51. Vaseashta, A.; Dimova-Malinovska, D. Nanostructured and Nanoscale Devices, Sensors and Detectors. *Sci. Technol. Adv. Mat.* **2005,** *6,* 312–318.

52. Andreiotelli, M.; Wenz, H. J.; Kohal, R. J. Are Ceramic Implants a Viable Alternative to Titanium Implants? A systematic literature review. *Clin. Oral. Implants Res.* **2009,** *20,* 32–47.

53. Blagosklonny, M. V. Analysis of FDA Approved Anticancer Drugs Reveals the Future of Cancer Therapy. *Cell Cycle* **2004,** *3,* 1035–1042.

54. Fritzsche, W.; Taton, T. A. Metal Nanoparticles as Labels for Heterogeneous, Chip-based DNA Detection. *Nanotechnology* **2003,** *14,* R63–R73.

55. Haun, J. B.; Yoon, T.; Lee, H. J.; Weissleder, R. Magnetic Nanoparticle Biosensors. *Wiley Interdisciplinary Reviews: Nanomed. Nanobiotechnol.* **2010,** *2,* 291–304.

56. Lacerda, L.; Soundararajan, A.; Singh, R.; Pastorin, G.; Al-Jamal, K. T.; Turton, J., et al. Dynamic Imaging of Functionalized Multi-Walled Carbon Nanotube Systemic Circulation and Urinary Excretion. *Adv. Mater.* **2008,** *20,* 225–230.

57. Lee, H.; Yoon, T.; Figueiredo, J.; Swirski, F. K.; Weissleder, R. Rapid Detection and Profiling of Cancer Cells in Fine-Needle Aspirates. *PNAS* **2009,** *106,* 12459–12464.

58. Lee, T. M. H.; Cai, H.; Hsing, I. M. Effects of Gold Nanoparticle and Electrode Surface Properties on Electrocatalytic Silver Deposition for Electrochemical DNA Hybridization Detection. *Analyst* **2005,** *130,* 364–369.

59. Merkoci, A. Nanoparticles-Based Strategies for DNA, Protein and Cell Sensors. *Biosens. Bioelectron.* **2010,** *26,* 1164–1177.

60. Runge, V. M. *Contrast Agents Safety Profile.* 2008 June 18, 2012. Available from: http://www.clinical-mri.com/pdf/Contrast%20Agents/Contrast%20Agents%20-%20Safety%20Profile%20amended%20table.pdf.

61. Kehoe, S.; Zhang, X. F.; Boyd, D. FDA Approved Guidance Conduits and Wraps for Peripheral Nerve Injury: A Review of Materials and Efficacy. *Injury* **2012,** *43*(5), 553–572.

62. Lepoittevin, B.; Devolkenaere, M.; Alexandre, M.; Pantoustier, N.; Calberg, C.; Jerome, R.; Dubois, P. Poly(e-caprolactone)/clay Nanocomposites Prepared by Melt Intercalation: Mechanical, Thermal and Rheological Properties. *Polymer* **2002,** *43,* 4017–4023.

63. Couvreur, P.; Vauthier, C. Nanotechnology: Intelligent Design to Treat Complex Disease. *Pharm. Res.* **2006,** *23,* 1417–1450.

64. Ben-Yakar, A.; Bourgeois, F. Ultrafast Laser Nanosurgery in Microfluidics for Genome-Wide Screenings. *Curr. Opin. Biotechnol.* **2009,** *20,* 1–6.

65. Vogel, A.; Noack, J.; Huttmann, G.; Paltauf, G. Mechanism of Femtosecond Laser Nanosurgery of Cells and Tissues. *Biophys. J.* **2005,** *90,* 3762–3773.

66. Han, S. W.; Nakamura, C.; Obataya, I.; Nakamura, N.; MIyake, J. A Molecular Delivery System by using AFM and Nanoneedle. *Biosens. Bioelectron.* **2005,** *20,* 2120–2125.

67. Kirson, E. D.; Yaari, Y. A Novel Technique for Micro-Dissection of Neuronal Processes. *J. Neurosci. Methods* **2000,** *98,* 119–122.

68. Kohli, V.; Elezzabi, A. Y.; Acker, J. P. Cell Nanosurgery using Ultrashort (Femtosecond) Laser Pulses: Applications to Membrane Surgery and Cell Isolation. *Lasers. Surg. Med.* **2005,** *37,* 227–230.

69. Sacconi, L.; Tolic-Norrelykke, I. M.; Antolini, R.; Pavone, F. S. Combined Intracellular Three-Dimensional Imaging and Selective Nanosurgery by a Nonlinear Microscope. *J. Biomed. Opt.* **2005,** *10,* 14002.

70. Tirlapur, U. K.; Konig, K. Femtosecond Near-Infrared Laser Pulses as a Versatile Non-Invasive Tool for Intra-Tissue Nanoprocessing in Plants without Compromising Viability. *Plant. J.* **2002,** *31,* 365–374.

71. Konig, R.; Rieman, I.; Fischer, P.; Halbhuber, K. J. Intracellular Nanosurgery with Near Infrared Femtosecond Laser Pulses. *Cell. Mol. Biol.* **1999,** *45,* 195–201.

72. Firtel, M.; Henderson, G.; Sokolov, I. Nanosurgery: Observation of Peptidoglycan Strands in Lactobacillus Helveticus Cell Walls. *Ultramicroscopy* **2004,** *101,* 105–109.

73. Ishiyama, K.; Sendoh, M.; Arai, K. I. Magnetic Micromachined for Medical Applications. *Biomed. Mater. Eng.* **2002,** *15,* 367–374.

74. Mathieu, J. B.; Martel, S.; Yahia, L.; Soulez, G.; Beaudoin, G. Preliminary Investigation of the Feasibility of Magnetic Propulsion for Future Microdevices in Blood Vessels. *Biomed. Mater. Eng.* **2002,** *15,* 367–374.

75. Martel, S.; Mathieu, J. B.; Felfoul, O.; Chanu, A.; Aboussouan, E.; Tamaz, S., et al. Automatic Navigation of an Untethered Device in the Artery of a Living Animal Using a Conventional Clinical Magnetic Resonance Imaging System. *Appl. Phys. Lett.* **2007,** *114105,* 90.

76. Yesin, K. B.; Exner, P.; Vollmers, K.; Nelson, B. J. Design and control of in-vivo magnetic microrobots, Duncan, J. S.; Gerig, G., Eds.; Proceedings of the 8th international conference on medical image computing and computer-assisted intervention (MICCAI 2005). Springer: Berlin, Germany, 2005, 819–826.

77. NIH. *National Institutes of Health Roadmap: Nanomedicine.* Available from: http://nihroadmap. nih.gov/nanomedicine/index.asp. Accessed on May 27, 2012.

78. Thomas, T. P.; Shukla, R.; Majoros, I. J.; Myc, A.; Baker, R. J. Polyamidoamine dendrimer-based multifunctional nanoparticles. In *Nanobiotechnology II: More concepts and applications*; Mirkin, C. A.; Niemeyer, C. M., Eds.; Wiley-VCH Press: Hoboken, NJ, 2007, Chapter 16.

79. Monroe, D. Micromedicine to the Rescue. *Commun. ACM* **2009,** *52,* 13–15.

80. Koo, O. M.; Rubinstein, I.; Onyuksel, H. Role of Nanotechnology in Targeted Drug Delivery and Imaging: A Concise Review. *Nanomedicine* **2005,** *1,* 193–212.

81. Vo Dinh, T.; Kasili, P.; Wabuyele, M. Nanoprobes and Nanobiosensors for Monitoring and Imaging Individual Living Cells. *Nanomedicine* **2006,** *2,* 22–30.

82. Aguilar, Z.; Aguilar, Y.; Xu, H.; Jones, B.; Dixon, J.; Xu, H.; Wang, A. Nanomaterials in Medicine. *Electrochem. Soc. Trans.* **2010,** *33,* 69–74.

83. Sekhon, B.; Kamboj, S. Inorganic Nanomedicine: Part 1. *Nanomed. Nanotechnol. Biol. Med.* **2010,** *6,* 516–522.

84. Park, J. -H.; von Maltzahn, G.; Zhang, L.; Derfus, A. M.; Simberg, D.; Harris, T. J.; Ruoslahti, E.; Bhatia, S. N.; Sailor, M. J. Systematic Surface Engineering of Magnetic Nanoworms for In vivo Tumor Targeting. *Small* **2009,** *5,* 694–700.

85. Akerman, M. E.; Chan, W. C.; Laakkonen, P.; Bhatia, S. N.; Ruoslahti, E. Nanocrystal Targeting In Vivo. *PNAS USA* **2002,** *99,* 12617–12621.

86. Yang, L.; Peng, X.; Wang, Y.; Wang, X.; Cao, Z.; Ni, C.; Karna, P.; Zhang, X.; Wood, W.; Gao, X.; Nie, S.; Mao, H. Receptor-Targeted Nanoparticles for In Vivo Imaging of Breast Cancer. *Clin. Cancer. Res.* **2009,** *15,* 4722–4732.

87. Das, S.; Jagan, L.; Isiah, R.; Rajech, B.; Backianathan, S.; Subhashini, J. Nanotechnology in Oncology: Characterization and *In Vitro* Release Kinetics of Cisplatin-Loaded Albumin Nanoparticles: Implications in Anticancer Drug Delivery. *Indian J. Pharmacol.* **2011,** *43,* 409–413.

88. Yang, S.; Zhu, J.; Lu, Y.; Liang, B.; Yang, C. Body Distribution of Camptothecin Solid Lipid Nanoparticles after Oral Administration. *Pharm. Res.* **1999**, *16*, 751–757.

89. Morgen, M.; Lu, G. W.; Dub, D.; Stehle, R.; Lembke, F.; Cervantes, J.; Ciotti, S.; Haskell, R.; Smithey, D.; Haley, K.; Fan, C. Targeted Delivery of a Poorly Water-Soluble Compound to Hair Follicles using Polymeric Nanoparticle Suspensions. *Int. J. Pharm.* **2011**, *416*(1), 314–322.

90. Allen, T. M.; Mumbengegwi, D. R.; Charrois, G. J. Anti-CD19-Targeted Liposomal Doxorubicin Improves the Therapeutic Efficacy in Murine B-Cell Lymphoma and Ameliorates the Toxicity of Liposomes with Varying Drug Release Rates. *Clin. Cancer Res.* **2005**, *11*, 3567–3573.

91. Chauhan, A.; Sridevi, S.; Chalasani, K.; Jain, A.; Jain, S.; Jain, N.; Diwan, P. Dendrimer-Mediated Transdermal Delivery: Enhanced Bioavailability of Indomethacin. *J. Control Release* **2003**, *90*, 335.

92. Chen, X.; Schluesener, H. J. Nanosilver: A Nanoproduct in Medical Application. *Toxicol. Lett.* **2008**, *176*, 1–12.

93. Labhasetwar, V. Nanotechnology for Drug and Gene Therapy: The Importance of Understanding Molecular Mechanisms of Delivery. *Curr. Opin. Biotechnol.* **2005**, *16*, 674–680.

94. Tiwari, S. B.; Amiji, M. M. A Review of Nanocarrier-Based CNS Delivery Systems. *Curr. Drug. Deliv.* **2006**, *3*, 219–232.

95. Liversidge, G. Controlled Release and Nanotechnologies: Recent Advances and Future Opportunities. *Drug Dev. and Deliv.* **2011**, *11*, 1.

96. Panagiotou, T.; Fisher, R. J. Enhanced Transport Capabilities via Nanotechnologies: Impacting Bioefficacy, Controlled Release Strategies, and Novel Chaperones. *J. Drug. Deliv.* **2011**, 1–14.

97. Singh, R.; James, W.; Lillard, J. Nanoparticle-Based Targeted Drug Delivery. *Exp. Mol. Pathol* **2009**, *86*, 215–223.

98. Yang, L.; Cao, Z.; Sajja, H.; Mao, H.; Wang, L.; Geng, H.; Xu, H.; Jiang, T.; Wood, W.; Nie, S.; Wang, A. Development of Receptor Targeted Iron Oxide Nanoparticles for Efficient Drug Delivery and Tumor Imaging. *J. Biomed. Nanotech.* **2008**, *4*, 1–11.

99. Tomalia, D.; Reyna, L.; Svenson, S. Dendrimers as Multi-Purpose Nanodevices for Oncology Drug Delivery and Diagnostic Imaging. *Biochem. Soc. Trans.* **2007**, *35*, 61.

100. Zhang, J. A.; Anyarambhatla, G.; Ma, L.; Ugwu, S.; Xuan, T.; Sardone, T.; Ahmad, I. Development and Characterization of a Novel Cremophor® EL Free Liposome-Based Paclitaxel (LEP-ETU) Formulation. *Eur. J. Pharm. Biopharm.* **2005**, *59*, 177–187.

101. Brigger, I.; Dubernet, C.; Couvreur, P. Nanoparticles in Cancer Therapy and Diagnosis. *Adv. Drug Deliv. Rev.* **2002**, *54*, 631–651.

102. Medina, O. P.; Pillarsettya, N.; Glekasa, A.; Punzalan, B.; Longo, V.; Gonen, M.; Zanzonico, P.; Smith-Jones, P.; Larson, S. M. Optimizing Tumor Targeting of the Lipophilic EGFR-Binding Radiotracer SKI 243 using a Liposomal Nanoparticle Delivery System. *J. Control Release* **2011**, *149*, 292–298.

103. Ruenraroengsak, P.; Cook, J. M.; Florence, A. T. Nanosystem Drug Targeting: Facing up to Complex Realities. *J. Control Release* **2010**, *141*, 265–276.

104. Kateb, B.; Chiu, K.; Black, K.; Yamamoto, V.; Khalsa, B.; Ljubimova, J.; Ding, H.; Patil, R.; Portilla-Arias, J.; Modo, M.; Moore, D.; Farahani, K.; Okun, M.; Prakash, N.; Neman, J.; Ahdoot, D.; Grundfest, W.; Nikzad, S.; Heiss, J. Nanoplatforms for Constructing New Approaches to Cancer Treatment, Imaging, and Drug Delivery: What Should be the Policy? *NeuroImage* **2011**, *54*, S106–S124.

105. Koo, O.; Rubinstein, I.; Onyuksel, H. Camptothecin in Sterically Stabilized Phospholipid Micelles: A Novel Nanomedicine. *Nanomedicine* **2005**, *1*, 77–84.
106. Patil, Y. B.; Swaminathan, S. K.; Sadhukha, T.; Panyam, J. The Use of Nanoparticle-Mediated Gene Silencing and Drug Delivery to Overcome Tumor Drug Resistance. *Biomaterials* **2010**, *31*, 358–365.
107. Hessler, T.; Mecke, A.; Banaszak-Holl, M.; Orr, B. G.; Uppuluri, S.; Tomalia, D. A., et al. Tapping Mode Atomic Force Microscopy Investigation of poly(Amidoamine) Core-Shell Tecto(Dendrimers) using Carbon Nanoprobes. *Langmuir* **2002**, *18*, 3127–3133.
108. Freitas, R. A. Pharmacytes: An Ideal Vehicle for Targeted Drug Delivery. *J. Nanosci. Nanotechnol.* **2006**, *6*, 2769–2775.
109. Wang, S. Y.; Williams, R. S., Eds.; *Nanoelectronics*, Springer: New York, 2005.
110. Sajja, H.; East, M.; Mao, H.; Wang, Y.; Nie, S.; Yang, L. Development of Multifunctional Nanoparticles for Targeted Drug Delivery and Noninvasive Imaging of Therapeutic Effect. *Curr. Drug Discov. Technol.* **2009**, *6*, 43–51.
111. Pusic, K.; Xu, H.; Stridiron, A.; Aguilar, Z.; Wang, A. Z.; Hui, H. Blood Stage Merozoite Surface Protein Conjugated to Nanoparticles Induce Potent Parasite Inhibitory Antibodies. *Vaccine* **2011**, *29*, 8898–8908.
112. Liu, H.; Webster, T. J. Review: Nanomedicine for implants: A Review of Studies and Necessary Experimental Tools, Cellular and Molecular Biology Techniques for Biomaterials Evaluation. *Biomaterials* **2007**, *28*, 354–369.
113. Lopes, M. A.; Saramago, B.; Santos, J. D.; Monteiro, F. J. Hydrophobicity, Surface Tension, and Zeta Potential of Glass Reinforced Hydroxyapatite Composites. *J. Biomed. Mater. Res.* **1999**, *45*, 370–375.
114. Vidal, G.; Delord, B.; Neri, W.; Gounel, S.; Roubeau, O.; Bartholome, C.; Ly, I.; Poulin, P.; Labrugere, C.; Sellier, E.; Durrieu, M. -C.; Amedee, J.; Salvetat, J. -P. The Effect of Surface Energy, Adsorbed RGD Peptides and Fibronectin on the Attachment and Spreading of Cells on Multiwalled Carbon Nanotube Papers. *Carbon* **2011**, *49*, 2318–2333.
115. Evans, E. A.; Calderwood, D. A. Forces and Bond Dynamics in Cell Adhesion. *Science*, 316, 1148–1153
116. Bruinsma, R.; Behrisch, A.; Sackmann, E. Adhesive Switching of Membranes: Experiment and Theory. *Phys. Rev. E* **2000**, *61*, 4253–4267.
117. Liu, X.; Lim, J. Y.; Donahue, H. J.; Dhurjati, R.; Mastro, A. M.; Vogler, E. A. Influence of Substratum Surface Chemistry/Energy and Topography on the Human Fetal Osteoblastic Cell Line hFOB 1.19: Phenotypic and Genotypic Responses Observed In Vitro. *Biomaterials* **2007**, *28*, 4535–4550.
118. Discher, D. E.; Janmey, P.; Wang, Y. L. Tissue Cells Feel and Respond to the Stiffness of their Substrate. *Science* **2005**, *310*, 1139–1143.
119. Underwood, P. A.; Bennet, t. F. A. A Comparison of the Biological Activities of the Cell-Adhesive Proteins Vitronectin and Fibronectin. *J. Cell. Sci.* **1989**, *93*, 641–649.
120. Curtis, A. S.; Forrester, J. V.; McInnes, C.; Lawrie, F. Adhesion of Cells to Polystyrene Surfaces. *J. Cell. Biol.* **1983**, *97*, 1500–1506.
121. Rho, J. Y.; Kuhn-Spearing, L.; Zioupos, P. Mechanical Properties and the Hierarchical Structure of Bone. *Med. Eng. Phys.* **1998**, *20*, 92–102.
122. Laschke, M. W.; Strohe, A.; Menger, M. D.; Alini, M.; Eglin, D. In Vitro and In Vivo Evaluation of a Novel Nanosize Hydroxyapatite Particles/Poly(Ester-Urethane) Composite Scaffold for Bone Tissue Engineering. *Acta. Biomater.* **2010**, *6*, 2020–2027.
123. Kennedy, I. M.; Wilson, D.; Barakat, A. I. Uptake and Inflammatory Effects of Nanoparticles in a Human Vascular Endothelial Cell Line. *Res. Rep. Health Eff. Inst.* **2009**, *136*, 3–21.

124. Park, E. J.; Yoon, J.; Choi, K.; Yi, J.; Park, K. Induction of Chronic Inflammation in Mice Treated with Titanium Dioxide Nanoparticles by Intratracheal Instillation. *Toxicology* **2009,** *260,* 37–46.

125. Wagner, E. M.; Sanchez, J.; McClintock, J. Y.; Jenkins, J.; Moldobaeva, A. Inflammation and Ischemia-Induced Lung Angiogenesis. *Am. J. Physiol. Lung Cell Mol. Physiol.* **2008,** *294,* L351–L357.

126. Boissard, C. I.; Bourban, P. E.; Tami, A. E.; Alini, M.; Eglin, D. Nanohydroxyapatite/Poly-(Ester-Urethane) Scaffold for Bone Tissue Engineering. *Acta. Biomater.* **2009,** *5,* 3316–3327.

127. Armentano, I.; Dottori, M.; Fortunati, E.; Mattioli, S.; Kenny, J. M. Biodegradable Polymer Matrix Nanocomposites for Tissue Engineering: A Review. *Polym. Degrad. Stab.* **2010,** *95,* 2126–2146.

128. Nejati, E.; Mirzadeh, H.; Zandi, M. Synthesis and Characterization of Nanohydroxyapatite Rods/Poly(L-Lactide Acid) Composite Scaffolds for Bone Tissue Engineering. *Compos. Part A* **2008,** *39,* 1589–1596.

129. Wie, G.; Ma, P. X. Structure and Properties of Nano-Hydroxyapatite/Polymer Composite Scaffolds for Bone Tissue Engineering. *Biomaterials* **2004,** *25,* 4749–4757.

130. Smith, I. O.; Liu, X. H.; Smith, L. A.; Ma, P. X. Nanostructured Polymer Scaffold for Tissue Engineering and Regenerative Medicine. *Interdiscip. Rev. Nanomed. Nanobiotechnol.* **2009,** *1,* 226–236.

131. Shuai, C.; Gao, C.; Nie, Y.; Hu, H.; Zhou, Y.; Peng, S. Structure and Properties of Nano-Hydroxypatite Scaffolds for Bone Tissue Engineering with a Selective Laser Sintering System. *Nanotechnology* **2011,** *22,* 285703.

132. Behneke, A.; Behneke, N.; D'hoedt, B. A 5-year Longitudinal Study of the Clinical Effectiveness of ITI Solid-Screw Implants in the Treatment of Mandibular Edentulism. *Int. J. Oral. Maxillofac. Implants* **2002,** *17,* 799–810.

133. Webster, T. J.; Siegel, R. W.; Bizios, R. Osteoblast Adhesion on Nanophase Ceramics. *Biomaterials* **1999,** *20,* 1221–1227.

134. Webster, T. J.; Ergun, C.; Doremus, R. H. Enhanced Functions of Osteoblasts on Nanophase Ceramics. *Biomaterials* **2000,** *21,* 1803–1810.

135. Gutwein, L. G.; Tepper, F.; Webster, T. J. Increased viable osteoblast cell density in the presence of nanophase compared to conventional alumina and titania particles. *Biomaterials* **2004,** *25,* 4175–4183.

136. Albrektsson, T.; Wennerberg, A. Oral Implant Surfaces: Part 1-Review Focusing on Topographic and Chemical Properties of Different Surfaces and In Vivo Responses to Them. *Int. J. Prosthodont.* **2004,** *7,* 536–543.

137. Liu, H.; Slamovich, E. B.; Webster, T. J. Increased Osteoblast Functions among Nanophase Titania/Poly(lactide-co-glycolide) Composites of the Highest Nanometer Surface Roughness. *J. Biomed. Mater. Res.* **2006,** *78,* 798–807.

138. Medonca, G.; Medonca, D. B. S.; Aragao, F. J. L.; Cooper, L. F. Review: Advancing Dental Implant Surface Technology - From Micron- to Nanotopography. *Biomaterials* **2008,** *29,* 3822–3835.

139. Webster, T. J.; Ejiofor, J. U. Increased Osteoblast Adhesion on Nanophase Metals: Ti, Ti_6Al_4V, and CoCrMo. *Biomaterials* **2004,** *25,* 4731–4739.

140. Scotchford, C. A.; Gilmore, C. P.; Cooper, E.; Leggett, G. J.; Downes, S. Protein Adsorption and Human Osteoblast-Like Cell Attachment and Growth on Alkylthiol on Gold Self-Assembled Monolayers. *J. Biomed. Mater. Res.* **2002,** *59,* 84–99.

141. Germanier, Y.; Tosatti, S.; Broggini, N.; Textor, M.; Buser, D. Enhanced Bone Apposition Around Biofunctionalized Sandblasted and Acid-Etched Titanium Implants Surfaces. A histomorphometric study in Miniature pigs. *Clin. Oral. Implants Res.* **2006,** *17,* 251–257.

142. Zhou, J.; Chang, C.; Zang, R.; Zhnag, L. Hydrogels Prepared from Unsubstituted Cellulose in NaOH/urea Aqueous Solution. *Macromol. Biosci.* **2007,** *7,* 804–809.

143. Kim, H. M.; Kokubo, T.; Fujibayashi, S.; Nishiguchi, S.; Nakamura, T. Bioactive Macroporous Titanium Surface Layer on Titanium Substrate. *Biomed. Mater. Res.* **2000,** *5,* 553–337.

144. Wang, X. X.; Hayakawa, S.; Tsuru, K.; Osaka, A. A Comparative Study of In Vitro Apatite Deposition on Heat-, H(2)O(2)-, and NaOH-Treated Titanium Surfaces. *J. Biomed. Mater. Res.* **2001,** *54,* 172–178.

145. Uchida, M.; Kim, H. M.; Miyaji, F.; Kokubo, T.; Nakamura, T. Apatite Formation on Zirconium Metal Treated with Aqueous NaOH. *Biomaterials* **2002,** *23,* 313–317.

146. Wang, X. X.; Hayakawa, S.; Tsuru, K.; Osaka, A. Bioactive Titania-Gel Layers formed by Chemical Treatment of Ti Substrate with a H_2O_2/HCl Solution. *Biomaterials* **2002,** *23,* 1353–1357.

147. Mante, F. K.; Little, K.; Mante, M. O.; Rawle, C.; Baran, G. R. Oxidation of Titanium, RGD Peptide Attachment, and Matrix Mineralization Rat Bone Marrow Stromal Cells. *J. Oral. Implantol.* **2004,** *30,* 343–349.

148. Ellingsen, J. E.; Thomsen, P.; Lyngstadaas, S. P. Advances in Dental Implants Materials and Tissue Regeneration. *Periodontology* **2004,** *41,* 136–156.

149. Isa, Z. M.; Schneider, G. B.; Zaharias, R.; Seabold, D.; Stanford, C. M. Effects of Fluoride Modified Titanium Surfaces on Osteoblast Proliferation and Gene Expression. *Int. J. Oral. Maxillofac. Implants* **2006,** *21,* 203–211.

150. Guo, J.; Padilla, R. J.; Ambrose, W.; DeKok, I. J.; Cooper, L. F. Modification of TiO_2 Grit Blasted Titanium Implants by Hydrofluoric Acid Treatment Alters Adherent Osteoblast Gene Expression In Vitro and In Vivo. *Biomaterials* **2007,** *28,* 5418–5425.

151. Ellingsen, J. E.; Johansson, C. B.; Wennerberg, A.; Holmen, A. Improved Retention and Bone-to-Implants Contact with Fluoride-Modified Titanium Implants. *Int. J. Oral. Implants* **2004,** *19,* 659–666.

152. Liu, D. M.; Troczynski, T.; Tseng, w. J. Water-based Sol-Gel Synthesis of Hydroxyapatite: Process Development. *Biomaterials* **2001,** *22,* 1721–1730.

153. Kim, H. W.; Koh, Y. H.; Li, L. H.; Lee, S.; Kim, H. E. Hydroxyapatite Coating on Titanium Substrate with Titania Buffer Layer Processed by Sol-Gel Method. *Biomaterials* **2004,** *25,* 2533–2538.

154. Piveteau, L. D.; Gasser, B.; Schlapbach, L. Evaluating Mechanical Adhesion of Sol-Gel Titanium Dioxide Coatings Containing Calcium Phosphate for Metal Implant Application. *Biomaterials* **2000,** *21,* 2193–2201.

155. Choi, A. H.; Ben-Nissan, B. Sol-gel Production of Bioactive Nanocoatings for Medical Applications. Part II: Current Research and Development. *Nanomedicine* **2007,** *2,* 51–61.

156. Nishimura, I.; Huang, Y.; Butz, F.; Ogawa, T.; Li, L.; Jake Wang, C. Discrete Deposition of Hydroxyapatite Nanoparticles on a Titanium Implant with Predisposing Substrate Microtopography Accelerated Osseointegration. *Nanotechnology* **2007,** *18,* 25101, (25109pp).

157. Ueno, T.; Tsukimura, N.; Yamada, M.; Ogawa, T. Enhanced Bone-Integration Capability of Alkali- and Heat-Treated Nanopolymorphic Titanium in Micro-to-Nanoscale Hierarchy. *Biomaterials* **2011,** *32,* 7297–7308.

158. Smith, G. C.; Chamberlain, L.; Faxius, L.; Johnston, G. W.; Jin, S.; Bjursten, L. M. Soft Tissue Response to Titanium Dioxide Nanotube Modified Implants. *Acta. Biomater.* **2011,** *7,* 3209–3215.

159. Dion, I.; Rouais, F.; Baquey, C.; Lahaye, M.; Salmon, R.; Trut, L.; Cazorla, J. P.; Huong, P. V.; Monties, J. R.; Havlik, P. Physico-Chemistry and Cytotoxicity of Ceramics. Part I. Characterization of Ceramic Powders. *J. Mater. Sci. Mater. Med.* **1997,** *8,* 325–332.

160. Christel, P.; Meunier, A.; Heller, M.; Torre, J. P.; Peille, C. N. Mechanical Properties and Short-Term In-Vivo Evaluation of Yttrium-Oxide-Partially-Stabilized Zirconia. *J. Biomed. Mater. Res.* **1989**, *23*, 45–61.

161. Piconi, C.; Burger, W.; Richter, H. G.; Cittadini, A.; Maccauro, G.; Covacci, V.; Bruzzese, N.; Ricci, G. A.; Marmo, E. Y-TZP Ceramics for Artificial Joint Replacements. *Biomaterials* **1998**, *19*, 1489–1494.

162. Webster, T. J.; Schadler, L. S.; Siegel, R. W.; Bizios, R. Mechanisms of Enhanced Osteoblast Adhesionon Nanophase Alumina Involve Vitronectin. *Tissue Eng.* **2001**, *7*, 291–301.

163. Webster, T. J.; Ergun, C.; Doremus, R. H.; Siegel, R. W.; Bizios, R. Specific Proteins Mediate Enhanced Osteoblast Adhesion on Nanophase Ceramics. *J. Biomed. Mater. Res.* **2000**, *51*, 475–483.

164. Webster, T. J.; Ergun, C. D.; Siegel, R. W.; Bizios, R. Enhanced Functions of Osteoclast-Like Cells on Nanophase Ceramics. *Biomaterials* **2001**, *22*, 1327–1333.

165. Li, P. Biomimetic Nano-Apatite Coating Capable of Promoting Bone in Growth. *J. Biomed. Mater. Res.* **2003**, *66*, 79–85.

166. Thapa, A.; Webster, T. J.; Haberstroh, K. M. Polymers with Nano-Dimensional Surface Features Enhance Bladder Smooth Muscle Cell Adhesion. *J. Biomed. Mater. Res.* **2003**, *67A*, 1374–1383.

167. Schift, H.; Heyderman, L. J.; Padeste, C.; Gobrecht, J. Chemical Nano-Patterning Using Hot Embossing Lithography. *Microelectron. Eng.* **2002**, *61-62*, 423–428.

168. Palin, E.; Liu, H.; Webster, T. J. Mimicking the Nanofeatures of Bone Increases Bone-Forming Cell Adhesion and Proliferation. *Nanotechnology* **2005**, *16*, 1828–1835.

169. Thapa, A.; Miller, D. C.; Webster, T. J.; Haberstroh, K. M. Nano-Structured Polymers Enhance Smooth Muscle Cell Function. *Biomaterials* **2003**, *24*, 2915–2926.

170. Athanasiou, A.; Niederauer, G. G.; agrawal, C. M. Sterilization, Toxicity, Biocompatibility and Clinical Applications of Polylactic Acid/Polyglycolic Acid Copolymers. *Biomaterials* **1996**, *17*, 93–102.

171. Qian, D.; Dickey, E. C.; Andrews, R.; Rantell, T. Load Transfer and Deformation Mechanisms in Carbon Nanotube-Polystyrene Composites. *Appl. Phys. Lett.* **2000**, *76*, 2868–2870.

172. Erik, T. T.; Tsu-Wei, C. Aligned Multi-Walled Carbon Nanotube-Reinforced Composites: Processing and Mechanical Characterization. *J. Phys. D. Appl. Phys.* **2002**, *35*, L77.

173. Cadek, M.; Coleman, J. N.; Barron, V.; Hedicke, K.; Blau, W. J. Morphological and Mechanical Properties of Carbon-Nanotube-Reinforced Semicrystalline and Amorphous Polymer Composites. *Appl. Phys. Lett.* **2002**, *81*, 5123–5125.

174. Balani, K.; Anderson, R.; Laha, T.; Andara, M.; Tercero, J.; Crumpler, E.; Agarwal, A. Plasma-Sprayed Carbon Nanotube Reinforced Hydroxyapatite Coatings and their Interaction with Human Osteoblasts In Vitro. *Biomaterials* **2007**, *28*, 618–624.

175. Iijima, S.; Brabec, C.; Maiti, A.; Bernholc, J. Structural flexibility of Carbon Nanotubes. *J. Chem. Phys.* **1996**, *104*, 2089–2092.

176. Treacy, M. M. J.; Ebbesen, T. W.; Gibson, J. M. Exceptionally High Young's Modulus Observed for Individual Carbon Nanotubes. *Nature* **1996**, *381*, 678–680.

177. Price, R. L.; Waid, M. C.; Haberstroh, K. M.; Webster, T. J. Selective Bone Cell Adhesion on Formulations Containing Carbon Nanofibers. *Biomaterials* **2003**, *24*, 1877–1887.

178. Zhao, B.; Hu, H.; Mandall, S. K.; Haddon, R. C. A Bone Mimic based on the Self-Assembly of Hydroxyapatite on Chemically Functionalized Single-Walled Carbon Nanotubes. *Chem. Mater.* **2005**, *17*, 3235–3241.

179. Zanello, L. P.; Zhao, B.; Hu, H.; Haddon, R. C. Bone Cell Proliferation on Carbon Nanotubes. *Nano. Lett.* **2006**, *6*, 562–567.

180. Shi, X.; Hudson, J. L.; Spicer, P. P.; Tour, J. M.; Krishnamoorti, R.; Mikos, A. G. Injectable Nanocomposites of Single-Walled Carbon Nanotubes and Biodegradable Polymers for Bone Tissue Engineering. *Biomacromolecules* **2006,** *7,* 2237–2242.

181. Khang, D.; Kim, S. Y.; Liu-Snyder, P.; Palmore, G. T. R.; Durbin, S. M.; Webster, T. J. Enhanced fibronectin Adsorption on Carbon Nanotube/Poly(Carbonate) Urethane: Independent Role of Surface Nano-Roughness and Associated Surface Energy. *Biomaterials* **2007,** *28,* 4756–4768.

182. Khang, D.; Lu, J.; Yao, C.; Haberstroh, K. M.; Webster, T. J. The role of Nanometer and Sub-Micron Surface Features on Vascular and Bone Cell Adhesion on Titanium. *Biomaterials* **2008,** *29,* 970–983.

183. Hallab, N. J.; Bundy, K. J.; O'Connor, K.; Moses, R. L.; Jacobs, J. J. Evaluation of Metallic and Polymeric Biomaterial Surface Energy and Surface Roughness Characteristics for Directed Cell Adhesion. *Tissue Eng.* **2001,** *7,* 55–71.

184. Price, R. L.; Waid, M. C.; Haberstroh, K. M.; Webster, T. J. Selective Bone Cell Adhesion on Formulations Containing Carbon Nanofibers. *Biomaterials* **2003,** *24,* 1877–1887.

185. Cales, B.; Stefani, Y. Mechanical Properties and Surface Analysis of Retrieved Zirconia Hip Joint Heads after an Implantation Time of Two to Three Years. *J. Mater. Sci. Mater. Med.* **1994,** *5,* 376–380.

186. Kohal, R. J.; Papavasiliou, G.; Kamposiora, P.; Tripodakis, A.; Strub, J. R. Three-Dimensional Computerized Stress Analysis of Commercially Pure Titanium and Yttrium-Partially Stabilized Zirconia Implants. *Int. J. Prosthodont.* **2002,** *15,* 189–194.

187. Lacefield, W. R. Materials Characteristics of Uncoated/Ceramic-Coated Implant Materials. *Adv. Dent. Res.* **1999,** *13,* 21–26.

188. Akagawa, Y.; Ichikawa, Y.; Nikai, H.; Tsuru, H. Interface Histology of Unloaded and Early Loaded Partially Stabilized Zirconia Endosseous Implant in Initial Bone Healing. *J. Prosthet. Dent.* **1993,** *69,* 599–604.

189. Tamai, N.; Myoui, A.; Hirao, M. A New Biotechnology for Articular Cartilage Repair: Subchondral Implantation of a Composite of Interconnected Porous Hydroxyapatite, Synthetic Polymer (PLA-PEG), and Bone Morphogenetic Protein-2 (rhBMP-2). *Osteoarthritis Cartilage* **2005,** *13,* 405–417.

190. Langer, R.; Vacanti, J. P. Tissue Engineering. *Science* **1993,** *260,* 9220–9926.

191. Wang, P.; Hu, J.; Ma, P. X. The Engineering of Patient-Specific, Anatomically Shaped, Digits. *Biomaterials* **2009,** *30,* 2735–2740.

192. Liu, X.; Jin, X.; Ma, P. X. Nanofibrous Hollow Microspheres Self-Assembled from Star-Shaped Polymers as Injectable Cell Carriers for Knee Repair. *Nat. Mater.* **2011,** *10,* 398–406.

193. Elisseeff, J.; Anseth, K.; Sims, D.; McIntosh, W.; Randolph, M.; Langer, R. Transdermal Photopolymerization for Minimally Invasive Implantation. *PNAS* **1999,** *96,* 3104–3107.

194. Kloxin, A. M.; Kasko, A. M.; Salinas, C. N.; Anseth, K. S. Photodegradable Hydrogels for Dynamic Tuning of Physical and Chemical Properties. *Science* **2009,** *324,* 59–63.

195. Rice, M. A.; Waters, K. R.; Anseth, K. S. Ultrasound Monitoring of Cartilaginous Matrix Evolution in Degradable PEG Hydrogels. *Acta. Biomater.* **2009,** *5,* 152–161.

196. Wang, D. A.; Varghese, S.; Sharma, B.; Strehin, I.; Fermanian, S.; Gorham, J.; Fairbrother, D. H.; Cascio, B.; Elisseeff, J. H. Multifunctional Chondroitin Sulphate for Cartilage Tissue-Biomaterial Integration. *Nat. Mater.* **2007,** *6,* 385–392.

197. Benoit, D. S.; Schwartz, M. P.; Durney, A. R.; Anseth, K. S. Small Functional Groups for Controlled Differentiation of Hydrogel-Encapsulated Human Mesenchymal Stem Cells. *Nat. Mater.* **2008,** *7,* 816–823.

198. Strehin, I.; Nahas, Z.; Arora, K.; Nguyen, T.; Elisseeff, J. A Versatile pH Sensitive Chondroitin Sulfate-PEG Tissue Adhesive and Hydrogel. *Biomaterials* **2010,** *31,* 2788–2797.

199. Li, W. J.; Cooper, J. A. J.; Mauck, R. L.; Tuan, R. S. Fabrication and Characterization of Six Electrospun Poly(alpha-hydroxy ester)-based Fibrous Scaffolds for Tissue Engineering Applications. *Acta. Biomater.* **2006,** *2,* 377–385.

200. Thorvaldsson, A.; Stenhamre, H.; Gatenholm, P.; Walkenstrom, P. Electrospinning of Highly Porous Scaffolds for Cartilage Regeneration. *Biomacromolecules* **2008,** *9,* 1044–1049.

201. Li, W. J.; Danielson, K. G.; Alexander, P. G.; Tuan, R. S. Biological Response of Chondrocytes Cultured in Three-Dimensional Nanofibrous Poly(epsilon-caprolactone) Scaffolds. *J. Biomed. Mater. Res. A* **2003,** *67,* 1105–1114.

202. Ma, Z.; Kotaki, M.; Inai, R.; Ramakrishna, S. Potential of Nanofiber Matrix as Tissue-Engineering Scaffolds. *Tissue Eng.* **2005,** *11,* 101–109.

203. Yao, C.; Slamovich, E. B.; Webster, T. J. Improved bone cell adhesion on nanophase titanium and Ti6Al4V. In *American Ceramic Society Conference Proceedings*, 2005, January 23–28, Cocoa Beach, FL.

204. Miller, D. C.; Thapa, A.; Haberstroh, K. M.; Webster, T. J. Endothelial and Vascular Smooth Muscle Cell Function on Poly(lactic-co-glycolic acid) with Nano Structured Surface Features. *Biomaterials* **2004,** *25,* 53–61.

205. Choudhary, S.; Haberstroh, K. M.; Webster, T. J. Greater Endothelial Cell Responses to Nanophase Metals. *Int. J. Nanomed.* **2006,** *1,* 37–47.

206. Zhao, L.; He, C.; Zhang, D. M.; Chang, J.; Cui, L. Comparison of Electrospun PBSU and PLGA Scaffolds Applied in Vascular Tissue Engineering. *J. Biomim. Biomater. Tissue Eng.* **2009,** *2,* 27–38.

207. Pattison, M. A.; Wurster, S.; Webster, T. J.; Haberstroh, K. M. Three-Dimensional, Nano-Structured PLGA Scaffolds for Bladder Tissue Replacement Applications. *Biomaterials* **2005,** *26*(15), 2491–2500.

208. Webster, T. J.; Waid, M. C.; McKenzie, J. L.; Price, R. L.; Ejiofor, J. U. Nano-Biotechnology: Carbon Nanofibres as Improved Neural and Orthopaedic Implants. *Nanotechnology* **2004,** *15,* 48.

209. Seil, J. T.; Webster, T. J. Electrically Active Nanomaterials as Improved Neural Tissue Regeneration Scaffolds. *Wiley Interdiscip. Nanomed Rev. Nanobiotechnol Rev.* **2010,** *2,* 635–647.

210. Johnson, C. *Getting an Artificial Leg up.* 2000 June 13, 2012. Available from: http://www.abc. net.au/science/slab/leg/default.htm.

211. Smith, G. C.; Plettenburg, D. H. Efficiency of Voluntary Closing Hand and Hook Prostheses. *Prosthet. Orthot. Int.* **2010,** *34,* 411–427.

212. Tang, S. F. T.; Chen, C. P. C.; Chen, M. J. L.; Chen, W. P.; Leong, C. P.; Chu, N. K. Transmetatarsal Amputation Prosthesis with Carbon-Fiber Plate: Enhanced Gait Function. *Am. J. Phys. Med. Rehabil.* **2004,** *83,* 124–130.

213. Boriani, S.; Bandiera, S.; Biagini, R.; De Iure, F.; Giunti, A. The use of the Carbon-Fiber Reinforced Modular Implant for the Reconstruction of the Anterior Column of the Spine. A Clinical and Experimental Study Conducted on 42 Cases. *Chir. Organic. Mov.* **2000,** *85,* 309–335.

214. Nguyen-Vu, T. D. B.; Chen, H.; Cassell, A. M.; Andrews, R.; Meyyappan, M.; Li, J. Vertically Aligned Carbon Nanofiber Arrays: An Advance Towards Electrial-Neural Interfaces. *Small* **2006,** *2,* 89–94.

215. McKnight, T. E.; Melechko, A. V.; Fletcher, B. I.; Jones, S. W.; Hensley, D. K.; Peckys, D. B.; Griffin, G. D.; Simpson, M. I.; Ericson, M. N. Resident Neuroelectrochemical Interfacing using Carbon Nanofiber Arrays. *J. Phys. Chem. B* **2006,** *110,* 15317–15327.

216. Shalak, R.; Fox, C. F., Eds.; *Tissue Engineering*, Liss, New York, 1988.

217. Jagur-Grodzinski, J. Polymers for Tissue Engineering, Medical Devices, and Regenerative Medicine. Concise General Review of Recent Studies. *Polymer. Adv. Technol.* **2006,** *17,* 395–418.

218. Ma, P. X. Scaffold for Tissue Engineering. *Mater. Today* **2004,** *7,* 30–40.

219. Guarino, V.; Ambrosio, L. The Synergic Effect of Polylactide Fiber and Calcium Phosphate Particle Reinforcement in poly e-caprolactone-based Composite Scaffolds. *Acta. Biomater.* **2008,** *4,* 1778–1787.

220. Christenson, E.; Anseth, K. S.; van den Beucken Jeroen, J. J. P.; Chan, C. K.; Ercan, B.; Jansen, J. A., et al. Nanobiomaterial Applications in Orthopedics. *J. Orthop. Res.* **2007,** *25,* 11–22.

221. Gleiter, H. Nanostructured Materials, Basic Concepts and Microstructure. *Acta. Mater.* **2000,** *48,* 1–12.

222. Saranya, N.; Saravanan, S.; Moorthi, A.; Ramyakrishna, B.; Selvamurugan, N. Enhanced Osteoblast Adhesion on Polymeric Nano-Scaffolds for Bone Tissue Engineering. *J. Biomed. Nanotech.* **2011,** *7,* 238–244.

223. Armentano, I.; Dottori, M.; Puglia, D.; Kenny, J. M. Effects of Carbon Nanotubes (CNTs) on the Processing and In-Vitro Degradation of Poly(DL-lactide-coglycolide)/CNT Films. *J. Mater. Sci. Mater. Med.* **2008,** *19,* 2377–2387.

224. Armentano, I.; Del Gaudio, C.; Bianco, A.; Dottori, M.; Nanni, F.; Fortunati, E., et al. Processing and Properties of Poly(e-caprolactone)/Carbon Nanofibre Composite Mats and Films Obtained by Electrospinning and Solvent Casting. *J. Mater. Sci.* **2009,** *44,* 4789–4795.

225. Bulte, J. W.; Douglas, T.; Witwer, B.; Zhang, S. C.; Strable, E.; Lewis, B. K., et al. Magneto-dendrimers Allow Endosomal Magnetic Labeling and In Vivo Tracking of Stem Cells. *Nat. Biotechnol.* **2001,** *19,* 1141–1147.

226. Harrison, B. S.; Atala, A. Review, Carbon Nanotube Applications for Tissue Engineering. *Biomaterials* **2007,** *28,* 344–353.

227. Gorrasi, G.; Vittoria, V.; Murariu, M.; Ferreira, A. D. S.; Alexandre, M.; Dubois, P. Effect of Filler Content and Size on Transport Properties of Water Vapor in PLA/ Calcium Sulfate Composites. *Compos. Sci. Technol.* **2008,** *9,* 627–632.

228. Peponi, L.; Tercjak, A.; Torre, L.; Mondragon, I.; Kenny, J. M. Nanostructured Physical Gel of SBS Block Copolymer and Ag/DT/SBS Nanocomposites. *J. Mater. Sci.* **2009,** *44,* 1287–1293.

229. Oiao, R.; Robinson, L. C. Simulation of Intherphase Percolation and Gradients in Polymer Nanocomposites. *Compos. Sci. Technol.* **2009,** *69,* 491–499.

230. Tiong, S. C. Structural and Mechanical Properties of Polymer Nanocomposites. *Mater. Sci. Eng.* **2006,** *53,* 73–97.

231. Murugan, R.; Ramakrishna, S. Development of Nanocomposites for Bone Grafting. *Compos. Sci. Technol.* **2005,** *65,* 2385–2406.

232. Hule, R. A.; Pochan, D. J. Polymer Nanocomposites for Biomedical Applications. *MRS Bull.* **2007,** *32,* 354–358.

233. Li, J.; Lu, X. L.; Zheng, Y. F. Effect of Surface Modified Hydroxyapatite on the Tensile Property Improvement of HA/PLA Composite. *Appl. Surf. Sci.* **2008,** *255,* 494–497.

234. Borum-Nicholas, L.; Wilson, J. O. C. Surface Modification of Hydroxyapatite. Part I. Dodecyl Alcohol. *Biomaterials* **2003,** *24,* 367–369.

235. Hong, Z. K.; Qui, X. Y.; Sun, J. R.; Deng, M. X.; Chen, X. S.; Jing, X. B. Grafting Polymerization of L-Lactide on the Surface of Hydroxyapatite Nano-Crystal. *Polymer* **2004,** *45,* 6705–6713.

236. Shin, H.; Jo, S.; Mikos, A. G. Biomimetic Materials for Tissue Engineering. *Biomaterials* **2003,** *24,* 4353–4364.

237. Wen, X.; Tresco, P. A. Fabrication and Characterization of Permeable Degradable Poly(DL-lactide-co-glycolide) (PLGA) Hollow Fiber Phase Inversion Membranes for Use as Nerve Tract Guidance Channels. *Biomaterials* **2006,** *27,* 3800–38009.

238. Koegler, W. S.; Griffith, L. G. Osteoblast Response to PLGA Tissue Engineering Scaffolds with PEO Modified Surface Chemistries and Demonstration of Patterned Cell Response. *Biomaterials* **2004**, *25*, 2819–2830.

239. Bolland, B. J.; Kanczler, J. M.; Ginty, P. J.; Howdle, S. M.; Shakessheff, K. M.; Dunlop, D. G.; Oreffo, R. O. C. The Application of Human Bone Marrow Stromal Cells and Poly(dl-lactic acid) as a Biological Bone Graft Extender in Impaction Bone Grafting. *Biomaterials* **2008**, *29*, 3221–3227.

240. Zhang, R.; Ma, P. X., Eds.; *Processing of Polymer Scaffolds: Phase Separation*; Academic Press: San Diego, 2001.

241. Lin, A. S. P.; Barrows, T. H.; Cartmell, S. H.; Guldberg, R. E. Microarchitectural and Mechanical Characterization of Oriented Porous Polymer Scaffolds. *Biomaterials* **2003**, *24*, 481–489.

242. Li, S. Hydrolytic Degradation Characteristics of Aliphatic Polyesters Derived from Lactic and Glycolic Acids. *J. Biomed. Mater. Res. Part B Appl. Biomater.* **1999**, *48*, 342–353.

243. Ma, P. X.; Langer, R., Eds.; *Degradation, Structure and Properties of Fibrous Poly(glycolic acid) Scaffolds for Tissue Engineering*; Materials Research Society: Penssylvania, 1995.

244. Kuo, Y. C.; Leou, S. N. Effects of Composition, Solvent, and Salt Particles on the Physicochemical Properties of Polyglycolide/Poly(lactide-co-glycolide) Scaffolds. *Biotechnol. Prog.* **2006**, *22*, 1664–1670.

245. Sarazin, P.; Li, G.; Orts, W. J.; Favis, B. D. Binary and Ternary Blends of Polylactide, Polycaprolactone and Thermoplastic Starch. *Polymers* **2008**, *49*, 569–609.

246. Bleach, N. C.; Nazhat, S. N.; Tanner, K. E.; Kellomaki, M.; Tormala, P. Effect of Filler Content on Mechanical and Dynamic Mechanical Properties of Particulate Biphasic Calcium Phosphate Polylactide Composites. *Biomaterials* **2002**, *23*, 1579–1585.

247. Wie, G.; Ma, P. X. Structure and Properties of Nano-Hydroxyapatite/Polymer Composite Scaffolds for Bone Tissue Engineering. *Biomaterials* **2004**, *25*, 4749–4757.

248. Sun, B.; Ranganathan, B.; Feng, S. S. Multifunctional Poly(D, L-lactide-co-glycolide)/Montmorillonite (PLGA/MMT) Nanoparticles Decorated by Trastuzumab for Targeted Chemotherapy of Breast Cancer. *Biomaterials* **2008**, *29*, 475–486.

249. Park, G. E.; Pattison, M. A.; Park, K.; Webster, T. J. Accelerated Chondrocyte Functions on NaOH-Treated PLGA Scaffolds. *Biomaterials* **2005**, *26*, 3075–3086.

250. Wang, Y.; Challa, P.; Epstein, D. L.; Yuan, F. Controlled Release of Ethacrynic Acid from Poly(lactide-co-glycolide) Films for Glaucoma Treatment. *Biomaterials* **2004**, *25*, 4279–4285.

251. Donlan, R. M.; Costerton, J. W. Biofilms: Survival Mechanisms of Clinically Relevant Microorganisms. *Clin. Microbiol. Rev.* **2002**, 167–193.

252. Bendix, D. Chemical Synthesis of Polylactide and its Copolymers for Medical Application. *Polym. Degrad. Stab.* **2008**, *59*, 129–135.

253. Li, G.; Gill, T. J.; De Frate, L. E.; Zayontz, S.; Glatt, V.; Zarins, B. Biomechanical Consequences of PCL Deficiency in the Knee Under Simulated Muscle Loads: An In Vitro Experimental Study. *J. Orthop. Res.* **2002**, *20*, 887–892.

254. Kang, X.; Xie, Y.; Powell, H. M.; Lee, L. J.; Belury, M. A.; Lannutti, J. J.; Kniss, D. A. Adipogenesis of Murine Embryonic Stem Cells in a Three-Dimensional Culture System using Electrospun Polymer Scaffolds. *Biomaterials* **2007**, *28*, 450–458.

255. Choi, S. H.; Park, T. G. Synthesis and Characterization of Elastic PLGA/PCL/PLGA Tri-Block Copolymers. *J. Biomater. Sci. Polym. Ed.* **2002**, *13*, 1163–1174.

256. Chew, S. Y.; Hufnagel, T. C.; Lim, C. T.; Leong, K. W. Mechanical Properties of Single Electrospun Drug-Encapsulated Nanofiber. *Nanotechnology* **2006**, *17*, 3880–3891.

257. Yang, F.; Sanne, K. B.; Yang, X.; Wallboomers, X. F.; Jansen, J. A., et al. Development of an Electrospun Nano-Apatite/PCL Composite Membrane for GTR/GBR Application. *Acta. Biomater.* **2009,** *5,* 3295–3304.

258. Pektok, E.; Nottelet, B.; Tille, J. C.; Gurny, R.; Kalangos, A.; Moeller, M., et al. Degradation and Healing Characteristics of Small-Diameter Poly(3-caprolactone) Vascular Grafts in the Rat Systemic Arterial. *Circulation* **2008,** *118,* 2563–2570.

259. Aishwarya, S.; Mahalakshmi, S.; Sehgal, P. K. Collagen-Coated Polycaprolactone Microparticles as a Controlled Drug Delivery System. *J. Microencapsul.* **2008,** *25,* 298–306.

260. Freed, L. E.; Novakovic, G. V.; Biron, R. J.; Eagles, D. B.; Lesnoy, D. C.; Barlow, S. K., et al. Biodegradable Polymer Scaffolds for Tissue Engineering. *Biotechnology* **1994,** *12,* 689–693.

261. Ferraz, M. P.; Monteriro, F. J.; Manuel, C. M. Hydroxyapatite Nanoparticles: A Review of Preparation Methodologies. *J. Appl. Biomater. Biomech.* **2004,** *2,* 74–80.

262. Woodard, R.; Hilldore, A. J.; Lan, S. K.; Park, C. J.; Morgan, A. W.; Eurell, J. A. C., et al. The Mechanical Properties and Osteoconductivity of Hydroxyapatite Bone Scaffolds with Multi-Scale Porosità. *Biomaterials* **2007,** *28,* 45–54.

263. Webster, T. J.; Ergun, C.; Doremus, R. H.; Siegel, R. W.; Bizios, R. Enahnced Functions if Osteoblasts on Nanophase Ceramics. *Biomaterials* **2000,** *2,* 1803–1810.

264. Liao, S. S.; F.Z., C.; Zhu, Y. Osteoblasts Adherence and Migration through Threedimensional Porous Mineralized Collagen based Composite: nHAC/PLA. *J. Bioact. Compat. Polym.* **2004,** *19,* 117–130.

265. Hench, L. L.; Polak, J. M. Third-Generation Biomedical Materials. *Science* **2002,** *295,* 1014–1017.

266. Kretlow, J. D.; Mikos, A. G. Review: Mineralization of Synthetic Polymer Scaffolds for Bone Tissue Engineering. *Tissue Eng* **2007,** *13,* 927–938.

267. Dresselhaus, M. S.; Dresselhaus, G.; Eklund, P. C. *Science of Fullerenes and Carbon Nanotubes*; Academic Press: San Diego, 2001.

268. Lee, C. J.; Park, J.; Kang, S. Y.; Lee, J. H. Growth and Field Electron Emission of Vertically Aligned Multiwalled Carbon Nanotubes. *Chem. Phys. Lett.* **2000,** *326,* 175–180.

269. Sun, L. F.; Liu, Z. Q.; Ma, X. C.; Zhong, Z. Y.; Tang, S. B.; Xiong, Z. T., et al. Growth of Carbon Nanotube Arrays using the Existing Array as a Substrate and their Raman Characterization. *Chem. Phys. Lett.* **2001,** *340,* 222–226.

270. Thostenson, E. T.; Ren, Z.; Chou, T. Advances in the Science and Technology of Carbon Nanotubes and their Composites: A Review. *Compos. Sci. Technol.* **2001,** *61,* 899–1912.

271. Zhang, X.; Liu, T.; Sreekumar, T. V.; Kumar, S.; Moore, V. C.; Hauge, R. H., et al. Poly(vinylalcohol)/SWNT Composite Film. *Nano. Lett.* **2003,** *3,* 1285–1288.

272. Valentini, L.; Armentano, I.; Biagiotti, J.; Kenny, J. M.; Santucci, S. Frequency Dependent Electrical Transport between Conjugated Polymer and Singlewalled Carbon Nanotubes. *Diam. Relat. Mater.* **2003,** *12,* 1601–1609.

273. Chen, G. X.; Kim, H. S.; Park, B. H.; Yoon, J. S. Controlled Functionalization of Multiwalled Carbon Nanotubes with Various Molecular-Weight Poly(L-lactic acid). *J. Phys. Chem. B.* **2005,** *109,* 22237–22243.

274. Armentano, I.; Alvarez-Pérez, M. A.; Carmona-Rodríguez, B.; Gutiérrez-Ospina, I.; Kenny, J. M.; Arzate, H. Analysis of the Biomineralization Process on SWNTCOOH and F-SWNT Films. *Mater. Sci. Eng. C* **2008,** *28,* 1522–1529.

275. Dai, H.; Shim, M.; Chen, R. J.; Li, Y.; Kam, N. W. S. Functionalization of Carbon Nanotubes for Biocompatibility and Biomolecular Recognition. *Nano. Lett.* **2002,** *2,* 285–288.

276. Correa-Duarte, M. A.; Wagner, N.; Rojas-Chapana, J.; Morsczeck, C.; Thie, M.; Giersig, M. Fabrication and Biocompatibility of Carbon Nanotube-Based 3d Networks as Scaffolds for Cell Seeding and Growth. *Nano. Lett.* **2004,** *4,* 2233–2236.

277. Harrison, B. S.; Atala, A. Carbon Nanotube Applications for Tissue Engineering. *Biomaterials* **2007,** *28,* 344–353.

278. Dumortier, H.; Lacotte, S.; Pastorin, G.; Marega, R.; Wu, W.; Bonifazi, D., et al. Functionalized Carbon Nanotubes are Non-Cytotoxic and Preserve the Functionality of Primary Immune Cells. *Nano. Lett.* **2006,** *6,* 1522–1528.

279. Tian, F.; Cui, D.; Schwarz, H.; Estrada, G.; Kobayashic, H. Cytotoxicity of Singlewall Carbon Nanotubes on Human Fibroblasts. *Toxicol. In Vitro* **2006,** *20,* 1202–1212.

280. Mattson, M. P.; Haddon, R. C.; Rao, A. M. Molecular Functionalization of Carbon Nanotubes and use as Substrates for Neuronal Growth. *J. Mol. Neurosci.* **2000,** *14,* 175–182.

281. Lovat, V.; Pantarotto, D.; Lagostena, L.; Cacciari, B.; Grolfo, M.; Righi, M., et al. Nanotube Substrates Boost Neuronal Electrical Signaling. *Nano. Lett.* **2005,** *5,* 1107–1110.

282. Mwenifumbo, S.; Shaffer, M. S.; Stevens, M. M. Exploring Cellular Behaviour with Multi-Walled Carbon Nanotube Constructs. *J. Mater. Chem.* **2007,** *17,* 1894–1902.

283. Smart, S. K.; Cassady, A. I.; Lu, G. Q.; Martin, D. J. The Biocompatibility of Carbon Nanotubes. *Carbon* **2006,** *44,* 1034–1047.

284. Xiao, G. Solvent-Induced Changes on Corona-Discharge-Treated Polyolefin Surfaces Probed by Contact Angle Measurement. *J. Colloid Interface Sci.* **1995,** *171,* 200–204.

285. Otsuka, H.; Nagasaki, Y.; Kataoka, K. Dynamic Wettability Study on the Functionalized PEGylated Layer on a Polylactide Surface Constructed by Coating of Aldehyde-Ended Poly(ethylene glycol) (PEG)/Polylactide (PLA) Block Copolymer. *Sci. Technol. Adv. Mater.* **2000,** *1,* 21–29.

286. Tang, Z. G.; Black, R. A. Surface Properties and Biocompatibility of Solvent-Cast Poly[3-caprolactone] Films. *Biomaterials* **2004,** *25,* 4741–4748.

287. Song, W.; Zheg, Z.; Tang, W.; Wang, X. A Facile Approach to Covalently Functionalized Carbon Nanotubes with Biocompatible Polymer. *Polymer* **2007,** *48,* 3658–3663.

288. Hong, Z. K.; Zhang, P.; He, C.; Qiu, X.; Liu, A.; Chen, L., et al. Nano-Composite of Poly(Llactide) and Surface Grafted Hydroxyapatite: Mechanical Properties and Biocompatibility. *Biomaterials* **2005,** *26,* 6296–6304.

289. Zhang, D.; Kandadai, M. A.; Cech, J.; Roth, S.; Curran, S. A. Poly(L-lactide) (PLLA)/Multiwalled Carbon Nanotube (MWCNT) Composite: Characterization and Biocompatibility Evaluation. *J. Phys. Chem. B* **2006,** *110,* 1291–1295.

290. Paiva, M. C.; Zhou, B.; Fernando, K. A. S.; Lin, Y.; Kennedy, J. M.; Sun, Y. P. Mechanical and Morphological Characterization of Polymerecarbon Nanocomposites from Functionalized Carbon Nanotubes. *Carbon* **2004,** *42,* 2849–2854.

291. Mamedov, A. A.; Kotov, N. A.; Prato, M.; Guldi, D. M.; Wicksted, J. P.; Hirsch, A. Molecular Design of Strong Single-Wall Carbon Nanotube/Polyelectrolyte Multilayer Composites. *Nat. Mater.* **2002,** *1,* 190–194.

292. Wu, D.; Wu, L.; Sun, Y.; Zhang, M. *Rheological properties and crystallization behavior of multi-walled carbon nanotube/poly(3-caprolactone) composites* **2007,** *25,* 3137–3147.

293. Rai, M.; Yadav, A.; Gade, A. Recently, A Variety of Nanocomposites based on Polyester And-carbon Nanostructures have been Explored for Potential use Asscaffold Materials. *Biotechnol. Adv.* **2009,** *27,* 76–83.

294. Schneider, O. D.; Loher, S.; Brunner, T. J.; Schmidlin, P.; Stark, W. J. Flexible, Silver Containing Nanocomposites for the Repair of Bone Defects: Antimicrobial Effect Against *E. coli* Infection and Comparison to Tetracycline Containing Scaffolds. *J. Mater. Chem.* **2008,** *18,* 2679–2684.

295. Xu, X.; Yang, Q.; Bai, J.; Lu, T.; Li, Y.; Jing, X. Fabrication of Biodegradable Electrospun Poly(L-lactide-co-glycolide) Fibers with Antimicrobial Nanosilver Particles. *J. Nanosci. Nanotechnol.* **2008,** *8,* 5066–5070.

296. Xu, X.; Yang, Q.; Wang, Y.; Yu, H.; Chen, X.; Jing, X. Biodegradable Electrospun Poly (l-lactide) Fibers Containing Antibacterial Silver Nanoparticles. *Eur. Polym. J.* **2006,** *42,* 2081–2087.

297. Lee, J. Y.; Nagahata, J. L. R.; Horiuchi, S. Effect of Metal Nanoparticles on Thermal Stabilization of Polymer/Metal Nanocomposites Prepared by a One-Step Dry Process. *Polymer* **2006,** *47,* 7970–7979.

298. Agarwal, A.; Weis, T. L.; Schurr, M. J.; Faith, N. G.; Czuprynski, C. J.; McAnulty, J. F., et al. Surfaces Modified with Nanometer-Thick Silver-Impregnated Polymeric Films that Kill Bacteria but Support Growth of Mammalian Cells. *Biomaterials* **2010,** *31,* 680–690.

299. Wang, J.; Li, J.; Ren, L.; Zhao, A.; Li, P.; Leng, Y., et al. Antibacterial Activity of Silver Surface Modified Polyethylene Terephthalate by Filtered Cathodic Vacuum Arc Method. *Surf. Coat. Technol.* **2007,** *201,* 6893–6796.

300. Katsikogianni, M.; Missirlis, Y. F. Concise Review of Mechanics of Bacterial Adhesion to Biomaterials and of Techniques used in Estimating Bacteriamaterial Interactions. *Eur. Cell. Mater.* **2004,** *8,* 37–57.

301. Ramage, G.; Tunney, M. M.; Patrick, S.; Gorman, S. P.; Nixon, J. R. Formation of Propionibacterium Acnes Biofilms on Orthopaedic Biomaterials and their Susceptibility to Antimicrobials. *Biomaterials* **2003,** *24,* 3221–3227.

302. Guo, P. RNA Nanotechnology: Engineering, Assembly and Applications in Detection, Gene Delivery and Therapy. *J. Nanosci. Nanotechnol.* **2005,** *5,* 1964–1982.

303. Drexler, E. *Engines of Creation: The Coming Era of Nanotechnology*; Knopf Doubleday Publishing Group, 1987.

304. Sajja, H. K.; East, M. P.; Mao, H.; Wang, A. Y.; Nie, S.; Yang, L. Development of Multifunctional Nanoparticles for Targeted Drug Delivery and Non-invasive Imaging of Therapeutic Effect. *Curr. Drug Discov. Technol.* **2009,** *6,* 43–51, http://www.ncbi.nlm.nih.gov/entrez/eutils/elink.fcgi?dbfrom=pubmed&retmode=ref&cmd=prlinks&id=19275541.

305. Beyerle, A.; Merkel, O.; Stoeger, T.; Kissel, T. PEGylation Affects Cytotoxicity and Cell-Compatibility of Poly(ethylene imine) for Lung Application: Structurefunction Relationships. *Toxicol. Appl. Pharmacol.* **2010,** *242,* 146–154.

306. Geish, K. Enhanced Permeability and Retention Effect of Macromolecular Drugs in Solid Tumors: A Royal Gate for Targeted Anticancer Medicines. *J. Drug Target.* **2007,** *15,* 457–464.

307. Moghimi, S. M.; Szebeni, J. Stealth Liposomes and Long Circulating Nanoparticles: Critical Issues in Pharmacokinetics, Opsonization and Protein-Binding Properties. *Prog. Lipid. Res.* **2003,** *42,* 463–478.

308. Soma, C. E.; Dubernet, C.; Bentolila, D.; Benita, S.; Couvreur, P. Reversion of Multidrug Resistance by Co-Encapsulation of Doxorubicin and Cyclosporin a in Polyalkylcyanoacrylate Nanoparticles. *Biomaterials* **2000,** *21,* 1–7.

309. Vauthier, C.; Dubernet, C.; Chauvierre, C.; Brigger, I.; Couvreur, P. Drug Delivery to Resistant Tumors: The Potential of Poly(alkyl cyanoacrylate) Nanoparticles. *J. Control. Release* **2003,** *93,* 151–160.

310. Wang, Y. -C.; Wu, Y. -T.; Huang, H. -Y.; Lin, -I.; Lo, L. -W.; Tzeng, S. -F.; Yang, C. -S. Sustained Intraspinal Delivery of Neurotrophic Factor Encapsulated in Biodegradable Nanoparticles following Contusive Spinal Cord Injury. *Biomaterials* **2008,** *29,* 4546–4553.

311. THomas, C. E.; Ehrhardt, A.; Kay, M. A. Progress and Problems with the use of Viral Vectors for Gene Therapy. *Nat. Rev. Genet.* **2003,** *4,* 346–358.

312. Park, T. G.; Jeong, J. H.; Kim, S. W. Current Status of Polymeric Gene Delivery Systems. *Adv. Drug. Deliv. Rev.* **2006,** *58,* 467–486.

313. Dang, J. M.; Leong, K. W. Natural Polymers for Gene Delivery and Tissue Engineering. *Adv. Drug Deliv. Rev.* **2006,** *58,* 487–499.

314. Singh, R.; Pamtarotto, D.; McCarthy, D.; Chaloin, O.; Hoebeke, J.; Partidos, C. D.; Briand, J. P.; Prato, M.; Bianco, A.; Kostarelos, K. Binding and Condensation of Plasmid DNA onto Functionalized Carbon Nanotubes: Toward the Construction of Nanotube-Based Gene Delivery Vectors. *J. Am. Chem. Soc.* **2005**, *127*, 4388–4396.

315. Bonadio, J. Tissue Engineering via Local Gene Delivery: Update and Future Prospects for Enhancing the Technology. *Adv. Drug Deliv. Rev.* **2000**, *44*, 185–194.

316. Wan, A. C. A.; Ying, J. Y. Nanomaterials for in situ Cell Delivery and Tissue Regeneration. *Adv. Drug Del. Rev.* **2010**, *62*, 731–740, http://www.sciencedirect.com/science/journal/0169409X. Accessed May 26, 2012.

317. Schillinger, U.; Wexel, G.; Hacker, C.; Kullmer, M.; Koch, C.; Gerg, M.; Vogt, S.; Ueblacker, P.; Tischer, T.; Hensler, D.; Wilisch, J.; Aigner, J.; Walch, A.; Stemberger, A.; Plank, C. A Fibrin Glue Composition as Carrier for Nucleic Acid Vectors. *Pharm. Res.* **2008**, *25*, 2946–2962.

318. Quick, D. J.; Anseth, K. S. Gene Delivery in Tissue Engineering: A Photopolymer Platform to Coencapsulate Cells and Plasmid. *Pharm. Res.* **2003**, *20*, 1730–1737.

319. de Laporte, L.; Yan, A. L.; Shea, L. D. Local Gene Delivery from ECM-Coated Poly(lactide-co-glycolide) Multiple Channel Bridges after Spinal Cord Injury. *Biomaterials* **2009**, *30*, 2361–2368.

320. Mattson, M. P.; Haddon, R. C.; Rao, A. M. Molecular Functionalization of Carbon Nanotubes and use as Substrates for Neuronal Growth. *J. Mol. Neurosci.* **2000**, *14*, 175–182.

321. Fab, h.; Lu, Y.; Stump, A., et al. Rapid Prototyping of Patterned Functional Nanostructures. *Nature* **2000**, *405*, 56–60.

322. Lim, S. H.; Liao, I. C.; Leong, K. W. Nonviral Gene Delivery from Nonwoven Fibrous Scaffolds Fabricated by Interfacial Complexation of Polyelectrolytes. *Mol. Ther.* **2006**, *13*, 1163–1172.

323. Madduri, S.; Gander, B. Growth Factor Delivery Systems and Repair Strategies for Damaged Peripheral Nerves. *J. Control Release* **2011**.

324. Kingham, P. J.; Terenghi, G. Bioengineered Nerve Regeneration and Muscle Reinnervation. *J. Anat.* **2006**, *209*, 511–526.

325. Stang, F.; Fansa, H.; Wolf, G.; Reppin, M.; Keilhoff, G. Structural Parameters of Collagen Nerve Grafts Influence Peripheral Nerve Regeneration. *Biomaterials* **2005**, *26*, 3083–3091.

326. Kannan, R. Y.; Salacinski, H. J.; Butler, P. E.; Seifalian, A. M. Artificial Nerve Conduits in Peripheral-Nerve Repair. *Biotechnol. Appl. Biochem.* **2005**, *41* (Pt3), 193–200.

327. Johnson, E. O.; Zoubos, A. B.; Saucacos, P. N. Regeneration and Repair of Peripheral Nerves. *Injury* **2005**, *36*, S24–S29.

328. Belkas, J. S.; Schoichet, M. S.; Midha, R. Peripheral Nerve Regeneration through Guidance Tubes. *Neurolog. Res.* **2004**, *26*, 151–160.

329. Wellescent. *Peripheral Neuropathy is more than the Loss of Touch.* 2011 June 13, 2012. Available from: http://wellescent.com/health_blog/.

330. Noble, J.; Munro, C. A.; Prasad, V. S. S.V.; Midha, R. Analysis of Upper and Lower Extremity Peripheral Nerve Injuries in a Population of Patients with Multiple Injuries. *J. Trauma* **1998**, *45*, 116–122.

331. de Ruiter, G. C. W.; Malessy, M. J. A.; Yszemski, M. J.; Windebank, A. J.; Spinner, R. J. Designing Ideal Conduits for Peripheral Nerve Repair. *Neurosurg. Focus* **2009**, *26*, 1–9.

332. Bellamkonda, R. V. Peripheral Nerve Regeneration: An Opinion on Channels, Scaffolds and Anisotropy. *Biomaterials* **2006**, *27*, 3515–3518.

333. Ruiter, G. C. W.; Malessy, M. J. A.; Yszemski, M. J.; Windebank, A. J.; Spinner, R. J. Designing Ideal Conduits for Peripheral Nerve Repair. *Neurosurg. Focus* **2009**, *26*, 1–9.

334. Wang, D. Y.; Huang, Y. Y. Fabricate Coaxial Stacked Nerve Conduits through Soft Lithography and Molding Processes. *J. Biomed. Mater. Res. Part A* **2008**, *85*, 434–438.

335. Xie, F.; Qing, F. L.; Gu, B.; Liu, K.; Guo, X. S. In Vitro and In Vivo Evaluation of a Biodegradable Chitosan-PLA Composite Peripheral Nerve Guide Conduit Material. *Microsurgery* **2008**, *28*, 471–479.

336. Alluin, O.; Wittman, C.; Wittman, C. Functional Recovery after Peripheral Nerve Injury and Implantation of a Collagen Guide. *Biomaterials* **2009**, *30*, 363–373.

337. Hu, X.; Huang, J.; Huang, J. A Novel Scaffold with Longitudinally Oriented Microchannels Promotes Peripheral Nerve Regeneration. *Tissue Eng. Part A* **2009**, *15*, 3927–3308.

338. Leach, J. B.; Schmidt, C. E. Characterization of Protein Release from Photo-Crosslinkable Hyaluronic Acid-Polyethylene Glycol Hydrogel Tissue Engineering Scaffolds. *Biomaterials* **2005**, *26*, 125–135.

339. Chang, Y.; Ho, T. Y.; Lee, H. C.; Lai, Y. L.; Lu, M. C.; Yao, C. H.; Chen, Y. S. Highly Permeable Genipin-Cross-Linked Gelatin Conduits Enhance Peripheral Nerve Regeneration. *Artif. Organs* **2009**, *33*, 1075–1085.

340. Madduri, S.; Papaloizos, M.; Gander, B. Trophically and Topographically Functionalized Silk Fibroin Nerve Conduits for Guided Peripheral Nerve Regeneration. *Biomaterials* **2010**, *31*, 2323–2334.

341. Chiono, V.; Tonda-Turo, C.; Ciardelli, G. Artificial Scaffolds for Peripheral Nerve Reconstruction. *Int. Rev. Neurobiol.* **2009**, *87*, 173–198.

342. Nisbet, D. R.; Crompton, K. E.; Horne, M. K.; Finkelstein, D. I.; Forsythe, J. S. Neural Tissue Engineering of the CNS using Hydrogels. *J. Biome. Mater. Res. Part B* **2008**, *87*, 251–263.

343. Ciardelli, G.; Chiono, V. Materials for Peripheral Nerve Regeneration. *Macromol. Biosci.* **2006**, *6*, 13–26.

344. Wang, W.; Itoh, S.; Iyoh, S. Enhanced Nerve Regeneration through a Bilayered Chitosan Tube: The Effect of Introduction of Glycine Spacer into the CYIGSR Sequence.. *J. Biome. Mater. Res. Part B* **2008**, *85*, 919–928.

345. Wang, S.; Cai, L. Polymers for fabricating nerve conduits. *Int J Polymer Sci* **2010**, 1–20.

346. Ahmed, M. R.; Vairamuthu, S.; Shafiuzama, M. D.; Basha, S. H.; Jayakumar, R. Microwave Irradiated Collagen Tubes as a Better Matrix for Peripheral Nerve Regeneration. *Brain Res.* **2005**, *1046*, 55–67.

347. Lu, M. C.; Hsiang, S. W.; Lai, T. Y.; Yao, C. H.; Lin, L. Y.; Chen, Y. S. Influence of Cross-Linking Degree of a Biodegradable Genipin-Cross-Linked Gelatin Guide on Peripheral Nerve Regeneration. *J. Biomater. Sci. Polym. Ed.* **2007**, *18*, 843–863.

348. Place, E. S.; Evans, N. D.; Stevens, M. M. Complexity in Biomaterials for Tissue Engineering. *Nat. Mater.* **2009**, *8*, 457–470.

349. Kehoe, S.; Zhang, X. F.; Boyd, D. FDA Approved Guidance Conduits and Wraps for Peripheral Nerve Injury: A Review of Materials and Efficacy. *Injury* **2012**, *43*(5), 553–572.

350. Muratoglu, O. K.; Spielberg, S. H.; Ruberti, J. W.; Abt, N. *PVA Hydrogel* **2007**, US Patent Application Number *235*, 592.

351. Meek, M. F.; Coert, J. H. US Food and Drug Administration/Conformit Europe-Approved Absorbable Nerve Conduits for Clinical Repair of Peripheral and Cranial Nerves. *Annals* **2006**, *60*, 110–116.

352. NIH. *Stem Cell Basics.* cited January 5, 2012. Available from: http://stemcells.nih.gov/info/basics/basics1.asp.

353. Pittenger, M.; Mackay, A.; Beck, S.; Jaiswal, R. K.; Douglas, R.; Mosca, J. D.; Moorman, M. A.; Simonetti, D. W.; Craig, S.; Marshak, D. R. Multilineage Potential of Adult Human Mesenchymal Stem Cells. *Science* **1999**, *284*, 143–147.

354. Zhang, G.; Hu, Q.; Braunlin, E. A.; Suggs, L. J.; Zhang, J. A. Enhancing Efficacy of Stem Cell Transplantation to the Heart with a PEGylated Fibrin Biomatrix. *Tissue Eng. Part A* **2008,** *14,* 1025–1036.

355. Zhang, D.; Drinnan, C. T.; Geuss, L. R.; Suggs, L. J. Vascular Differentiation of Bone Marrow Stem Cells is Directed by a Tunable Three-Dimensional Matrix. *Acta. Biomater.* **2010,** *3,* 3395–3403.

356. Zhang, g.; Wang, X.; Wang, Z.; Zhang, J. A.; Suggs, L. A PEGylated Fibrin Patch for Mesenchymal Stem Cell Delivery. *Tissue Eng.* **2006,** *12,* 9–19.

357. Valarmati, M.; Davis, J.; Yost, M.; Goodwin, R.; Potts, J. A Three-Dimensional Model of Vasculogenesis. *Biomaterials* **2009,** *30,* 1098–1112.

358. Al-Khalid, A.; Elipoulod, N.; Martineau, D., et al. Postnatal Bone Marrow Stromal Cells Elicit a Potent VEGF-Dependent Neoangiogenic Response In Vivo. *Gene. Ther.* **2003,** *10,* 621–629.

359. Guzman, R.; Uchida, N.; Bliss, T., et al. Long-Term Monitoring of Transplanted Human Neural Stem Cells in Developmental and Pathological Contexts with MRI. *PNAS USA* **2007,** *104,* 10211–10216.

360. Chen, R.; Huang, G.; Ke, P. Calcium-Enhanced Exocytosis of Gold Nanoparticles. *Appl. Phys. Lett.* **2010,** *97,* 093706.

361. Chithrani, B.; Chan, W. Elucidating the Mechanisms of Cellular uptake and Removal or Protein-Coated Gold Nanoparticles of Different Sizes and Shapes. *Nano. Lett.* **2007,** *7,* 1542–1550.

Chapter 7

Nanopharmacology

Chapter Outline

7.1 INTRODUCTION

Nanoparticles (NPs) can be engineered to diagnose conditions and recognize pathogens; identify ideal pharmaceutical agents to treat the condition or pathogens; fuel high-yield production of matched pharmaceuticals (potentially in

Nanomaterials for Medical Applications. http://dx.doi.org/10.1016/B978-0-12-385089-8.00007-8

vivo); locate, attach or enter target tissue, structures or pathogens; and dispense the ideal mass of matched biological compound to the target regions.

The application of nanotechnology for drug design and drug delivery to selected targets for improved pharmacodynamics and kinetic profiles toward safer and effective treatment is the area today that is known as nanopharmacology.[1] It encompasses proper drug engineering design, development, and manufacture of the nanostructured drug or drug carrier for nanoscale molecular targets, drug formulation, and drug release. Nanotechnology promises to revolutionize the area of pharmacology owing to the unique size and properties of nanomaterials (NMs). NMs hold promise in improving the curative abilities of various conventional drugs. This chapter is dedicated to the applications of NMs in nanopharmacology.

7.2 CURRENT ISSUES AND STATUS OF NANOPHARMACOLOGY

Nanopharmacology is complicated by the need to establish the behavior of nanoparticles (NPs) such as quantum dots (QDs), carbon nanotubes (CNTs), gold nanoparticles (AuNPs), iron oxide magnetic nanoparticles (IOMNPs), and many more within the traditional pharmacological parameters of absorption, distribution, metabolism and excretion (ADME). Nanoconstructs, in many cases, have limited metabolism and excretion and persist in biological systems, which gains importance when containing toxic atoms such as cadmium. This poses a need to carefully examine our common ADME parameters and revise them if necessary.

Absorption into the host system is generally the first hurdle to be overcome which is dependent on route of delivery (Figure 7.1). To date, research has established that various NPs can enter an organism through skin absorption, inhalation, oral delivery, and parenteral administration. For QDs, the most important route of delivery at present appears to be systemic distribution through parenteral delivery, although occupational and environmental exposures via dermal and inhalation routes are also possible. What few studies are available on QD absorption at the organism level primarily utilize parenteral IV delivery. QD targeting studies have shown that QDs with targeting functional groups can be accumulated in selected target tissues upon IV administration. However, distribution to non-target tissues in an organism has not been examined and is an area where information is critically needed. Due to the high fluorescence of QDs and the metallic cores, particle deposition within an organism should be readily measurable.

During the past decade, there are more than 26 FDA approved anticancer drugs for clinical use[2] on top of other therapeutic agents for various conditions from cardiovascular disease to inflammation.[3] These conventional drugs exhibit therapeutic potential but various limitations hinder clinical translation and success. These limitations include the physico-chemical properties of the agents that prevent them from being efficiently administered in the molecular form.[3] Majority of the drugs are polycyclic making them insoluble in water.[4] Paclitaxel and dexamethasone, for example, have low water solubility values of $0.0015\,mg/mL$[5] and $0.1\,mg/mL$,[6] respectively, making them unacceptable for aqueous intravenous injection.[3] A major obstacle which prevents the drug from reaching its target is its highly unspecific distribution with only 1 in 10,000 to 1 in 100,000 molecules reaching their intended site of action.[7] As a result, a much higher dose needs to be administered to obtain the desired therapeutic effect which in turn could lead closer to the toxic dose[8] as exemplified by doxorubicin which exhibits prominent cardiotoxicity.[9] Considering these factors, it is desirable to modify the drug with features that would pharmacologically guarantee increased stability, solubility, and specific targeting to the site of action.[3] To this end, nanotechnology promises to revolutionize the area of pharmacology. Owing to their unique size and properties, NMs hold promise in improving the curative abilities of various conventional drugs.

Nanotechnology has prominently contributed the most to oncology[3] during the last 15 years. Nanocarriers occupied an important area in the treatment of cancer with liposomes being the first commercially available drug nanocarrier for injectable therapeutics.[10,11,12] In 1990, liposomal doxorubicin has been granted with FDA approval for use against Kaposi's sarcoma.[3] It was also later approved for metastatic breast cancer and recurrent ovarian cancer therapy. To date, a variety of nanocarrier based drug-delivery systems with various compositions, physicochemical characteristics, geometry, and surface functionalizations have been generated and are in different stages of development.[13,14]

Various nanocarriers that can be used for specific drugs and many more conditions are currently undergoing development.[3] These nanocarriers can be classified into three main categories.[10,13,15] The first category includes nanomaterials (NMs) that reaches the disease through passive mechanism.[15] The liposomes[16] belong to this category where in cancer, they utilize the enhanced permeability of the neovasculature to localize into the disease site through enhanced permeation and retention (EPR) mechanism [17,18] including those in clinical applications. In various cases of cancer, liposomes utilize the enhanced permeability of the neovasculature as the mechanism to localize into the disease site through so called the EPR mechanism.[17,18]

Extravasation of NMs is favored because of the presence of large (several hundred nanometers) vascular fenestrations on newly formed angiogenic vessels. The carriers can have surface modifications with materials such as a polyethylene glycol (PEG) that make the nanovectors "stealth" thereby preventing their uptake by the reticuloendothelial system (RES). "Stealth" particles have sufficient prolonged circulation time that increases the likelihood of homing in on tumor.[19–21] Significant success in chemistry and materials science have yielded several other NMs for drug delivery, including polymer–drug conjugates,[22] polymer micelles,[23–28] and dendrimers.[23,24,26,29–33] Thus, at the onset of studies, NMs-delivery systems for drugs had no active mechanisms of disease site location and therapy, the second generation involves nanodrug-delivery systems with targeting functionality [34-48]. The targeting functionality may be attributed to (1) specific molecular recognition moieties on the nanovector to receptors overexpressed on the tumor cells or adjacent blood vessels (such as Ab conjugated NMs) or (2) a possibility for active/triggered release of the payload at the diseased location (e.g. magnetic nanoparticles (MNPs)).[49,50] Thus, the NMs are superior to their precursors through the use of targeting moieties, remote activation, and environmentally sensitive components, bringing additional degrees of sophistication in design that promises increased success in accomplishing the intentions. Additional sophistication through the design of logic embedded vectors (LEVs) is envisioned as the natural successor for more effective accomplishment of the intended applications.[51] LEVs are therapeutic multicomponent nanostructures that are specifically engineered to avoid biological barriers, where the functions of biorecognition, cytotoxicity and no susceptibility to biobarrier are decoupled with efficacious operational harmony.[3] Ideally, this chemotherapeutic strategy will be capable of navigating through the vasculature after intravenous administration, to reach the desired tumor site at full concentration, and to selectively kill cancer cells with a cocktail of agents and at the same time have minimal harmful side effects. These can be used also for advanced therapy and imaging with immense potential for enhanced drug delivery that will bear a high impact on the future of personalized medicine (Figure 7.1).

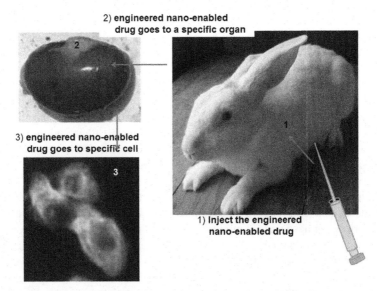

FIGURE 7.1 Schematic of targeted drug delivery using engineered NMs. *(For color version of this figure, the reader is referred to the online version of this book)*

7.3 NMs FOR GENE DELIVERY

One of the most promising applications of NMs is gene delivery. NMs-mediated gene delivery holds promise to cure many inheritable or acquired diseases that are currently considered incurable.[52] NMs can be packed with DNA strands or fragments very easily through the various conjugation or attachments methods discussed in Chapter 3. In addition, because of the highly negative phosphate backbone of DNA, it can easily be attached to positively charged NMs through charge–charge interactions.

A number of NMs have been used as gene carriers[53] for both in vitro[54,55] and in vivo gene delivery[56] that can theoretically reach a target site because of their size and charge.[57] NMs can be used to conjugate[54,55] or to encapsulate[58] various genetic materials in the form of DNA plasmids, RNA, and siRNA.

The group of Kneuer developed an approach to create positively charged silica NPs through the simultaneous hydrolysis of tetraethoxysilane and N-($â$-aminoethyl)-$ç$-aminopropyltyiethoxysilane in a water-in-oil microemulsion process.[55] The modification with amine active groups in silane resulted in silica NPs that were 10–100 nm in diameter with zeta potential at +7 to +31 mV at pH 7.4. The protonation of the amine surface resulted in positive charge on the surface of the NMs that allowed for the linking of plasmid DNA (pDNA) through electrostatic binding.[53] The DNA that was captured as DNA~NMs complex can be released at alkaline pH (>10) or in the presence of high salt concentrations (>2 mol/L NaCl)[59]. The same process was used by the group of Bharali[60] to deliver a plasmid encoding enhanced green fluorescent protein (EGFP) into mouse ventral midbrain and lateral ventricle. The presence of the EGFP allowed fluorescent visualization of the successful transfection of neuron-like cells. They also exhibited the application of the amino-modified silica NPs for selective delivery of a nucleus-targeting fibroblast growth factor receptor type 1 into mouse brain that led to significant inhibition of the incorporation of bromodeoxyuridine into the subventricular zone and the adjacent rostral migratory stream.[60]

Studies encapsulating DNA or RNA inside biodegradable polymeric NPs for controlled gene release have also been reported.[61–63] The encapsulation protects the nucleic acids (NAs) from enzymatic digestion during transit in systemic circulation, thereby allowing targeting to specific tissues or cells through the surface functionalization of the NMs.[53] The encapsulation also provides protection that avoids uptake of the NAs by the mononuclear phagocytic system because of the presence of the NMs.[58] An approach using PEGylated gelatin NMs by the acidic or basic hydrolysis of collagen[64] to encapsulate NAs have been used to exhibit the delivery of a pDNA into NIH 3T3 murine fibroblast cells.[65]

Targeted gene delivery has been made with ligands conjugated with antibodies on biodegradable NMs encapsulating DNA. A DNA-polycation complex was formed by mixing pDNA with Polyetheylene imine (PEI) at different ratios[66]. Monoclonal antibody against the human epidermal growth factor receptor-2 (HER-2) using trastuzumab (herceptin) was conjugated to the DNA/polycation complexes to target tumor cells. The studies indicated that the surface functionalized complexes had up to 20-fold higher transfection activity compared with non-cationic polymer based gene transfer in breast cancer cells. This is a significant improvement that promises possible chemotherapeutic applications of the DNA/polycation complexes against cancer cells.

Studies have also indicated that the size of the NMs can significantly impact gene transfer efficiency in vivo.[67] Optimization of particle size has been observed to improve the clearance behavior of intravenously injected NMs as well as their tissue distribution and therefore, the efficiency of drug or gene delivery is also improved.[68,69] Studies have also indicated that smaller poly-(D,L-lactide-*co*-glycolide) (PLGA) about 70 ± 2 nm in diameter carrying a pDNA exhibited 27-fold higher transfection than larger-sized NPs in the HEK-293 cell line.[67]

NMs have been used for the delivery of small interfering RNA (siRNA) as a potential therapeutic approach for genetic diseases.[53] NMs have been used to stabilize siRNA in physiological fluids and to improve their intracellular uptake.[70] Chitosan coated polyisohexylcyanoacrylate (PIHCA) NMs that encapsulated anti-RhoA siRNA in nude mice with breast cancer showed 90% inhibition of tumor growth without toxic effect.[71] PEI that was complexed with siRNA (PEI-complexed siRNA) targeting the HER-2 receptor that was intraperitoneally injected in mice resulted in the delivery of the intact siRNA into the tumors that exhibited reduction in tumor growth.[72,73]

Today, liposomes are clinically more advanced than other NMs as drug-delivery systems because of their inherent properties that includes biocompatibility, high drug payload, and easy drug-encapsulation capability.[16,52] Barriers to its widespread acceptability requires improved efficiency and lower cytotoxicity which may behave toward opposite directions such that to improve efficiency may require higher levels of the liposome but this level may lead to higher toxicity. Optimization conditions may be achieved through a balance between these two conditions. New NMs for gene-delivery systems that provide precise physical and chemical engineering of nanoscale structures have emerged in the last few years which address these issues.[74,75]

7.3.1 Gene Delivery with Inorganic NMs

Research has demonstrated that the use of AuNPs serve as excellent systems for the delivery of genetic materials into cells.[76,77] AuNPs as gene-delivery vehicles are especially attractive because the particles are easily conjugated with biomolecules[78] and allows high gene packing density that facilitates better delivery efficiency as well as improved enzymatic degradation of DNA strands.[52] In addition, AuNPs are non-toxic and not immunogenic.[79,80] In one of the more recent studies, liposomes and AuNPs were combined in an attempt to combine the advantageous properties of both types of NMs, Rhim and collaborators[52] developed a lipid–DNA–AuNP (L–DNA–AuNP) hybrid-based gene-delivery system. In their study, the L–DNA–AuNP was used for improved transfection efficiency and reduced cytotoxicity. DNA strands were loaded onto the AuNPs to increase the payload per delivery event that enhances transfection efficiency. But, negatively charged DNA strands that are exposed in this system deteriorates during contact between DNA–AuNPs and cells because the cell membrane itself carries a weak negative charge. This phenomenon is overcome by attaching a cationic lipid layer to DNA-modified AuNP that neutralizes the negative charge thereby, facilitating cell membrane penetration of DNA-modified AuNPs as well as protecting the modified DNA.

7.3.1.1 Protocol for Loading DNA in AuNP and Encapsulating with Liposome[52]

The modification of the AuNP is based on electrostatic interaction with the DNA at a controlled pH. The process involved adjusting the pH of the citrate AuNPs to 9 and exposure to the pDNA followed by subsequent modification with the lipids.

(1) Centrifuge the citrate-stabilized AuNPs (15, 30,50, and 80 nm) and collect the pellet.
(2) Dilute the pDNA to 20 ng/uL (in 10 mM phosphate buffer at pH 9).
(3) Measure the concentration of the pDNA using a UV/Vis absorbance at 260 nm.
(4) Add the pDNA to the AuNPs and mix vigorously. The negatively charged phosphates backbone of the pDNA chain facilitates the exchange with the citrate to form pDNA~AuNP which leads to the formation of the higher bonding energy between Au and phosphates compared with that between Au and carboxylates in citrates.[81]
(5) Incubate this mixture in an orbital shaker at 300 rpm at 37 °C overnight.
(6) Centrifuge the pDNA-loaded AuNPs and separate the supernatant from the residue.
(7) Measure the amount of unreacted pDNA from the supernatant by taking the absorbance at 260 nm.
(8) Calculate the amount of pDNA loaded per AuNP particle by subtracting the amount that was unreacted from the original concentration. The reacted pDNA is divided by the number of AuNPs used during the pDNA loading.
(9) Check the stability of the pDNA–AuNPs by adding 200 nM NaCl salt concentration to 50 mM AuNP. During this saline addition, color change from reddish wine to purple means aggregation of AuNPs due to unstable or incomplete binding of the pDNA to the AuNPs.
(10) Mix the pDNA–AuNP with 1.5 uL or 3 uL liposomes and incubate at 25 °C for 20 min with vigorous shaking.

Results from the studies of Rhim and collaborators that published this protocol[52] showed that the AuNPs had 10–100 pDNA strands per particle depending on the size. Zeta potential measurements indicated that the AuNPs contained the pDNA strands as shown by the enhanced negative charge. The high DNA-loading on the AuNPs is expected to improve gene delivery without the need for increasing the dosage. Because the AuNPs are modified a dense quantity of pDNA strands are less likely to be degraded by cell nuclei before delivering the payload.[82,83] Furthermore, the complexation with cationic liposomes masks the negative charge that helps the pDNA–AuNP complexes to penetrate the partially negative cell membranes. In addition, the liposomes are expected to impart structural stability to the AuNP gene-delivery platform.

The L–DNA–AuNP system was used in a transfection study using DNA (pEGFP-N1) which triggers EGFP expression that was delivered to mammalian cells with various gene-delivery vehicles (RHIM). When pDNA was delivered in the absence of the AuNPs and the lipids, negligible green fluorescence was detected compared with the L–pDNA–AuNP. The results suggest that pDNA transfection was mainly facilitated by L–pDNA–AuNP hybrids. The studies suggested that less lipid is needed in the L–pDNA–AuNP system for efficient pDNA delivery than in the lipid–pDNA system without the AuNP.

7.3.2 Gene Delivery with Biodegradable Polymers

Delivery of genes using biodegradable non-viral systems such as liposomes and cationic lipid or polymer forming DNA~NMs complexes is usually transient that requires multiple delivery of the expression vector to maintain a therapeutic level of the expressed protein in the target tissue.[84–86] The number of doses needed would be dependent upon the needs of the disease, the efficiency of gene expression, and the stability of the protein that is expressed in the tissue.[84,87] Toxicity of the vector may come as a consequence of repeated delivery and the therapy may lose potency. Repeated delivery of the vector may cause toxicity, and the therapy may not be effective.[84,88] Alternatives to avoid these issues include various sustained release gene-delivery systems including polymeric implants, gels, and other materials are being studied.[63,89]

The use of biodegradable polymers, PLGA and polylactide (PLA), as gene-delivery systems have recently gained attention.[61,62,90] These NMs have been investigated extensively as a carrier for various therapeutic agents, including macromolecules such as proteins and peptides. Studies have reported the rapid escape (within 10 min) of these NMS from the endolysosomal compartment to the cytoplasmic compartment after intracellular uptake via an endocytic process[91] that was attributed to the reversal of their surface charge from anionic to cationic in the acidic pH of the endolysosomal compartment. This results in the NMs interaction with the endolysosomal membrane allowing their escape into the cytoplasmic compartment.[84] This rapid escape from the endolysosomal compartment is potentially advantageous for the protection of the NMs encapsulated DNA from degradation prior to delivery of the gene. Once localized in the cytoplasmic compartment, the encapsulated DNA can be slowly released allowing for sustained gene expression that can be used for a chronic gene delivery for therapeutic efficacy.[87]

Biodegradable NMs, ~200 nm in diameter biocompatible polymer, PLGA have the potential for sustained gene delivery have been reported.[84] The wild-type (wt) p53 gene (DNA) was loaded in NMs (PLGA~DNA) and used in a breast cancer cell line to determine its antiproliferative activity.[84] The PLGA~DNA were formulated using a multiple-emulsion-solvent evaporation technique before these were used for cell transfection. Cells transfected with wt-p53 DNA that were loaded in the PLGA NMs demonstrated higher sustained antiproliferative effect than those with naked wt-p53 DNA or wt-p53 DNA complexed with a commercially available transfecting agent (Lipofectamine).[84] The breast cancer cells that were transfected with wt-p53 DNA-loaded PLGA NMs showed sustained levels of p53 mRNA compared with cells which were transfected with naked wt-p53 DNA or the wt-p53 DNA–Lipofectamine complex. Further studies using fluorescent labeled DNA under a confocal microscopy and quantitative analyses with a microplate reader also indicated sustained intracellular localization of PLGA~DNA which suggested the slow release of DNA from the NMs that were localized inside the cells. The loading of the DNA in PLGA is described in the protocol below.

7.3.2.1 Protocol for Gene Delivery with Biodegradable Polymers PLGA[84]

(1) Dissolve 1 mg DNA and 2 mg of nuclease free Bovine serum albumin (BSA) in 200 uL of Tris-EDTA, pH 8.
(2) Prepare the primary emulsion by sonicating 30 mg of PLGA 50:50 (intrinsic viscosity of 1.32 g/dL, Birmingham Polymers) in 1 mL of chloroform with the above DNA solution for 2 min over an ice bath using a probe sonicator set at 55 W of energy output.
(3) Emulsify the result further into a 2% w/v polyvinyl alcohol (PVA, 30–70 kDa, Sigma) solution for 5 min to form a multiple (water-in-oil-in-water) emulsion.
(4) Stir this emulsion overnight on a magnetic stir plate that is kept in a vacuum desiccator for 1 h to evaporate chloroform.
(5) Separate the NMs using ultracentrifugation at 35,000 rpm for 20 min at 4 °C.
(6) Wash twice to remove PVA and unencapsulated DNA.
(7) Resuspend the pellet in 5 mL of sterile water by sonication for 30 s.
(8) Lyophilize the suspension (−80 °C and <10 umHg) for 48 h.
(9) Collect all washing of the PLGA~DNA.
(10) Measure the OD at 260 nm.
(11) Compare with original DNA that is not exposed to PLGA and calculate the amount of DNA loaded on the PLGA.
(12) Take a 0.1 mg/mL suspension of the PLGA~DNA and sonicate in ice bath for 30 s.
(13) Measure the size of the NMs in a particle size analyzer.
(14) Establish the zeta potential before and after the DNA loading.

The studies of Prabha[84] used the wild-type p53-gene loaded in PLGA NMs for the transfection of breast cancer cell MDA MB231, a cell line that is derived from a human ductal carcinoma from patient with metastatic disease and had not been subjected to chemotherapy.[92] The p53 gene rearrangement in this cell line causes a reduced level of expression of p53 making it suitable for studying the effect of p53 gene therapy.[93] Using multiple-emulsion-solvent evaporation technique, wild-type p53-gene was loaded in PLGA NMs to determine the gene's antiproliferative activity in a breast cancer cell line. The intracellular trafficking of both the NPs and the nanoparticle-entrapped DNA were monitored through the use of coumarin and luciferase labeled genes. The results[93] indicated that cells transfected with wt-p53 DNA-loaded NPs showed significantly greater antiproliferative effect than those with naked wt-p53 DNA or wt-p53 DNA complexed with a commercially available transfecting agent (Lipofectamine). The cells transfected with wt-p53 DNA-loaded NPs also showed sustained p53 mRNA levels compared to cells which were transfected with naked wt-p53 DNA exhibiting the sustained antiproliferative activity of NPs. Microscope examination of cells transfected with fluorescently labeled DNA indicated intracellular localization of DNA with NMs that may be interpreted as a result of the slow release of DNA from NMs localized inside the cells. Thus, this study showed that nanoparticle-mediated wt-p53 gene delivery resulted in antiproliferative activity, that can be used for cancer therapy.

Chitosan nanoparticles (cNPs) have also been demonstrated as effective gene-delivery vehicles.[73] pDNAs were transported in cNPs and expressed in the lung epithelium of mice. The results indicated that intranasal delivery of plasmids by cNPs resulted in sustained expression of the encoded protein in the lung which led to an effective supply therapeutic or prophylactic levels of an immunomodulatory molecule.

7.3.3 Electrostatic Loading of DNA in NMs

The negative nature of the DNA backbone is advantageous in linking with positively charged NMs leading to a DNA~NMs complexes that are formed through electrostatic binding between the positive charges of the NMs and the negative charges of the DNA (Figure 7.2). This electrostatic interaction is strong enough and is very easy to carry out in any laboratory. The 30 nm IOMNPs that are modified with amines exhibit an positive charge at low pH <5. When exposed to single strands of DNA (ssDNA), the IOMNPs easily form ssDNA~IOMNP complex. When the ssDNA~IOMNP complex is exposed to the complementary ssDNA, the double stranded DNA (dsDNA are formed on the surface of the IOMNP resulting in dsDNA~IOMNP. The formation of the dsDNA~IOMNP complex is verified with a dye that intercalates with dsDNA but not with a ssDNA. Acridine orange can intercalate with the dsDNA~IOMNP complex. The same process has also been used in liposome and other polymer-mediated gene transfer.[55,56,94] At Ocean NanoTech, 30 nm IOMNPs were used to capture dsDNA from lysed breast cancer cell line SK-BR3 as described below.

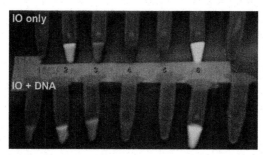

FIGURE 7.2 Amine functionalized IOMNP were used to capture dsDNA that was from lysed SK-BR3 cells. (Legend: 1-IO after dsDNA extraction, 2-supernatant 1 (SUP1) after capture and acridine orange (AO) addition, 3-SUP2 after capture+AO, 4-SUP3 after capture+AO, 5- SUP4 after capture+AO, 6-AO +buffer, 7-buffer). *Courtesy of Ocean NanoTech. (For color version of this figure, the reader is referred to the online version of this book)*

7.3.3.1 Protocol for the Electrostatic Loading of dsDNA in IOMNPs

The following protocol is used to prepare and verify the formation of dsDNA~IOMNP complex. The dsDNA was prepared from SK-BR3 breast cancer cell lines.

(1) Grow the SK-BR3 cells following manufacturer's protocol.

(2) When the cells reach 70–80% confluence, harvest following the manufacturer's protocol.

(3) Place 100,000 cells in a microcentrifuge tube.

(4) Centrifuge at 4000 rpm to precipitate the cells.

(5) Remove the supernatant and add 100 uL of Dulbecco's Phosphate-Buffered Saline (DPBS).

(6) Lyze the cells with lysozyme or sonicate for 15 min to rupture the cells.

(7) Take 0.5 mg of 30 nm IOMNPs that are amine functionalized (Ocean NanoTech Catalog # SHA30).

(8) Magnetize to isolate the IOMNPs from solution.

(9) Disperse in 100 uL deionized water (DI) water and adjust the pH to 5.

(10) Add the lyzed cells into the IOMNPs and vortex.

(11) Incubate in a slow shaker for 1 h.

(12) Centrifuge at 5000 rpm for 10 min.

(13) Discard the supernatant and save the pellet which consists of the IOMNP~dsDNA.

(14) Wash the IOMNP~dDNA three times with sodium citrate buffer (1×SSC).

(15) Reconstitute with 150 uL DI water.

(16) Add 50 uL of acridine orange.

(17) Put in a shaker for 20–30 min.

(18) Centrifuge at 5000 rpm for 10 min.

(19) Discard the supernatant and save the pellet which consists of the IOMNP~dsDNA+acridine orange.

(20) Wash the IOMNP~dDNA three times with sodium citrate buffer (1XSSC).

(21) Reconstitute with 1× SSC.

(22) Observe under UV light.

In the presence of dsDNA, intercalated acridine orange (AO) gives a yellow coloration to the otherwise black IOMNPs (Figure 7.2). This is exhibited by the tube 1 at the bottom of the picture that is labeled IO+DNA. After 4 times of washing, the supernatant did not exhibit the presence of AO anymore while the IOMNPs exposed to the lysed SK-BR3 still gave a yellow color. The IO that was not exposed to the lysed SK-BR3, and therefore, did not capture dsDNA remained black as shown in tube 1 on top labeled IO only.

7.4 NANOIMMUNOTHERAPY

The part of the human system which deals with antigens (foreign substances that stimulate antibody generation) is the immune system (IS). The IS consist of a dynamic network of cells that undergoes a process whereby it must recognize and deal with antigens or highly conserved structural motifs expressed by microbial pathogens, called pathogen-associated microbial patterns.[95] These processes involve adaptive (acquired or humoral) events on the surface of antigen-presenting cells (APCs) which perform the function of displaying antigens coupled with the major histocompatibility complex (MHC)[95] that are recognized by T-cells using their T-cell receptor (TCR) complexes. Recognition by APCs (macrophages, dendritic cells (DCs), and B cells) elicit an early innate immune response by cytokine communication. This steers the differentiation of T-helper (Th) cells into Th1 or Th2 subsets[96] that activate other cells of the immune system such as cytotoxic T cells and macrophages.[97] The DCs are responsible for connecting innate and adaptive immune responses and have particular functions at different stages of maturation.[95] Before activation, DCs are found in peripheral tissues as immature cells that capture self-antigens.[98] After the antigen is processed forming an antigen-loaded mature DC it moves to the secondary lymphoid organs where it induces antigen-specific immunity by presenting the antigen to T cells. This initiates T cell-mediated immunity through intracellular signaling that is mediated by the MHC and co-stimulatory molecules.[95]

NMs can modulate cellular and humoral immune responses and would be potentially useful as effective vaccine adjuvants for the therapy of infectious diseases and cancer.[99] NMs can be engineered with specific physical properties and chemical composition to be used as vehicles for specific DC targeting. Different strategies and approaches are available to use NMs as effective vehicles, including conjugation to antigens that are recognized by specific receptors; encapsulating antigens within NMs that potentially protect the antigen from degradation; and labeling NMs to be recognized by specific receptors and allow tracking of their journey in the host system.[95] These various approaches can be leveraged for various medical applications such as cancer immunotherapy, allergen therapy, and vaccine delivery to manipulate the immune system for enhanced therapeutic benefits as well as minimize side effects. In addition, different NMs are suitable for tracking that also allows the tracking of any material that is loaded in them to evaluate the correct migration of the NMs to its target.

Antigen interactions with different engineered NMs such as dendrimers, polymer, metallic NMs, MNMs, and QDs are important considerations in designing their particular medical applications. Thus, this chapter will focus on several NMs that will be used for immunotherapy. Two particular areas that will be discussed are nanoimmunotherapy for allergy and for cancer.

The oral route for allergen degradation is the most often used route because of convenience, safety, and because it is the least expensive. However, the disadvantages of oral immunotherapy for allergen degradation within the gut results from the gastric acidity or to the presence of proteolytic enzymes.[100] Clinical trials applying oral immunotherapy techniques for allergens were very poor.[101,102] Although some studies have shown a significant improvement of the allergic symptoms,[103,104] they had to administer high doses of allergen to observe successful treatment. At a lower dose of allergen, it would be essential to use an appropriate adjuvant to increase the immune response and prevent the allergen degradation in the gastrointestinal tract.[105]

The only adjuvant that is currently approved for human use is alum which had been demonstrated to have no capacity to elicit sufficient mucosal immune response and it is ineffective when administered by oral route.[105,106] Some mucosal adjuvants have been described such as monophosphoryl lipid A (MPL), CpG oligonucleotides or particulate mucosal delivery adjuvants such as immune-stimulating complexes (ISCOMs)[105,106] but these have limited efficacy when administered orally.[107–109] The use of adjuvants for delivery system with controlled release delivery systems in the form of micro[110] or NPs[111] as adjuvant have been proposed because they can potentially: (i) protect the loaded antigen from enzymatic degradation in the gastrointestinal tract, (ii) prolong immune response, (iii) enhance the delivery to the cells and gut associated lymphoid tissue (GALT), (iv) reduce the number of dosage.[111,112]

Several groups have studied the use of various NPs for immunotherapeutic applications.[61,67,73,84,95,105,111,113–116] The group of Salam used poly(methyl vinyl ether-comaleic anhydride, MW 200,000 to demonstrate bioadhesive capacity and high affinity toward normal mucosal tissue and Peyer's patches.[117] The group of Gomez[105] studied the immunotherapeutic effect when administered by oral route to a model of sensitized mice and demonstrated that poly(methyl vinyl ether-comaleic anhydride (Gantrez® AN)) NPs protected the sensitized mice from death by anaphylactic shock by using OVA complexed with NMs.

Chitosan, a cationic polysaccharide derived from the crustacean shell chitin is biocompatible[118,119] and in the form of NPs (100–200 nm), it has been used to deliver plasmids.[94,120] Chitosan has wound healing,[121] stimulation of the immune system,[122] anticoagulant,[123] antimicrobial,[124] and is non-toxic in humans.[73] In humans, it is non-hemolytic, weakly immunogenic, and slowly biodegradable that is why it has been used widely for controlled drug delivery.[125–127] Its muco-adhesive properties increase transcellular and paracellular transport across the mucosal epithelium that potentially facilitates gene delivery to mucosa- and bronchus-associated lymphoid tissue[128] making it an ideal agent for gene-delivery agent for effective gene expression therapy.[73]

cNPs have also been demonstrated as effective gene-delivery vehicles.[73] pDNAs were transported in cNPs and expressed in the lung epithelium of mice. The results indicated that intranasal delivery of plasmids by with cNPs resulted in sustained expression of the encoded protein in the lung which led to an effective supply of therapeutic or prophylactic levels of an immunomodulatory molecule. The group of Kong demonstrated treatment with chitosan interferon-γ (IFN-γ) plasmid deoxyribonucleic acid (DNA) NPs (chitosan interferon-γ nanogene [CIN or cIFN]) led to in situ production of IFN-γ and a reduction in inflammation and airway reactivity in mice. Recently, the effect of cIFN treatment on the immune responses of CD8+ T cells and dendritic cells was examined in a BALB/c mouse model of ovalbumin (OVA)-induced allergic asthma. Examination of dendritic cells from lung and lymph nodes indicated that cIFN treatment decreased their antigen-presenting activity that was shown from the lower CD80 and CD86 expression. In addition, the cIFN treatment reduced the level of CD11c+b+ dendritic cells in lymph nodes which possibly indicates that endogenous IFN-γ expression may immunomodulate dendritic cell migration and activation. The cIFN therapy resulted in the reduced levels of pro-inflammatory CD8+ T cells and antigen-presenting activity of dendritic cells.

Interferon-γ (IFN-γ) has been extensively studied for immunomodulatory and antiviral activity since its discovery.[73] Studies have shown that mice lacking the IFN-γ receptor exhibit a T-helper (Th)2-like cytokine profile that suggests that IFN-γ may play a role as a key cytokine in asthma.[129] IFN-γ delivers the stimulatory signal for interleukin (IL)-12,[129] which induces the Th1 response and inhibits Th2 cells by down-regulating the production of IL-4 and IL-5.[73] The interleukin IL-18 that induces IFN-γ also shifts the immune response from a Th2 to a Th1 state.[130] The interferons, IFN-α, IFN-β, and IFN-γ, inhibit leukotriene C_4 production in murine macrophages[131] while IFN-γ treatment of guinea pigs released prostanoids and nitric oxide that affected the airway epithelium that modified airway smooth muscle responses.[132] The production of IFN-γ and IFN-γ-dependent IL-12 in whole blood cultures is lower in patients with allergic asthma after stimulation with a mitogen.[133] As a result of the reciprocal regulation of T-helper cells, it was projected that IFN-γ level increases with the use of IFN-γ in cNPs (chitosan interferon-γ nanogene [cIFN]) would promote a Th1 response by blocking Th2 cytokine production.[73] Because the IFN-γ upregulates the IL-13Rα2 decoy receptor this causes diminished IL-13 signaling[134] as well as decreased goblet cell hyperplasia and eosinophilia.[135] In allergic individuals, IFN-γ inhibits the release of leukotrienes from peripheral blood leukocytes (PBLs) after wasp venom immunotherapy.[136] IFN-γ performs other functions that includes down-regulation of transforming growth factor β and procollagen I and III and decreases fibrosis in a mouse model of bleomycin-induced lung injury.[137] These cytokines, IFN-γ, IL-12, and IL-18, have limitations in vivo at moderate to high doses that can cause adverse effects[138] limiting their therapeutic applications.

Using the cloned cytokine complementary deoxyribonucleic acid (cDNA) under the regulation of a constitutive promoter, these have been applied as a means of boosting in vivo production of specific cytokines. For example, IFN-γ and IL-12 have proven effective as prophylactics and adjuncts in therapy against diverse human diseases.[139] The transfer of an expression of IL-12 gene in mouse airway cured airway eosinophilia and immunoglobulin E (IgE) synthesis.[140] Many other benefits from the use of IFN-γ, IL-12, and IL-18 gene therapy have been shown in different animal models[141,142] but the use of lipofectamine to transduce plasmids in mice are not directly applicable to humans because of issues of toxicity.[73]

Kong and collaborators[73] investigated the mechanism of cIFN-mediated immunomodulation using the mouse OVA-allergic asthma model. The summary of some of the studies they performed are given below.

7.4.1 Protocol for the Preparation of Chitosan IFN-γ pDNA NPs and Green Fluorescent Protein Test of Expression

In this study, Kong and collaborators,[73] used mouse IFN-γ cDNA that was cloned in the mammalian expression vector pVAX (Invitrogen, San Diego, CA) which was complexed with chitosan as previously described.[143] The stepwise process is as follows.

(1) Plasmids in 25 mM Na_2SO_4 and chitosan (Vanson, Redmond, WA) that was dissolved in 25 mM Na acetate, pH 5.4, to a final concentration of 0.02% were separately heated for 10 min at 55 °C.

(2) After heating mix the chitosan and the DNA (plasmid-encoding green fluorescent protein [pEGFP]).

(3) Vortex the mixture vigorously for 20–30 s.

(4) Store at room temperature until use.

(5) Take the Transmission electron microscopy (TEM) and Dynamic Light Scattering (DLS) to verify that the NMs are 200–300 nm diameter.

(6) Administer 10 μg of pEGFP intranasally to mice.

(7) After 1, 3, and 7 days, euthanize the mice.

(8) Collect the lungs and fix in buffered formalin.

(9) Embed the whole lungs in paraffin, section, and examine for GFP by fluorescent microscopy.

(10) Estimate the approximate percentage of GFP-positive cells.

In the same study, mice were allergen-sensitized by intraperitoneal injection of 50 μg of OVA (ovalbumin) adsorbed to 2 mg of alum which was followed by an intranasal challenge with 50 μg of OVA after 1 or 2 weeks.[73] Boosting

IFN-γ production on allergen sensitization was also tested by giving the mice an intranasal treatment of 10 µg of cIFN that constituted the prophylactic cIFN regimen. Some mice were given cIFN treatments after OVA sensitization as a therapeutic regimen. In both the prophylactic and therapeutic treatments, a final challenge with OVA were given before the mice were euthanized, and the lungs were perfused in situ with phosphate-buffered saline (PBS), removed, and fixed in 4% buffered formalin. From each group, lungs were left unfixed and homogenized for lymphocyte isolation.[73] The whole lungs that were for-malin-fixed were paraffin-embedded and sectioned into 15-micron portions. From each mouse two sections were dewaxed, rehydrated, and labeled with either anti-IL-12Rb2-fluorescein isothiocyanate (FITC) (Th1) or anti-T1/ST2L-rhodamine (Th2) that were examined with a Nikon TE300 fluorescence microscope.

7.4.2 The Use of Ceramic Core NPs as Delivery Systems for Immunotherapy

The group of Pandey[111] evaluated carbohydrate modified ultrafine ceramic core based NPs (aquasomes) as delivery systems (adjuvants) for immunotherapy with ovalbumin (OVA) as model allergen. Both humoral and cellular-induced immune responses were studied in BALB/c mice using aquasomes and alumi-num hydroxide as allergen-delivery systems following the protocol described below.

7.4.2.1 Preparation of Hydroxyapatite NMs

The hydroxyapatite (HA) core was first prepared following published protocols using the self-precipitation method.[144] The process is as follows:

(1) Add $0.5 M \cdot (NH_4)_2HPO_4$ to $0.5 M$ $Ca(NO_3)_2 \cdot 4H_2O$ ethanol solution with vigorous stirring. The pH of both solutions has to be 10 by adding NH_4OH drop wise.

(2) Stir the mixture vigorously for 1 h using mechanical stirrer (REMI C-24, Mumbai, India).

(3) Dry the mixture at 40 °C in oven overnight.

(4) Collect and wash the precipitated hydroxyapatite (ceramic) particles with ethanol and then with distilled DI water.

(5) Dry the washed ceramic particles overnight at 40 °C.

(6) Use Fourier transformed infrared spectroscopy (FT-IR) for structure analy-sis. Prepare the KBr sample disk using 1% (w/w) of hydroxyapatite pow-der and dry at 100 °C. Record the spectra at 4000 to 400 cm^{-1} (resolution 4.0 cm^{-1}).

(7) Perform phase analysis using X-ray diffraction (XRD) with Cu Kα radia-tion ($45 kV \times 40 mA$) in a wide-angle X-ray diffractometer (XRD-6000, Shimadzu, Japan).

(8) Take the TEM for shape and size analysis. Place one drop of aqueous dispersion over a 400-mesh carbon-coated copper grid followed by negative staining with phosphotungstic acid (3%, w/v, adjusted to pH 4.7 with KOH) and place at the accelerating voltage of 80 kV.

(9) Record the mean hydrodynamic diameter, polydispersity and zeta potential of core by photon correlation spectroscopy (PCS) using Zeta Nano ZS 90 (Malvern, UK) after appropriate dilution (1:200) with PBS pH 7.4 prior to analysis.

Aquasomes are prepared using tin oxide, hydroxyapatite (HA), diamond and brushite (calcium phosphate dihydrate).[145–147] Hydroxyapatite is biodegradable, inexpensive, stable, and safe. It is used for tissue engineering, implants, as well as for drug and antigen delivery[148–159] and particularly useful for protein delivery because of high adsorption capability.[160]

HA particles prepared following the above process were smaller in size and crystalline in nature.[111] The Fourier transform infrared spectroscopy (FTIR) bands for PO_4^{-3} of the calcined powder were observed at 507, 604, 945, 964, 1024, and 1184 cm^{-1}, whereas the medium sharp peak at 633, 2910, and 3570 cm^{-1} was due to the OH^{-1} bending deformation (Figure 7.3).[111]

The X-ray diffraction patterns of HA showed characteristic intense absorption peaks at 31–32, 49–50, 25–27 (2θ angle) which are indicative of the crystalline behavior (Figure 7.4).[111] The ultrafine nanosize spherical morphology of the HA core is shown in the TEM image. The DLS results supported the TEM data with 39 nm particle diameter having a polydispersity index of 0.28.[111]

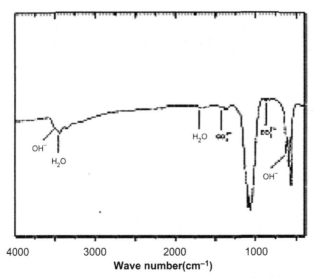

FIGURE 7.3   The FTIR spectra of hydroxyapatite core particles obtained from the mixture of calcium nitrate and di-ammonium hydrogen phosphate. *From Pandey 2011.*

7.4.2.2 Preparation and Characterization of OVA Adsorbed Aquasomes

The OVA loaded hydroxyapatite NMs were prepared with slight modifications of a reported process.[111,146] The process is described below.

(1) Mix 15 mg of hydroxyapatite into a beaker with 30 mL of 29.2 mM trehalose with vigorous stirring.

(2) Sonicate the suspension for 10 min at approximately 20 kHz at 25 °C using a probe sonicator (Soniweld India Ltd., Mumbai, India).

(3) Centrifuge the dispersion at 10,000 rpm for 20 min at 4 °C.

(4) Discard any remaining pellets.

(5) Lyophilize the supernatant at a condenser temperature of −82 °C and pressure of less than 10−1 mbar using trehalose as stabilizer.

(6) Dissolve in 20 mL of 25 mM phosphate buffer, pH 7.4.

(7) Remove excess trehalose centrifugation.

(8) Take 10 mg of the trehalose coated NMs (ceramic/carbohydrate based biocompatible and biodegradable nanoparticulate system called "aquasomes") and disperse in 8 mg/mL OVA in PBS pH 7.4 OVA.

(9) Incubate the solution at 4 °C overnight.

(10) Wash the OVA adsorbed aquasomes with DI water.

(11) Centrifuge at 10,000 rpm for 30 min.

(12) Repeat the washing three times and store at 4 °C.

(13) Characterize as in the previous section.

(14) Establish the sugar content on surface of hydroxyapatite following the anthrone method161 using glucose as standard.

(15) Establish the integrity of the OVA by SDS-PAGE under non-denaturing condition.[111] Extract the OVA out by dissolving the aquasomes in 2 mL of 5% (w/v) SDS in 0.1 N HCl. Use Coomassie blue staining for the protein bands.

The results indicated that the aquasome formulations were spherical and elongated in shape. Photon correlation spectroscopy (PCS) confirmed the nanometer

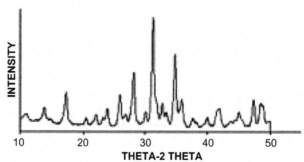

FIGURE 7.4   X-ray diffraction pattern of hydroxyapatite core particles obtained from the mixture of calcium nitrate and di-ammonium hydrogen phosphate. *From Pandey, 2011.*

size of the aquasomes. The results of both TEM (Figure 7.5) and PCS indicated that the aquasomes were about 47 ± 19 nm with a polydispersity of 0.32. The OVA loading was estimated at 60 ± 2 ug/mg.[111]

7.4.2.3 Adsorption Efficiency and OVA Release from Aquasomes

The percent efficiency of OVA adsorption on aquasomes is determined as follows[146]:

(1) Weigh out 200 mg of OVA adsorbed aquasome formulations and suspended in Triton-X 100 (0.01%, w/v).
(2) Incubate in a wrist action shaker for 1 h.
(3) Centrifuge at 14,000 rpm for 15 min.
(4) Collect the supernatant and perform micro BCA method for protein analysis using aquasome formulation treated in the same manner as blank.
(5) For in vitro release studies, take 200 mg of OVA adsorbed aquasomes and suspend in phosphate buffer (pH 7.4, 10 mL) with slow magnetic stirring. Withdraw 1 mL samples every 15 min followed by centrifugation (1700 rpm for 10 min at 4 °C).

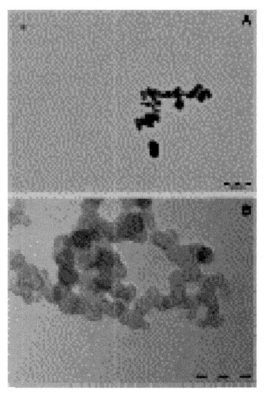

FIGURE 7.5   TEM image of antigen-loaded formulation of: (A) plain hydroxyapatite ceramic core and (B) OVA adsorbed aquasomes. *From Pandey, 2011.*

(6) Measure the protein released in the supernatant by BCA protein assay at various times. Add equal quantity of fresh buffer after each sampling to maintain the sink conditions. Take the volume and protein quantity from the portions that were removed at each time point into consideration during calculations.

The freeze dry coating with trehalose indicated that HA core adsorbed 2.9% of the trehalose giving a slightly negative zeta potential which confirmed the coating of sugar layer.[111] Adsorption loading of OVA gave negative zeta potential value of -11.34 ± 1.4 mV. The release of OVA every 10 min shown indicated that about 40% of the absorbed OVA was released into the medium. After 30 min, subsequent release of OVA was small and decreased over time giving a cumulative OVA release in 50 min at about 90%.[111]

7.4.2.4 In Vivo Immunological Response

The aquasomes prepared in the previous section can be used to harness immunological response in female BALB/c mice (age 7–9 weeks; weight 15–20 g). The mice have to be properly housed (23 ± 2 °C; RH: 60%) with 12 h light–dark cycle controlled animal quarters in group of six ($n = 6$) and fed standard rodent pellet and have free access to drinking water. Immunizations can follow after one week of acclimatization with the environment. This process was published and implemented by Pandey's group[111] involved no food intake 3 h before immunization. Animal immunizations regimen are described below.

(1) The animals are immunized by two intradermal injections with two weeks interval, i.e. at day 0 (priming) and at day 14 (boosting) with one of the following: (i) free OVA (10 μg per mouse) in 50 μl of PBS; (ii) blank aquasomes 100 μg in 50 μl of PBS; (iii) OVA aquasomes (equivalent of 10 μg of OVA per mouse); and (iv) OVA in alum (OVA alum) and (v) sterile PBS 50 μl only. OVA alum are prepared by dissolving the protein (50 μg/mL) in PBS (pH 7.4, 0.01 M) and subsequently mixing by sonication with aluminum hydroxide gel (1 mg/mL).

(2) Blood from the saphenous vein of mice (under mild ether anesthesia) are collected at day 0 (pre-immune sera, 3 h before immunization), 14 days and 42 days (terminal samples) of priming.

(3) Terminal blood samples are taken by cardiac puncture post euthanasia.

(4) The serum is separated by centrifugation at 1500×g for 5 min after coagulation for 30 min at room temperature.

(5) Serum samples are stored at -22 °C until use.

(6) The spleen of three mice from each group are surgically removed for the cytokine assay.

7.4.2.5 Measurement of Humoral Response

The immune response in terms of level of OVA-specific IgG antibodies and isotypes is established using indirect immunoassay. The assay is performed in a 96-well plate.

(1) Coat each well (NUNC-Immune Plate® Fb96 Maxisorb, Nunc, India) with 100 uL of antigen (100 µg/mL, 50 µg/mL, 25 µg/mL OVA in bicarbonate buffer, pH 9.6).

(2) Seal the plate and incubate at 4 °C overnight.

(3) Wash the plate three times with PBS-Tween 20 (PBS-T, 0.05%, v/v).

(4) Block with 150 µL of 3% gelatin in PBS for 90 min at 37 °C.

(5) Wash three times with PBS-T.

(6) Place 100 µL of serum (1:800) in gelatin in PBS-T20.

(7) Incubate at RT for 90 min and wash again three times.

(8) Put 100 µL of horse radish peroxidase (HRP) labeled goat anti-mouse IgG, IgG2a or IgG1 (1:1000) in each well.

(9) Seal the plates and incubate for 1 h at RT.

(10) Repeat the washing step.

(11) Place 100 µL of substrate O-phenylenediamine dihydrochloride (OPD) (prepared in citrate buffer $+ H_2O_2$) or tetramethyl benzidene (TMB) enzyme substrate.

(12) Incubate for at least 10 min at RT or until color development ensues.

(13) When full color is developed, add 25 µL of 2.5 M H_2SO_4 to stop the reaction.

(14) Measure the absorbance at 492 nm. The OD at 492 or at 450 is a measure of the level of immune response. The response is directly proportional to the level of the IgG, IgG2, or IgG1 when the horse radish peroxidase (HRP) is attached to goat anti-mouse IgG, IgG2a or IgG1, respectively. A calibration curve for each of these antibodies must be established to quantify the signals.

7.4.2.6 Estimation of Cytokine Levels

The effect of the OVA and the NMs were evaluated by Pandey[111] in terms of the levels of IL-4 and IFN-γ in mouse spleen homogenates using ELISA kits for cytokines.[116] This process involved the following protocol.

(1) Separate and weigh the individual spleens from euthanized mice.

(2) Homogenize the spleens in ice-cold RPMI containing 1% 3-(cholamido-propyl-o-dimethylammonio)-1-propanesulphonate (CHAPS; Sigma) in a micro tissue homogenizer.

(3) Store the 10% (w/v) homogenates for 1 h at 2–4 °C.

(4) Centrifuge at 2000×g for 20 min to remove insoluble debris.

(5) Apply the mouse cytokine assay kit from eBioscience (San Diego, CA) to determine the levels of cytokines following the manufacturer's instructions.

(6) Use the standard curve provided by the manufacturer for IL-4 and IFN-γ to estimate the levels that are expressed in pg/mL.

Fifteen days after therapy, animals were challenged with OVA and different signs of anaphylactic shock were evaluated. Developed aquasomes possessed a negative zeta potential (−11.3 mV) and an average size of 47 nm with OVA adsorption efficiency of ~60.2 µg mg⁻¹ of hydroxyapatite core. In vivo immune response after two intradermal injections with OVA adsorbed aquasomes resulted in a mixed Th1/Th2-type immune response. OVA-sensitized mice model, treatment with OVA adsorbed aquasomes elicited lower levels of IgE ($p < 0.05$), serum histamine and higher survival rate in comparison with alum adsorbed OVA. Symptoms of anaphylactic shock in OVA aquasome-treated mice were weaker than the one induced in the alum adsorbed OVA group. Results from their studies demonstrated the valuable use of aquasomes in allergen immunotherapy.[111]

7.4.3 NMs for Tumor Immunotherapy

Tumors induce local immune suppression as a mechanism to avoid detection and elimination by the host immune system and also elicit immune responses against tumor-associated self-antigens.[115,162,163] Strategies to combat such immunosuppression using non-cell-based therapies such as cytokines, immune receptor-targeting monoclonal antibodies, or Toll-like Receptor (TLR) agonists to break tumor-associated tolerance, by blocking tumor-induced suppressive factors or directly providing the co-stimulatory signals have been studied prime an anti-tumor immune response.[164–168] However, the side effects of these immune-agonists dampen their clinical value to achieve therapeutic efficacy while avoiding excessive systemic exposure.[169–171]

Two immunostimulatory agents that exhibit the two edged action of immunotherapy are anti-CD40 antibodies and CpG oligonucleotides.[115] The CD40 signaling triggered through the anti-CD40 ligation leads to strong activating signals to APCs providing them the capacity to prime strong anti-tumor cytotoxic T-cell responses.[172,173] The efficacy of anti-CD40 therapy against a wide variety of tumor models, either as a monotherapy[174,175] and combined with chemotherapy,[176] or combined with other immunostimulants such as interleukin (IL)-2[177] have been documented in pre-clinical studies. The application of anti-CD40 therapy in phase I clinical trials for human patients have also been reported for non-Hodgkins lymphoma, multiple myeloma, and other solid malignancies.[178–180] These achieved moderate levels of therapeutic efficacy but the maximum tolerated dose for human therapy has been limited by inflammation in non-target organs.[178,180,181] Intravenous administration of anti-CD40 leads to systemic exposure to the immuno-agonist that causes various symptoms of cytokine release syndrome (such as fever, headaches, nausea, chills), ocular inflammation, elevated hepatic enzymes (indicative of liver damage), and hematologic toxicities including T-cell depletion.[115] Inflammatory effects in the liver, lungs, and gut have been documented in mice including evidence of systemic cytokine release.[182–184] Most of the reported side effects were transient but long-term immunosuppression following anti-CD40 therapy that was possibly related to the activation-induced apoptosis of CD4+ or CD8+ T-cells has been reported in mice.[185]

The CpG oligonucleotides, ligands for Toll-like receptor (TLR) 9 expressed by APCs belong to another class of potent immunostimulatory factors that has been tested against a wide variety of tumor models in mice showing tumor inhibition or regression.[166,186,187] In combinations of CD40 agonists and TLR ligands, highly potent anti-tumor responses were stimulated in vivo.[188,189] But, systemic overexposure to CpG with dangerous side effects such as lymphoid follicle destruction and the suppression of adaptive T-cell immunity via indoleamine 2,3-dioxygenase (IDO) induction in the spleen and have been reported.[190–192]

As a result of the dangers of systemic immunostimulatory therapy, intratumoral or peritumoral treatments have been studied to reduce the level of side effects.[115] Local immunotherapy has been proposed for the treatment of unresectable tumors or for post-surgical therapy to prevent local recurrence.[193,194] Anti-CD40[175], CpG,[195] target antibody-cytokine (IL-2) fusion proteins,[196] or other immunostimulants[167,197,198] that successfully inhibited the growth of distal untreated tumors when used as local therapies applied at a single tumor site.[115] Recently in a phase I clinical trial, the intratumoral injection of CpG against B-cell lymphoma in humans exhibited anti-lymphoma clinical responses at distant, untreated tumor sites in some patients.[199] But despite such therapeutic benefits, it has been established in pre-clinical and clinical studies that local injection of soluble agonists[200,201] or controlled release of drugs from a local injection site[202,203] does not prevent such agonists from entering the systemic circulation and dispersing to distal organs through drainage through lymphatics to the thoracic duct or via direct entry into the bloodstream from leaky tumor vessels. Subcutaneous or intratumoral administrations of cytokines IL-2[204] or IL-12/GM-CSF[205] in mice showed rapid clearance within minutes after injection. In human patients, intratumoral/subcutaneous injection showed high circulating levels of IL-12[206] or IL-2[201] within 30 min or 3 h (respectively). Thus, the undesired widespread exposure and off-target inflammatory symptoms may still limit the maximum tolerated dose in local immunotherapy.[115]

A biomaterial-based delivery strategy for immunostimulatory factors that could retain injected therapeutics at a local tumor site, limit the tissue drainage, and maintain their potent therapeutic efficacy in activating an anti-tumor immune response will be ideal for immunotherapy. With this as a goal, the group of Kwong[115] coupled anti-CD40 and CpG to the surface of PEGylated unilamellar liposomes, for simultaneous co-delivery. Attaching both molecules to liposomal carriers for a more confined biodistribution after intratumoral injection would enhance local retention while maintaining bioactivity. The studied carried out to achieve their goal are presented and their protocols may be applied to other immunotherapeutic ensembles and NPs.

7.4.3.1 Protocol for the Synthesis of Liposome-anchored Anti-CD40 and CpG[115]

The liposomes that are synthesized using this protocol are specifically designed for the anti-CD40 and CpG. The process may also be used for other biomolecules with respective optimization of the various parameters.

(1) Liposomes with a composition of cholesterol/DOPC/maleimide-PEG-DSPE/PEG-DSPE 35/50/5/10 by mol% is synthesized.

(2) A 0.5 mol% of fluorescent rhodamine-labeled DOPE is also incorporated for biodistribution experiments (histology and flow cytometry).

(3) The lipids are vacuum-dried, rehydrated in PBS at 15 μmol/mL.

(4) Sonicate the lipids for 4 min (alternating 5–7 Watts) using a Misonix probe-tip sonicator (Qsonica, Newtown, CT) to form unilamellar liposomes.

(5) Prepare the anti-CD40 with exposed free hinge region thiols by mixing anti-CD40 (12–15 mg/mL) with a 25× molar excess of DTT for 20 min at 25 °C in the presence of 10 mm EDTA in PBS.

(6) Pass the mildly reduced anti-CD40 through a desalting column to remove DTT.

(7) Immediately mix with maleimide-functionalized liposomes at a ratio of 1 mg Ab:2.5 μmol liposomes for covalent coupling in the presence of 10 mm EDTA.

(8) Allow the maleimide–thiol reaction to proceed for at least 10 h at 25 °C.

(9) Centrifuge the resulting liposome aggregates and wash multiple times with PBS to remove unbound antibody.

(10) Syringe extrude the anti-CD40-liposomes 25× through 100 nm polycarbonate filter membranes (Avanti Polar Lipids).

Lipid-conjugated CpG can be prepared as previously described.[207] In this process, the liposome phosphoramidite is added to the CpG during synthesis for 15 min, using the DNA synthesizer. After synthesis, CpG and CpG-PEG-lipid conjugates are purified by reverse phase HPLC. The liposomes bearing anti-CD40 + CpG are prepared by post-insertion approach to insert the purified CpG-lipid conjugate onto the surface of anti-CD40-conjugated liposomes. This process is as follows:

(1) Mix ~3 nmol CpG-lipid with 1 umol anti-CD40-liposomes for 2 h at 25 °C.

(2) Centrifuge the resulting combination liposomes and wash multiple times with PBS.

(3) Syringe extrude to remove unimer or micellar CpG-lipid through a 200 nm polycarbonate filter membranes (Avanti).

(4) Characterize the liposome size distributions by dynamic light scattering.

(5) Store in PBS at 4 °C until use.

7.4.3.2 Quantification of Anti-CD40 and CpG on Liposomes[115]

An ELISA assay is used to quantify the amount of anti-CD40 or CpG on the liposomes. To carry this out, the following protocol is followed.

(1) Mix the anti-CD40-conjugated to liposomes with PBS containing 0.5% Tween 20 surfactant to solubilize the lipids.

(2) Coat standard 96-well plates with 2 μg/mL of goat anti-human IgG antibody.

(3) Add 100 ng/mL recombinant mouse CD40/human Fc fusion protein. Use of recombinant CD40 as the capture agent for lipid-anchored anti-CD40 ensured that only bioactive anti-CD40 still capable of binding its target receptor would be quantified.

(4) Add the solubilized anti-CD40+liposomes with PBS containing 0.5% Tween 20 and incubate for 2 h.

(5) Wash three times with PBS containing 0.5% Tween 20.

(6) Add 200 ng/mL of HRP-conjugated goat anti-rat IgG and incubate for 1 h.

(7) Wash three times with PBS containing 0.5% Tween 20.

(8) Place 100 uL HRP-anti goat IgG and incubate for 30 min or until color development is complete.

(9) Stop the reaction with 3 N HCl.

(10) Measure the absorbance at 492 nm.

(11) Determine the anti-CD40 concentration against a standard.

(12) The CpG and CpG-lipid were both tracked using a fluorescent FAM label on the 3′ end. The fluorescence was measure at 480ex and 520em wavelengths.

7.4.4 Release of Anti-CD40 and CpG from Liposomes In vitro[115]

To measure the *in vitro* release of anti-CD40 or CpG-lipid from combination liposomes, dialysis cassettes (1 mL capacity) with a 300 kD MWCO membrane were used (Float-a-lyzer G2, Spectrum Labs, Rancho Dominguez, CA). 400 μL samples were dialyzed against 20 mL PBS containing 10% fetal calf serum, with gentle agitation, at 37 °C. Samples and dialysis buffers were collected at each indicated time point; anti-CD40 was measured by sandwich ELISA and CpG was measured by its fluorescent label FAM. All samples were mixed with 0.5% Tween 20 to disrupt intact liposomes prior to the anti-CD40 ELISA.

The stability of anti-CD40 and CpG complexed with PEGylated liposomes were measured in terms of the release of the immunostimulatory ligands *in vitro* in the presence of serum. The combination liposomes carrying anti-CD40 and CpG were dialyzed (300 kD MWCO membrane in PBS pH 7.4 containing 10% fetal calf serum) at 37 °C. The release of ligands into the dialysis buffer indicated that anti-CD40 and CpG both diffused freely into the buffer with substantial release in <5 h. In contrast, the PEG-DSPE-anchored anti-CD40 only showed <10% released over 7 days. The CpG-lipid inserted into combination liposomes was retained by the vesicles inefficiently allowing ~80% release in 24 h that was complete in ~7 days. The release materials were confirmed with gel electrophoresis.

When used with live animals, the anti-CD40-liposomes did not directly exert cytotoxic effects on B16 tumor cells during *in vitro* culture[115] with minimal nonspecific binding of immunoliposomes to the tumor cells. During *in vivo* studies, locally administered soluble anti-CD40 strongly inhibited B16 tumor growth, while the anti-CD40-liposomes slowed tumor growth by ~50% as effectively as the soluble antibody. In terms of systemic effects, the locally administered soluble anti-CD40 caused a significant weight loss in mice for several days after initiation of therapy.[115] On the other hand, the anti-CD40-liposomes treatment did not cause significant weight loss relative to PBS-treated controls at any time point.[115] Circulating serum levels of IL-6 provided indication of systemic inflammation in response to immunostimulant therapy. The anti-CD40 that was intratumorally injected caused a significant increase in serum IL-6 within 24 h but the anti-CD40-liposomes induced levels in serum were insignificant compared with the control mice. The studies of Kwong indicated the potential benefits of liposome anchoring but it inhibited the anti-tumor efficacy of anti-CD40 monotherapy.

The anti-tumor efficacy of liposomal combination anti-CD40/CpG in the B16 model showed a delay in tumor growth compared to untreated animals but eventually all succumbed.[115] The combination of soluble CpG with soluble anti-CD40 provided only a modest enhancement over soluble anti-CD40 alone. No significant difference in survival benefit was observed between either regimen of soluble therapy ($p = 0.33$, n.s. by log-rank test).

In contrast, the liposomal anti-CD40/CpG showed a significant increase in the time to progression for partial responders from a mean of 27.8 ± 1.4 days for soluble treatment to 33.4 ± 1.8 days for liposomal anti-CD40/CpG.[115] The liposome-anti-CD40/CpG therapy prolonged the survival of tumor-bearing mice and exhibited a longer survival period. Additionally, the combinatorial liposome therapy demonstrated a significant increase in potency compared with liposomal anti-CD40 alone.[115] A synergistic effect in the particle-mediated co-delivery of both immunostimulants can be inferred from these observations.

The use of biomaterial systems for the local delivery of anti-CD40, CpG, and immunomodulatory cytokines have been described using liposomes and NPs to larger microspheres and hydrogels. A variety of biomaterial carriers demonstrated significant anti-tumor effects of IL-2, IL-12, and/or GM-CSF in therapeutic challenge models, but the systemic inflammatory effects were not examined.[204,205,208] In the setting of prophylactic vaccinations (or pre-tumor challenge), Hatzifoti et al.[209] demonstrated that liposomal entrapment decreased anti-CD40-induced toxicity (as measured by splenomegaly), while another study[200] showed that subcutaneous injection of cationic gelatin NMs complexed with CpG DNA and vaccine antigens reduced systemic cytokine induction relative to soluble injections of the agonist (via decreased systemic exposure to nanoparticle-bound CpG compared to unencapsulated CpG).[115] In another study, when De Jong et al.[203] used liposomes to encapsulate CpG DNA they found that subcutaneous liposomal delivery significantly increased plasma levels of inflammatory cytokine compared with subcutaneous free CpG. These observations might reflect differences in the stability of agonist entrapment in the various carriers since soluble drugs or immuno-agonists released from locally-injected carriers have been shown to reach the systemic circulation as early as 6 h post-injection.[202,205] These observations amplify the benefits of physically anchoring immunomodulatory compounds to the carriers compared to more commonly used encapsulation/release strategies.[115]

Various leukocyte cell populations have been implicated in mediating the anti-tumor effects of anti-CD40 and CpG therapies.[115] Activation of APCs such as dendritic cells, macrophages, and B cells with TLR9 is known to potentiate antigen cross-priming, the production of T_H1-skewed cytokines, and the induction of potent CTL and NK-cell responses.[210] Different studies have suggested DCs, macrophages, B cells, or combinations thereof as the primary cells responsible for priming potent CTL or NK-cell activity[173,174,211] or T-cell independent[212] immune responses but the mechanisms of anti-CD40 tumor inhibition are currently less well defined.[115] Analysis indicated that DCs and macrophages had taken up CpG and rhodamine-labeled liposomes following the injection of combination liposomes which indicated that the liposomal carriers had not prevented them from reaching target APCs[115] and the tumor-draining lymph node at a higher level than soluble free CpG.

The studies reported by Kwong's group showed that liposome NPs were effective in carrying both the anti-CD40 and the CpG.[115] Coupling of these ligands to the liposome surface retains them at a high level in the tumor and the surrounding tissues following intratumoral injection, allowing presentation to APCs at the tumor and the tumor-draining lymph node and at the same time, restricting them from entering systemic circulation or reaching distal lymphoid organs.[115]

7.4.5 NMs for Vaccine Delivery

Recently, the use of <15 nm, water soluble, inorganic NPs as a vaccine-delivery system for a blood stage malaria vaccine has been reported.[213] Amphiphilic polymer-coated QD CdSe/ZnS NPs were modified with recombinant proteins, rMSP1, via surface carboxyl groups to form rMSP1-QDs. In mice injected with the rMSP1-QDs, the anti-MSP1 antibody responses were found to have 2–3 log higher titers than those obtained with rMSP1 administered with the conventional vaccine adjuvants, Montanide ISA51 and CFA (Figure 7.6).[213] In addition, the immune response (IL-4 and IFN-γ) (Figure 7.7)[213] and induction of parasite inhibitory antibodies were significantly higher in mice injected with rMSP1-QDs. Antibody titers using the rMSP1-QDs were not affected by route of injection such as intraperitoneal (i.p.), intramuscular (i.m.), and subcutaneous (s.c.) (Figure 7.7).[213] The high level of immunogenicity exhibited by the rMSP1-QDs was achieved without further addition of other adjuvant components.

Bone marrow derived dendritic cells (BMDCs) were shown to efficiently take up the NPs leading to their activation and the expression/secretion of key cytokines, suggesting that this may be a mode of action for the enhanced immunogenicity.[213] The RT-PCR quantification of expression of six cytokine genes in QD-stimulated dendritic cells expressed and secreted markedly high levels of pro-inflammatory cytokines (IL-6, IL-1a, TNF-a) and chemokines (CCL3, CCL4, CXCL1) necessary for efficient immune responses, especially toward a TH1-mediated immunity.[213] The level of chemokines produced showed that

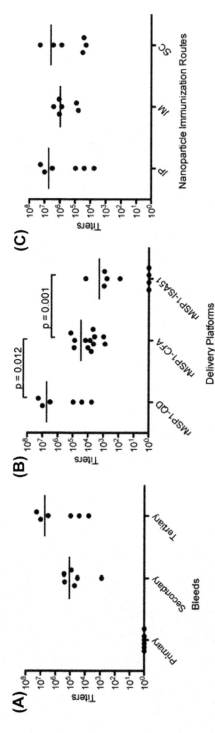

FIGURE 7.6 Antibody response in Swiss Webster mice. Antibody titers from (A) mice vaccinated (IP) with rMSP1-QD and (B) mice vaccinated with different adjuvant/delivery platforms (rMSP1-QD, rMSP1-CFA, and rMSP1-ISA51). (C) Tertiary bleed antibody response in mice vaccinated with rMSP1-QD via different routes (i.p., i.m., and s.c.). Horizontal bars indicate mean antibody titers. Significant differences in ELISA titers among vaccination groups are indicated with *p*-values (Mann–Whitney test). *From Pusic, 2011.*

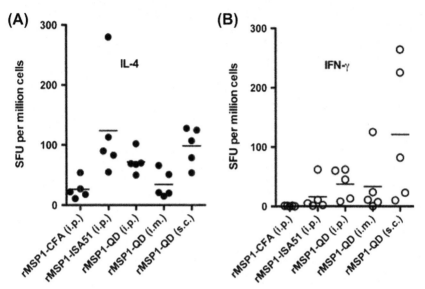

FIGURE 7.7   IL-4 and IFN-γ responses induced by rMSP1-QD and other adjuvants. A) MSP1-specific IL-4 and B) IFN-γ as determined by ELISPOT. Horizontal bars indicate mean SFU. Mouse splenocytes were harvested 21 days after the last immunization. *Courtesy of Pusic et al., 2011.*

stimulation of BMDCs by QDs enhance the migratory characteristics of these immune cells resulting in more efficient antigen presentation and/or T cell activation. The QDs showed induction of the production of some chemokines (CCL3/CCL4) at levels similar to those that are induced by LPS stimulated BMDCs which indicated their potential to activate a strong immune response as shown in Figure 7.8.[213]

When the purified tertiary bleed mouse antibodies were pooled and tested for parasite inhibition in vitro, the antibodies produced using QD-based delivery inhibited parasite growth from 73% to 81% (Table 7.1). The antibodies produced using the QD-based vaccine delivery were more potent in inhibiting the *Plasmodium falciparum* growth compared with the antibodies induced by commercial adjuvants, CFA, and Montanide ISA51.[213] The study provides promising results for water soluble, inorganic NPs (<15 nm) as platforms to enhance the immunogenicity of peptide vaccine candidates in adjuvant-free immunizations.

7.5 NMs FOR THERMAL ABLATION

For patients with unresectable malignancies, the standard of care is chemotherapy and external beam radiation.[3] When these do not work out, alternative treatments are needed. Currently, local thermal ablation under ultrasound or computed tomography guidance are used as alternative methods.[214,215] Thermal ablation uses heat treatment to destroy a tissue or to impair its function. This method has been routinely used for the treatment of uterine bleeding, atrial fibrillation primary lung

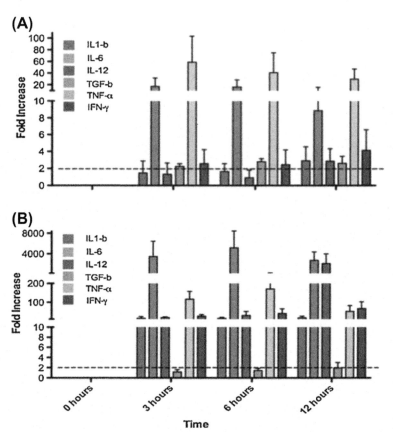

FIGURE 7.8 RT-PCR quantification of expression of six cytokine genes in QD-stimulated dendritic cells (A) and LPS-stimulated dendritic cells (B) over a 12-h period. Data were normalized to GAPDH and fold changes were calculated based on "0 h" samples. *From Pusic et al., 2011. (For color version of this figure, the reader is referred to the online version of this book)*

TABLE 7.1 In vitro *P. falciparum* Growth Inhibition by Antibodies of Mouse Immunized with Various MSP1 Formulations

Tertiary Bleed	% Growth Inhibition
rMSP1-QD (i.p.)	81
rMSP1-QD (i.m.)	73
rMSP1-QD (s.c.)	78
rMSP1-QD (s.c.)	17
rMSP1-ISA51 (i.p.)	0

and liver cancers and liver metastasis.[216] Thermal ablation is achieved by using different sources of heating, like laser light, focused ultrasound, microwaves, radiofrequency field, and magnetic resonance.[3] The most common traditional method is radiofrequency ablation (RFA) which utilize the natural differences in properties of the normal and carcinogenic tissues to achieve differential heat deposition.[3] RFA has low side effects in the treatment of primary and metastatic liver tumors[3] even though it requires targeting of each individual lesion. In RFA therapy, complete destruction of the entire tumor with at least a 0.5 cm margin by heating the tissue between 50–100 °C, forming "coagulation necrosis" is the ultimate goal. Radio waves produce heat through resistive forces by ionic agitation as they travel from the implanted electrode tip to the ground source placed outside the body. RF energy has been shown to have low tissue specific absorption rates (SAR) allowing for excellent whole body tissue penetration with documented safety in humans exposed to an RF field for 10 min up to several hours. But, the difference in sensitivity between normal and abnormal tissues is too small, so normal tissue can be damaged under RF irradiation.[3] Furthermore, the heterogeneity of electrical conductivity of tissues does not allow selective heating.

To solve these issues, NMs are being studied to increase the contrast between the two tissues for effective treatment.[3] The use of submicron particles to enable cellular uptake that cause intracellular hyperthermia has been suggested to increase the selectivity of the thermal destruction. The use of NMs introduce advantages such as increased sensitivity to radiofrequency energy, lower required doses and exposure times, selective delivery, and improved homogeneity of heat induction.[3] Currently, the NMs being studied for thermal ablation therapies include superparamagnetic iron oxide nanoparticles (SPIONs), paramagnetic copper–nickel alloy NPs, magnetite cationic liposomes, carbon particles (single walled carbon nanotubes and fullerenes), AuNPs and nanoshells.[3]

7.5.1 Thermal Ablation Using MNPs

An approach to thermal ablation involves seeding the tumor with MNPs for selective generation of heat in the tumor.[3] Iron oxide nanoparticles (IONPs) have very good magnetic properties that allow them to heat up when placed in an alternating magnetic field by hysteresis loss, induced eddy currents and Neel relaxation.[217] NMs composed of Fe_3O_4 were tested for heat induction in human breast cancer xenografts in immunodeficient mice by loading the tumors with 7.7 ± 2.3 mg magnetite per 100 mg tissue.[218] When the mice were exposed to an AC magnetic field for 4 min at an amplitude of 6.5 kA/m and frequency of 400 kHz using a circular coil applicator,[3] the results showed elevated temperatures between 18 and 55 °C at sites containing magnetite agglomerates but there were heterogeneous particle distribution. Furthermore, migration of particles from the tumor tissue that were similar to those observed in human Phase I studies for the treatment of prostate cancer were recorded.[219] These situations must be addressed during further developments for tumor applications.

In a study involving rabbits with malignant kidney tumors, SPIONs using CT guided placement were implanted[218] which were later exposed to an alternating electromagnetic field (0.32 kA/m) for 15 min. The tumor necrosis was verified with CT perfusion imaging and histological evaluation. They also studied the effect of a single injection of SPIONs (8–10 nm) compared with continuous infusion during exposure to the magnetic field.[220] They showed that continuous infusion of SPIONs resulted in a larger zone of necrosis compared with the single injection, but, non-uniform ferrofluid distribution led to highly variable size coagulation necrosis.[220]

Studies involving AuNPs and nanoshells that can be remotely activated by near infrared light (NIR, 650–950 nm) are very interesting because they are generally biocompatible and biologically non-toxic.[221,222] The application of molecular targeting using AuNOs to cancer cells to create RF induced hyperthermic cytotoxicity has several advantages that include 1) low cost and ease of production; 2) optical absorption for characterization; 3) active manipulation of surface chemistry with respect to charge and shape; 4) straight forward attachment of targeting molecules, such as antibodies, nucleotides, peptides, or pharmacologic agents; and 5) small size (5–10 nm diameter) diameter can effectively penetrate through pores and fenestrations in the neovasculature of solid tumors.[223] Having these properties, targeted AuNPs easily access the surface of cancer cells and bind to target receptors. This is followed by internalization into the cytoplasm of the cells[224] and activation by remote RF energy to release sufficient heat to produce thermal cytotoxicity in the cancer cells.[3] AuNPs present the added advantage of current clinical use to treat some patients with severe rheumatoid arthritis and is known to have a low toxicity profile. Gold coated nanoshells with silica core offer versatility in that they can absorb in the NIR region for selective ablation[225,226] causing 100% regression of tumors after photothermal treatment. With the use of the non-targeted nanoshells, these are passively localized in the tumor based on EPR mechanism.[3]

Tissue thermal ablation using NMs that are functionalized to serve as specific thermal agents, offer great potential for the treatment of unresectable tumors with which can be personalized based on the recognition molecule attached to the particle surface. After intravenous administration the targeted NMs, in an ideal situation, they will be capable of navigating into the vasculature to reach the desired site at full concentration and to selectively kill the cancer cells with energy that is applied from a remote source. These kinds of pharmacological agents are much needed to improve cancer therapeutics. Enormous research are currently making progress toward partially achieving this goal in the very near future.

7.5.2 Thermal Ablation and NMs Combination Therapeutics

The limitations of thermal ablation discussed in the previous section, combined with the development and availability of chemotherapeutic drugs that are encapsulated in nanoparticle delivery vehicles, led to the incorporation of adjuvant liposomal doxorubicin (Doxil) into the combination therapy.[215,227] Liposome NPs are completely biocompatible with very little toxic or antigenic reaction and are biologically inert.[216] While water-soluble drugs can be trapped in the inner aqueous compartment, hydrophobic compounds may be located into the liposomal hydrophobic layer thereby protecting the drugs from the destructive environment in vivo.[216] The disadvantage of liposomal preparations are their elimination from the systemic circulation by the RES due to rapid opsonization[228] has been overcome by surface-modification with flexible hydrophilic polymers such as PEG[228–230] that eliminates plasma protein absorption on liposome surfaces that causes subsequent recognition and uptake of liposomes by the RES.[216] The benefits of using liposomes to encapsulate chemotherapeutic agents include escape from systemic phagocytosis resulting in prolonged circulation time, selective agent delivery through the leaky tumor endothelium (enhanced permeability and retention effect), as well as reduced toxicity profiles.[229] Thus, the liposome- doxorubicin formulation is widely accepted for clinical practice.[231,232] Subsequent studies combining RF ablation with adjuvant liposomal doxorubicin demonstrated significant increases in mean tumor coagulation diameter from combination RF/Doxil therapy (13.1 mm) compared to RF alone (6.7 mm) in rats.[233] Other animal models also exhibited the same observations in overall ablation-induced tumor coagulation during confirmatory studies.[215,227,233,234] The results of small and large animal models demonstrated up to 5.6 fold increase in intratumoral doxorubicin accumulation following RF ablation with: (1) the greatest amount of intratumoral doxorubicin in the zone immediately peripheral to the central RF area, and (2) smaller amounts of doxorubicin in the central RF-coagulated area suggesting drug deposition in areas with residual, patent vasculature[235] which explains why liposomal doxorubicin is complementary to RF ablation.[216] Majority of the liposomes were deposited in an area immediately peripheral to the section coagulated by RF heating and within the region where non-lethal hyperthermia and increased destruction is observed.[216,235] Furthermore, the penetration of liposomes into the coagulation zone is evidence of infiltration of chemotherapy into the coagulated focus (possibly through residual patent vessels) that may lead to the completeness of tumor destruction.[216] Finally, improved intratumoral drug accumulation as well as tumor coagulation led into gains in both animal survival/tumor growth studies and in preliminary clinical studies.[216]

Results of a pilot clinical study where RF ablation (internally cooled electrode) was combined with adjuvant liposomal doxorubicin, 10 patients with 18 intrahepatic tumors were randomized to receive either liposomal doxorubicin (20 mg Doxil) 24 h prior to RF ablation or RF ablation alone (mean tumor size undergoing ablation was 4.0 ± 1.8 cm).[236] There was no difference in the amount of tumor destruction between groups immediately following RF but after 2–4 weeks, patients receiving liposomal doxorubicin had an increase in tumor destruction of 24–342% volumetric increase (median 32%) compared to a decrease of 76–88% for treated with RF alone.[236] In the combination therapy group, increased diameter of the treatment effect for multiple tumor types, improved completeness of tumor destruction particularly adjacent to intratumoral vessels, and increased treatment effect including the peritumoral liver parenchyma (suggesting a contribution to achieving an adequate ablative margin) were observed.

7.6 NMS AS CONTRAST AGENTS

The recent advances in instrumentation and molecular profiling of diseases have motivated the development of specific contrast agents to facilitate the noninvasive detection and visualization of morphological and biochemical changes that influence disease and/or its response to therapy.[3] The advances in this area has been focused largely in oncology, from the identification of specific molecular pathways associated with tumorigenesis to the clinical monitoring of cancer biomarkers before and after treatment. The discovery and integration of new and improved highly specific contrast agents with existing conventional as well as upcoming diagnostic imaging techniques can have a major impact on the detection, diagnosis, and decision making for personalized molecular-based treatment.

Today, molecular specific imaging in the clinics is already in practice.[3] Magnetic resonance imaging (MRI), positron emission tomography (PET), and single photon emission computed tomography (SPECT) are some of the first clinical imaging modalities capable of generating images with molecular specificity.[3] These technologies take advantage of the use of different exogenously administered contrast agents to monitor and collect information about tissue anatomy, physiology, and metabolism. New improved and specific contrast agents for these and other imaging techniques are continually being introduced to enhance clinical care. Probably this century's most promising platform for clinical imaging techniques are NMs which offer high contrast, tunable size, shape, and surface properties, ease of integrating multiple functionalities, and long circulation times.[237,238] Various NMs including superparamagnetic materials, metal NPs, dendrimers, polymers, liposomes, and more are currently being developed for a wide range of clinical indications. These different platforms offer varying degrees in bioavailability, pharmacokinetics, toxicity, immunogenicity, and specificity. Hence, it is more than likely that a variety of different and specialized NMs platforms will be suited for targeting different diseases and processes. A number of NMs based contrast agents are already in the market and additional products are currently undergoing clinical testing or entering the pipeline.[3]

The nanoparticle-based contrast agents developments were initially focused to compete with gadolium (Gd) based contrast agents for MRI.[3] Today, the SPIONs based contrast agents are already in clinical use.[3]

7.6.1 NMs Contrast Agents in Clinical Use

There are two intravenous formulations of SPIONs in clinical use and one formulation has been approved for oral use[3] (Table 7.2). The first NMs to be clinically approved for in vivo imaging are the SPIONs.[3] The first clinically available brand is Feridex I.V.® (ferumoxides injectable solution) which was introduced as the world's first organ specific MR contrast agent in 1996.[3] It was followed by Resovist® (ferucarbotran injectable solution) that was approved in the European Union (EU), Australia, and Japan for the detection and evaluation liver lesions using MRI.[3] Resovist consists of 80 nm particles while Feridex is about 50-180 nm.[239] These two iron-based NMs, Feridex I.V.® and Resovist®, have iron content that produces strong local disruptions in the magnetic field of MRI scanners, causing an increased $T2^*$ relaxation and decreased signal intensity in the areas where the NMs accumulate.[3] As a result, they are considered "negative" contrast agents. Both of these contrast agents rely on passive targeting strategies to detect alterations in the RES, making normal liver, spleen, bone marrow, and lymph nodes appear dark.[3] Processes that reduce the uptake of SPIONs such as inflammation, scarring, and most focal lesions of the liver produce localized regions of signal.[240] In comparison with other heavy metals that are harmful, the key advantage of SPIONs as MRI contrast agents is their ability to integrate physiologically as the iron and iron oxides are metabolized, stored in intracellular pools as ferritin, and incorporated into hemoglobin.[3] In rodent models, dose escalation studies using a dose well above that used for MRI procedures (<5 mg/kg) showed no identifiable side effects even at 100 mg iron/kg.[241] The iron NMs, based on radiotracer and histological studies in rodents, becomes part of the body iron pool, first accumulating in the RES and then slowly disappearing over the course of 14–28 days.[242,243] Intravenous administration of semisynthetic carbohydrates coated IO NMs was found to safely increase mean blood hemoglobin concentrations by about 1.0 g/dL over a 35 day period in humans.[244] Based on these studies, in June 2009, Feraheme™

TABLE 7.2 Clinically Approved Nanomaterials

Brand/Name	Composition	Size	Use
Feridex™	Dextran coated SPIO	50–180 nm	MRI Contrast
Resovist™	Carboxydextran coated SPIO	80 nm	MRI Contrast
Feraheme™	Polyglucose sorbitol Carboxy-methylether coated SPIO	17–31 nm	Iron deficiency anemia

(ferumoxytol injectable solution) was approved for the treatment of iron deficiency anemia in adult patients with chronic kidney disease.[3] The suitability of ferumoxytol as an MRI contrast agent for the nervous system disease, brain neoplasms, and peripheral artery disease are ongoing in clinical trials.[3]

SPIONs, unlike the gadolinium-based MR contrast agents engineered to target liver hepatocytes, are selectively taken up by Kupffer cells in the RES primarily in the liver and exert their effects on both T2- and T1-relaxation times.[239] Both Feridex (Endorem) and Resovist are approved specifically for liver MR imaging but Resovist is provided as a ready-to-use formulation that can be administered as a rapid bolus that is used with both dynamic and delayed imaging while Feridex has to be administered as a slow infusion for delayed phase imaging.[245] The side effects from Feridex reports an incidence of adverse events of 9.4% (114/1535 subjects) with back and leg pain being the most common events reported (3.6%). Severe pain that cause interruption or discontinuation of the infusion was reported in 55/2240 (2.5%) of patients.[245] In the case of Resovist the overall incidence of adverse events was 7.1% (75/1053 subjects) with vasodilation and paraesthesia as the most common (<2%).[245]

These SPIONs will likely play an important role in advancing personalized medicine being the first two NMs for human use.[3] Feridex I.V.® is well suited for the detection of small focal lesions with high accuracy, particularly when images are collected before and after contrast agent injection because it is administered as a slow infusion in conjunction with delayed phase imaging.[246,247] On the other hand, Resovist® can be administered as a rapid bolus making it useful for dynamic imaging to produce higher liver to tumor contrast.[248] Other applications of these two contrast agents are being actively pursued, including the preoperative staging of pancreatic cancer (currently in Stage IV clinical trials), monitoring of tissue margins following radiofrequency ablation to predict tumor recurrence,[249] non-invasive differentiation of hepatocellular cancer grades,[250] and the monitoring of macrophage infiltration into other pathologic tissues,[251] Interest in using SPIONs to track cell movement in vivo following transplantation[252] for the long-term goal of developing and monitoring personalized cell based therapies is also an area of interest.[3]

An increase in the numbers of NMs are currently undergoing clinical trials[3] (Table 7.3) but the most advanced NPs for human use are still based on the IOMNP platform which vary in surface coating, size, and function.[3] Currently under investigation is the first molecular specific, nanoparticle-based injectable contrast agent. These contrast agents include Combidex® (ferumoxtran10) which is an ultrasmall (20 nm diameter) SPION (USPIO) coated with low molecular weight dextrans for lymph node imaging. After intravenous administration, these NMs are internalized by macrophages through phagocytosis and accumulate in benign lymph nodes.[3] Alterations in lymph flow and/or nodal architecture as a result of injury or disease cause abnormal patterns of NMs accumulation that can be detected by MRI.[253]

TABLE 7.3 Nanomaterials as MRI Contrast Agents in Clinical Trials

Chemical composition/ name	Brand name	Application	Company	Status
Dextran coated superparamagnetic iron oxide, SPIO (ferumoxtran-10)	Combidex/Sinerem	Cancerous lymph node	AMAG Pharmaceuticals, Inc	Phase III
Carboxy dextran-coated SPIO (ferucarbotran)	Supravist	Blood pooling detection with MRA	Bayer Schering Pharm AG	Phase III
Polyglucose sorbitol carboxymethyl ether-coated SPIO (ferumoxytol)	–	Nervous system disease; brain neoplasm; peripheral artery disease	AMAG Pharmaceuticals, Inc	Phase II
Citrate coated very small SPIO	VSOP-C184	Blood pooling detection with MRA	Charite-Universitatsmedizin Berlin	Phase I
Radiolabeled HER-2 antibody	ABY-025	Breast cancer	Antibody Holding AB	Phase I

Although Combidex® has been approved for use in some EU countries, it has had difficulty gaining widespread regulatory approval due to a high false positive rate.[3] In a recent multicenter study that evaluated the use of Combidex® for MRI to identify lymph node metastases occurring outside the normal area, pelvic lymph node dissection in 296 patients with prostate cancer[254] resulted in a 24.1% false positive rate causing unnecessary surgical interventions.[3] Following FDA advice, Combidex® is currently undergoing additional clinical trials in an attempt to improve the safety and accuracy for specific applications.[3] These potential applications include the screening and assessment of therapeutic response to "anti-inflammatory" interventions,[255] the imaging of brain and pelvic neoplasms, lymph node staging in prostate cancer, and the prediction of abdominal aortic aneurysm instability.[3] Two SPIONs are under clinical investigation as contrast agents for MR angiography (MRA). Supravist® (Ferucarbotran), which is a T1 weighted reformulation of Resovist® that has been developed for "positive" detection of blood pooling.[3] Supravist® has shown promising results using both first pass and steady state angiography after bolus injection[256] and are comparable to those achieved using gadolinium(Gd) based contrast agents.[257] Phase III clinical trials in patients with peripheral artery disease and renal vascular disease have been completed but not yet published.[258] A 7 nm citrate coated

SPION formulation (VSOPC184) has also generated first pass images that are equivalent to those taken using Gd based agents.[259] The results of the Phase I clinical trials have demonstrated acceptable safety, tolerability, and data that exhibited efficacy.[260] The NMs that are being evaluated as MRA agents have long half-life in the plasma making them suitable for detection of small vessels with slow and/or complex flow; and may be able to advance angiography as an imaging tool for personalized medicine.[261] The potential applications of these NMs as MRA agents that are being tested in humans and/or animals include functional imaging,[262] perfusion imaging,[263] dynamic detection of bleeding,[264] and the characterization of tumor related angiogenesis.[265]

The first molecular specific NM based contrast agent binds to HER2, a growth factor whose overexpression is associated with more aggressive and malignant breast cancer phenotypes.[266,267] This NMs-based contrast agent is an engineered compact three-helix bundle (i.e. affibody®) that entered Phase I clinical trials in August 2009 when AffibodyAG obtained the final approval and funding for a Phase I study of its ABY025 compound.[3] Results from a Phase 1 first-in-human clinical trial in seven HER2-positive or -negative females with metastasized breast cancer, assessing safety of use, tissue distribution of ABY-025 and possibilities to discriminate low/high HER2- expression in lesions.[268] The results gave excellent quality SPECT images and full body scans that were recorded and analyzed for tissue distribution. Evidence for differences in uptake and kinetics between low/high HER2-expressing lesions were reported. There were no observed drug induced adverse reactions and no induced formation of antibodies against ABY-025. Their results indicated that ABY-025 can be used safely in humans for whole body HER2-receptor molecular imaging capabilities as noted with a previous generation Affibody molecule. These clinical trial results provided promising indications of in vivo HER2-receptor status assessment capabilities and the potential to guide treatment in cancer patients.[268]

7.6.2 NMs as Imaging Contrast Agents in Preclinical Development

The success in human applications of the NMs-based imaging contrast agents has spurred the upsurge in the development of more efficient and complex nanoparticle systems. The NIH Molecular Imaging and Contrast Agent Database (MICAD) reveals over 50 nanoparticle-based systems that are currently undergoing preclinical development.[269] A few of these NMs are shown in Table 7.4.

Some of these NMs are being used for in vitro studies. Mesenchymal stem cells (MSCs), were labeled with commercially available FluidMAG iron nanoparticles.[270] FluidMAG nanoparticles are ferrofluids consisting of an aqueous dispersion of magnetic IOs that have hydrodynamic diameter of 200 nm and a starch coating. Loebinger, et al. showed that the FlluidMag labeled cells retained their MSC characteristics and the ability to differentiate into stromal

TABLE 7.4 A few of the Nanoparticle-based Contrast Agents from the NIH MICAD

NAME	NMs	Detection	Disease
FluidMag	IOMNP	MRI	Tumor
FANPs	Au–Fe$_3$O$_4$	NIR	Tumor, atherosclerosis, etc
GD4C/Cy5.5–Fn–^{64}Cu nanocages	Cu	PET, NIRF	Tumor
VEGF$_{121}$/rGel-MNPs	Mn–Fe$_2$O$_4$	MRI	Tumor
Gd$_2$O$_3$@SiO$_2$	Gd$_2$O$_3$–SiO$_2$	MRI	Tumor
Fn-Fe nanocages	Iron oxide	MRI	Atherosclerosis
USPIO-PEG-OCT	Iron oxide	MRI	Tumors
USPIO-anti-CD20 MAb	Iron oxide	MRI	Malignant B cells
VINP-28 NP	Iron oxide	MRI	Atherosclerosis
EuPFC	Eu, PFC	MRI	Thrombosis

tissues.[270] The labeled and unlabeled MSCs had equivalent *in vitro* tumor homing (104.4±5.6 vs 113.1±16.1 cells per ×10 magnification field; $p>0.05$) in transwell migration studies.[270] As shown by MTS NAD(P)H-dependent proliferation assay, or on cell viability, that was exhibited by annexin V flow cytometry apoptosis assay (33.0±4.2% vs 29.4±2.1% dead or apoptotic cells without and with labeling), the NMs label had no effect on the MSCs. They also showed that intravenously injected labeled cells could be tracked in vivo to home to multiple lung metastases.[270]

MSCs that were used in the FluidMag studies represent a heterogeneous subset of pluripotent stromal cells that can be isolated from different adult tissues including adipose tissue, liver, muscle, amniotic fluid, placenta, umbilical cord blood, and dental pulp, although the bone marrow remains the principal source for most preclinical and clinical studies.[271,272] MSCs have the potential to differentiate into cells of diverse lineages such as adipocytes, chondrocytes, osteocytes, myoblasts, cardiomyocytes, neurons, and astrocytes. One of the most important characteristics of MSCs is their ability to home in to tumors making them useful vehicles for directed cancer delivery.[273,274] Although the specific chemokines responsible for MSC migration are poorly characterized,[273,274] homing to tumors have been confirmed with traditional immunohistochemistry and other methods. This was used by Loebinger et al. with FluidMAG labeled MSCs that were imaged to home in tumor with MRI.[270]

One of the nanoparticle-based contrast agents undergoing developments on the MICAD list is called FANPs (flower-like gold nanoparticles). The FANPs consists of Cy5.5–Gly–Pro–Leu–Gly–Val–Arg–Gly–(Lys–TDOPA)$_3$-flower-like gold–Fe$_3$O$_4$ optical NPs and have been evaluated for imaging protease expression *in vivo*. The peptide sequence with a Cy5.5 NIR dye molecule is attached to AuNPs to form fluorescence-quenched NPs (Cy5.5–Gly–Pro–Leu–Gly–Val–Arg–Gly–Cys–AuNPs (Cy5.5-MMP–AuNPs or GANPs)). The presence of Cy5.5 molecules in close proximity result in fluorescence quenching from the efficient fluorescence resonance energy transfer to Au.[275] When the Leu–Gly bond is cleaved by matrix metalloproteinases (MMPs), the NIR fluorescence signal from the Cy5.5 will increase as the Cy5.5-containing fragments is released. The Cy5.5 has a NIR absorbance maximum at 675 nm, an emission maximum at 694 nm, and an extinction coefficient of 250,000 M^{-1}cm^{-1}. The FANPs are being developed for NIR fluorescence imaging of MMPs that are expressed in tumors, atherosclerosis, myocardial infarction, and other diseases.[276] Xie et al.[276] modified the FANPs by replacing the AuNP with Au–Fe$_3$O$_4$, to induce a fluorescently quenched state to the overall nanostructure. The composite NP which is shaped like a flower has three IO "petals" on each AuNP. The gold surface was passivated with a thiolated PEG (SH-PEG$_{5000}$) while the MMP peptide was covalently linked to the Lys-tridihydrophenylalanine (Lys-TDOPA) on the surface of the IO NMs. This Cy5.5–Gly–Pro–Leu–Gly–Val–Arg–Gly–(Lys–TDOPA)$_3$-flower-like gold–Fe$_3$O$_4$ optical NPs (FANPs) have been evaluated for imaging protease expression in vivo. The following process was used in the synthesis of the FANPs.

(1) The Fe$_3$O$_4$ was allowed to grow on the surface of AuNPs (8 nm) through pyrolysis of Fe(CO)$_5$ for 10 min at 220 °C to form flower-like gold–Fe$_3$O$_4$ NPs.
(2) Standard solid-phase peptide synthesis was used to prepare the Gly–Pro–Leu–Gly–Val–Arg–Gly–(Lys–TDOPA)$_3$.
(3) Standard methods of conjugation was applied to attach the Cy5.5 to the *N*-terminus of Gly–Pro–Leu–Gly–Val–Arg–Gly–(Lys–TDOPA)$_3$ to produce Cy5.5–Gly–Pro–Leu–Gly–Val–Arg–Gly–(Lys–TDOPA)$_3$.
(4) To 0.4 mg of the Cy5.5–Gly–Pro–Leu–Gly–Val–Arg–Gly–(Lys–TDOPA)$_3$ and 25 mg SH–PEG$_{5000}$ in 0.9 mL DMSO was added to 2 mL gold–Fe$_3$O$_4$ NPs (27 mg) in CHCl$_3$.
(5) The mixture was incubated at room temperature for ~18 h to form the FANPs.
(6) The mixture was centrifuged and the FANPs pellet was collected.
(7) This pellet was reconstituted and characterized.

The IO "petals" showed a diameter of 13.4 ± 3.5 nm.[276] The overall diameter of FANPs was 40.0 ± 4.3 nm, as determined with dynamic light scattering. There were 152 ± 12 molecules of Cy5.5–Gly–Pro–Leu–Gly–Val–Arg–Gly–(Lys–TDOPA)$_3$ per FANP and the quenching efficiency of a single FANP for the Cy5.5 was estimated to be >95%.[276] Stability of the FANPs were observed in phosphate-buffered saline, 10 mM dithiothreitol (DTT) solution, and fetal bovine serum containing medium after 2–3 h of incubation at 37 °C.

Similar to the FANPs in optical fluorescence concept are the RGD4C/Cy5.5–Fn–^{64}Cu nanocages.[277] These nanocages were prepared by genetically grafting $\alpha_v\beta_3$-targeted peptide (RDCRGDCFC, RGD4C) onto heavy chain ferritin (RGD4C–Fn) and chemically coupling Cy5.5 onto the heavy chain ferritin to form Cy5.5–Fn. Hybridization of RGD4C–Fn and Cy5.5–Fn (1:1) in the presence of ^{64}CuCl$_2$ resulted in the formation of RGD4C/Cy5.5-ferritin ^{64}Cu-loaded nanocages (RGD4C/Cy5.5–Fn–^{64}Cu nanocages).[277] These nanocages have been developed for positron emission tomography and NIRF multimodality imaging of tumor vasculature to study in vivo biodistribution of the tracer in tumor-bearing mice. RGD4C/Cy5.5–Fn–^{64}Cu nanocages have been shown to have a high accumulation in the tumor vasculature and a predominant liver accumulation.

Another contrast agent that is undergoing development as contrast agent is the VEGF$_{121}$/rGel–MNP.[278] This agent is a combination of the vascular endothelial growth factor A isoform 121 (VEGF$_{121}$)-gelonin fusion protein (VEGF$_{121}$/rGel) that was conjugated with manganese ferrite (MnFe$_2$O$_4$) nanoparticle (NP). It is a VEGF receptor (VEGFR)-targeted contrast agent for monitoring the targeting efficiency and treatment efficacy of the VEGF$_{121}$/rGel immunotoxin.[278] In vitro studies showed that in PAE/KDR cells (porcine aortic endothelial cells transfected with cDNA of VEGFR2) exhibited >105 times and >108 times more VEGFR2 expression than did HUVEC cells and 253JB-V cells (a human bladder cancer cell line), respectively. Using this NMs, it was shown that binding in cells over expressing the T2-weighted magnetic resonance imaging (MRI) at 1.5 T exhibited a dose-dependent enhancement of signal intensity over the concentration range of 0.04–5.0 µg for the PAE/KDR cells but not for the control.[278] The NMs were predominantly found in the cytoplasm. The VEGF$_{121}$/rGel-MNPs were tested in vivo in male BALB/c nude mice bearing 253JB-V tumor xenografts in the bladder dome.[278] MRI signal enhancement was identified initially after injection in the vessels surrounding the bladder and later in the intratumoral vessels. In endothelial cells, the targeted delivery of VEGF$_{121}$/rGel-MNPs to intratumoral vessels was further verified with immunofluorescence.[278] This is a promising development because VEGFs are potent inducers of cell migration, invasion, vascular permeability, and neovascular formation[279] via the tyrosine kinase receptor.[280] On the surface of endothelial cells of tumor neovasculature, these receptors are overexpressed and are almost undetectable in the endothelium of adjacent normal tissues. Sequestration of these receptors to inhibit neovascular formation is one key step in preventing tumor development.

The Gd$_2$O$_3$@SiO$_2$ NPs are non-targeted MRI contrast agents that are very stable.[281] The in vitro T1-weighted phantom images exhibited that Gd$_2$O$_3$@SiO$_2$·NPs had a higher signal intensity and had a larger T1 relaxivity than commercial Gd-labeled diethylene triaminepentaacetic acid (Gd-DTPA) at 1.5 T[281]. These NMs were used in MRI of mice bearing subcutaneous xenografts of CNE-2 tumor cells (nasopharyngeal carcinoma cells). The results of the T1-weighted images exhibited significant signal enhancement in the livers from mice treated with $Gd_2O_3@SiO_2$ NPs from 15 min after injection and the signal enhancement lasted for >24 h. The tumor xenografts exhibited increased signal intensity starting at 30 min after injection.

Majority of the NMs undergoing development for applications as contrast agents are made of IO NMs as shown in Table 7.4. They differ from one another by composition such as the presence of one or more contrast generating materials (para/superparamagnetic, electron density, or fluorescence), the bioactive targeting molecules (peptides, antibodies, growth factors, receptors, NAs, etc), the biocompatibility coating (carbohydrates, polymers, peptides, etc.), and other surface functionalization. These NMs are generally designed and engineered modularly to allow various desirable properties to be incorporated at the best ratios. The most common nanoparticle platforms as contrast agents include IOMNPs, non-magnetic metals such as gold, liposomes, synthetic carbon structures, polymeric NMs, and emulsions.[3] New classes are emerging with better biocompatibility, improved targeting efficiency, higher signal, and lower levels of toxicity.

7.7 MAGNETIC IO NP-MEDIATED CIRCULATING TUMOR CELL ISOLATION

Cancer causes 1 in 4 deaths in the US with a total of 1,529,560 new cancer cases annually.[282] In 2010, the 3 most commonly diagnosed types of cancer among women in 2010 were cancer of the breast, lung, and bronchus, and colon/rectum; accounting for 52% of estimated cancer cases in women. Breast cancer was expected to account for 28% (207,090) of all new cancer cases in women and it is the second leading cause of cancer death in women in the US.[282]

Reports have indicated that circulating tumor cells (CTCs) can be found in patients before the primary tumor is detected.[283,284] In the presence of billions of normal white blood cells (WBCs) and red blood cells (RBCs), a few CTCs may be present in the peripheral blood during the early stage when the primary tumor is not detectable by currently available methods.[285] Early detection of CTCs can be sued to guide therapeutic strategies for treatment at the early stages of cancer. But, the biggest hurdle in the detection of CTCs is their extremely low concentration and the difficulty of separation. Human blood consists of WBCs ($3–10 \times 10^6$ mL^{-1}), RBCs ($3–9 \times 10^9$ mL^{-1}), and platelets ($2.5–4 \times 10^8$ mL^{-1}) while the number of CTCs in blood from a cancer patient may range from 0 to 50 mL^{-1} of blood[286] which means 0–50 CTCs in 10B blood cells.[285] Because of the low levels of CTCs in blood, existing immunomagnetic cell separation techniques lack the ability to separate the CTCs from untreated whole blood.[285] Hence, the group of Xu[285] investigated the use of IOMNPs at 30 nm diameter (Figure 7.9) as substitute for the currently used micron sized magnetic beads (microbead). The IOMNPs

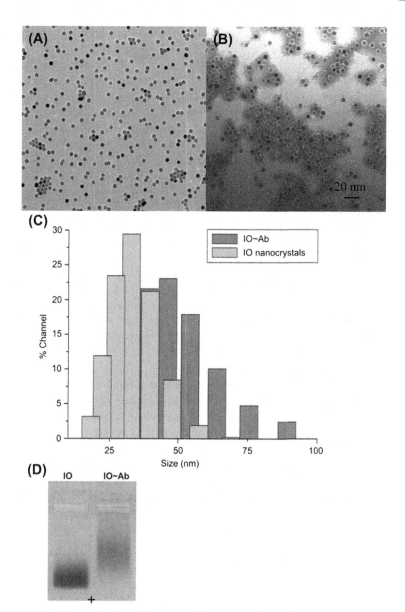

FIGURE 7.9   Characterization of IO nanoparticles. (A) TEM image of the hydrophobic inorganic core of the IO NPs, showing a diameter around 27 ± 5 nm (relative standard deviation of 9.5% for $n = 50$); (B) TEM image of antibody conjugated biocompatible water-soluble IO, IO–Ab, using phosphotungstic acid for background staining; (C) light scattering properties of biocompatible water-soluble IO showing a hydrodynamic size around 33 nm with a zeta potential of −51 mV, and IO–Ab showing a hydrodynamic size around 41 nm and a zeta potential of −36 mV; (D) agarose gel electrophoresis of biocompatible water soluble IO (on left) and IO–Ab (on right), the electric pole is negative for top and positive for the bottom. *Courtesy of Xu, et al.*[285] *(For color version of this figure, the reader is referred to the online version of this book)*

were modified with specific antibodies that targeted the cell surface proteins that are overexpressed in cancer cells.[287] The IOMNPs offer high surface to volume ratio causing higher binding capacity and higher efficiency for CTC. Compared with microbeads, a decrease in the size of the capture particles from micrometers to nanometers increases the available adsorptive areas by 100–1000 times. While the interaction between microparticles and target cells is a quasi–heterogeneous reaction, those between the IOMNPs and CTCs is almost entirely homogeneous because of the small NMs size making capture faster in suspension. Additionally, magnetic microbeads are not efficient for the separation of target cells in whole blood because of high viscosity, high cell density, high protein content, and its generally complex composition preventing efficient contact with the cell surface antigen.[288] Microbead magnetic separation of CTCs is controlled by aggregation when a large number of microbeads accumulate on the cells causing cell detection to be difficult especially with flow cytometry, because the size of the aggregated cells that are captured with the microbeads affect light scattering.[289] To improve the microbead capture of CTCs, complicated pre-treatment of blood such buffy coat preparation and lysis of the RBCs, are necessary for success but such preparation steps can destroy the cells, resulting in decreased number of CTCs making the diagnosis unreliable.[285] These challenges and issues in magnetic-microbead based capture of CTCs may be solved with the use of NPs which are three orders of magnitude smaller in size.

NPs are small providing a higher surface to volume ratio that allows a more efficient contact with the surface of the cells.[285] The nanoscale size allows multiple NPs to attach on the cell surface without cell aggregation as shown in Figure 7.10. With these concepts, Xu and his group demonstrated the separation of circulating cancer cells using an antibody conjugated IO NPs (IO–Ab) under a low magnetic field gradient.[285] Using these demonstrated the ability of the IO–Ab to capture cancer cells in spiked fresh human whole blood without a pre-treatment process. Some of the evaluation processes during SK-BR3 capture with IO–Ab in fresh whole human blood are described below.

7.7.1 IO–Ab Separation of Cancer Cells in Spiked Fresh Human Whole Blood[285]

The cells were first grown following the manufacturer's recommendation or as described in Chapter 4 Section 6.1. The fresh female whole blood was purchased from Biological Specialty Corporation (Colmar, PA) certified with no hepatitis or HIV contamination. IO–Ab conjugation is as described in Chapter 3 Section 3.1. The following steps are recommended to perform IO–Ab capture of cells that are spiked in fresh human whole blood. All the experiments involving human blood must be performed in a BSL2 laboratory.

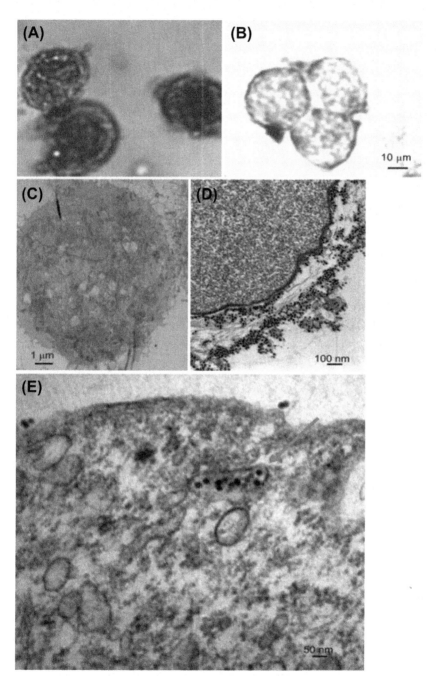

FIGURE 7.10   Detection of IOMNPs in SK-BR3 cells (A) exposed to IOMNP-Ab, (B) IOMNP only. TEM of IOMNP-Ab (C) whole cell section under low magnifications, (D) partially magnified cell membrane exposed to IO–Ab; and (E) IO–Ab taken up by the cell. *From Xu, et al.*[285] *(For color version of this figure, the reader is referred to the online version of this book)*

7.7.1.1 Preparation of the Whole Blood

Dilute the whole blood with DPBS. Expose the blood to acridine orange (AO) to convert the WBCs nuclei to pinkish yellow color without affecting the RBCs in order to establish the number of WBCs and RBCs.

(1) Dilute 10 µL of whole blood at 1:100 with DPBS and mix with the AO at a ratio of 1:1.
(2) Incubate the mixture for 10 min at room temperature.
(3) Centrifuge the cells at 5000 rpm for 5 min.
(4) Collect the pelleted cells.
(5) Wash two times with DPBS to remove excess AO.
(6) Count the stained cells with a hemocytometer under a fluorescence microscope.

7.7.1.2 Capture of the SK-BR3 Cells with IO–Ab

In order to make easy visualization of capture, the freshly harvested SK-BR3 cells are pre-stained with a live cell staining fluorescent dye CMFDA (5-chloromethylfluorescein diacetate, Invitrogen, Carlsbad, CA) that converts the cells to greenish yellow color following the manufacture's staining protocol.[285]

(1) Count the cells and spike in 1 mL whole blood sample.
(2) Add 0.05 mL of IO–Ab NPs at 2 mg Fe/mL.
(3) Swirl gently to mix at room temperature for 1 h to form IO–Ab + cells.
(4) Place the mixture in a SuperMag™ separator for 1 h to allow magnetic isolation of the IO–Ab + cells.
(5) Withdraw the supernatant gently with a pipettor making sure not to disturb the captured IO–Ab + cells that stuck on the wall of the tube where the magnetic field is strongest.
(6) Resuspend the captured pellet containing the IO–Ab + cells in 100 µL DPBS for cell inspection and counting.

7.7.1.3 Protocol for the Prussian Blue Staining of the IO–Ab Captured SK-BR3 Cells

To confirm the IO–Ab tagging of the SK-BR3, the cells were stained with potassium ferrocyanide/HCl mixture.[285] The potassium ferrocyanide and HCl mixture converts the IO from the IO–Ab accumulated on the cells into $KFe^{III}[Fe^{II}(CN)_6]$ which is blue in color.

(1) Take the SK-BR3 cells grown in a 6-well cell culture plate out of the cell medium (description of cell culture is described Chapter------).
(2) Fix the IO–Ab with ice-cold 95% EtOH for 15 min.
(3) Add the IO–Ab (as 0.5 mg Fe) or IO (as 0.5 mg Fe) NPs in the binding buffer (20 mm Tris, 150 mm NaCl, 2 mm $CaCl_2$, 1 mm $MnCl_2$, 1 mm $MgCl_2$, 0.1% (wt/vol) BSA; pH 7.4).

(4) Incubate at room temperature for 1 h with gentle shaking.

(5) Wash with DPBS three times to remove excess reagents.

(6) Incubate the with Prussian blue staining solution (equal volumes of 20% HCl and 10% potassium ferrocyanide aqueous solution) for 40 min at room temperature.

(7) Wash the cells twice with DPBS buffer.

(8) Place under the microscope for inspection.

The studies done by the group of Xu at Ocean NanoTech[285] demonstrated the effectiveness of IO–Ab mediated CTCs capture in fresh human whole blood. The results shown in Figure 7.10A indicated the presence of IO on the cell surface through the Prussian blue staining which was not observed in the cells that were exposed to IO alone (Figure 7.10B).[285] The TEM images shown in Figure 7.10 C,D also proved the attachment of the IO–Ab on the cell surface even after the cells were washed multiple times with DPBS.[285] In this study, only 300 of the CMFDA pre-stained SK-BR3 cells were added to 1 mL whole blood in a ratio of cancer cells to blood cells (WBCs and RBCs) at about 1:10,000,000. The IO–Ab caused the formation of IO–Ab + SK-BR3 cells which were resuspended in 100 µL DPBS. The CMFDA stained SK-BR3 cells appeared greenish yellow in color which were bigger in diameter than the WBCs and RBCs as show in Figure 7.11A. An enrichment factor was calculated at 1:10,000,000 based on the number of WBCs and RBCs in the spiked whole blood.[285] The unique properties of the hydrophilic biocompatible polymer coating on the IO NPs contributed to the high capture rate in fresh human whole blood. This system holds promise for the specific isolation CTCs in fresh human whole blood that can have the way for early diagnosis and treatment of cancer.

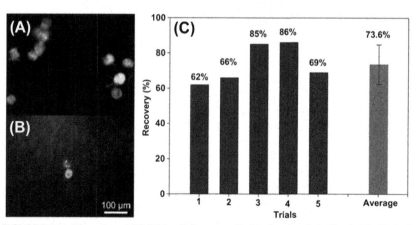

FIGURE 7.11 Separation of SK-BR3 cell that was spiked in female whole blood. (A) SK-BR3 cell pre-stained with CMFDA, (B) isolated CMFDA pre-stained SK-BR3 cells from whole blood, (C) IO–Ab captured cell from spiked whole blood. *Courtesy of Xu, et al.*[285] *(For color version of this figure, the reader is referred to the online version of this book)*

Xu and his group[285] demonstrated a process using IOMNPs with conjugated specific antibodies for the capture and separation of tumor cells in fresh whole blood. The amphiphilic polymer coated 30 nm IOMNPs were modified with antibodies against human epithelial growth factor receptor 2 (anti-HER2 or anti-HER2/neu) forming the IO–Ab. The IO–Ab captured and separated 73.6% ($N = 5$, enrichment of 84%) of SK-BR3 cells that were spiked in 1 mL of fresh human whole blood.[285] The IO–Ab preferentially captured the SK-BR3 cells over the normal cells found in blood due to the high level of HER2/neu receptor on the cancer cell surfaces exhibiting 1:10,000,000 enrichment of cancer cells over normal cells in the presence of a magnetic field gradient of 100 T/m.[285] This is a very promising strategy for the diagnosis and treatment at the early stages of cancer when only a few CTCs are found in the blood that the current methods cannot detect.

7.8 DESIGN TRENDS FOR INDIVIDUALIZED MEDICINE

The new NMs systems in development for nanopharmacological applications contain active targeting molecules aside from the chemotherapeutic payloads. These molecules are used to improve the specific function of the NPs as well as to enhance their ability for gene delivery, immunotherapy, and imaging. Targeting materials for NMs in gene delivery are important so that repair of damaged nucleotides can be immediately carried out at the desired locations. Targeting materials are desired in nanoimmunotherapy so that the immune system can be modulated at the site where the disease most need the immune modulation. Finally, targeting molecules are desired in the contrast agents so that the NMs can be delivered and accumulated at the site where the diseased tissue needs to be visually located. All these are applications of the NMs in nanopharmacology both for the delivery of desired treatment at well as for the measurement of the degree of treatment. The NPs have revolutionized pharmacology in the sense that now there is hope that chemotherapeutic agents can be brought to the desired tissue as well as be detected whether it performs the desired treatment or not.

The specificity of the nanopharmacologically relevant NMs are ensured by the discovery of various targeting molecules which are now a part of our vast knowledge in science and medicine. A few of the most commonly used targeting molecules include cancer biomarkers (e.g. Her2, EGFR, VEGF, integrin $\alpha v \beta 3$, PSMA, CD20), inflammatory biomarkers (e.g. Eselectin, ICAM1, VCAM1, IL-12), apoptosis markers, and many others. A molecular specific targeting molecule used for in vivo imaging was provided by Weissleder et al. used monocrystalline IO functionalized with antimyosin Fab fragments to detect myocardial infarcts in rats.[290]

Nowadays, because many NMs have been tested for biocompatibility and for delivery functions, attention and effort has been directed toward the rational design of targeting moiety attachment.[291] The knowledge that NMs can accommodate multiple small ligands that enable multivalent targeting to one or more biomarkers, new designs are emerging which allow increased target affinity for individual probes. Molecular specific modified NMs have more detailed ability to provide specific information that is not possible using conventional methods.

The most simple possible application of targeted NMs in nanopharmacology is the intravenous injection of contrast agent that could be used to non-invasively detect the expression of biomarkers that are important for disease diagnosis and the treatment selection, eliminating the need for invasive biopsy. The design of many of the new nanoparticle-based contrast agents in preclinical testing today are designed with this principle as a goal aside from improved biocompatibility, long circulation times, less repeat administration of contrast, dynamic monitoring of biomarker expression behavior and levels with time and medication, all of which are essential for determining disease progression and response to therapy.[3]

Smarter NMs designed for probing disease states and progression through the collection of important information from specific molecular targets before, during, and after treatment may further revolutionize the current state of medicine. For example, elevated telomerase activity is associated with poor prognosis and increased risk of recurrence of cancer.[292] Such capabilities coupled with the knowledge about other prognostic proteins or nucleotide levels could be used for a more informed decision on the selection of personalized therapy. The use of multimodal nanoparticles that can be used for delivery of multiple agents as well as be detected in multiple ways can find essential information about disease state and treatment efficacy simultaneously. This is shown by the new NMs designed by Xie et al.[276] which contains both AuNP and Fe_3O_4. The AuNP can be used for X-ray contrast while the Fe_3O_4 can be used in magnetic imaging modality. In addition, the Cy5.5 label is a very sensitive dye for NIR fluorescence in the FANPs. The NIR fluorescence is quenched until the cleavage of the Leu–Gly bond releases the Cy5.5 containing fragments which exhibit the signal.

The group of Pandey and coworkers[293] investigated the possibility of delivering contrast agents to living tumor cells by conjugating gadolinium complexes to hexylether derivative of pyropheophorbide, HPPH, a tumor-avid chlorophyll derivative at Phase II clinical trials. Up to six Gd^{3+} aminobenzyl DTPA complexes were coupled to HPPH that had enhanced tumor-imaging potential, which increased with a larger number of Gd^{3+} units. The three Gd^{+3} aminobenzyl DTPA conjugates that showed the best PDT activity in vitro showed higher accumulation in the tumor at 24 h post-injection[293] compared with that in blood, muscle, and most organs.

A lot of research has come up in the areas where multifunctional NMs are used as a combination of detection and therapeutic functions. This integration that is called "theranostics" is attractive because it allows the imaging detection of therapeutic delivery and at the same time performs informed observation to assess the treatment efficacy. Theranostics offers the possibility of allowing imaging to be performed before, after, and during a treatment regimen. The NMs that are already used as imaging agents can be readily adopted to the theranostic agents category by loading therapeutic agents and/or functions on them. The driving force behind this combination is that imaging and therapy both require sufficient accumulation of agents in diseased tissues. Combining both the targeting and therapeutic requirement brings the two research areas closer and since many techniques to enhance imaging can theoretically be readily transferred to the therapeutic domain, and vice versa.[294]

One of the most versatile and medically useful NMs is the IOMNP because of all the properties that have been previously mentioned. As such, along with its ease of synthesis and use, it has been well characterized and studied for theranostic applications. The group of Namiki[295] used polymer- and lipid-coated magnetic nanocrystals, LipoMag, to deliver silencing RNA that was magnetically guided to deliver and silence genes in cells and tumors in mice. This LipoMag was made of an oleic acid-coated magnetic NM core with a cationic lipid shell. The LipoMag displayed was used for gene silencing in 9 of 13 cell lines with improved anti-tumor effects in mice bearing gastric tumors by delivering a sequence of silencing RNA that targeted the epidermal growth factor receptor of tumor vessels without adverse immune reaction or side effects.

The theranostic capability of properly designed and engineered NMs has been captured in the study of perfluorocarbonated materials to target various atherosclerotic plaque lesion components including the $\alpha v \beta 3$ integrin[296] and fibrin.[297] In their studies, they applied gadolinium containing lipids on a perfluorocarbon core that uses both ^{19}F and conventional MRI.[3] In the animal studies where they administered $\alpha v \beta 3$ targeted NMs containing the drug fumagillin, the theranostic showed significant accumulation at the atherosclerotic lesions during the first week but which was not observed on the second round of theranostic injection in the second week.

This is a good example of NMs applications for a combination of detection, targeted therapy, and therapy assessment all with a single nanoparticle agent. A list of theranostic NPs that are currently being studied include siRNA molecular beacons,[298] polymer coated IOMNPs,[295] and those found in a review by Xie.[294]

7.9 CONCLUSIONS

Pharmacology has definitely been revolutionized by the coming of the nanotechnology era that has seen a boost at the end of the twentieth century and toward the beginning of the twentyfirst century. NMs have been and research and development continue to engineer various types of NMs to diagnose disease and health conditions; to recognize pathogenic infections; to locate, attach, and penetrate target tissue or structures or pathogens; and dispense the payload of drugs or biological compound to the targeted regions of the body. This is the area now known as nanopharmacology.

Nanopharmacology, although still in its early stages, has witnessed an over-hauling of the conventional pharmacology through changes in drug engineering design and development, manufacture of nano-enabled drug or drug carrier, and the application of nanoscale molecular species in drug formulations and drug release. All these are geared toward achieving the promise of NMs in improving the curative capabilities of conventional drugs as well as to harness the diagnostic efficacy of modern diagnostic instruments. To date, multiple NMs have been complexed to drugs and various biomolecules with the goal of improving the diagnostic and therapeutic capabilities for various diseases.

A portion of nanopharmacology that is still in its infancy, is the area of "theranostics" that refers to the combination of diagnostics and therapeutics. Research on the multifunctional capabilities of NMs are on-going to combine the detection and therapeutic functions in a single nanoparticle. This integration allows the imaging detection of therapeutic delivery as well as perform informed observation to assess the treatment efficacy. Although research in this area has barely just begun, the NMs that are already used as imaging agents that can be readily adopted to the theranostics agents category by loading therapeutic agents and/or functions on them. Combining both the targeting and therapeutic requirements using especially designed and engineered NMs brings the two individual areas together that will eventually bring the benefit to the patient.

REFERENCES

1. Lal, R.; Ramachandran, S.; Arnsdorf, M. F. Multidimensional Atomic Force Microscopy: A Versatile Novel Technology for Nanopharmacology Research. *AAPS J.* **2010,** *12,* 716–728.
2. Blagosklonny, M. V. Analysis of FDA Approved Anticancer Drugs Reveals the Future of Cancer Therapy. *Cell Cycle* **2004,** *3,* 1035–1042.
3. Sakamoto, J. H.; van de Ven, A. L.; Godin, B.; Blanco, E.; Serda, R. E.; Grattoni, A.; Ziemys, A.; Bouamrani, A.; Hu, T.; Ranganathan, S. I.; De Rosa, E.; Martinez, J. O.; Smid, C. A.; Buchanan, R.; Lee, S. Y.; Srinivasan, S.; Landry, M.; Meyn, A.; Tasciotti, E.; Li, X.; Decuzzi, P.; Ferrari, M. Review: Enabling Individualized Therapy Through Nanotechnology. *Pharm. Res.* **2010,** *62,* 57–89.
4. Hatefi, A.; Amsden, B. Camptothecin Delivery Methods. *Pharm. Res.* **2002,** *19,* 1389–1399.
5. Sutton, D.; Nasongkla, N.; Blanco, E.; Gao, J. Functionalized Micellar Systems for Cancer Targeted Drug Delivery. *Pharm. Res.* **2007,** *24,* 1029–1046.
6. Huuskonen, J.; Salo, M.; Taskinen, J. Neural Network Modeling for Estimation of the Aqueous Solubility of Structurally Related Drugs. *J. Pharm. Sci.* **1997,** *86,* 450–454.
7. Ferrari, M. Nanovector Therapeutics. *Curr. Opin. Chem. Biol.* **2005,** *9,* 343–346.
8. Canal, P.; Gamelin, E.; Vassal, G.; Robert, J. Benefits of Pharmacological Knowledge in the Design and Monitoring of Cancer Chemotherapy. *Pathol. Oncol. Res.* **1998,** *4,* 171–178.
9. Tallaj, J. A.; Franco, V.; Rayburn, B. K.; Pinderski, L.; Benza, R. L.; Pamboukian, S., et al. Response of Doxorubicininduced Cardiomyopathy to the Current Management Strategy of Heart Failure. *J. Heart Lung Transplant.* **2005,** *24,* 196–201.
10. Heath, J. R.; Davis, M. E. Nanotechnology and Cancer. *Annu. Med. Rev.* **2008,** *59,* 251–265.
11. Wang, M. D.; Shin, D. M.; Simons, J. W.; Nie, S. Nanotechnology for Targeted Cancer Therapy. *Expert Rev. Anticancer Ther.* **2007,** *7,* 833–837.

12. Riehemann, K.; Schneider, S. W.; Luger, T. A.; Godin, B.; Ferrari, M.; Fuchs, H. Nanomedicine-challenge and Perspectives. *Angew. Chem. Int. Ed. Engl.* **2009**, *48,* 872–897.

13. Ferrari, M. Cancer Nanotechnology: Opportunities and Challenges. *Nat. Rev. Cancer* **2005**, *5,* 161–171.

14. Wagner, W.; Dullaart, A.; Bock, A. K.; Zweck, A. The Emerging Nanomedicine Landscape. *Nat. Biotechnol.* **2006**, *24,* 1211–1217.

15. Sanhai, W. R.; Sakamoto, J. H.; Canady, R.; Ferrari, M. Seven Challenges for Nanomedicine. *Nat. Nanotechnol.* **2008**, *3,* 242–244.

16. Torchilin, V. P. Recent Advances with Liposomes as Pharmaceutical Carriers. *Nat. Rev. Drug Discov.* **2005**, *4,* 145–160.

17. Hashizume, H.; Baluk, P.; Morikawa, S.; McLean, J. W.; Thurston, G.; Roberge, S., et al. Openings between Defective Endothelial Cells Explain Tumor Vessel Leakiness. *Am. J. Pathol.* **2000**, *156,* 1363–1380.

18. Maeda, H. The Enhanced Permeability and Retention (EPR) Effect in Tumor Vasculature: The Key Role of Tumor-Selective Macromolecular Drug Targeting. *Adv. Enzyme Regul.* **2001**, *41,* 189–207.

19. Harris, C. M. Liquid Array Single-handedly Detects Bounty of BW Agents. *Anal. Chem.* **2003**.

20. Maeda, H.; Bharate, G. Y.; Daruwalla, J. Polymeric Drugs for Efficient Tumortargeted Drug Delivery Based on EPR Effect. *Eur. J. Pharm. Biopharm.* **2009**, *71,* 409–419.

21. Duncan, R. Polymer Conjugates as Anticancer Nanomedicines. *Nat. Rev. Cancer* **2006**, *6,* 688–701.

22. Duncan, R. The Dawning era of Polymer Therapeutics. *Nat. Rev. Drug Discov.* **2003**, *2,* 347–360.

23. Akerman, M. E.; Chan, W. C.; Laakkonen, P.; Bhatia, S. N.; Ruoslahti, E. Nanocrystal Targeting In vivo. *PNAS U.S.A.* **2002**, *99,* 12617–12621.

24. Ballou, B.; Lagerholm, B. C.; Ernst, L. A.; Bruchez, M. P.; Waggoner, A. S. Noninvasive Imaging of Quantum Dots in Mice. *Bioconjugate Chem.* **2004**, *15,* 79–86.

25. Dabholkar, R. D.; Sawant, R. M.; Mongayt, D. A. Polyethylene Glycol-phosphatidylethanol-amine Conjugate (PEG-PE)-based Mixed Micelles: Some Properties, Loading with Paclitaxel, and Modulation of P-glycoprotein-mediated Efflux. *Int. J. Pharm.* **2006**, *315,* 148–157.

26. Gao, X.; Cui, Y.; Levenson, R. M.; Chung, L. W. K.; Nie, S. In vivo Cancer Targeting and Imaging with Semiconductor Quantum Dots. *Nat. Biotechnol.* **2004**, *22,* 969–976.

27. Koo, O.; Rubinstein, I.; Onyuksel, H. Camptothecin in Sterically Stabilized Phospholipid Micelles: A Novel Nanomedicine. *Nanomedicine* **2005**, *1,* 77–84.

28. van Nostrum, C. Polymeric Micelles to Deliver Photosensitizers for Photodynamic Therapy. *Adv. Drug. Delivery Rev.* **2004**, *56,* 9–12.

29. Chauhan, A.; Sridevi, S.; Chalasani, K.; Jain, A.; Jain, S.; Jain, N.; Diwan, P. Dendrimer-mediated Transdermal Delivery: Enhanced Bioavailability of Indomethacin. *J. Controlled Release* **2003**, *90,* 335.

30. Barrett, T.; Ravizzini, G.; Choyke, P.; Kobayashi, H. Dendrimers in Medical Nanotechnology. *IEEE Eng. Med. Biol. Mag.* **2009**, *28,* 12–22.

31. Battah, S.; Balaratnam, S.; Casas, A.; O'Neill, S.; Edwards, C.; Batlle, A.; Dobbin, P.; MacRobert, A. Macromolecular Delivery of 5-aminolaevulinic Acid for Photodynamic Therapy Using Dendrimer Conjugates. *Mol. Cancer Ther.* **2007**, *6,* 876.

32. Bharali, D.; Khalil, M.; Gurbuz, M.; Simone, T.; Mousa, S. Nanoparticles and Cancer Therapy: A Concise Review with Emphasis on Dendrimers. *Int. J. Nanomed.* **2009**, *4,* 1–7.

33. Dufes, C.; Uchegbu, I.; Schatzlein, A. Dendrimers in Gene Delivery. *Adv. Drug Deliv. Rev.* **2005,** *57,* 2177.

34. Allen, T. M.; Mumbengegwi, D. R.; Charrois, G. J. Anti-CD19-targeted Liposomal Doxorubicin Improves the Therapeutic Efficacy in Murine B-cell Lymphoma and Ameliorates the Toxicity of Liposomes with Varying Drug Release Rates. *Clin. Cancer Res.* **2005,** *11,* 3567–3573.

35. Barreiro, A.; Rurali, R.; Harnandez, E. R.; Moser, J.; Pichler, T. F.; L., et al. Subnanometer Motion of Cargos Driven by Thermal Gradients Along Carbon Nanotubes. *Science* **2008,** *320,* 775–778.

36. Bertholon, I.; Ponchel, G.; Labarre, D.; Couvreur, P.; Vauthier, C. Bioadhesive Properties of Poly(alkylcyanoacrylate) Nanoparticles Coated with Polysaccharide. *J. Nanosci. Nanotechnol.* **2006,** *6,* 3102–3109.

37. Beyerle, A.; Merkel, O.; Stoeger, T.; Kissel, T. PEGylation Affects Cytotoxicity and Cell-compatibility of Poly(ethylene imine) for Lung Application: Structure Function Relationships. *Toxicol. Appl. Pharmacol.* **2010,** *242,* 146–154.

38. Blum, J. L.; Savin, M. A.; Edelman, G.; Pippen, J. E.; Robert, N. J.; geister, B. V.; Kirby, R. L.; Clawson, A.; O'shaughnessy, J. A. Phase II Study of Weekly Albumin-bound Paclitaxel for Patients with Metastatic Breast Cancer Heavily Pretreated with Taxanes. *Clin. Breast Cancer* **2007,** *7,* 850–856.

39. Brigger, I.; Dubernet, C.; Couvreur, P. Nanoparticles in Cancer Therapy and Diagnosis. *Adv. Drug Del. Rev.* **2002,** *54,* 631–651.

40. Calvo, P.; Remuñan-López, C.; Vila-Jato, J. L.; Alonso, M. J. Chitosan and Chitosan/Ethylene Oxide-propylene Oxide Block copolymer Nanoparticles as Novel Carriers for Proteins and Vaccines. *Pharm. Res.* **1997,** *14,* 1431–1436.

41. Chen, Y.; McCulloch, R. K.; Gray, B. N. Synthesis of Albumin-Dextran Sulfate Microspheres Possessing Favourable Loading and Release Characteristics for the Anticancer Drug Doxorubicin. *J Controlled Release* **1994,** *31,* 49–54.

42. Couvreur, P.; Barratt, G.; Fattal, E.; Legrand, P.; Vauthier, C. Nanocapsule Technology: A Review. *Crit. Rev. Ther. Drug Carrier Syst.* **2002,** *19,* 99134.

43. Dang, J. M.; Leong, K. W. Natural Polymers for Gene Delivery and Tissue Engineering. *Adv. Drug Deliv. Rev.* **2006,** *58,* 487–499.

44. Kreyling, W. G.; Möller, W.; Semmler-Behnke, M.; Oberdörster, G. In *Particle Toxicology*; Born, D. K., Ed.; CRC Press: Boca Raton, 2007.

45. Linhardt, R. J. In *Controlled Release of Drugs*; Rosoff, M., Ed.; VCH Publishers: New York, 1989; pp 53–95.

46. Muller, R. H.; Mader, K.; Gohla, S. Solid Lipid Nanoparticles (SLN) for controlled Drug Delivery ± A Review of the State of the Art. *Eur. J. Pharm. Biopharm.* **2000,** *50,* 161–177.

47. Panyam, J.; Labhasetwar, V. Biodegradable Nanoparticles for Drug and Gene Delivery to Cells and Tissue. *Adv. Drug Deliv. Rev.* **2003,** *12,* 329–347.

48. Redhead, H. M.; Davis, S. S.; Illum, L. Drug Delivery in Poly(lactide-co-glycolide) Nanoparticles Surface Modified with Poloxamer 407 and Poloxamine 908: In vitro Characterisation and In vivo Evaluation. *J. Controlled Release* **2001,** *70,* 353–363.

49. Yang, L.; Cao, Z.; Sajja, H.; Mao, H.; Wang, L.; Geng, H.; Xu, H.; Jiang, T.; Wood, W.; Nie, S.; Wang, A. Development of Receptor Targeted Iron Oxide Nanoparticles for Efficient Drug Delivery and Tumor imaging. *J. Biomed. Nanotech.* **2008,** *4,* 1–11.

50. Yang, L.; Peng, X.; Wang, Y.; Wang, X.; Cao, Z.; Ni, C.; Karna, P.; Zhang, X.; Wood, W.; Gao, X.; Nie, S.; Mao, H. Receptor-targeted Nanoparticles for In vivo Imaging of Breast Cancer. *Clin. Cancer Res.* **2009,** *15,* 4722–4732.

51. Ferrari, M. Frontiers in Cancer Nanomedicine: Directing Mass Transport Through Biological Barriers. *Trends Biotechnol.* **2010,** *786,* 1–8.

52. Rhim, W. -K.; Kim, J. -S.; Nam, J. -M. From Lipid–Gold–Nanoparticle Hybrid-based Gene Delivery. *Small* **2008,** *4,* 1651–1655.

53. Jin, S.; Ye, K. Nanoparticle-Mediated Drug Delivery and Gene Therapy. *Biotechnol. Prog.* **2007,** *23,* 32–41.

54. Tan, W.; Wang, K.; He, X.; Zhao, X. J.; Drake, T.; Wang, L.; Bagwe, R. P. Bionanotechnology Based on Silica Nanoparticles. *Med. Res. Rev.* **2004,** *24,* 621–638.

55. Kneuer, C.; Sameti, M.; Bakowsky, U.; Schiestel, T.; Schirra, H.; Schmidt, H.; Lehr, C. M. A Nonviral DNA Delivery System Based on Surface Modified Silica-nanoparticles can Efficiently Transfect Cells In vitro. *Bioconjugate Chem.* **2000,** *11,* 926–932.

56. Singh, M.; Briones, M.; Ott, G.; O'Hagan, D. Cationic Microparticles: A Potent Delivery System for DNA Vaccines. *Proc. Natl. Acad. Sci. U.S.A.* **2000,** *97,* 811–816.

57. Nomura, T.; Koreeda, N.; Yamashita, F.; Takakura, Y.; Hashida, M. Effect of Particle Size and Charge on the Disposition of Lipid Carriers After Intratumoral Injection into Tissue-isolated Tumors. *Pharm. Res.* **1998,** *15,* 128–132.

58. Kaul, G.; Amiji, M. Tumor-targeted Gene Delivery Using Poly-(ethylene glycol)-modified Gelatin Nanoparticles: In vitro and In vivo Studies. *Pharm. Res.* **2005,** *22,* 951–961.

59. He, X.; Wang, K.; Tan, W.; Liu, B.; Liu, X.; Huang, S.; Li, D.; He, C.; Li, J. A Novel Gene Carrier Based on Amino-Modified Silica Nanoparticles. *Chin. Sci. Bull.* **2003,** *48,* 223–228.

60. Bharali, D. J.; Klejbor, I.; Stachowiak, E. K.; Dutta, P.; Roy, I.; Kaur, N.; Bergey, E. J.; Prasad, P. N.; Stachowiak, M. K. Organically Modified Silica Nanoparticles: A Nonviral Vector for In vivo Gene Delivery and Expression in the Brain. *Proc. Natl. Acad. Sci. U.S.A.* **2005,** *102,* 11539–11544.

61. Prabha, S.; Labhasetwar, V. Critical Determinants in PLGA/PLA Nanoparticle-mediated Gene Expression. *Pharm. Res.* **2004,** *21,* 354–3363.

62. Cohen, H.; Levy, R. J.; Gao, J.; Fishbein, I.; Kousaev, V.; Sosnowski, S.; Slomkowski, S.; Golomb, G. Sustained Delivery and Expression of DNA Encapsulated in Polymeric Nanoparticles. *Gene Ther.* **2000,** *7,* 1896–1905.

63. Lim, Y. B.; Han, S. O.; Kong, H. U.; Lee, Y.; Park, J. S.; Jeong, B.; Kim, S. W. Biodegradable Polyester, Poly[R-(4-aminobutyl)-L-glycolic acid], as a Non-toxic Gene Carrier. *Pharm. Res.* **2000,** *17,* 811–816.

64. Kaul, G.; Amiji, M. In *Polymeric Gene Delivery: Principles and Applications*; Amiji, M., Ed.; CRC Press: Boca Raton, FL, 2004; pp 429–447.

65. Kaul, G.; Amiji, M. Cellular Interactions and In vitro DNA Transfection Studies with Poly(ethylene glycol)-modified Gelatin Nanoparticles. *J. Pharm. Sci.* **2005,** *94,* 184–198.

66. Chiu, S. J.; Ueno, N. T.; Lee, R. J. Tumor-targeted Gene Delivery via anti-HER2 Antibody (trastuzumab, Herceptin) Conjugated Polyethylenimine. *J. Controlled Release* **2004,** *97,* 357–369.

67. Prabha, S.; Zhou, W. Z.; Panyam, J.; Labhasetwar, V. Size Dependency of Nanoparticle-mediated Gene Transfection: Studies with Fractionated Nanoparticles. *Int. J. Pharm.* **2002,** *211,* 105–115.

68. Ahl, P. L.; Bhatia, S. K.; Meers, P.; Roberts, P.; Stevens, R.; Dause, R.; Perkins, W. R.; Janoff, A. S. Enhancement of the In vivo Circulation Lifetime of L-alpha-Distearoylphosphatidylcholine Liposomes: Importance of Liposomal Aggregation Versus Complement Opsonization. *Biochim. Biophys. Acta* **1997,** *1329,* 370–382.

69. Kong, G. A.; Braun, R. D.; Dewhirst, M. W. Hyperthermia Enables Tumor-specific Nanoparticle Delivery: Effect of Particle Size. *Cancer Res.* **2000,** *60,* 4440–4445.

70. Toub, N.; Malvy, C.; Fattal, E. Innovative Nanotechnologies for the Delivery of Oligonucleotides and siRNA. *Biomed. Pharmacother.* **2006**, *60*, 607–620.

71. Pille, J. Y.; Li, H.; Blot, E.; Bertrand, J. R.; Pritchard, L. L.; Opolon, P.; Maksimenko, A.; Lu, H.; Vannier, J. P.; Soria, J.; Malvy, C.; Soria, C. Intravenous Delivery of Anti-RhoA Small Interfering NA Loaded in Nanoparticles of Chitosan in Mice: Safety and Efficacy in Xenografted Aggressive Breast Cancer. *Hum. Gene. Ther.* **2006**, *17*, 1019–1026.

72. Urban-Klein, B.; Werth, S.; Abuharbeid, S.; Czubayko, F.; Aigner, A. RNAi-mediated Gene-targeting Through Systemic Application Of Polyethylenimine (PEI)-complexed siRNA In vivo. *Gene Ther.* **2005**, *12*, 461–466.

73. Kong, X.; Hellermann, G. R.; Zhang, W.; Jenna, P.; Kumar, M. N.; Behera, A.; Behera, S.; Lockeey, R.; Mohapatra, S. S. Chitosan Interferon-γ Nanogene Therapy for Lung Disease: Modulation of T-Cell and Dendritic Cell Immune Responses. *Allergy Asthma Clin. Immunol.* **2008**, *4*, 95–105.

74. Park, T. G.; Jeong, J. H.; Kim, S. W. Current Status of Polymeric Gene Delivery Systems. *Adv. Drug Deliv. Rev.* **2006**, *58*, 467–486.

75. SHi, X.; Wang, S. X.; Meshinchi, S.; Van Antwerp, M. E.; Bi, X.; Lee, I.; Baker, J. R. J. Dendrimer-entrapped Gold Nanoparticles as a Platform for Cancer-Cell Targeting and Imaging. *Small* **2007**, *3*, 1245–1252.

76. Rosi, N. L.; Giljohann, D. A.; Thaxton, C. S.; Lytton-Jean, A. K. R.; Han, M. S.; Mirkin, C. A. Oligonucleotidemodified Gold Nanoparticles for Infracellular Gene Regulation. *Science* **2006**, *312*, 1020–1027.

77. Sullivan, M. M. O.; Green, J. J.; Przybycien, T. M. Development of a Novel Gene Delivery Scaffold Utilizing Colloidal Gold-polyethylenimine Conjugates for DNA Condensation. *Gene Ther.* **2003**, *22*, 1882–1890.

78. Mirkin, C. A.; Letsinger, R. L.; Mucic, R. C.; Storhoff, J. J. A DNA-based Method for Rationally Assembling Nanoparticles into Macroscopic Materials. *Nature* **1996**, *382*, 607–609.

79. Paciotti, G. F.; Myer; Weinreich, D.; Goia; Pavel; McLaughlin, E.; Tamarkin, L. Colloidal Gold: A Novel Nanoparticle Vector for Tumor Directed Drug Delivery. *Drug Deliv.* **2004**, *11*, 169–183

80. Connor, E. E.; Mwamuka, J.; Gole, A.; Murphy, C. J.; Wyatt, M. D. Gold Nanoparticles are Taken Up by Human Cells But Do Not Cause Acute Cytotoxicity. *Small* **2005**, *1*, 325.

81. Andrews, P. R.; Craik, D. J.; Martin, J. L. Functional Group Contributions to Drug-Receptor Interactions. *J. Med. Chem.* **1984**, *27*, 1648–1657.

82. Jin, R.; Wu, G.; Li, Z.; Mirkin, C. A.; Schatz, G. C. What Controls the Melting Properties of DNA-linked Gold Nanoparticle Assemblies? *JACS* **2003**, *125*, 1643–1654.

83. Akamatsu, K.; Kimura, M.; Shibata, Y.; Nakano, S.; Miyoshi, D.; Nawafune, H.; Sugimoto, N. A DNA Duplex with Extremely Enhanced Thermal Stability Based on Controlled Immobilization on Gold Nanoparticles. *Nano Lett.* **2006**, *6*, 491–495.

84. Prabha, S.; Labhasetwar, V. Nanoparticle-mediated Wild-type p53 Gene Delivery Results in Sustained Antiproliferative Activity in Breast Cancer Cells. *Mol. Pharm.* **2004**, *1*.

85. Li, S.; Huang, L. Nonviral Gene Therapy: Promises and Challenges. *Gene Ther.* **2000**, *7*, 31–34.

86. Brown, M. D.; Schatzlein, A. G.; Uchegbu, I. F. Gene Delivery with Synthetic (Non Viral) Carriers. *Int. J. Pharm.* **2000**, *229*, 1–21.

87. Bonadio, J.; Smiley, E.; Patil, P.; Goldstein, S. Localized, Direct Plasmid Gene Delivery In vivo: Prolonged Therapy Results in Reproducible Tissue Regeneration. *Nat Med.* **1999**, *5*, 753–759.

88. Maheshwari, A.; Han, S.; Mahato, R. I.; Kim, S. W. Biodegradable Polymer-based Interleukin-12 gene Delivery: Role of Induced Cytokines, Tumor Infiltrating Cells and Nitric Oxide in Anti-Tumor Activity. *Gene Ther.* **2002**, *9*, 1075–1084.

89. Luo, D.; Woodrow-Mumford, K.; Belcheva, N.; Saltzman, W. M. Controlled DNA Delivery Systems. *Pharm. Res.* **1999**, *16*, 1300–1308.

90. Labhasetwar, V.; Bonadio, J.; Goldstein, S. A.; Levy, R. J. Gene Transfection Using Biodegradable Nanospheres: Results in Tissue Culture and a Rat Osteotomy Mode. *Colloids Surf. Biointerfaces* **1999**, *16*, 281–290.

91. Panyam, J.; Zhou, W. Z.; Prabha, S.; Sahoo, S. K.; Labhasetwar, V. Rapid Endo-lysosomal Escape of Poly(DL-lactide-*co*-glycolide) Nanoparticles: Implications for Drug and Gene Delivery. *FASEB* **2002**, *16*, 1217–1226.

92. Cailleau, R.; Young, R.; Olive, M.; Reeves, W. J. Breast Tumor Cell Lines from Pleural Effusions. *J. Natl. Cancer Inst.* **1974**, *53*, 661–674.

93. Runnebaum, I. B.; Nagarajan, M.; Bowman, M.; Soto, D.; Sukumar, S. Mutations in p53 as Potential Molecular Markers for Human Breast Cancer. *Proc. Natl. Acad. Sci. U.S.A.* **1991**, *88*, 10657–10661.

94. Erbacher, P.; Zou, S.; Bettinger, T.; Steffan, A. M.; Remy, J. S. Chitosan-based Vector/DNA Complexes for Gene Delivery: Biophysical Characteristics and Transfection Ability. *Pharm. Res.* **1998**, *15*, 1332–1339.

95. Klippstein, R.; Pozo, D. Nanotechnology-based Manipulation of Dendritic Cells for Enhanced Immunotherapy Strategies. *Nanomed. Nanotechnol. Biol. Med.* **2010**, *6*, 523–529.

96. Maldonaro-Lopez, R.; Moser, M. Dendritic Cell Subsets and the Regulation of Th1/Th2 Responses. *Semin. Immunol.* **2001**, *13*, 275–282.

97. Guermonprez, P.; Valladeau, J.; Zitvogel, L.; Thery, C.; Amigorena, S. Antigen Presentation and T cell Stimulation by Dendritic Cells. *Annu. Rev. Immunol.* **2002**, *20*, 621–667.

98. Banchereau, J.; Steinman, R. M. Dendritic Cells and the Control of Immunity. *Nature* **1998**, *392*, 245–252.

99. Banchereau, J.; Palucka, A. K. Dendritic Cells as therapeutic Vaccines Against Cancer. *Nat. Rev. Immunol.* **2005**, *5*, 296–306.

100. Hori, M.; Onishi, H.; Machida, Y. Evaluation of Eudragit-coated Chitosan Microparticles as an Oral Immune Delivery System. *Int. J. Pharm.* **2005**, *297*, 223–234.

101. Oppenheimer, J.; A., J.; Nelson, H. S. Safety and Efficacy Of Oral Immunotherapy with standardized Cat Extract. *J. Allergy Clin. Immunol.* **1994**, *93*, 61–67.

102. Van Deusen, M. A.; Angelini, B. L.; Cordoro, K. M.; Seiler, B. A.; Wood, L.; Skoner, D. P. Efficacy and Safety of oral Immunotherapy with short Ragweed Extract. *Ann. Allergy Asthma Immunol.* **1997**, *78*, 753–780.

103. Mosbech, H.; Dreborg, S.; Madsen, F.; Ohlsson, H.; Stahl Skov, P.; Taudorf, E., et al. High Dose Grass Pollen Tablets used for Hyposensitization in Hay Fever Patients. A One-year Double Blind Placebo-controlled Study. *Allergy* **1987**, *42*, 451–455.

104. Moller, C.; Dreborg, S.; Lanner, A.; Bjorksten, B. Oral Immunotherapy of Children with Rhinoconjunctivitis due to Birch Pollen Allergy. A Double Blind Study. *Allergy* **1986**, *41*, 271–279.

105. Gomez, S.; Gamazo, C.; San Roman, B.; Ferrer, M.; Sanz, M. L.; Irache, J. M. Gantrez AN Nanoparticles as an Adjuvant for Oral Immunotherapy with Allergens. *Vaccine* **2007**, *25*, 5263–5271.

106. Petrovsky, N.; Aguilar, J. C. Vaccine Adjuvants: Current State and Future Trends. *Immunol Cell Biol.* **2004**, *82*, 488–496.

107. Sanders, M. T.; Brown, L. E.; Deliyannis, G.; Pearse, M. J. ISCOM-based Vaccines: The Second Decade. *Immunol. Cell. Biol.* **2005**, *83*, 119–128.

108. Childers, N. K.; Miller, K. L.; Tong, G.; Llarena, J. C.; Greenway, T.; Ulrich, J. T., et al. Adjuvant Activity of Monophosphoryl Lipid A for nasal and Oral Immunization with Soluble or Liposome-associated Antigen. *Infect. Immun.* **2000,** *68,* 5509–5516.

109. Doherty, T. M.; Olsen, A. W.; van Pinxteren, L.; Andersen, P. Oral Vaccination with Subunit Vaccines Protects Animals Against Aerosol Infection with *Mycobacterium tuberculosis.* *Infect. Immun.* **2002,** *70,* 3111–3121.

110. O'Hagan, D. T.; Singh, M. Microparticles as Vaccine Adjuvants and Delivery Systems. *Expert Rev. Vaccines* **2003,** *2,* 269–283.

111. Pandey, R. S.; Sahu, S.; Sudheesh, M. S.; Madan, J.; Kumar, M.; Dixit, V. K. Carbohydrate Modified Ultrafine Ceramic Nanoparticles for Allergen Immunotherapy. *Int. Immunopharm.* **2011,** *11,* 925–931.

112. Van Der Lubben, I. M.; Konings, F. A.; Borchard, G.; Verhoef, J. C.; Junginger-He, C. In vivo Uptake Of Chitosan Microparticles by Murine Peyer's Patches: Visualization Studies Using Confocal Laser Scanning Microscopy and Immunohistochemistry. *J. Drug Target.* **2001,** *9,* 39–47.

113. Canon, M. J.; O'Brien, T. J.; Underwood, L. J.; Crew, M. D.; Bondurant, K. L.; Santin, A. D. Novel Target Antigens for Dendritic Cell-based Immunotherapy Against Ovarian Cancer. *Expert Rev. Anticancer Ther.* **2002,** *2.*

114. Nowakowski, A.; Wang, C.; Powers, D. B.; Amersdorfer, P.; Smith, T. J.; Montgomery, V. A.; Sheridan, R.; Blake, R.; Smith, L. A.; Marks, J. D. Potent Neutralization of Botulinum Neurotoxin by Recombinant Oligoclonal Antibody. *PNAS* **2002,** *99,* 11346–11350.

115. Kwong, B.; Liu, H.; Irvine, D. J. Induction of Potent Anti-tumor Responses While Eliminating Systemic Side Effects via Liposome-anchored Combinatorial Immunotherapy. *Biomaterials* **2011,** *32,* 5134–5147.

116. Pandey, R. S.; Dixit, V. K. Evaluation of ISCOM Vaccines for Mucosal Immunization Against Hepatitis B. *J. Drug Del.* **2010,** *18,* 282–291.

117. Salman, H. H.; Gamazo, C.; Campanero, M. A.; Irache, J. M. Salmonella-like Bioadhesive Nanoparticles. *J. Controlled Release* **2005,** *106,* 1–13.

118. Qurashi, T.; Blair, H. S.; Allen, S. J. Studies on Modified Chitosan Membranes. I. Preparation and Characterization. *J. Appl. Polym. Sci.* **1992,** *46,* 255–261.

119. Shin, H.; Jo, S.; Mikos, A. G. Biomimetic Materials for Tissue Engineering. *Biomaterials* **2003,** *24,* 4353–4364.

120. Richardson, S. C.; Kolbe, H. V.; Duncan, R. Potential of Low Molecular Mass Chitosan as a DNA Delivery System: Biocompatibility, Body Distribution and Ability to Complex and protect DNA. *Int. J. Pharm.* **1999,** *178.*

121. Muzzarelli, R.; Baldassarre, V.; Conti, F. Biological Activity of Chitosan: Ultrastructural Study.*Biomaterials* **1988,** *9,* 247–252.

122. Nishimura, K.; Nishimura, S.; Nishi, N. Immunological Activity of Chitin and its Derivatives. *Vaccine* **1984,** *2,* 93–99.

123. Otterlei, M.; Varum, K. M.; Ryan, L.; Espevik, T. Characterization of Binding and TNF-alpha-inducing Ability of Chitosans on Monocytes: The Involvement of CD14. *Vaccine* **1994,** *12,* 232–285.

124. Pappineau, A.; Hoover, D.; Knoor, D.; Farkas, D. *Food Biotechnology*; Marcel and Dekker: New York, 1991.

125. Lee, K. Y.; Kwon, I. C.; Kim, Y. H. Preparation of Chitosan Self-aggregates as a Gene Delivery System. *J. Controlled Release* **1998,** *51,* 213–220.

126. Aspden, T. J.; Mason, J. D.; Jones, N. S. Chitosan as a Nasal Delivery System: The Effect of Chitosan Solutions on In vitro and In vivo Mucociliary Transport Rates in Human Turbinates and Volunteers. *J. Pharm. Sci.* **1997,** *86,* 509–513.

127. Illum, L.; Farraj, N. F.; Davis, S. S. Chitosan as a Novel Nasal Delivery System for Peptide Drugs. *Pharm. Res.* **1994,** *11,* 1186–1189.

128. Artursson, P.; Lindmark, T.; Davis, S. S.; Illum, L. Effect of Chitosan on the Permeability of Monolayers of Intestinal Epithelial Cells (Caco-2). *Pharm. Res.* **1994,** *11,* 1358–1361.

129. Coyle, A. J.; Tsuyuki, S.; Bertrand, C. Mice Lacking the IFN-gamma Receptor have Impaired Ability to Resolve a Lung Eosinophilic Inflammatory Response Associated with a Prolonged Capacity of T Cells to Exhibit a Th_2 Cytokine Profile. *J. Immunol.* **1996,** *156,* 2680–2685.

130. Szeto, C.; Gillespie, K. M.; Mathieson, P. W. Levamisole Induces Interleukin-18 and Shifts Type 1/type 2 Cytokine Balance. *Immunology* **2000,** *100,* 217–224.

131. Boraschi, D.; Censini, S.; Bartalini, M. Interferons Inhibit LTC4 Production in Murine Macrophages. *J. Immunol.* **1987,** *138,* 4341–4346.

132. Chen, H.; Munakata, M.; Amishima, M. Gamma-interferon Modifies Guinea Pig Airway Functions In vitro. *Eur. Respir. J.* **1994,** *7,* 74–80.

133. Pouw Kraan, T. C. v.; Boeije, L. C.; de Groot, E. R. Reduced Production of IL-12 and IL-12-dependent IFN-gamma Release in Patients with Allergic Asthma. *J. Immunol.* **1997,** *158,* 5560–5565.

134. Daines, M. O.; Hershey, G. K. A Novel Mechanism by which Interferon-gamma can Regulate Interleukin (IL)-13 Responses. Evidence for Intracellular Stores of IL-13 Receptor alpha-2 and Their Rapid Mobilization by Interferon-gamma. *J. Biol. Chem.* **2002,** *277,* 10387–10393.

135. Ford, J. G.; Rennick, D.; Donaldson, D. D. IL-13 and IFN-gamma: Interactions in Lung Inflammation. *J. Immunol.* **2001,** *167,* 1769–1777.

136. Krasnowska, M.; Medrala, W.; Malolepszy, J.; Krasnowski, R. Effect of Recombinant IFN-gamma on IgE-dependent Leukotriene Generation by Peripheral Blood Leukocytes in Patients with Pollinosis and Asthma. *Arch. Immunol. Ther. Exp. (Warsz)* **2000,** *48,* 287–292.

137. Gurujeyalakshmi, G.; Giri, S. N. Molecular Mechanisms of Antifibrotic Effect of Interferon Gamma in Bleomycin-mouse Model of Lung Fibrosis: Downregulation of TGF-beta and Procollagen I and III Gene Expression. *Exp. Lung Res.* **1995,** *21,* 791–808.

138. Cohen, J. IL-12 Deaths: Explanation and a Puzzle. *Science* **1995,** *270,* 908.

139. Hogan, S. P.; Foster, P. S.; Tan, X.; Ramsay, A. J. Mucosal IL-12 Gene Delivery Inhibits Allergic Airways Disease and Restores Local Antiviral Immunity. *Eur. J. Immunol.* **1998,** *28,* 413–4123.

140. Sur, S.; Lam, J.; Bouchard, P. Immunomodulatory Effects of IL-12 on Allergic Lung Inflammation Depend on Timing of Doses. *J. Immunol.* **1996,** *157,* 4173–4180.

141. Dow, S. W.; Schwarze, J.; Heath, T. D. Systemic and Local Interferon Gamma Gene Delivery to the Lungs for Treatment of Allergen-induced Airway Hyperresponsiveness in Mice. *Hum. Gene Ther.* **1999,** *10,* 1905–1914.

142. Okubo, T.; Hagiwara, E.; Ohno, S. Administration of an IL-12-encoding DNA Plasmid Prevents the Development of Chronic graft-versus-host disease (GVHD). *J. Immunol.* **1999,** *162,* 4013–4017.

143. Kumar, M.; Behera, A. K.; Lockey, R. F. Intranasal Gene Transfer by Chitosan-DNA Nanospheres Protects BALB/c Mice Against Acute Respiratory Syncytial Virus Infection. *Hum. Gene Ther.* **2002,** *13,* 1415–1425.

144. Zhang, Y. J.; Lu, J. J. A Simple Method to Tailor Spherical Nanocrystal Hydroxyapatite at Low Temperature. *J. Nanopart. Res.* **2007,** *9,* 589–594.

145. Goyal, A. K.; Khatri, K.; Mishra, N.; Mehta, A.; Vaidya, B.; Tiwari, S., et al. Aquasomes-a Nanoparticulate Approach for the Delivery of Antigen. *Drug Dev. Ind. Pharm.* **2008,** *34,* 1297–1305.

146. Goyal, A. K.; Rawat, A.; Mahor, P. N.; Khatri, k.; Vyas, S. P. Nanodecoy System: A Novel Approach to Design Hepatitis B Vaccine for Immunopotentiation. *Int. J. Pharm.* **2006,** *309,* 227–233.

147. Kossovsky, N.; Gelman, A.; Sponsler, E. E.; Hnatyszyn, H. J.; Rajguru, S.; Torres, M., et al. Surface Modified Nanocrystalline Ceramics for Drug Delivery Applications. *Biomaterials* **1994,** *15,* 1201–1207.

148. Ferraz, M. P.; Monteriro, F. J.; Manuel, C. M. Hydroxyapatite Nanoparticles: A Review of Preparation Methodologies. *J. Appl. Biomater. Biomech.* **2004,** *2,* 74–80.

149. Freed, L. E.; Novakovic, G. V.; Biron, R. J.; Eagles, D. B.; Lesnoy, D. C.; Barlow, S. K., et al. Biodegradable polymer Scaffolds for Tissue Engineering. *Biotechnology* **1994,** *12,* 689–693.

150. Hench, L. L.; Polak, J. M. Third-generation Biomedical Materials. *Science* **2002,** *295,* 1014–1017.

151. Hong, Z. K.; Qui, X. Y.; Sun, J. R.; Deng, M. X.; Chen, X. S.; Jing, X. B. Grafting Polymerization of L-Lactide on the Surface of Hydroxyapatite Nano-crystal. *Polymer* **2004,** *45,* 6705–6713.

152. Kim, H. W.; Koh, Y. H.; Li, L. L.; Lee, S.; Kim, H. E. Hydroxyapatite Coating on Titanium Substrate with Titania Buffer Layer Processed by Sol-Gel Method. *Biomaterials* **2004,** *25,* 2533–2538.

153. Klein, C. P. A.T.; Driessen, A. A.; de Groot, K.; van den Hooff, A. Biodegradation Behaviour of various Calcium Phosphate Materials in Bone Tissue. *J. Biomed. Mater. Res.* **2004,** *17,* 769–784.

154. Liao, S. S.; F.Z., C.; Zhu, Y. Osteoblasts Adherence and Migration Through Three Dimensional Porous Mineralized Collagen Based Composite: nHAC/PLA. *J. Bioact. Compat. Polym.* **2004,** *19,* 117–130.

155. Rezwan, K.; Chen, Q. Z.; Blaker, J. J.; Boccaccini, A. R. Biodegradable and Bioactive Porous Polymer/Inorganic Composite Scaffolds for Bone Tissue Engineering. *Biomaterials* **2006,** *27.*

156. Webster, T. J.; Ergun, C.; Doremus, R. H.; Siegel, R. W.; Bizios, R. Enahnced Functions if Osteoblasts on Nanophase Ceramics. *Biomaterials* **2000,** *2,* 1803–1810.

157. Webster, T. J.; Schadler, L. S.; Siegel, R. W.; Bizios, R. Mechanisms of Enhanced Osteoblast Adhesion on Nanophase Alumina Involve Vitronectin. *Tissue Eng.* **2001,** *7,* 291–301.

158. Webster, T. J.; Siegel, R. W.; Bizios, R. Osteoblast Adhesion on Nanophase Ceramics. *Biomaterials* **1999,** *20,* 1221–1227.

159. Paul, W.; Sharma, C. P. Ceramic Drug Delivery: A Perspective. *J. Biomater. Appl.* **2003,** *17,* 253–264.

160. Barroug, A.; Lernoux, E.; Lemaitre, J.; Rouxhet, P. G. Adsorption of Catalase on Hydroxyapatite. *J. Colloid Interface Sci.* **1998,** *208,* 147–152.

161. Hedge, J. E.; Hofreiter, B. T. In *Methods in Carbohydrate Chemistry*; Whistler, R. L., Be Miller, J. N., Eds.; Academic Press: New York, 1962.

162. Whiteside, T. L. The Tumor Microenvironment and its Role in Promoting Tumor Growth. *Oncogene* **2008,** *27,* 5904–5912.

163. Swann, J. B.; Smyth, M. J. Immune Surveillance of Tumors. *J. Clin. Invest.* **2007,** *117,* 1137–1146.

164. Kortylewski, M.; Swiderski, P.; Herrmann, A.; Wang, L.; Kowolik, C.; Kujawski, M., et al. In vivo Delivery of siRNA to Immune Cells by Conjugation to a TLR9 Against Enhances Antitumor Immune Responses. *Nat. Biotechnol.* **2009,** *27,* 925–932.

165. Yang, Y.; Huang, C. T.; Huang, X.; Pardoll, D. M. Persistent Toll-like Receptor Signals are Required for Reversal of Regulatory T Cell-mediated CD8 Tolerance. *Nat. Immunol.* **2004,** *5,* 508–515.

166. Houot, R.; Levy, R. T-cell Modulation Combined with Intratumoral CpG cures Lymphoma in a Mouse Model Without the Need for Chemotherapy. *Blood* **2009,** *113,* 3546–3552.

167. Jackaman, C.; Lew, A. M.; Zhan, Y.; Allan, J. E.; Koloska, B.; Graham, P. T., et al. Deliberately Provoking Local Inflammation Drives Tumors to Become Their Own Protective Vaccine Site. *Int. Immunol.* **2008,** *20,* 1467–1479.

168. Curran, M. A.; Montalvo, W.; Yagita, H.; Allison, J. P. PD-1 and CTLA-4 Combination Block-ade Expands Infiltrating T Cells and Reduces Regulatory T and Myeloid Cells Within B16 Melanoma Tumors. *Proc. Natl. Acad. Sci. U.S.A.* **2010,** *107,* 4275–4280.

169. Elgueta, R.; Benson, M. J.; de Vries, V. C.; Wasiuk, A.; Guo, Y.; Noelle, R. J. Molecular Mechanism and Function of CD40/CD40L Engagement in the Immune System. *Immunol. Rev.* **2009,** *229,* 152–173.

170. Carson, W. E.; Dierksheide, J. E.; Jabbour, S.; Anghelina, M.; Bouchard, P.; Ku, G., et al. Coad-ministration of Interleukin-18 and Interleukin-12 Induces a Fatal Inflammatory Response in Mice: Critical Role of Natural Killer Cell Interferon-gamma Production and STAT-mediated Signal Transduction. *Blood* **2000,** *96,* 1465–1473.

171. Phan, G. Q.; Yang, J. C.; Sherry, R. M.; Hwu, P.; Topalian, S. L.; Schwartzentruber, D. J., et al. Cancer Regression and Autoimmunity Induced by Cytotoxic T Lymphocyte-associated Antigen 4 Blockade in Patients with Metastatic Melanoma. *Proc. Natl. Acad. Sci. U.S.A.* **2003,** *100,* 8372–8377.

172. French, R. R.; Chan, H. T.; Tutt, A. L.; Glennie, M. J. CD40 Antibody Evokes a Cytotoxic T-cell Response that Eradicates Lymphoma and Bypasses T-cell Help. *Nat. Med.* **1999,** *5,* 548–553.

173. Sotomayor, E. M.; Borrello, I.; Tubb, E.; Rattis, F. M.; Bien, H.; Lu, Z., et al. Conversion of Tumor-specific CD4+ T-cell Tolerance to T-cell Priming Through In vivo Ligation of CD40. *Nat. Med.* **1999,** *5,* 780–787.

174. Tutt, A. L.; O'Brien, L.; Hussain, A.; Crowther, G. R.; French, R. R.; Glennie, M. J. T Cell Immunity to Lymphoma Following Treatment with Anti-CD40 Monoclonal Antibody. *J. Immunol.* **2002,** *168,* 2720–2728.

175. van Mierlo, G. J.; den Boer, A. T.; Medema, J. P.; van der Voort, E. I.; Fransen, M. F.; Offringa, R., et al. CD40 Stimulation Leads to Effective Therapy of CD40(−) Tumors Through Induc-tion of Strong Systemic Cytotoxic T Lymphocyte Immunity. *Proc. Natl. Acad. Sci. U.S.A.* **2002,** *99,* 5561–5566.

176. Nowak, A. K.; Robinson, B. W.; Lake, R. A. Synergy between Chemotherapy and Immu-notherapy in the Treatment of Established Murine Solid Tumors. *Cancer Res.* **2003,** *63,* 4490–4496.

177. Hamzah, J.; Nelson, D.; Moldenhauer, G.; Arnold, B.; Hammerling, G. J.; Ganss, r Vascular Targeting of Anti-CD40 Antibodies and IL-2 into Autochthonous Tumors Enhances Immuno-therapy in Mice. *J. Clin. Invest.* **2008,** *118,* 1691–1699.

178. Vonderheide, R. H.; Flaherty, K. T.; Khalil, M.; Stumacher, M. S.; Bajor, D. L.; Hutnick, N. A., et al. Clinical Activity and Immune Modulation in Cancer Patients Treated with CP-870,893, a Novel CD40 Agonist Monoclonal Antibody. *J. Clin. Oncol.* **2007,** *25,* 876–883.

179. Ruter, J.; Antonia, S. J.; Burris, H. A.; Huhn, R. D.; Vonderheide, R. H. Immune Modula-tion with Weekly Dosing of an Agonist CD40 Antibody in a Phase I Study of Patients with Advanced Solid Tumors. *Cancer Biol. Ther.* **2010,** *10,* 983–993.

180. Hussein, M.; Berenson, J. R.; Niesvizky, R.; Munshi, N.; Matous, J.; Sobecks, R., et al. A Phase I Multidose Study of Dacetuzumab (SGN-40; Humanized anti-CD40 Monoclonal Anti-body) in Patients with Multiple Myeloma. *Haematologica* **2010,** *95,* 845–848.

181. Advani, R.; Forero-Torres, A.; Furman, R. R.; Rosenblatt, J. D.; Younes, A.; Ren, H., et al. Phase I Study of the Humanized Anti-CD40 Monoclonal Antibody Dacetuzumab in Refrac-tory or Recurrent Non-Hodgkin's Lymphoma. *J. Clin. Oncol.* **2009,** *27,* 4371–4377.

182. Kimura, K.; Moriwaki, H.; Nagaki, M.; Saio, M.; Nakamoto, Y.; Naito, M., et al. Pathogenic Role of B cells in Anti-CD40-induced Necroinflammatory Liver Disease. *Am. J. Pathol.* **2006,** *168,* 786–795.

183. Gendelman, M.; Halligan, N.; Komorowski, R.; Logan, B.; Murphy, W. J.; Blazar, B. R., et al. Alpha Phenyl-tert-butyl nitrone (PBN) Protects Syngeneic Marrow Transplant Recipients from the Lethal Cytokine Syndrome Occurring After Agonistic CD40 Antibody Administration. *Blood* **2005,** *105,* 428–431.

184. Hixon, J. A.; Anver, M. R.; Blazar, B. R.; Panoskaltsis-Mortari, A.; Wiltrout, R. H.; Murphy, W. J. Administration of Either anti-CD40 or Interleukin- 12 Following Lethal Total Body Irradiation Induces Acute Lethal Toxicity Affecting the Gut. *Biol. Blood Marrow Transplant* **2002,** *8,* 316–325.

185. Bartholdy, C.; Kauffmann, S. O.; Christensen, J. P.; Thomsen, A. R. Agonistic Anti-CD40 Antibody Profoundly Suppresses the Immune Response to Infection with Lymphocytic Choriomeningitis Virus. *J. Immunol.* **2007,** *178,* 1662–1670.

186. Lonsdorf, A. S.; Kuekrek, H.; Stern, B. V.; Boehm, B. O.; Lehmann, P. V.; Tary-Lehmann, M. Intratumor CpG-oligodeoxynucleotide Injection Induces Protective Antitumor T cell Immunity. *J. Immunol.* **2003,** *171,* 3941–3946.

187. Baines, J.; Celis, E. Immune-mediated Tumor Regression Induced by CpG-Containing Oligodeoxynucleotides. *Clin. Cancer Res.* **2003,** *9,* 2693–2700.

188. Scarlett, U. K.; Cubillos-Ruiz, J. R.; Nesbeth, Y. C.; M, D. G.; Engle, X.; Gewirtz, A. T., et al. In situ Stimulation of CD40 and Toll-like Receptor 3 Transforms Ovarian Cancer-infiltrating Dendritic Cells from Immunosuppressive to Immunostimulatory Cells. *Cancer Res.* **2009,** *69,* 7329–7337.

189. Stone, G. W.; Barzee, S.; Snarsky, V.; Santucci, C.; Tran, B.; Langer, R., et al. Nanoparticle-delivered Multimeric Soluble CD40L DNA Combined with Toll-Like Receptor Agonists as a Treatment for Melanoma. *PLoS One* **2009,** *4,* e7334.

190. Wingender, G.; Garbi, N.; Schumak, B.; Jungerkes, F.; Endl, E.; von Bubnoff, D., et al. Systemic Application of CpG-rich DNA Suppresses Adaptive T Cell Immunity Via Induction of IDO. *Eur. J. Immunol.* **2006,** *36,* 12–20.

191. Mellor, A. L.; Baban, B.; Chandler, P. R.; Manlapat, A.; Kahler, D. J.; Munn, D. H. Cutting Edge: CpG Oligonucleotides Induce Splenic CD19+ Dendritic Cells to Acquire Potent Indoleamine 2,3-dioxygenase-dependent T Cell Regulatory Functions Via IFN Type 1 Signaling. *J. Immunol.* **2005,** *175,* 5601–5605.

192. Heikenwalder, M.; Polymenidou, M.; Junt, T.; Sigurdson, C.; Wagner, H.; Akira, S., et al. Lymphoid Follicle Destruction and Immunosuppression After Repeated CpG Oligodeoxynucleotide Administration. *Nat. Med.* **2004,** *10,* 187–192.

193. Gimbel, M. I.; Delman, K. A.; Zager, J. S. Therapy for Unresectable Recurrent and In-Transit Extremity Melanoma. *Cancer Control* **2008,** *15,* 225–232.

194. Den Otter, W.; Jacobs, J. J.; Battermann, J. J.; Hordijk, G. J.; Krastev, Z.; Moiseeva, E. V., et al. Local Therapy of Cancer with Free IL-2. *Cancer Immunol. Immunother.* **2008,** *57,* 931–950.

195. Heckelsmiller, K.; Rall, K.; Beck, S.; Schlamp, A.; Seiderer, J.; Jahrsdorfer, B., et al. Peritumoral CpG DNA Elicits a Coordinated Response of CD8 T Cells and Innate Effectors to Cure Established Tumors in a Murine Colon Carcinoma Model. *J. Immunol.* **2002,** *169,* 3892–3899.

196. Johnson, E. E.; Lum, H. D.; Rakhmilevich, A. L.; Schmidt, B. E.; Furlong, M.; Buhtoiarov, I. N., et al. Intratumoral Immunocytokine Treatment Results in Enhanced Antitumor Effects. *Cancer Immunol. Immunother.* **2008,** *57,* 1891–1902.

197. Simmons, A. D.; Moskalenko, M.; Creson, J.; Fang, J.; Yi, S.; Van roey, M. J., et al. Local Secretion of Anti-CTLA-4 Enhances the Therapeutic Efficacy of a Cancer Immunotherapy with Reduced Evidence of Systemic Autoimmunity. *Cancer Immunol. Immunother.* **2008,** *57,* 1263–1270.

198. Galili, U.; Wigglesworth, K.; Abdel-Motal, U. M. Intratumoral Injection of Alpha-gal Glyco-lipids Induces Xenograft-like Destruction and Conversion of Lesions Into Endogenous Vac-cines. *J. Immunol.* **2007,** *182,* 5217–5224.

199. Brody, J. D.; Ai, W. Z.; Czerwinski, D. K.; Torchia, J. A.; Levy, M.; Advan, R. H., et al. In situ Vaccination with a TLR9 Agonist Induces Systemic Lymphoma Regression: A Phase I/II Study. *J. Clin. Oncol.* **2010,** *28,* 4324–4332.

200. Bourquin, C.; Anz, D.; Zwiorek, K.; Lanz, A. L.; Fuchs, S.; Weigel, S., et al. Targeting CpG Oligonucleotides to the Lymph Node by Nanoparticles Elicits Efficient Antitumoral Immu-nity. *J. Immunol.* **2008,** *181,* 2990–2998.

201. Eton, O.; Rosenblum, M. G.; Legha, S. S.; Zhang, W.; Jo East, M.; Bedikian, A., et al. Phase I Trial of Subcutaneous Recombinant Human Interleukin-2 in Patients with Metastatic Mela-noma. *Cancer* **2002,** *95,* 127–134.

202. Hori, Y.; Stern, P. J.; Hynes, R. O.; Irvine, D. J. Engulfing Tumors with Synthetic Extracellular Matrices for Cancer Immunotherapy. *Biomaterials* **2009,** *30,* 6757–6767.

203. de Jong, S.; Chikh, G.; Sekirov, L.; Raney, S.; Semple, S.; Klimuk, S., et al. Encapsulation in Liposomal Nanoparticles Enhances the Immunostimulatory, Adjuvant and Anti-tumor Activ-ity of Subcutaneously Administered CpG ODN. *Cancer Immunol. Immunother.* **2007,** *56,* 1251–1264.

204. Hanes, J.; Sills, A.; Zhao, Z.; Suh, K. W.; Tyler, B.; DiMeco, F., et al. Controlled Local Deliv-ery of Interleukin-2 by Biodegradable Polymers Protects Animals from Experimental Brain Tumors and Liver Tumors. *Pharm. Res.* **2001,** *18,* 899–906.

205. Hill, H. C.; Conway, T. F., Jr.; Sabel, M. S.; Jong, Y. S.; Mathiowitz, E.; R.B., B., et al. Cancer Immunotherapy with Interleukin 12 and Granulocyte-Macrophage Colony-stimulating Fac-tor-encapsulated Microspheres: Coinduction of Innate and Adaptive Antitumor Immunity and Cure of Disseminated Disease. *Cancer Res.* **2002,** *62,* 7254–7263.

206. Van Herpen, C. M.; Huijbens, R.; Looman, M.; De Vries, J.; Marres, H.; Van De Ven, J., et al. Pharmacokinetics and Immunological Aspects of a Phase Ib Study with Intratumoral Admin-istration of Recombinant Human Interleukin-12 in Patients with Head and Neck Squamous Cell Carcinoma: A Decrease of T-bet in Peripheral Blood Mononuclear Cells. *Clin. Cancer Res.* **2003,** *9,* 2950–2956.

207. Liu, H.; Zhu, Z.; Kang, H.; Wu, Y.; Sefan, K.; Tan, W. DNA-based Micelles: Synthesis, Micel-lar Properties and Size-dependent Cell Permeability. *Chemistry* **2010,** *16,* 3791–3797.

208. Sabel, M. S.; Arora, K.; Su, G.; Mathiowitz, E.; Reineke, J. J.; Chang, A. E. Synergistic Effect of Intratumoral IL-12 and TNF-a Microspheres: Systemic Anti-tumor Immunity is Mediated by Both CD8+ CTL and NK Cells. *Surgery* **2007,** *142,* 749–760.

209. Hatzifoti, C.; Bacon, A.; Marriott, H.; Laing, P.; Heath, A. W. Liposomal Co-entrapment of CD40mAb Induces Enhanced IgG Responses Against Bacterial Polysaccharide and Protein. *PLoS One* **2008,** *3,* e2368.

210. Klinman, D. M. Immunotherapeutic Uses of CpG Oligodeoxynucleotides. *Nat. Rev. Immunol.* **2004,** *4,* 249–258.

211. Stumbles, P. A.; Himbeck, R.; Frelinger, J. A.; Collins, E. J.; Lake, R. A.; Robinson, B. W. Cutting Edge: Tumor-specific CTL are Constitutively Cross-armed in Draining Lymph Nodes and Transiently Disseminate to Mediate Tumor Regression Following Systemic CD40 Activation. *J. Immunol.* **2004,** *173,* 5923–5928.

212. Rakhmilevich, A. L.; Buhtoiarov, I. N.; Malkovsky, M.; Sondel, P. M. CD40 Ligation In vivo Can Induce T Cell Independent Antitumor Effects Even Against Immunogenic Tumors. *Cancer Immunol. Immunother.* **2008,** *57,* 1151–1160.

213. Pusic, K.; Xu, H.; Stridiron, A.; Aguilar, Z.; Wang, A. Z.; Hui, H. Blood Stage Merozoite Surface Protein Conjugated to Nanoparticles Induce Potent Parasite Inhibitory Antibodies. *Vaccine* **2011**, *29*, 8898–8908.

214. Sengupta, S.; Eavarone, D.; Capila, I.; Zhao, G.; Watson, N.; Kiziltepe, T., et al. Temporal Targeting of Tumour Cells and Neovasculature with a Nanoscale Delivery System. *Nature* **2005**, *436*, 568–572.

215. Ahmed, M.; Lukyanov, A.; Torchilin, V.; Tournier, H.; Schneider, A. N.; Godlberg, A. N. Combined Radiofrequency Ablation and Adjuvant Liposomal Chemotherapy: Effect of Chemotherapeutic Agent, Nanoparticle Size, and Circulation Time. *J. Vasc. Interv. Radiol.* **2005**, *16*, 1365–1371.

216. Ahmed, M.; Moussa, M.; Goldberg, S. N. Synergy in Cancer Treatment Between Liposomal Chemotherapeutics and Thermal Ablation. *Chem. Phys. Lipids* **2012**. Doi:10.1016/j.chemphyslip.2011.12.002.

217. Adair, E. R.; Blick, D. W.; Allen, S. J.; Mylacraine, K. S.; Ziriax, J. M.; Scholl, D. M. Thermophysiological Responses of Human Volunteers to Whole Body RF exposure at 220 MHz. *Bioelectromagnetics* **2005**, *26*, 448–461.

218. Hilger, I.; Hiergeist, R.; Hergt, R.; Winnefeld, K.; Schubert, H.; Kaiser, W. A. Thermal Ablation of Tumors Using Magnetic Nanoparticles: An In Vivo Feasibility Study. *Invest. Radiol.* **2002**, *37*, 580–586.

219. Han, S. K.; Kim, R. S.; Lee, J. H.; Tae, G.; Cho, S. H.; Yuk, S. H. In *Nanomaterials for Medical Diagnosis and Therapy*; Kumar, C., Ed.; Wiley, VCH: Darmstadt, Germany, 2009; pp 143–189.

220. Johanssen, M.; Gneveckow, U.; Taymoorian, K.; Cho, C. H.; Thiesen, B.; Scholz, R., et al. Thermal Therapy of Prostate Cancer Using Magnetic Nanoparticles. *Actas Urol. Esp.* **2007**, *31*, 660–667.

221. Brunners, P.; Hodenius, M.; Baumann, M.; Oversohl, J.; Gunther, R. W.; SchmidtzRoe, T., et al. Magnetic Thermal Ablation Using Ferrofluids: Influence of Administration Mode on Biological Effect in Different Porcine tissues. *Cardiovasc. Intervent. Radiol.* **2008**, *31*, 1193–1199.

222. Zhang, X. D.; Guo, M. L.; Wu, H. Y.; Sun, Y. M.; Ding, Y. Q.; Feng, X., et al. Irradiation Stability and Cytotoxicity of Gold Nanoparticles for Radiotherapy. *Int. J. Nanomed.* **2009**, *4*, 165–173.

223. Gannon, C. J.; Patra, C. R.; Bhattacharya, R.; Mukherjee, P.; Curley, S. A. Intracellular Gold Nanoparticles Enhance Noninvasive Radiofrequency Thermal Destruction of Human Gastrointestinal Cancer Cells. *J. Nanobiotechnol.* **2008**, *6*, 2.

224. Loo, C.; Hirsch, I.; Lee, M. H.; Chang, E.; West, J. L.; Halas, N. J., et al. Gold Nanoshell Bioconjugates for Molecular Imaging in Living Cells. *Opt. Lett.* **2005**, *30*, 1012–1014.

225. Loo, C.; Lin, A. S. P.; Hirsch, I.; Lee, M. H.; Barton, J.; Halas, N. J., et al. Nanoshellenabled Photonicsbased Imaging and Therapy Of Cancer. *Technol. Cancer Res. Treat.* **2004**, *3*, 33–40.

226. Gobin, A. M.; Lee, M. H.; Halas, N. J.; James, W. D.; Drezek, R. A.; West, J. L. Nearinfrared Resonant Nanoshells for Combined Optical Imaging and Photothermal Cancer Therapy. *Nano Lett.* **2007**, *7*, 1929–1934.

227. Ahmed, M.; Goldberg, S. N. Combination Radiofrequency Thermal Ablation and Adjuvant IV Liposomal Doxorubicin Increases Tissue Coagulation and Intratumoural Drug Accumulation. *Int. J. Hyperthermia* **2004**, *20*, 781–802.

228. Senior, J. H. Combination radiofrequency thermal ablation and adjuvant IV liposomal doxorubicin increases tissue coagulation and intratumoural drug accumulation. *Crit. Rev. Ther. Drug Carrier Syst.* **1987**, *3*, 123–193.

229. Schroeder, A.; Honen, R.; Turjeman, K.; Gabizon, A.; Kost, J.; Barenholz, Y. Ultrasound Triggered Release of Cisplatin from Liposomes in Murine Tumors. *J. Controlled Release* **2009**, *37*, 63–68.

230. Zhao, H.; Li, G. L.; Wang, R. Z.; Li, S. F.; Wei, J. J.; Feng, M., et al. A Comparative Study of Transfection Efficiency between Liposomes, Immunoliposomes and Brain-specific Immunoliposomes. *J. Int. Med. Res.* **2010**, *38*, 957–966.

231. Gordon, A. N.; Granai, C. O.; Rose, P. G.; Hainsworth, J.; Lopez, A.; Weissman, C., et al. Phase II Study of Liposomal Doxorubicin in Platinum- and Paclitaxelrefractory Epithelial Ovarian Cancer. *J. Clin. Oncol.* **2000**, *18*, 3093–3100.

232. Ranson, M. R.; Carmichael, J.; O'Byrne, K.; Stewart, S.; Smith, D.; Howell, A. Treatment of Advanced Breast Cancer with Sterically Stabilized Liposomal Dox-orubicin: Results of a Multicenter Phase II Trial. *J. Clin. Oncol.* **1997**, *15*, 3185–3191.

233. Ahmed, M.; Monsky, W. E.; Girnun, G.; Lukyanov, A.; D'Ippolito, G.; Kruskal, J. B., et al. Radiofrequency Thermal Ablation Sharply Increases Intratumoral Liposomal Doxorubicin Accumulation and Tumor Coagulation. *Cancer Res.* **2003**, *63*, 6327–6333.

234. Ahmed, F.; Pakunlu, R. I.; Srinivas, G.; Brannan, A.; Bates, F.; Klein, M. L.; Minko, T.; Discher, D. E. Shrinkage of a Rapidly Growing Tumor by Drug-loaded Polymersomes: pH-triggered Release Through Copolymer Degradation. *Mol. Pharm.* **2006**, *3*, 340–350.

235. Monsky, W. L.; Kruskal, J. B.; Lukyanov, A. N.; Girnun, G. D.; Ahmed, M.; Gazelle, G. S., et al. Radio-frequency Ablation Increases Intratumoral Liposomal Doxorubicin Accumulation in a Rat Breast Tumor Model. *Radiology* **2002**, *224*, 823–829.

236. Goldberg, S. N.; Kamel, I. R.; Kruskal, J. B.; Reynolds, K.; Monsky, W. L.; Stuart, K. E., et al. Radiofrequency Ablation of Hepatic Tumors: Increased Tumor Destruction with Adjuvant Liposomal Doxorubicin Therapy. *Am. J. Roentgenol.* **2002**, *179*, 93–101.

237. Brantley Sieders, D.; Schmidt, S.; Parker, M.; Chen, J. Eph Receptor Tyrosinekinases in Tumor and Tumor Microenvironment. *Curr. Pharm. Des.* **2004**, *20*, 3431–3442.

238. Brindle, K. New Approaches for Imaging Tumour Responses to Treatment. *Nat. Rev. Cancer* **2008**, *8*, 94–107.

239. Kirchin, M. A.; Runge, V. M. Contrast Agents for Magnetic Resonance Imaging: Safety Update. *Top Magn. Reson. Imaging* **2003**, *14*, 426–435.

240. Emerich, D. F.; Thanos, C. G.; Emerich, D. F.; Thanos, C. G. Targeted Nanoparticle Based Drug Delivery and Diagnosis. *J. Drug Target.* **2007**, *15*, 163–183.

241. Groneberg, D. A.; Giersig, M.; Welte, T.; Pison, U. Nanoparticle Based Diagnosis and Therapy. *Curr. Drug Target.* **2006**, *7*, 643–648.

242. Jain, T. K.; Reddy, M. K.; Morales, M. A.; LesliePelecky, D. L.; Labhasetwar, V. Biodistribution, Clearance, and Biocompatibility of Iron Oxide Magnetic Nanoparticles in Rats. *Mol. Pharm.* **2008**, *5*, 316–327.

243. Simonsen, C. Z.; Ostergaard, L.; VestergaardPoulsen, P.; Rohl, L.; Bjornerud, A.; Gyldensted, C. CBF and CBV Measurements by USPIO Bolus Tracking: Reproducibility and Comparison with Gd Based Values. *J. Magn. Reson. Imaging* **1999**, *9*, 342–347.

244. Okon, E.; Pouliquen, D.; Okon, P.; Kovaleva, Z. V.; Stepanova, T. P.; Lavit, S. G.; Kudryavtsev, B. N.; Jallet, P. Biodegradation of Magnetite Dextran Nanoparticles in the Rat: a Histologic and Biophysical Study. *Am. J. Roentgenol.* **1994**, *71*, 895–903.

245. Runge, V. M. *Contrast Agents Safety Profile*, 2008 (accessed jun 18, 2012) Available from: http://www.clinical-mri.com/pdf/Contrast%20Agents/Contrast%20Agents%20-%20Safety%20Profile%20amended%20table.pdf.

246. Coyne, D. W. Ferumoxytol for Treatment of Iron Deficiency Anemia in Patients with Chronic Kidney Disease. *Expert Opin. Pharmacother.* **2009**, *10*, 2563–2568.

247. Weissleder, R.; Stark, D. D.; Engelstad, B. L.; Bacon, B. R.; Compton, C. C.; White, D. L.; Jacobs, P.; Lewis, J. Superparamagnatic Iron Oxide: Pharmacokinetics and Toxicity. *Am. J. Roentgenol.* **1989,** *152,* 167–173.

248. Kim, Y. K.; Lee, J. M.; Kim, C. S.; Chung, G. H.; Kim, C. Y.; Kim, I. H. Detection of Liver Metastases: Gadobenate Dimeglumine Enhanced Three Dimensional Dynamic Phases and One Hour Delayed Phase MR Imaging Versus Superparamagnetic Iron Oxide Enhanced MR Imaging. *Eur. Radiol.* **2005,** *15,* 220–228.

249. Seneterre, E.; Taourel, P.; Bouvier, Y.; Pradel, J.; Van Beers, B.; Daures, J. P., et al. Detection of Hepatic Metastases: Ferumoxides Enhanced MR Imaging Versus Unenhanced MR Imaging and CT During Arterial Portography. *Radiology* **1996,** *200,* 785–792.

250. Schnorr, J.; Wagner, S.; Abramjuk, C.; Drees, R.; Schink, T.; Schellenberger, E. A., et al. Focal Liver Lesions: SPIO, Gadolinium, and Ferucarbotran Enhanced Dynamic T1 Weighted and Delayed T2 Weighted MR Imaging in Rabbits. *Radiology* **2006,** *240,* 90–100.

251. Mori, K.; Fukuda, K.; Asaoka, H.; Ueda, T.; Kunimatsu, A.; Okamoto, Y., et al. Radiofrequency Ablation of the Liver: Determination of Ablative Margin at MR Imaging with Impaired Clearance of Ferucarbotran-feasibility Study. *Radiology* **2009,** *251,* 557–565.

252. Chen, R. C.; Lii, J. M.; Chou, C. T.; Chang, T. A.; Chen, W. T.; Li, C. S., et al. T2 Weighted and T1 Weighted Dynamic Superparamagnetic Iron Oxide (ferucarbotran) Enhanced MRI of Hepatocellular Carcinoma and Hyperplastic Nodules. *J. Formos Med. Assoc.* **2008,** *107,* 798–805.

253. Kim, H. J.; Kim, K. W.; Byun, J. H.; Won, H. J.; Shin, Y. M.; Kim, P. N., et al. Comparison of Mangafodipir Trisodium and Ferucarbotran Enhanced MRI for Detection and Characterization Of Hepatic Metastases in Colorectal Cancer Patients. *Am. J. Roentgenol.* **2006,** *186,* 1059–1066.

254. Rogers, W. J.; Meyer, C. H.; Kramer, C. M. Technology Insight: In vivo Cell Tracking by Use of MRI. *Nat. Clin. Pract. Cardiovasc. Med.* **2006,** *3,* 554–562.

255. Islam, T.; Harisinghani, M. G. Overview of Nanoparticle Use in Cancer Imaging. *Cancer Biomarkers* **2009,** *5,* 61–67.

256. Heesakkers, R. A.; Jager, G. J.; Hovels, A. M.; de Hoop, B.; van den Bosch, H. C.; Raat, F., et al. Prostate Cancer: Detection of Lymph Node Metastases Outside the Routine Surgical Area with Ferumoxtran10 Enhanced MR Imaging. *Radiology* **2009,** *251,* 408–414.

257. Tang, T. Y.; Howarth, S. P.; Miller, S. R.; Graves, M. J.; Patterson, A. J.; UKingIm, J. M., et al. The ATHEROMA (Atorvastatin Therapy: Effects on Reduction of Macrophage Activity) Study. Evaluation using ultrasmall superparamagnetic iron oxideenhanced magnetic resonance imaging in carotid disease. *J. Am. Coll. Cardiol.* **2009,** *53,* 2039–2050.

258. Reimer, P.; Bremer, C.; Allkemper, T.; Engelhardt, M.; Mahler, M.; Ebert, W., et al. Myocardial perfusion and MR angiography of chest with SH U 555 C: results of placebo controlled clinical phase i study. *Radiology* **2004,** *231,* 474–481.

259. Wyttenbach, R.; Gianella, S.; Alerci, M.; Braghetti, A.; Cozzi, L.; Gallino, A. Prospective Blinded Evaluation of GdDOTA Versus GdBOPTA Enhanced Peripheral MR Angiography, As Compared with Digital Subtraction Angiography. *Radiology* **2003,** *227,* 261–269.

260. Bremerich, J.; Bilecen, D.; Reimer, P. MR Angiography with Blood Pool Contrast Agents. *Eur. Radiol.* **2007,** *17,* 3017–3024.

261. Schnorr, J.; Wagner, S.; Abramjuk, C.; Wojner, I.; Schink, T.; Kroencke, T. J., et al. Comparison of the Iron Oxide Based Blood Pool Contrast Medium VSOPC184 with Gadopentetate Dimeglumine for First Pass Magnetic Resonance Angiography of the Aorta and Renal Arteries in Pigs. *Invest. Radiol.* **2004,** *39,* 546–553.

262. Allkemper, T.; Bremer, C.; Matuszewski, L.; Ebert, W.; Reimer, P. Contrast Enhanced Blood Pool MR Angiography with Optimized Iron Oxides: Effect of Size and Dose on Vascular Contrast Enhancement in Rabbits. *Radiology* **2002**, *223*, 432–438.

263. Taupitz, M.; Wagner, S.; Schnorr, J.; Kravec, I.; Pilgrimm, H.; Bergmann Fritsch, H., et al. Phase I Clinical Evaluation of Citrate Coated Monocrystalline Very Small Superparamagnetic Iron Oxide Particles as a New Contrast Medium for Magnetic Resonance Imaging. *Invest. Radiol.* **2004**, *39*, 394–405.

264. Schoenberg, S. O.; Aumann, S.; Just, A.; Bock, M.; Knopp, M. V.; Johansson, L. O., et al. Quantification of Renal Perfusion Abnormalities Using an Intravascular Contrast Agent (part 2): Results in Animals and Humans with Renal Artery Stenosis. *Magn. Reson. Med.* **2003**, *49*, 288–298.

265. Karczmar, G. S.; Fan, X.; AlHallaq, H.; River, J. N.; Tarlo, K.; Kellar, K. E., et al. Functional and Anatomic Imaging of Tumor Vasculature: High Resolution MR Spectroscopic Imaging Combined with a Superparamagnetic Contrast Agent. *Acad. Radiol.* **2002**, *9*, S115–S118.

266. Weishaupt, D.; Hetzer, F. H.; Ruehm, S. G.; Patak, M. A.; Schmidt, M.; Debatin, J. F. Three Dimensional Contrast Enhanced MRI Using an Intravascular Contrast Agent for Detection of Traumatic Intra-abdominal Hemorrhage and Abdominal Parenchymal Injuries: An Experimental Study. *Eur. Radiol.* **2000**, *10*, 1958–1964.

267. Gambarota, G.; Leenders, W.; Maass, C.; Wesseling, P.; van der Kogel, B.; van Tellingen, O., et al. Characterisation of Tumour Vasculature in Mouse Brain by USPIO Contrast Enhanced MRI. *Br. J. Cancer* **2008**, *98*, 1784–1789.

268. Affibody *First in Human Whole-body HER2-receptor Mapping Using Affibody Molecular Imaging with ABY-025*, 2011 Available from: http://www.affibody.com/en/News/News/First-in-Human-Whole-Body-HER2-Receptor-Mapping-Using-Affibody-Molecular-Imaging-with-ABY-025/.

269. NIH; NCBI, Ed.; NCBI: Bethesda, 2004–2011.

270. Loebinger, M. R.; Kyrtatos, P. G.; Turmaine, M.; Price, A. N.; Pankhurst, Q.; Lythgoe, M. F.; Janes, S. M. Magnetic Resonance Imaging Of Mesenchymal Stem Cells Homing to Pulmonary Metastases Using Biocompatible Magnetic Nanoparticles. *Cancer Res.* **2009**, *69*, 2267–8862.

271. Mathiasen, A. B.; Haack-Sorensen, M.; Kastrup, J. Mesenchymal Stromal Cells for Cardiovascular Repair: Current Status and Future Challenges. *Future Cardiol.* **2009**, *5*, 605–617.

272. Sadan, O.; Melamed, E.; Offen, D. Bone-marrow-derived Mesenchymal Stem Cell Therapy for Neurodegenerative Diseases. *Expert Opin. Drug Del.* **2009**, *9*, 1487–1497.

273. Kuhn, N. Z.; Tuan, R. S. Regulation of Stemness and Stem Cell Niche of Mesenchymal Stem Cells: Implications in Tumorigenesis and Metastasis. *J. Cell Phys.* **2010**, *222*, 268–277.

274. Feng, B.; Chen, L. Review of Mesenchymal Stem Cells and Tumors: Executioner or Coconspirator? *Cancer Biother. Radiopharm.* **2009**, *24*, 717–721.

275. Lee, S.; Cha, E. J.; Park, K.; Lee, S. Y.; J.K., H.; Sun, I. C.; Kim, S. Y.; Choi, K.; Kwon, I. C.; Kim, K.; Ahn, C. H. A Near-infrared-fluorescence-Quenched Gold-nanoparticle Imaging Probe for In vivo Drug Screening and Protease Activity Determination. *Angew. Chem. Int. Ed. Engl.* **2008**, *47*, 2804–2807.

276. Xie, J.; Zhang, F.; Aronova, M.; Zhu, L.; Lin, X.; Quan, Q.; Liu, G.; Zhang, G.; Choi, K. Y.; Kim, K.; Sun, X.; Lee, S.; Sun, S.; Leapman, R.; Chen, X. Manipulating the Power of an Additional Phase: A Flower-like Au-Fe_3O_4 Optical Nanosensor for Imaging Protease Expressions In vivo. *ACS Nano.* **2011**, *5*, 3043–3051.

277. Lin, X.; Xie, J.; Niu, G.; Zhang, F.; Gao, H.; Yang, M.; Quan, Q.; Aronova, M. A.; Zhang, G.; Lee, S.; Leapman, R.; X., C. Chimeric Ferritin Nanocages for Multiple Function Loading and Multimodal Imaging. *Nano Lett.* **2011**, *11*, 814–819.

278. Cho, E. J.; Yang, J.; Mohamedali, K. A.; Lim, E. K.; Kim, E. J.; Farhangfar, C. J.; Suh, J. S.; Haam, S.; Rosenblum, M. G.; Y.M., H. Sensitive Angiogenesis Imaging of Orthotopic Bladder Tumors in Mice Using a Selective Magnetic Resonance Imaging Contrast Agent Containing VEGF121/rGel. *Invest. Radiol.* **2011,** *46,* 441–449.

279. Koch, S.; Tugues, S.; Li, X.; Gualandi, L.; Claesson-Welsh, L. Signal Transduction by Vascular Endothelial Growth Factor Receptors. *Biochem. J.* **2011,** *437,* 169–183.

280. Press, M. F.; Lenz, H. J. EGFR, HER2 and VEGF Pathways: Validated Targets for Cancer Treatment. *Drugs* **2007,** *67,* 2045–2075.

281. Shao, Y. Z.; Liu, L. Z.; Song, S. Q.; Cao, R. H.; Liu, H.; Cui, C. Y.; Li, X.; Bie, M. J.; Li, L. A Novel One-step Synthesis of Gd3+-incorporated Mesoporous SiO$_2$ Nanoparticles for Use as an Efficient MRI Contrast Agent. *Contrast Media Mol. Imaging* **2011,** *6,* 110–118.

282. Jemal, A.; Siegel, R. W.; Xu, J.; Ward, E. Cancer Statistics. *Cancer J. Clin.* **2010,** *60,* 277–300.

283. Meng, S.; Tripathy, D.; Frenkel, E. P.; Shete, S.; Naftalis, E. Z.; Huth, J. F., et al. Circulating Tumor Cells in Patients with Breast Cancer Dormancy. *Clin. Cancer Res.* **2004,** *10,* 8152–8162.

284. Peierga, J. Y.; Bonneton, C.; Vincetn-Salomon, A.; de Cremoux, P.; Nos, C.; Blin, N., et al. Clinical Significance of Immunocytochemical Detection of Tumor Cells Using Digital Microscopy in Peripheral Blood and Bone Marrow of Breast Cancer Patients. *Clin. Cancer Res.* **2004,** *10,* 1392–1400.

285. Xu, H.; Aguilar, Z. P.; Yang, L.; Kuang, M.; Duan, H.; Xiong, Y.; Wei, H.; Wang, A. Y. Antibody Conjugated Magnetic Iron Oxide Nanoparticles for Cancer Cell Separation in Fresh Whole Blood. *Biomaterials* **2011,** *32,* 9758–9765.

286. Allard, W. J.; Matera, J.; Miller, M. C.; Repollet, M.; Connelly, M. C.; Rao, C., et al. Tumor Cells Circulate in the Peripheral Blood of all Major Carcinomas but not in Healthy Subjects or Patients with Nonmalignant Diseases. *Clin. Cancer Res.* **2004,** *10,* 6897–6904.

287. Miltenyi, S.; Muller, W.; Weichel, W.; Radbruch, A. High Gradient Magnetic Cell Separation with MACS. *Cytometry* **1990,** *11,* 231–238.

288. Pamme, N.; Wilhelm, C. Continuous Sorting of Magnetic Cells Via On-chip Freeflow Magnetophoresis. *Lab Chip* **2006,** *6,* 974–980.

289. Xu, R. *Particle Characterization: Light Scattering Methods*; Kluwer Academic Publishers: Dordrecht, 2001.

290. Weissleder, R.; Kelly, K.; Sun, E. Y.; Shtatland, T.; Josephson, L. Cell-specific Targeting of Nanoparticles by Multivalent Attachment of Small Molecules. *Nat. Biotechnol.* **2005,** *23,* 1418–1423.

291. Decuzzi, P.; Pasqualini, R.; Arap, W.; Ferrari, M. Intravascular Delivery of Particulate Systems: Does Geometry Really Matter? *Pharm. Res.* **2009,** *26,* 235–243.

292. Bautista, C. V.; Felis, C. P.; Espinet, J. M.; Garcia, J. B.; Salas, J. V. Telomerase Activity is a Prognostic Factor for Recurrence and Survival in Rectal Cancer. *Dis. Colon Rectum* **2007,** *50,* 611–620.

293. Spernyak, J. A.; White, W. H.; Ethirajan, M.; Patel, N. J.; Goswami, L.; Chen, Y. H.; Turowski, S.; Missert, J. R.; Batt, C.; Mazurchuk, R.; Pandey, R. K. Hexylether Derivative of Pyropheophorbide-a (HPPH) on Conjugating with 3gadolinium(III) Aminobenzyldiethylenetriaminepentaacetic acid shows Potential for In vivo Tumor Imaging (MR, fluorescence) and Photodynamic Therapy. *Bioconjugate Chem.* **2010,** *21,* 828–835.

294. Xie, J.; Lee, S.; Chen, X. Nanoparticle-based Theranostic Agents. *Adv. Drug Deliv. Rev.* **2010,** *62,* 1064–1079.

295. Namiki, Y.; Namiki, T.; Yoshida, H.; Ishii, Y.; Tsubota, A.; Koido, S.; Nariai, K.; Mitsunaga, M.; Yanagisawa, S.; Kashiwagi, H.; Mabashi, Y.; Yumoto, Y.; Hoshin, S.; Fujise, K.; Tada, N. A Novel Magnetic Crystal Lipid Nanostructure for Magnetically Guided In vivo Gene Delivery. *Nat. Nanotechnol.* **2009,** *4,* 598–606.

296. Winter, P. M.; Neubauer, A. M.; Caruthers, S. D.; Harris, T. D.; Robertson, J. D.; Williams, T. A., et al. Endothelial αvβ3 IntegrinTargeted Fumagillin Nanoparticles Inhibit Angiogenesis in Atherosclerosis. *Arterioscler Thromb. Vasc. Biol.* **2006,** *26,* 2103–2109.

297. Flacke, S.; Fischer, S.; Scott, M. J.; Fuhrhop, R. J.; Allen, J. S.; McLean, M., et al. Novel MRI Contrast Agent for Molecular Imaging of Fibrin: Implications for Detecting Vulnerable Plaques. *Circulation* **2001,** *104,* 1280–1285.

298. Bryson, J. M.; Fichter, K. M.; W.J., C.; Lee, J. H.; Li, J.; Madsen, L. A. , et al. Polymer beacons for luminescence and magnetic resonance imaging of DNA delivery. *Proc. Natl. Acad. Sci. U.S.A.* **2009,** *106,* 16913–16918.

Nanotoxicology and Remediation

8.1 INTRODUCTION

Nanotoxicology is a new area of study that deals with the toxicological profiles of nanomaterials (NMs). Compared with the larger counterparts, the quantum size effects and large surface area to volume ratio brings NMs their unique properties that may or may not be toxic to living things. Thus, nanotoxicology deals with elucidating how different NMs affect living systems. Inert elements like gold become active at nanoscale dimensions. Nanotoxicity studies are intended to determine whether and to what extent the properties of gold and other materials in the nanoscale dimensions may pose a threat to the environment and to living things.

The nanotechnology industry has shown an industrial revolution over the last few years, a trend which is more than likely to continue into the future. Unfortunately, the exponential progress in nanotechnology has exceeded the advances of research on the impact of NMs on living systems especially on

Nanomaterials for Medical Applications. http://dx.doi.org/10.1016/B978-0-12-385089-8.00008-X

human health. To date, we have barely scratched the lessons to learn and to comprehend the effects of these tiny molecules on cells, tissues, and whole organisms. This chapter will focus on the current knowledge of nanotoxicity and highlight areas where new information is available and suggest directions for additional and future research.

To complete existing knowledge about the interactions between the NMs and the biological systems, nanotoxicology deals with the study of their toxic or biological effects. Because NMs belong to a new class of materials, progress in this new discipline relies largely on developing methodology to characterize NMs in biological samples, quantify them in living systems, study their uptake, translocation, biodistribution, accumulation, and chemical status in vitro and in vivo. In addition, the biochemical pathways and biomolecules that are directly or indirectly affected by their presence in a living system need to be established both short term and long term in order to understand possible consequences when they are used for medical applications. Appropriate analytical techniques and their application to the study of the toxicological activities of NMs need to be developed to provide appropriate and powerful means for characterizing the toxic effects or biological behaviors in biological systems.

Nanotoxicology addresses the toxicology profiles of NMs which appear to have unusual toxicity effects that are not observed with larger particles. The NMs of interest in this book are those which are deliberately produced for medical applications such as engineered carbon nanotubes,[1–3] quantum dots (QDs),[4–14] iron oxide magnetic nanoparticles (IOMNPs),[4,15–17] liposomes,[18–26] titanium oxide,[27] and many more. A few of these NMs such as gold,[28] silver,[29–31] titanium dioxide, alumina, metal oxides, liposomes, polymers,[32] and carbon nanotubes[33] have been studied in terms of toxicity in a limited manner. Some NMs exhibit size-dependent pathogenic effects that are different from larger particles.[29] NMs have larger surface area to mass ratios which may be responsible for the ease of penetration of the cells and tissues or cells that in some cases may lead to the release of immune response.[14,34–39] Some NMs exhibit the ability to translocate from solution into cells[14] or even transcend the blood brain barrier.[40] This accelerated the studies on nanoparticle toxicology study in the brain, blood, liver, skin, and gut.

The rapid growth of medical applications of NMs calls for concerns about the potential health and environmental risks related to the use and widespread production required by the demands to support this outburst in nanotechnology. Multiple areas of concern related with the usage of NMs including the deposition and clearing, biocompatibility, systemic translocation, and body distribution of NMs, intestinal tract involvement, and direct effects on the central nervous system have been studied so far.[41] The different physico-chemical and structural properties of NMs that result from their nanoscale size can be sued to account for a number of material interactions that can lead to toxic effects.[42] Studies have shown that NMs can have pronounced environmental effects even at very low aqueous concentrations.[43] As an example, the use of CdSe QDs in humans may be limited because these contain the heavy metals cadmium which are reportedly toxic to cells at concentrations as low as 10ug/mL.[44] The various properties of the QD such as its size, charge, concentration, capping material, functional groups, and mechanical stability have been studied as possible determining factors in toxicity.[45] Although toxicology is an area that is critical in medicine, there is currently a wide gap between research on NMs medical applications and nanotoxicology.[46]

Today, nanotechnology has begun to show its worth and possible contributions to the future of medicine and health care. In drug delivery, gene delivery, and immunotherapy, the ideal NMs can achieve high payload, biocompatibility, selective targeting, long circulation time, low immunogenicity, and efficient penetration of barriers to achieve timely arrival at the tissues of interest without clinical side effects.[47] The penetration of NMs into cells and eventually into the diseased tissues can open various applications as delivery vehicles in various disease therapies. But, different NMs of different compositions, sizes, surface topography, and other properties need to be scrutinized meticulously to establish the efficacy and safety for their use in humans.

Toxicity studies can begin with in vitro tests using various cell lines that play a vital role in predicting the response of animal and humans to a broad range of compounds.[48–51] In vitro studies are used as the first line for screening the toxic biological consequences of potential therapeutic compounds before in vivo testing.[52] Common conventional in vitro toxicity assays use colorimetric or fluorescent dyes as markers to determine cell viability assessing membrane integrity (i.e. neutral red, calcein AM) or cell metabolism (i.e. MTT, alamar Blue) (same source). However, although these assays provide reliable data for classic small molecule cytotoxicity studies, they have to be adapted for the assessment of NMs[51] to avoid inaccurate results. Existing technique need to be calibrated and/or new techniques need to be developed for accurate toxicity screening and evaluation of the toxicity and health risk potentials of NMs. The prediction that nanotechnology-based products will reach nearly 4T dollars by 2015 and will continue to grow[53] needs to be coupled with the growth on nanotoxicological research.[54]

This chapter on nanotoxicology and remediation will focus on finished and on-going various toxicity evaluations of various NMs that are used and currently being developed for medical applications. A few of commercially available NMs that are currently being developed for imaging, drug delivery, biosensors, and other medical applications will be featured in this chapter.

8.2 NMs EXHIBITING TOXICITY

Many of the NMs that have emerged to be useful in medicine have shown mild to no evidences of toxicity to date. However, both long- and short-term effects need to be evaluated in order to establish immediate and future damage from

NMs. Existing reports on the toxicological investigations of NMs imply that e.g. size, shape, chemical composition, surface charge, solubility, their ability to bind and affect biological sites as well as their metabolic fate and excretion influence the toxicity of NPs. The toxicity of the most common NMs will be discussed in this chapter.[55,56]

8.2.1 Carbon Nanotubes and Fullerenes

Carbon nanotubes (CNTs) are NMs made of the element carbon. CNTs are composed of carbon units that tend to aggregate due to strong van der Waals forces.[52] They are characterized by their electrical and mechanical properties especially their incredible tensile strength.[57-66] CNTs are needle-like fibers in appearance under TEM or SEM like asbestos. CNTs can come in the form of single-walled nanotubes (SWNTs), multiwall nanotubes (MWNTs), or as fullerenes (C_{60}).[3,54,58,62,65,67-69] CNTs have found varied applications from biosensors,[63,70,71] regenerative medicine,[61,72,73] cell growth,[66,74,75] electronic devices,[54] and electrocatalysis.[76] The unique properties of this well-studied class of NMs offers a full range of potential medical applications and more.

To harness the full potential of CNTs toxicological studies must go hand in hand with the development for medical applications. A clear acceptable framework for regulatory authorities and the public based on the toxicological and pharmacological studies must be presented and used as a basis for developing guidelines for the safe use of carbon nanotubes in medicine.[33]

A number of studies have focused on the potential toxicities of CNTs in various biological systems. A study that introduced carbon nanotubes into the abdominal cavity of mice showed long thin carbon nanotubes to be similar in effect as long thin asbestos fibers and as such, exposure to carbon nanotubes may lead to mesothelioma which is the cancer of the lining of the lungs that is caused by exposure to asbestos.[77] The similarities in shape and size between asbestos and CNTs have led to speculations of possible potential risks that require thorough and effective control as well as proper regulations under defined circumstances to evaluate the CNTs for safe handling and proper disposal.[78] CNTs have been shown to accumulate in cells of various types including macrophages (Figure 8.1).[79]

One of the studies conducted on CNTs have shown that these can enter human cells and accumulate in the cytoplasm leading to cell death.[80] The studies conducted on rodents indicated that regardless of the synthesis process to produce the CNTs and the types and amounts of metals they contained, the CNTs resulted in inflammation, granulomas, fibrosis, and toxicological changes in the lungs.[81] Studies that involved equal weights of tested materials showed that SWNTs were more toxic than the bulk material quartz.[82] In contrast, ultrafine carbon black was shown to produce minimal lung damage compared with CNTs (Figures 8.2).[79] A pilot study that exposed the mesothelial lining of the body cavity of mice to long MWNTs showed asbestos-like, length-dependent,

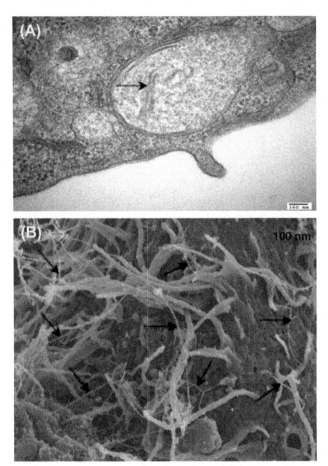

FIGURE 8.1 Representative transmission electron (A) and scanning electron (B) micrographs of RAW264.7 macrophages with engulfed PS-coated SWCNT. RAW264.7 macrophages (0.3×10^6 cells/ml) were incubated for 2 h with PS-coated SWCNT. Arrows indicate SWCNT. *From Shveda 2009. (For color version of this figure, the reader is referred to the online version of this book)*

cell damage that included inflammation and formation of lesions or granulomas.[77] This is contradictory to the assumptions that CNTs are less hazardous than graphite causing the research and business communities to invest heavily in carbon nanotubes for a wide range of products. Supporting data gathered in other studies also suggests that under certain conditions, such as those involving chronic exposure, CNTs can pose a serious risk to human health.[80,82,83] These in vivo studies suggested the need for extensive research before introducing CNTs-enabled products into the market to avoid long-term damage. The studies conducted are a good example of strategic, highly focused research for safe and responsible development of nanotechnology.

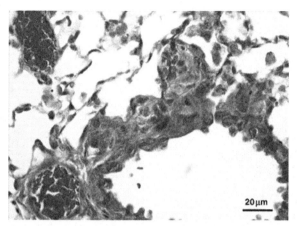

FIGURE 8.2 Representative image of lung section from the SWCNT inhalation study (5 mg/m³, 5 h/day, 4 days) depicting granuloma formation on day 28 post-treatment. Fibrosis is indicated by blue staining in this Masson's Trichrome stained section of the lung. *From Shveda 2009. (For color version of this figure, the reader is referred to the online version of this book)*

The C_{60} type of CNTs, also called fullerenes or bucky balls have been synthesized and their toxicity profile have also been investigated albeit not to a full extent. Formed by a graphite arc process, sixty carbon atoms combine into a stable spherical structure of twenty hexagons and twelve pentagons about 1 nm in diameter. To create a solution of C_{60}, it is suspended in the organic solvent tetrahydrofuran[85,86] or stirred in water over time.[87] The solid C_{60} have been studied by Oberdörster[88] who raised questions of potential cytotoxicity that had been shown by other groups to be likely caused by the tetrahydrofuran used in preparing the 30–100 nm particles of C_{60} used in the research.[86,89] Isakovic et al.[89] gave studies that showed that removal of THF from the C_{60} particles resulted in a loss of toxicity.[89] Similarly, Sayes et al. (2007), showed that C_{60} particles instilled intratracheally in rats caused no detectable inflammatory response after 3 months of observation[90] using quartz particles as control, which resulted in inflammatory response. Other studies indicated that nC_{60} are toxic in human fibroblasts and liver carcinoma cells,[86] human neuronal astrocytes,[91] and guinea pig alveolar macrophages.[92] Studies with human skin cells showed a decrease in viability at 24 h with an increase in nC_{60} concentration.[93] These in vitro tests have been used to conduct high throughput screening of nanoparticles (NPs) to help understand the mechanism of cellular interactions as well as to minimize animal use. The interactions of CNTs with cells in culture have been reported by many investigators to determine their in vitro effects on different cell types. Studies in human keratinocyte cells, HaCaT, and in human epidermal keratinocytes (HEK) suggested that SWCNTs are toxic.[94] Unmodified MWCNTs within the cytoplasmic vacuoles of HEK resulted in decreased cell viability and a dose-dependent increase in the levels of proinflammatory cytokine interleukin 8 (IL-8).[95]

However, a conflicting review of fullerenes beginning in the early 1990s to 2007 concluded that the evidence gathered overwhelmingly pointed to C_{60} being non-toxic.[96] A few more investigators found no cytotoxic effects from SWCNTs and MWCNTs in human umbilical vein endothelial cells,[97] rat alveolar macrophages,[98] human osteoblasts and fibroblasts,[99] and human lung and colon cells.[100] Studies have shown that these results may have been due to the ability of the CNTs to adsorb the dye (neutral red) or dye products (formazan) used in viability and cytokine assays as well as their ability to adsorb proteins and nutrients in the culture medium.[94,101] Hence, conventional indicator dyes are not appropriate for assessment of CNTs toxicity.[102]

In the most recent review written by Zhao and Liu,[84] the various routes for CNTs toxicity had been evaluated extensively, a summary of which is given on Table 8.1. In humans, the skin is the first line of defense against any toxic material. Mice exposed to unpurified CNTs exhibited oxidative stress, depletion of glutathione, increased dermal cell number, localized alopecia and skin thickening.[103,104] The lungs are the most likely route of exposure to CNTs because of the fiber like nature of CNTs which can be easily airborne and inhaled. The asbestos-like properties of CNTs have led to concern that inhalation of CNTs may cause similar lung pathologies.[105,106] Unlike asbestos, the MWCNTs were found to cause focal subpleural fibrosis and mononuclear cell aggregation.[107] The MWCNTs in vitro was shown to trigger cytotoxic effects in phagocytotic cells by rupturing the plasma membrane.[108] In other cell types, such as neurons and glial cells, SWCNTs significantly decreased the overall DNA content. Serum proteins were found adsorbed on CNTs and attenuated the inherent cytotoxicity of CNTs which increased with increasing amounts of serum proteins adsorbed on CNTs.[109]

8.2.2 Toxicity Evaluation of QDs

One of the most extensively exploited quantum dots for medical applications are the cadmium-based quantum dots. QDs are used as high-performance fluorescent bioprobes because of their high photoluminescence quantum yield (PLQY), broad absorption wavelength, narrow emission wavelength, and strong photostability.[110] Over the past few years, QDs have been used in immunofluorescence assays, labeling of fixed cells and tissues, immuno-staining of proteins, and many more.[4–6,10–13,111–118] QDs are brighter than organic dyes because of the extinction coefficients that are an order of magnitude larger than those of most dyes.[119,120] The main advantage of QDs reside in their resistance to bleaching over long periods of time (over six months in most cases) allowing long term acquisition of crisp images with good contrast.[110] One of the most useful properties of QDs for immunofluorescence imaging is the small number necessary to produce a signal.[121] The flickering of specimens under the microscope is a phenomenon due to the blinking of a small number of QDs[121,122] which demonstrates that single QDs can be observed in cells with an ultimate sensitivity

TABLE 8.1 CNTs Toxicity In vivo[84]

Organism	CNT size	Dosage	Damage	Reference
C57/BL/6J Mice	MWNTs L: 3.9 um D: 49 nm	10, 20, 40, 80 ug/mouse	Pharyngeal aspiration: penetration of alveolar macrophages	Mercer, 2010
SKH Mice	SWNTs	5 daily dosage of 40, 60, or 80 ug/mouse	Skin contact: stress, depletion of glutathione, oxidation of protein thiols, and carbonyls; skin thickening	Murray et al., 2009[104]
Balb c mice	SWNTs L: 10–20 um D: 100–150 nm	1 mg implanted in 1 cm incision	Skin contact: Localized alopecia	Koyama et al., 2009[103]
Wistar rats	MWNTs with defects L: 0.7 um D: 20–50 nm	2 mg/rat/day	Lung inhalation: pulmonary toxicity and genetoxicity	Muller, 2008
Wistar rats	MWNTs L: 0.1–10 um D: 5–15 nm	0.1, 0.5, 2 mg/m^3 at 6 h/day, M-F, 13 weeks	Lung inhalation: Inflammation and granuloma formation in lungs and associated lymph nodes	Ma-Hock, 2009
C57BL/6J mice	SWNTs D: 1–4 nm SA: 1040 m^2/g	0, 10, 20, 40 ug/mouse	Intratracheal instillation: acute inflammation, fibrosis, granuloma	Shvedova et al., 2005[79]
C57BL/6J mice	MWCNTs in BSA/saline dispersion D: 10–30 nm L: 2 um average	50 mg/mouse	Injection: asbestos-like inflammation, granuloma	Poland et al., 2008[77]

limit of one QD per target molecule. QDs are currently commercially available in a number of well-separated colors, all excitable by a single wavelength (Figure 8.3). Different kinds of QDs (e.g. CdSe/ZnS core-shell QDs, CdTe/CdS/ZnS core-shell-shell QDs) have been fabricated and utilized for applications including biosensing, bioimaging, and disease diagnosis.[4–6,10–13,111,112]

Just like other NMs, systematic toxicity assessment of QDs is critical for their practical medical and biological applications.[123] Many studies have been

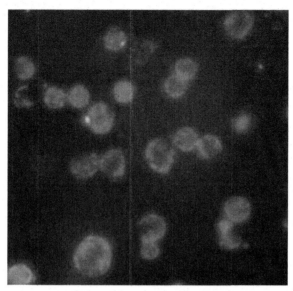

FIGURE 8.3   Breast cancer cell line SK-BR3 after exposure to QDs. *Courtesy of Ocean NanoTech.* *(For color version of this figure, the reader is referred to the online version of this book)*

conducted to evaluate the toxicity of QDs.[123,124] One study had shown that surface oxidation of QDs led to the reduction of Cd on the QD surface causing the release of free cadmium ions in solution causing cell death.[125] Another study showed that toxicity was caused by the nanocrystalline particles and by the molecules covering the surface of the QD molecules.[126] In addition to the release of Cd^{2+} ions from the surface of QDs, it was also reported that the precipitation of QDs on the cell surface impaired the cell growth.[127] When the QDs were only found in the medium surrounding the cells, they were less toxic than when the QDs were taken up by the cells.[127]

Various cell lines were used in the toxicity evaluation of CdTe, CdTe/CdS core-shell structured and CdTe/CdS/ZnS core-shell-shell structured QDs.[128] The results indicated high toxicity of the QDs to the various cell lines studied which was diminished with epitaxial growth of a CdS layer that reduced the release of Cd^{2+} ions. In addition, building a ZnS shell around the CdS or CdTe layer effectively prevented the Cd^{2+} release that essentially made the QDs compatible to cells.[128] In vivo studies indicated that the water-soluble QDs initially accumulated in liver after 0.5–4 h post-injection and absorbed by the kidney at 15–80 days in the blood.[129] The studies also showed that the biodistribution of aqueous QDs was size-dependent.

To evaluate the toxic effects of QDs on cells in vitro, direct counting of cell HEK293 population was used 3 days after treatment with CdTe QDs at various concentrations. The results indicated that the growth curve of HEK293 cells treated with 37.5 nM CdTe QDs was not significantly altered as compared to that of the control but 300 or 600 nM CdTe QDs nearly completely inhibited cell growth.

Exposure of breast cancer cells SK-BR3 to QDs leads to attachment of the QDs to the cell surface.[4,130] This occurs with or without receptor targeting especially when QDs with positive zeta potential are used. In Figure 8.3, the cells which accumulated the QDs show specks of fluorescent material on the cell surface when observed under the microscope.

In vitro studies on QD toxicity was carried out at Ocean NanoTech as part of a small business innovations research funded by the national Science Foundation (NSF, USA).[131] Although the project was focused on the use of NMs for the enhancement of antibody production through effective presentation of antigens to antigen presenting cells,[14,131,132] the effect of NMs on the viability of cells were evaluated (Figure 8.3). Two methods were used in evaluating QD toxicity in vitro as described in the succeeding sections.

8.2.2.1 Procedure for the Evaluation of QD Toxicity to Cancer Cell Lines, U937

The effect of QDs at various concentrations to the cell growth was evaluated using water-soluble QDs. The QDs were made of CdSe/ZnS or CuInS2 that were coated with amphiphilic polymer.[132]

(1) Grow the U937 cells from newly harvested suspension in culture flasks following the manufacturer's recommendation.
(2) Harvest the cells when they reach about 70–80% confluence.
(3) Place 10^5 cells from the newly harvested suspension in individual centrifuge tubes.
(4) Add enough QDs to each tube to attain the final concentrations of 0.025, 0.5, and 2 μM aqueous solutions using the medium as diluent.
(5) Incubate at 37 °C in 5% CO_2 for 1, 4, and 24 h.
(6) Spin the cells down at 3000 rpm for 3–4 min to collect the cells.
(7) Wash the cells three times with 1× DPBS (Dulbecco's Phosphate-Buffered Saline) to remove NPs.
(8) Resuspend the cells in 1× DPBS and place in a 96-well plate.
(9) Perform MTT assay following the manufacturer's recommendation.
(10) Dissolve the crystals formed in 50 uL of MTT buffer.
(11) Scan the solutions at 595 nm and subtract the background signal.

The MTT assay results in Table 8.2 indicated that the CdSe/ZnS with carboxyl on the surface showed toxicity to the cells even at concentrations down to 0.025 μM. Unlike the cadmium containing QDs, the $CuInS_2$ was very slightly toxic after 4 or 24 h of exposure to 0.05 μM concentration. However, the results were highly variable and some data had very low standard deviation while others had very high standard deviations. A confirmatory test was performed by actually counting the number of viable and non-viable cells after exposure to the QDs. The process is presented in the next section.

TABLE 8.2 MTT Assay Signals for QD Toxicity to U937 Cells

QD, µM	Cell-QD incubation period		
	1 h	4 h	24 h
CdSe/ZnS with COOH on the surface			
0.025	0.181 ± 0.029	0.185 ± 0.003	0.172 ± 0.035
0.5	0.171 ± 0.033	0.171 ± 0.012	0.165 ± 0.022
2	0.186 ± 0.021	0.150 ± 0.035	0.131 ± 0.007
CuInS2 with COOH on the surface			
0.025	0.213 ± 0.052	0.209 ± 0.040	0.237 ± 0.011
0.05	0.213 ± 0.051	0.215 ± 0.009	0.205 ± 0.007
1.25	0.239 ± 0.030	0.273 ± 0.026	0.210 ± 0.011
Control			
None	0.246 ± 0.004	0.220 ± 0.025	0.232 ± 0.051

8.2.2.2 Procedure for the Evaluation of QD Toxicity to U937 Cells using the DAPI Staining and Cell Count Method

In order to have a better idea of the toxic effects of QDs on cells, an alternative strategy that involves actual counting of cells, both viable and non-viable, can be used. Using (4',6-diamidino-2-phenylindole) DAPI stain, the dead cells absorb the dye whereas live cells do not. Briefly, the assay is performed as follows.

(1) Grow the cells on a glass cover slip inserted in a 6-well plate until they are 30–50% confluent.
(2) Replace the medium with a new medium to which the NPs are mixed to attain the desired NP concentrations.
(3) Incubate the plates for 24 h at 37 °C and 5% CO_2.
(4) Remove the medium with NPs.
(5) Add 1 mL of 1× DPBS to each well to wash the cells.
(6) Repeat the washing 2 more times.
(7) Add 1 mL of 1× DPBS to each well.
(8) Add 50 uL of DAPI solution.
(9) Incubate at 37 °C and 5% CO_2 for 5 min.
(10) Remove the DPBS with DAPI.
(11) Rinse the cells with 1× DPBS.
(12) Place 500 uL 1× DPBS and scan the cells under the microscope.

(13) Scan each cover slip under the microscope across one edge to the other over three sections in the middle to count the number of dead cells and the number of live cells (see Figure 8.4).

(14) Calculate the % of dead cells using:

$$\% \text{ dead cells} = \frac{\text{number of dead cells}}{\text{number of dead cells} + \text{number of live cells}} \times 100\,\%$$

The results in Table 8.3 indicated that the cadmium-free QDs, CuInS2 exhibited minimal cell death above 0.2 μM concentration while the CdSe/ZnS exhibited 4.77% cell death even at the lowest concentration used that was at 50 nM.[131] This is almost double the cell death that was observed in the control. In order to evaluate the effects of lower concentrations of QDs and those of different sizes, additional studies must be performed.

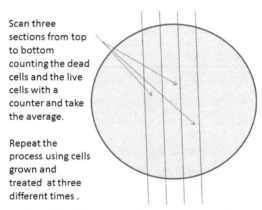

FIGURE 8.4 Basis of DAPI cell death assay. *(For color version of this figure, the reader is referred to the online version of this book)*

TABLE 8.3 % Cell Death from Exposure to QDs

QDs	Concentrations		
CdSe/ZnS w/ polymer~COOH coating	0.2 μM	0.1 μM	0.05 μM
% Cell death	25.24 ± 2.32	18.16 ± 3.75	4.77 ± 1.36
CuInS2 w/polymer~COOH coating	0.4 μM	0.2 μM	0.1 μM
% Cell death	12.01 ± 2.43	3.27 ± 0.61	1.81 ± 0.35
Control		2.89 ± 1.26	

Studies have shown that water-soluble QDs cause slow but long-term inhibition of cell proliferation that are speculated to result from reactive oxygen species (ROS) role in QD-induced cytotoxicity.[123] Previous studies have shown that cadmium-based QDs can generate free radicals including ROS.[133,134] that can cause oxidative stress[135] and mitochondrial damage that can result in loss of metabolic functions.[136] When the oxidative damages are not repaired, the cadmium-based QDs induced apoptotic changes in the IMR-32 human neuroblastoma cell including loss of mitochondrial membrane potential, mitochondrial release of cytochrome C, and activation of caspase-9 and caspase-3.[137]

The effect of cadmium-based QDs was investigated on HEK293 cells against $CdCl_2$. The results showed that the cell proliferation was inhibited but not stopped by $25\,\mu M$ solution of $CdCl_2$ but at higher concentrations, $50\,\mu M$ or $100\,\mu M$, the cell proliferation was completely inhibited.[135] Inductively coupled plasma-mass spectrometry (ICP-MS) showed that the concentrations of intracellular Cd^{2+} ions from the $10\,\mu M$ $CdCl_2$ resulted in significantly higher intracellular concentration of Cd^{2+} ion ($>20\,ng/10^5$ cells) than that with $150\,nM$ CdTe QDs ($<10\,ng/10^5$ cells).[128] In this study, it was shown that both cellular metabolic activity and proliferation rate suggested that treatment of cells with $150\,nM$ CdTe QDs caused stronger inhibition effects than that with $10\,\mu M$ $CdCl_2$. It was also shown that the cadmium-based QDs affected the various gene expressions from the HEK293 cells.[128] Treatment with different concentrations of CdTe QDs from $18.75\,nM$ to $300\,nM$ all caused similar induction levels of the mRNA transcripts.

Investigation of the distribution of QDs in the cell have also been reported to elucidate the toxicity of the QDs.[128] Optical fluorescence imaging has indicated that CdTe QDs were located predominantly in the cytoplasmic/perinuclear area ($200–300\,nm$ resolution).[123]

It is very important to study and to understand the effect of QDs on live cells, tissues, or organs in order to support its growing applications in medicine. In addition, it is equally important to determine the related mechanism of toxicity in order to evaluate the pros and cons for its applications in medical imaging, diagnostics, and therapy. At present, it is still a challenge to compare and draw unambiguous conclusion from reported studies because these studies have focused on a wide variety of QDs, cell lines, and analytic methods.[138,139] The synthesis and purification process, the chemical composition, size, shape, and the surface modifications of the QDs are factors that can affect its interactions with the cell membrane that may or may not lead to subsequent uptake into the cells.[14,140] In addition, different cell types have varying reactions and responses as well as different threshold to stimuli like the QDs making evaluations of toxicity much more challenging. The various ways to interpret cytotoxicity such as cell number, cell growth, apoptosis, cellular morphology or changes in metabolic activity complicate the interpretation of QD toxicity. Thus, a standard method for the evaluation of QD toxicity has yet to be written in order to have a consistent basis for predicting effects in living organisms.

8.2.3 Gold NMs Toxicity

Gold is one of the inert metals possessing many applications that has been used for centuries.[141] During the past couple of decades, gold nanoparticles (AuNPs) have been one of the most studied types of NPs for biomedical applications.[142] A variety of methods have been developed for reproducible synthesis of gold to produce a variety of morphologies with a narrow size distribution and precise characteristics.[143–145] Many of these properties are important for biomedical applications including targeted drug and gene delivery,[146–149] imaging diagnostics,[150,151] or photothermal therapy.[152] Gold nanorods have been applied to imaging cancer[150] and tumor ablation.[153]

One of the drawbacks of the use of NMs in biological systems are the adsorption of proteins and nucleic acids onto the nanoparticle surface. NMs used for targeted therapy depend on attached biomolecules with specific functions to allow them to carry out their functions and most NPMs typically adsorb blood serum proteins in an in vivo environment.[154–156] Thus, a comprehensive understanding of protein binding, structure, and function as influenced by nanoparticle characteristics including size, topography, crystal structure, and surface chemistry is important in order to understand how the NMs affect cells, tissues, organs, and organism.

A study reported by Gagner et al.[142] investigated the effect of gold nanosphere (AuNS) and gold nanorod (AuNR) morphology on the adsorbed proteins lysozyme (Lyz) and a-chymotrypsin (ChT). Both physical and spectroscopic techniques were used to characterize the changes in protein structure and activity upon adsorption, as well as the stability and morphology of the protein–nanoparticle conjugates. Their studies indicated that protein adsorption is affected by the AuNP morphology. Both lysozyme and chymotrypsin adsorbed to AuNPs with relatively low surface coverage with lysozyme forming a dense protein layer on the surface of the nanorods.[142] The lysozyme adsorption on the AuNPs resulted in conformational changes that led to conjugate aggregation.

In a separate study, it has been reported that AuNPs can bind specifically to heparin binding growth factors such as VEGF165 and bFGF, the two critical cytokines for the induction of angiogenesis, inhibit the cytokine activity in vitro, and inhibit VEGF-induced angiogenesis in vivo[157] but without toxicity observed in the study. This finding indicates that AuNPs may be excellent NMs for further modification and development of targeted drug or gene delivery. Gold needs to be formulated to generate a common platform that can be modified easily to conjugate different molecules for drug or gene delivery.

The interaction of AuNPs with cells in vitro was evaluated using two cancer cell lines (human T-cell leukemia Jurkat and human pancreatic carcinoma (PANC1)).[158] AuNPs at of 10, 25, 50, and 100 nm in diameter at a constant mass were exposed to the cells either in deionized (DI) water or in Dulbecco's Modified Eagle's Media (DMEM) supplemented with fetal calf serum (FCS). The zeta potential indicated that protein rich FCS increased the dispersion of the AuNPs. The Jurkat cells showed higher uptake for the 50 nm AuNPs than the PANC1 cell lines[158] as shown by inductively coupled plasma-mass spectroscopy. The AuNPs were observed to be non-toxic to Jurkat and PANC1 cells. Jurkat cells in the presence of 25 nm and 50 nm AuNPs at 10 µg/mL exhibited a viability of 102% and 93%, respectively at 24 h as compared with controls (100%); and 99% and 100%, respectively at 48 h.[158] The PANC1 cells showed viability of 107% and 124% compared with the controls when grown for 24 h in the presence of 25 nm and 50 nm AuNPs, and 91% and 83%, respectively at 48 h.[158] Thus, at 10 ug/mL concentration, the AuNPs were found to be non-toxic to the cells in vitro.[158] These observations are critical in the design of AuNPs for drug delivery or for delivery of NPs for other therapeutic purposes.

For practical purposes, the AuNPs of various shapes and sizes showed insignificant toxicity as exhibited by the various studies that had been cited.[142,143,145,146,148,150,153,155,157–159] These studies do not show conflicting results in both the in vitro and in vivo studies. However, it is still recommended to continue the toxicity studies in order to learn the possible long-term consequences of AuNPs in animals and in humans.

8.2.4 IOMNP Toxicity

One of the most rapidly growing areas of interest in nanotechnology is in IOM-NPs or superparamagnetic iorn oxide nanomaterials (SPIONs). The IOMNPs have found excellent applications in magnetic resonance imaging (MRI), magnetic isolation of cells, drug delivery, hyperthermia, and many more.[4,15–17,160–163] IOMNPs are excellent NMs for these applications because of their ease of manipulation with the use of permanent or electric magnets.[164]

IOMNPs are NMs that consist of iron oxide core materials that are usually coated with biocompatible materials for medical applications. The surfaces of the IOMNPs are easily modified to attach different molecules based on the desired function. The advantage of the IOMNPs over other NMs is the ease of manipulation with external magnets that can be targeted to the required area through external magnets.[165] Depending upon the size and the amount of magnetic material, the IOMNPs can exhibit properties that include superparamagnetism, high field irreversibility, high saturation field, and extra anisotropy contributions or shifted loops after field cooling.[166] Today, studies on the medical applications of the IOMNPs have gone to include reduction of the amount of cytotoxic drug for the systemic distribution thereby eliminating possible side effects and decreasing the drug through more efficient and localized delivery of the drug.

The IOMNPs come in two forms: 1) magnetic particle core composed of magnetite, Fe_3O_4, or maghemite, γ-Fe_2O_3, coated with a biocompatible polymer[132] or 2) a biocompatible polymer in which the IOMNPs are precipitated inside the pores.[165,167] The coating can be an amphiphilic polymer that is used to make the IOMNPs water soluble and at the same time protects the nanoparticle from the surrounding environment.[165] The coating can be functionalized by attaching antibodies, biotin, avidin, streptavidin, protein G, and other molecules.[4,15–17,131,132,165] Depending upon the molecule on the IOMNP surface, drugs, receptors, proteins, or nucleic acids can be coupled on the surface for various medical applications.

The various medical applications of IOMNPs include drug delivery, cellular labeling/cell separation, tissue repair, magnetic resonance imaging, magnetic hyperthermia and magnetofection.[4,15–17,160–163,165–174] These medical applications will ultimately involve humans or other animals, it is imperative to study toxicity of IOMNPs in appropriate models. A list of commercially available IOMNPs is given in Table 8.4.

The most important considerations in the successful applications of IOMNPs in medicine are their biocompatibility and toxicity. Various parameters to evaluate biocompatibility that include the size of the core and the coatings (shell), stability, and surface modification. For efficient applications, the IOMNPs must exhibit high magnetization in order for their translocation in a living system to be controlled as close as necessary to the targeted pathologic tissue with an external magnetic field.[175]

The other important consideration for the IOMNPs for medical applications is internalization into specific cells or cell uptake which may be compromised by (a) short blood half-life of the NPs, (b) non-specific targeting, and (c) low cell internalization efficiency.[176] Different studies have been reported on the control of the size and surface properties of IOMNPs to improve these areas.[165,170,177] The most common molecules used for stabilizing IOMPNs are surfactants such as oleic acid, lauric acid, alkane sulphonic acids, and alkane phosphonic acids.[178] A method to prepare hydrophobic IOMNPs is the use of alpha-cyclodextrin by host–guest interactions making the NMs able to disperse from organic to aqueous solution.[173] This is also achieved by using an amphiphilic polymer shell[179] such as poly (ethylene-co-vinyl acetate), polyvinylpyrrolidone (PVP), polylactic-co-glycolic acid (PLGA), polyethylene glycol (PEG), or polyvinyl alcohol (PVA) have also been used as coating materials in aqueous suspension.[174] The IOMNPs are coated with these amphiphilic polymers that introduce amines or carboxyl groups creating an internal hydrophobic structure enveloping the organic soluble iron oxide core and a hydrophilic outer layer making the IOMNPs water soluble. Other materials such as gelatin, dextran, polylactic acids, starch, albumin, liposomes, chitosan, and ethyl cellulose have been used in modifying IOMNPs for drug delivery.

Although iron oxide particles are known to be non-toxic, some of the coating materials used to make them water soluble could be toxic. For instance, silica is known to be biocompatible but not biodegradable.[165] Amorphous silica coating on magnetite NMs that results in silica-coated core–shell particles when dispersed in aqueous suspensions showed negative charge above the isoelectric point of silica which is at pH ~ 2.[171] The interactions of IOMNPs with biological fluids can lead to increased formation of free hydroxyl radicals and reactive

TABLE 8.4 Commercial Sources of IOMNPs *(Copyright from Mahmoudi[165])*

Company	URL	Applications
Stem Cell Technologies	www.stemcell.com	Immunomagnetic cell separation
Chemicell	www.chemicell.com	Biological separations and detection
Imego	www.imego.com	Medical diagnostics
Micromod	www.micromod.de	Drug delivery, biomagnetic separation, nucleic acid purification and protein separation
Magnisense	www.magnisense.com	Bioassays for human and animal diagnostics, food safety and environmental protection
Magsense	www.magsenselife.com	Bioseparation, diagnostic, immunoassay, and bioanalytical measurements
Diagnostic Biosensors	www.diagnosticbiosensors. com	Diagnostic biosensors
Dexter Magnetic Technologies	www.dextermag.com	Biological magnetic separation
AMAG Pharmaceuticals	www.amagpharma.com	MRI contrast agents; Diagnosis of cardiovascular disease and cancer
Magforce	www.magforce.de	Hyperthermia
NanoTherics, Ltd	www.nanotherics.com	Magnetic gene transfer
European Institute of Science	www.biotechniques.com	Hyperthermia
Miltenyi Biotec	www.miltenyibiotec.com	immunology, cell and molecular biology, bioinformatics, and stem cell reagents
EMD Chemicals	eshop.emdchemicals.com	Immunoassay and immunoreagent development
Ocean NanoTech	www.oceannanotech.com	Biosensors, cell separation, MRI contrast agent, and drug delivery reagents development

oxygen species (ROS) but can be prevented by coating the IOMNPs with gold[168] preventing the formation of large aggregates.

One of the advantages of using NMs that are <100 nm in diameter is their higher effective surface areas, lower sedimentation rates (or high stability in suspension) and improved diffusion in tissues.[165] Particles that are <100 nm can escape from the reticuloendothelial system (RES) more easily,[165] remain in the circulation after injection and are capable of passing through the capillary systems of organs and tissues avoiding vessel embolism.[165] The size of the NMs is equally important for achieving enhanced permeability and retention (EPR) effect because particles larger than 10 nm cannot penetrate the endothelium at physiological conditions but can pass in inflammation or tumor infiltration.[180] Systematic injection of drug-loaded NMs into the bloodstream may or may not be able to perform their designed function depending upon their size, morphology and surface charge. For instance, tissue macrophages (i.e. Kupffer cells in the liver) are highly sensitive to invading microorganism and NPMs.[165,181] In the bloodstream, the plasma proteins (opsonins) easily adsorb on the surface of NMs depending on their sizes, surface charge, and morphology.[165] Various authors have studied the protein adsorption on NPs either in vitro or in vivo.[176] Moghimi et al.[181] studied the opsonization process (adsorption of plasma protein) on NMs as a function of surface charge, size, and hydrophilicity/hydrophobicity. Their results showed that the smaller the size the higher the hydrophilicity of the NMs, the more inefficient is the opsonisation process. Zhang et al.[176] reported that PEG and folic acid coating are most efficient for inhibiting protein adsorption in vivo. The use of polymer coating, *Poly{3-(trimethoxy silyl propyl) methacrylate-r-polyethylene glycol methacrylate}*, on magnetite has been reported to generate a stable, protein-resistant magnetic resonance imaging probe.[182] They suggested that the polymer coating bestowed long-circulating properties to the SPIONs in plasma allowing their escape from RES uptake by macrophages.

RES uptake controls NMs with sizes above 200 nm or below 10 nm making them unsuitable for drug delivery. It has been reported that NMs of sizes between 10 and 100 nm can evade RES uptake and are therefore, most effective for drug delivery purposes.[183] Furthermore, SPIONs with a positive charge showed higher internalization into human breast cancer cells compared with negatively charged SPIONs but there was no difference in the degree of internalization into Human Umbilical Vein Endothelian Cells (HUVECs). This shows that the uptake pattern depends also on the cell type.[184]

Mouse fibroblast cells and human leukemia cells have been used to establish the cytotoxicity of PVA-coated SPIONs with different shapes and morphologies (e.g. nanospheres, nanorods, nanoworms, magnetite colloidal nanocrystal clusters, and nanobeads).[185] The results indicated that the SPIONs showed no or little toxicity. In another study using human lung cancer cell line, 20 and 40 µg/mL showed no DNA damage nor intracellular ROS (i.e. production of reactive oxygen species) were observed except for small oxidative DNA lesions.[186] One study reported that by staining with crystal violet dye, the existence of gas vesicles in SPIONs-treated cells were observed with increased granularity of the cells.[187] It was explained that such observation might have been the result of autophagy that caused cytotoxicity.

It has been suggested that the proteins, which adsorb on the surface of NMs including IOMNPs[188,189] can have significant impact on the NMs biological, biochemical, and cellular behavior.[188] This nanoparticle–protein interaction is now recognized as a key issue for defining the toxicity of NMs[188] because of unfavorable changes in protein configurations that can lead to fibrillation, exposure to new antigenic epitopes, and possible loss of protein function.[165,190] The protein adsorption on IOMNPs can cause denaturation that can lead to the exposure of new antigenic sites which can initiate a cascade of immune response.[190] Hence, the specific binding rates and affinities of different plasma proteins to NMs have been the subject of some investigations.[191] They used size-exclusion chromatography (SEC) to determine the affinity and stoichiometry of protein bonded to particles, surface plasmon resonance (SPR) to get the rates of protein association and dissociation; and isothermal titration calorimetry (ITC). The quantity of the proteins adsorbed to NMs was the subject of the study by Lynch et al.[192]

In an in vitro study, exposing IOMNPs to cell medium for a period of 24 h caused the proteins in the medium to coat the NMs creating the protein corona. These protein coated NMs were then used for cell toxicity studies.[187] The results indicated that the IOMNPs that were pre-coated with proteins from the cell medium had significantly lower toxicity. In a biological unit like a cell, organ, or tissue, the NMs are presented coated with the proteins that adsorbed along the way before the NMs reached their target.[193]

Another area of possible toxigenicity of IOMNPs as they move through narrow capillaries is agglomeration that may lead to clogging (embolizations) of small blood vessels. Thus, stabilization of IOMNPs is a critical matter in their function as drug delivery vehicles. Considerations of the isoelectric point around pH 7 which is same as that for biological fluids has to be taken into account during the applications of IOMNPs in vivo.[194] By carefully choosing the coating on the IOMNPs, colloidal stability can be imparted, thereby, increasing the blood circulation half-life.[165] In addition, the particle size, size distribution, shape, concentration/volume, stability of the drug/ferrofluid binding (desorption characteristics), method of administration (oral, intraperitoneal, intra-muscular, etc.), duration/rate of the injection/infusion, and strength/duration of the magnetic field applied are parameters to be considered as well.[165] For personal medical applications, various patient-related parameters such as weight, blood volume, cardiac output and systemic vascular resistance, and tumor-related parameters such as circulation time, tumor volume and location, vascular content of tumor, and blood flow in tumor must be taken into consideration.[195]

8.2.4.1 Procedure for In vitro Evaluation of IOMNP Toxicity using the MTT Assay[131,132]

The effect of amphiphilic polymer coated water-soluble IOMNPs at various concentrations to the growth of the cell line U937 was investigated.[132] The IOMNPs in the study were 5 and 10 nm in diameter.

(1) Grow the U937 cells from newly harvested suspension in culture flasks following the manufacturer's recommendation.
(2) Harvest the cells when they reach about 70–80% confluence.
(3) Place 10^5 cells from the newly harvested suspension in individual centrifuge tubes.
(4) Add enough IOMNPs to each tube to attain the final concentrations of 0.025, 0.5, and 2 µM aqueous solutions using the medium as diluent.
(5) Incubate at 37 °C in 5% CO_2 for 1, 4, and 24 h.
(6) Spin the cells down at 3000 rpm for 3–4 min to collect the cells.
(7) Wash the cells three times with 1× DPBS to remove NPs.
(8) Resuspend the cells in 1× DPBS and place in a 96-well plate.
(9) Perform MTT assay following the manufacturer's recommendation.
(10) Dissolve the crystals formed in 50 uL of MTT buffer.
(11) Scan the solutions at 595 nm and subtract the background signal.

The MTT assay evaluation of IOMNP toxicity did not exhibit toxic effects of both the 5 nm and 10 nm diameter particles that were coated with amphiphilic polymer[131] (Table 8.5). These results are important for the use of IOMNPs in animal studies for evaluations of their medical applications. However, because of the difficulty in reading the signals resulting from the presence of NMs in the cells that may have affected the results of the study, a more direct approach to cell death was used as an alternative method to MTT. This process is given below.

8.2.4.2 Procedure for the Evaluation of IOMNPs Toxicity to U937 Cells using the DAPI Staining and Cell Count Method

In order to have a better idea of the toxicity of IOMNP on cells, an alternative strategy that involves actual counting of cells, both viable and non-viable, can be used. Using DAPI stain, the dead cells absorb the dye whereas live cells do not. Briefly, the assay is performed as follows.

(1) Grow the cells on glass cover slip inserted in a 6-well plate until they are 30–50% confluent.
(2) Replace the medium with a new medium to which the IOMNPs are mixed to attain the desired concentrations.
(3) Incubate the plates for 24 h at 37 °C and 5% CO_2.
(4) Remove the medium with NPs.
(5) Add 1 mL of 1×DPBS to each well to wash the cells.
(6) Repeat the washing 2 more times.
(7) Add 1 mL of 1×DPBS to each well.

TABLE 8.5 MTT Assay for IOMNP Toxicity to U937 Cells

IOMNP, mg/mL	Cell-IOMNP incubation period		
	1 h	4 h	24 h
IOMNP with COOH on the surface, 5 nm diameter			
0.025	0.224 ± 0.038	0.216 ± 0.015	0.207 ± 0.020
0.5	0.235 ± 0.019	0.243 ± 0.043	0.214 ± 0.014
1	0.210 ± 0.025	0.261 ± 0.019	0.216 ± 0.021
IOMNP with COOH on the surface, 10 nm diameter			
0.025	0.282 ± 0.025	0.261 ± 0.015	0.237 ± 0.033
0.5	0.218 ± 0.016	0.243 ± 0.043	0.225 ± 0.015
2	0.211 ± 0.022	0.206 ± 0.019	0.217 ± 0.028
Control			
None	0.246 ± 0.004	0.220 ± 0.025	0.232 ± 0.051

(8) Add 50 uL of DAPI solution.
(9) Incubate at 37 °C and 5% CO_2 for 5 min.
(10) Remove the DPBS with DAPI.
(11) Rinse the cells with 1 × DPBS.
(12) Place 500 uL 1 × DPBS and scan the cells under the microscope.
(13) Scan each cover slip under the microscope across one edge to the other over three sections in the middle to count the number of dead cells and the number of live cells (see Figure 8.4).
(14) Calculate the % of dead cells.

The results in Table 8.6 indicated that both the 5 and 10 nm diameter IOMNPs showed % cell death at the highest concentration tested that are similar to those of the control that were not exposed to any NM.[131] This observation is significant for the growing applications of IOMNPs in medicine.

The alternative protocol for assessing NM toxicity in cells in vitro is easy to use and very inexpensive. Although it requires time, multiple scans of the cells over the glass cover slip can be performed for better sensitivity. The only instrument required is an optical microscope that can differentiate between blue stained cells and non-stained cells.

8.2.5 Silver NPs Toxicity

Silver nanoparticles (AgNPs) show low toxicity to human cells but they have effective broad-spectrum activity against bacteria and a far lesser probability

TABLE 8.6 % Cell Death from Exposure to IOMNPs

IOMNPs	Concentrations, mg/mL		
IOMNPs w/ polymer~COOH coating, 5 nm	0.2	0.1	0.05
% Cell death	2.04 ± 0.48	1.86 ± 0.36	0.50 ± 0.11
IOMNPs w/ polymer~COOH coating, 10 nm	0.2	0.1	0.05
% Cell death	2.05 ± 0.97	2.77 ± 1.06	1.45 ± 0.47
Control		2.80 ± 1.26	

to cause microorganism resistance than conventional antibiotics.[196,197] Because of these antimicrobial characteristics, AgNPs are used for water purification[198] and wound dressing to disinfect microorganisms.[198–200] AgNPs can be coated on common polyurethane foams through its interaction with the nitrogen atom of the polyurethane.[199] The wound dressing with AgNPs exhibited better wound healing capacity, improved cosmetic appearance, and scar-less healing in an animal model.[200]

A number of studies have shown that AgNPs have efficient antibacterial activity compared with their bulk counterpart due to high surface-to-volume ratio providing better contact with microorganisms.[201] TEM studies revealed that the majority of AgNPs get localized on cell membranes that appeared severely damaged as indicated by the presence of numerous pits and gaps.[202–204] AgNPs may also damage the permeability of bacterial membranes causing efflux of reducing sugars and proteins and depletion of intracellular adenosine triphosphate (ATP).[203,205] AgNPs can cause destabilization of the outer membrane causing the plasma membrane potential to collapse.[206] It has also been observed that expressions of several cell envelope proteins were stimulated after a short exposure to AgNPs.[205] It has also been claimed that AgNPs inside the bacterial cell attack the respiratory chain by interacting with thiol groups of essential enzymes that lead to their inactivation and also dephosphorylate peptides on tyrosine residues that could influence bacterial signal transduction which eventually leads to cell death.[207] All these studies had focused on the description of damage and mode of action of AgNPs on exposed bacteria, but the primary reason for the induced antimicrobial effects remains unclear.

Silver NPs (AgNPs) are, due to their antimicrobial properties, the most widely used NPs in commercial products. AgNPs are incorporated into medical products like bandages as well as textiles and household items.[208] AgNPs are also known to induce toxicity in many different species[209] and in humans, chronic exposure to silver causes argyria and/or argyrosis.[210] In vitro studies using different cell lines have shown the toxicity of AgNPs number of in vitro studies.[211–213] The size, shape, chemical composition, surface charge, solubility, and their ability to bind affect biological sites and their metabolic fate and excretion influence the toxicity of NPs.[55,56] The high surface area to volume ratio in metal NPs increases the potential release of metal ions in solution[214,215] but it is not clear if the toxicity of AgNPs results from released silver.[213] Some suggested that the AgNP toxicity is due to oxidative stress and independent of silver ions[213] while other indicated that measured silver ion content of the AgNP suspension could not fully explain the toxicity of the AgNPs in suspension.[212,216]

The studies conducted by Beer et al.[217] indicated that at low silver ion fractions (2.6% and below) the toxicity of the AgNP suspension was significantly higher than that of the supernatant, which could suggest an involvement of factors other than pure silver ions. The same observation was observed in a study on copper oxide NPs (CuONPs) that had a higher toxicity than dissolved copper ions.[218] In these studies the suspension of AgNP showed low amounts of silver ions and the ionic fraction of the AgNP suspension could not explain the observed toxicity. The Beer et al.[217] results indicated that there were no significant differences in the proportion of apoptotic or necrotic cells after treatment with AgNP suspension or AgNP supernatant. The study by Qu et al.[29] focused on evaluating the mechanism of the antimicrobial property of AgNPs. Their data indicated that the Ag^+ ions in solution could not be the only source of toxicity of the AgNPs. To elucidate the role of reactive oxygen species (ROS) in the antibacterial mechanism of AgNPs, the antibacterial activity of AgNPs was investigated in the presence of N-acetylcysteine (NAC) which is an effective antioxidant containing a mercapto group. If ROS is the cause of AgNP toxicity, the presence of NAC can prevent the oxidative damage induced by AgNPs. In the absence of NAC, AgNPs alone killed ~50% and almost 99% when used at 5 and 10 mg/L respectively. When combined with 10 mM NAC, cell death decreased to 20% and 40% in the presence of AgNPs at 5 and 10 mg/L, respectively. These results demonstrated that the antibacterial activity of AgNPs was attenuated in the presence of the antioxidant NAC which is in agreement with reports that NAC not only reduce the concentration of ROS in the culture medium as a ROS scavenger, but also induces the production of glutathione which is an important cellular antioxidant.[219] Thus, the presence of NAC as ROS scavenger may have been responsible for the reduced antimicrobial activity of the AgNPs or it is equally possible that NAC induced the production of glutathione.[29] These studies support the claim that ROS are partly responsible for the antibacterial activity of AgNPs. Similarly, Foldberg et al.[211] indicated that ionic and/or nanoparticulate silver induces ROS in A549 cells. In their studies, they concluded that the higher ROS production of cells treated with AgNP supernatant is most likely due to the higher amounts of silver ions to which the cells are exposed, where the same mass of silver was applied.

8.3 HANDLING, STORAGE, AND DISPOSAL OF NMs

The number of NMs and nano-enabled products in the shelves are rapidly increasing but the regulations for their proper handling, shipping, storage, and disposal are not yet in place. Currently, it is up to the manufacturers to recommend the levels of safety, proper handling, storage, and disposal of the NMs. It is imperative to have proper ventilation. The following general safety precautions are recommended for the handling, storage, and disposal of NMs.

8.3.1 Handling

(1) Always wear proper protective equipment (PPE) including laboratory gown, gloves, eye goggles, and closed shoes when handling, opening, pouring, or pipetting NMs in solution or in solid form.
(2) Wear a mask when handling NMs in powder form.
(3) Transfer solid NMs from one container to another inside a safety fume hood that is in good working condition.
(4) Pour NMs in organic solvents under a safety fume hood.
(5) Work in a well-ventilated area.
(6) Always carry large glass bottles of NMs using a safety bucket.

8.3.2 Storage

(1) Store NMs and nano-enabled products in appropriate temperature and pressure with proper ventilation. For example, biomolecule modified NMs must be stored at 2–4 °C.
(2) Store powder NMs in tightly closed vials at ambient room temperature (ART).
(3) Store aqueous solutions and organic solutions of NMs tightly closed vials at 2–8 °C.

8.3.3 Disposal

(1) Store used NMs and nano-enabled products in properly labeled appropriate hazardous waste containers for hazardous waste disposal.
(2) Have a separate hazardous waste container for aqueous NMs suspension and organic solvent NM suspensions.
(3) Collect all solids that have been exposed to NMs in a hazardous waste trash container for proper disposal. This includes vials of used QDs, pipet tips, paper towels, gloves, weighing boats, etc.
(4) NEVER dispose any used NMs down the drain.
(5) All waste solutions containing NMs and all solids exposed to NMs must be treated as hazardous waste just like ordinary hazardous chemicals.

Within the California Environmental Protection Agency (EPA), the Department of Toxic Substances Control (DTSC) published its intention to request information on analytical test methods, fate and transport in the environment, and other relevant information from manufacturers of NMs.[220] The request for information is intended to identify information gaps and to develop further knowledge about the health and safety of NMs. The Department has requested information on NMs such as nano silver, nano titanium dioxide, nano zerovalent iron, nano cerium oxide, quantum dots, and nano zinc oxide. The DTSC exercises its authority under California Health and Safety Code, Chapter 699, sections 57018–57020[220] which resulted from Assembly Bill AB 289 (2006). The DTSC intends to collect information on the fate and transport, detection and analysis, and other information on chemicals that are more available from those who manufacture or import the chemicals. A formal information request letter was sent to manufacturers who produce or import carbon nanotubes in California, or who may export carbon nanotubes into the State in January of 2009 and the information must be submitted within one year. This letter was the first formal implementation of the authorities resulting from AB 289 (2006) which is directed to manufacturers of carbon nanotubes, both industry and academia within the State, and to manufacturers outside California who export carbon nanotubes to California. In January 22, 2010, the manufacturers and importers of carbon nanotubes in California were required to submit their responses and the responses were posted by DTSC along with a list of companies that had failed to respond to the information request. DTSC also indicated interest in expanding the Specific Chemical Information Call-in to brominated flame retardants, methyl siloxanes, and other nanometals and nanometal oxides such as vanadium oxide, aluminum oxide, silicon dioxide, titanium dioxide, zinc oxide, cerium oxide, nano platinum, nano silver, and nano zerovalent iron. There is also a plan to include quantum dots, ocean plastics, and nanoclay in the list of chemicals of interest.

8.4 REMEDIATION IN CASE OF NMs SPILLS

NMs are currently being produced in small-scale synthesis processes in most laboratories. However, based on accumulated reports in the literature, some of the NMs are harmful and toxic to living organisms. Therefore, it is very important to handle NMs and their accidental spills in the work place and in the environment. In lieu of regulations for the proper handling of NMs spills, each laboratory is currently implementing their own remediation procedures. These procedures are based on the limited knowledge of how the NMs can affect the air, water, and ultimately the living organisms that eventually get exposed to the NMs either through inhalation, drinking contaminated water, or eating contaminated produce. In the event of a spill, the following protocol is recommended at small laboratories and/or small business manufacturing, packaging, and vending NMs.

8.4.1 Spills of NMs in solution

(1) Call the immediate supervisor if the personnel who spilled the NMs did not get contaminated with the NMs in any part of the body or garments.

(2) Allow the solution to soak in paper towels. There must be stacks of paper towels together with the caustic and acid spills kit.

(3) Collect the paper towels in NMs contaminated trash bins that are properly labeled with "hazardous materials".

(4) In the case of QD spills, immediately use cotton washcloth soaked in soap and water to clean up the area of the spill. In the case of IOMNPs, AuNPs, CNTs, and AgNPs, these are easier to remove from solid surfaces than QDs.

(5) To remove all traces of the spilled NMs solution, immediately scrub the spill area with a washcloth soaked in soap and water.

(6) Discard all used paper towels and wash clothes properly in hazardous waste containers.

8.4.2 Spills of NMs in Powder Form

All types of powders disperse through air movement very easily. Dangerous and hazardous powders such as the NMs must be handled inside a safety fume hood at all times.

(1) Always wear the PPE at all times.

(2) Make sure to handle all powder form NMs inside the fume hood.

(3) Place the fume hood window as low as the allowable level.

(4) In the event of a spill inside the fume hood, take damp paper towels and carefully place on top of the spilled powders to prevent escape into the air.

(5) Collect the NMs powder carefully with the damp paper towels avoiding any possible disturbance of the dry powder to prevent it from escaping into the atmosphere.

(6) In the case of QD spills, immediately use cotton washcloth soaked in soap and water to clean up the area of the spill.

(7) To remove all traces of the spilled NMs in powder form, immediately scrub the spill area with a washcloth soaked in soap and water.

(8) Discard all used paper towels and wash clothes properly in hazardous waste containers.

The best practice in dealing with NMs is to always assume that these are harmful. Hence, all personnel must were PPE at all times. Handle the NMs, whether in powder or in solution inside a safety fume hood and away from any part of the body. Make sure there is proper ventilation in the laboratory at all times. If a spill occurs, do not try to solve the problem if you are not trained to do so, especially in the event of powder spills. Call your immediate supervisor when in doubt of what to do after you spill any NMs.

8.5 NANOTOXICITY REGULATIONS

Nanotechnology awareness has slightly increased in 2009.[221] About three in ten (31%) Americans indicate hearing about nanotechnology and about 37% of adults still indicate that they have heard nothing about nanotechnology and 68% say they have heard just a little or nothing at all.[221] Similarly to the previous years reported, men say 42% heard a lot or some with men under 50 (48%), college graduates (45%), and individuals with an annual household income over $75,000 (46%) report the highest levels of awareness of nanotechnology.

The supporters of nanotechnology see it as a new industrial revolution which presents enormous economic potential as well as the possibility of applications in everything from materials to medicine to engineering to space travel.[222,223] But this is accompanied by nanotechnology's potential to present new risks to human health and to the environment. The various potential applications of nanotechnology offers the possibility to radically transform the quality of everyday life, therefore, their ethical and social significance must be thoroughly evaluated. In 2008, the UK Prime Minister Ian Pearson noted in a speech noted that Nanotechnology's development is 'an ethical as well as a scientific question, and the public's voice should be heard in answering it'.[222,223] In Europe, scientific research on nanotechnology has been accompanied by interest in its ethical implications, public awareness, and making its regulations more robust. In the past five years international policy discussions concerning the appropriate mechanisms for the governance and regulation of nanotechnology has emerged. This is intertwined with the dilemma between enhancing innovation while preventing potential risks to the environment and human health. This leads to 'anticipatory' governance because most people are unfamiliar with nanotechnology and have little exposure to factual knowledge of its nature and capabilities. Most nanotechnologies especially the NMs for medicine are at early or premarket stage of development that have not gone out of the bench top studies. Moreover, there are too many different kinds, types, sizes, shapes, etc. of existing and emerging NMs that there is considerable task to be accomplished before the risks to human and to the environment can begin to unfold.

The European Commission prepared and adopted the Code of Conduct for responsible nanosciences and nanotechnologies research.[224] This defined the code of conduct in the various research areas in the nanotechnology which have called the attention of policymakers and civil society organizations because of potential societal and environmental controversies that may be generated. Nanotechnology brings lots of hope on the potential benefits for human health, especially on those diseases which currently have no cure or prevention, the environment and the quality of life while at the same time they generate concerns about equal potential for risks to health and the environment. Ethical concerns and protection of fundamental rights from the upsurge of nano-enabled materials that have no established potential long-term effects can give rise to controversies that are inherent to the research process and to the uncertainties during the search for scientific knowledge. The interactions of NPs with bio-molecules to cells to tissues to organs and to whole organisms much less to humans and the environment is not yet fully understood and is utmost barely scratched on the surface, therefore, precautions are our best defense for now. On the other hand, research in nanotechnologies may lead to possible applications that are unacceptable to the present realm of human knowledge and may be rejected by the society. Thus, it is imperative that nanotechnology research be undertaken in a framework that is conducive to scientific excellence, innovation, and human morality providing equal opportunity among all races and countries in the world. Thus, the European Commission Competitiveness Council of 2008 adopted the"Regulatory aspects of nanomaterials", which reviewed the legisla-tion that covered in principle the potential health, safety and environmental risks in relation to NMs. In the 2004 reports of the Royal Society, they recommended a review of existing regulations to assess and control work place exposure to NPs and nanotubes. The report expressed particular concern for the inhalation of large quantities of NPs by workers involved in the manufacturing process.

In the US and other parts of the world, the on-going controversy on the implications of nanotechnology caused discussions on the needs to require spe-cial government regulations. This particularly focuses on the assessment of new substances before their release into the market, community, and the environ-ment.[225] In the UK, the Royal Society recognizes the huge potential of nano-technology to bring benefits to many areas of research and application, thereby, attracting rapidly increasing investments from Governments and from private entities worldwide.[226] The recognition of the new challenges in the safety, regulatory or ethical impacts, caused the government to commission the Royal Society and the Royal Academy of Engineering to carry out an independent study into current and future developments in nanotechnology. One of the most interesting content of their report stated that it is unlikely that new manufactured NMs can be introduced into humans in doses sufficient to cause similar health effects as those that have been associated with polluted air. However, they rec-ognized possible inhalation in the workplaces in significant amounts, therefore, steps should be taken to minimize exposure.[226]

The upsurge of nano-enabled products in the market from cosmetics to shirts, bicycles, tennis rackets, and electronic gadgets have triggered calls for increased community participation and effective evaluation, regulation, and improved gov-ernance of nanotechnologies.[227] Public and scientific debates have been called to anticipate and address the likely social, environmental, and ethical impacts of these new technologies. In Australia, the national science research organization, the Commonwealth Scientific and Industrial Research Organization (CSIRO) is carrying out scientific research at the nanoscale in various areas. Alongside the technical research, a small team of social scientists has focused on the local social implications and public perceptions of nanotechnologies in Australian context. The team has explored social perspectives on nanotechnology research and devel-opment with the goal to establish a discussion between CSIRO and 'interested public'[228] on the implications of the CSIRO-designated 'emerging science' of nanotechnology.[227] The second goal focused on exploring ways of integrating a broader range of perspectives on science and technology into research planning and assessment within CSIRO.[227] In this paper, the interested public consisted of not only scientific 'experts' but also 'lay unrecognized experts' including government, non-government, industry and community-based groups, plus general community members. This was to foster strategies and approaches that enable to bridge knowledge divides and to find common ground across conflicting values that may exist within a broadly-conceived 'public'. To date, these approaches have not led to successful comprehensive regulation to oversee research and the commercial application of nanotechnologies or to proper labeling of products that contain NMs or are derived from nanotechnologies.[229]

Various regulatory bodies such as the United States Environmental Protection Agency (US EPA), the Food and Drug Administration (US FDA) and the Health and Consumer Protection Directorate of the European Commission have initiated action regarding the potential risks from NMs. These regulatory bodies have concluded that NPs form the potential for an entirely new risk and that it is necessary to carry out an extensive analysis of the risk.

The challenge for regulation is whether a standard system of evaluating the risk to NMs can be developed to identify NMs and their formulations' toxicological properties or if it is more likely to test each particle or formulation separately. To date, engineered NMs and the products or materials that contain them are not subject to any special regulation during production, handling, or labeling. Currently, there is no authorized body to regulate nanotech-based products, there are also no nanotoxicity standards to follow, and no toxicity regulations in place to enforce. Most laboratories conducting nanotechnology-related studies perform their own toxicity assessments but even the existing cytotoxicity tests that are standardized for materials in bulk but not for NMs may fail and result in conflicting data.[52] Thus, it is urgently needed to develop standardized methods of assessing short- and long-term effects of NMs on cells, tissues, organs, and whole organisms.

There are non-nanotechnology specific regulatory agencies that cover some products and processes under existing regulations but there are insufficient regulations of the NMs which enable some nano-enabled products to be released without coverage by any regulations. This is particularly the case for titanium dioxide (TiO_2) that are used in sunscreen. The US FDA reviewed the immediate health effects of exposure but did not review its impacts for aquatic ecosystems when the sunscreen rubs off, nor did the EPA, or any other agency.[225] In similar context, the Australian Therapeutic Goods Administration (TGA)[230] approved the use of NPs in sunscreens (without inclusion in the package label) on the basis that although NMs TiO_2 and zinc oxide (ZnO) produce free radicals and oxidative DNA damage in vitro, these were unlikely to pass into the stratum corneum of human skin. This decision was short sighted because it did not consider prolonged use especially on children with cut skin, the elderly with thin skin, people with diseased skin or use over other skin imperfections.[231]

A more thorough investigation of the long-term effects of NMs on the skin shows that the uncoated anatase form of TiO_2 undergoes a photocatalytic reaction that degraded the surface of newly installed prepainted steel roofs in areas that came in contact with sunscreen coated hands of workers.[232] The rapid growth in nanotechnology and its fast upsurge of commercial products is more than likely to create more gaps in regulation such as these.

The nano-enabled drugs are just in the initial stages of the drug regulatory processes to date and within a few decades, have the potential to comprise a dominant group within the class of innovative pharmaceuticals and therapeutics. With the current apparent philosophy of regulators regarding the safety of NMs and their focus on cost-effectiveness of assessment and monitoring that these products give rise to few if any nano-specific issues it may take a few disastrous consequences before proper action is taken.[233] The increased research in the applications of NMs for medical purposes may create heightened policy challenges that will warrant attention to safety regulations.[234] These may lead to new models of safe drug discovery and development more systematically toward easing the burden of currently incurable diseases.[235]

The most recent news release from the US FDA concerning NMs was issued in April 20, 2012 and addresses the use of NMs in food and cosmetics.[236] The two draft guidance documents are entitled "Guidance for Industry: Assessing the Effects of Significant Manufacturing Process Changes, including Emerging Technologies, on the Safety and Regulatory Status of Food Ingredients and Food Contact Substances, Including Food Ingredients that are Color Additives" and "Guidance for Industry: Safety of Nanomaterials in Cosmetic Products." The draft on food gives the manufacturers the factors that should be considered when determining whether changes in manufacturing processes such as nanotechnology will result in a significant change that may affect the identity of the food substance, affect the safety of the use of the food substance, affect the regulatory status of the use of the food substance, or needs a regulatory submission to FDA.[236] Similarly, the draft guidance on cosmetics is focused on the safety assessment of NMs when used in cosmetic products. In this guidance, the legal requirements for nanomaterial-based cosmetics are the same as those for other cosmetics. Although cosmetics do not require premarket approval, companies and individuals who market cosmetics have legal responsibilities regarding the safety of their products which must be properly labeled.[236] The draft suggests the modification of existing methods or the development of new methods of safety assessments of cosmetic products containing NMs. Consultation with the agency are encouraged in both guidances before releasing their products to market so that FDA experts can help address questions related to the safety, other attributes, and the regulatory status of nanotechnology products.[236] The US FDA is investing in an FDA-wide nanotechnology regulatory science program to enhance its scientific capabilities and to develop necessary data and tools to identify properties of NMs as well as to assess possible impacts on products. "Understanding nanotechnology remains a top FDA priority. FDA is strengthening the scientific tools and methods for evaluating food products, cosmetics, drugs and medical devices," said FDA Commissioner Margaret A. Hamburg, MD.[236] "We are taking a prudent scientific approach to assess each product on its own merits and to not make broad, general assumptions about the safety of nanotechnology products." It must be noted that these two guidances on NMs for food and cosmetics uses are not intended for the use of NMs in other products including drugs or medical devices that are regulated by the FDA.

The draft of the guidance for cosmetic regulations recommends that the safety assessment for cosmetic products using NMs should address several important factors. These factors include[237]:

- the physico-chemical characteristics,
- agglomeration and size distribution of nanomaterials at the toxicity testing conditions which should correspond to those of a final product
- impurities
- potential product exposure levels, and the potential for agglomeration of NPs in the final product
- dosimetry for in vitro and in vivo toxicology studies
- in vitro and in vivo toxicological data on ingredients and their impurities, dermal penetration, irritation (skin and eye) and sensitization studies, mutagenicity/genotoxicity studies
- clinical studies to test the ingredient, or finished product, in human volunteers under controlled conditions.

The FDA expects that the science involving NMs will continue to evolve and lead to the development of new toxicity testing methods.[237] Thus, the safety cosmetic products containing NMs should be evaluated by analyzing the physico-chemical properties and the relevant toxicological effects of each ingredient as a result of expected exposure levels from the intended use of the finished product.[237]

The draft of the guidance for food the role of nanotechnology was based on its application in food manufacturing.[238] Traditional manufacturing of food substances may include particles in the nanometer range, but nanotechnology processes can be applied in the intentional production of food substances with nanometer particle size distributions that lead to new properties not seen in traditionally manufactured food substances[238] resulting attributes that differ from those of conventionally-manufactured products. The FDA does not judge all products containing NMs or involving nanotechnology as either benign or harmful but considers the characteristics of the finished product and its safety.[238] The FDA guidance for the evaluation of food additives, color additives, and food contact substances recommends rigorous safety assessments.[239]

In January of 2009, the European Commission Directorate General for Health and Consumers released their report.[239] The report recognized the current infancy of the procedures for assessing the potential risks of engineered NMs which can remain the same until sufficient scientific information becomes available to establish the possible harmful effects on humans and the environment.[239] The priority of concern is focused on the free and low solubility NMs because of inhalation exposures that may be natural and or accidental. Just as in the FDA draft guidances, the EC recognized the importance of proper character-ization of NMs to gather information that can be sued as the basis for the safety evaluation and the material safety data sheet (MSDS).[239] It is recommended that NMs be subject to biological systems for safety evaluation because they may be coated with proteins and other biomolecules that can considerably change their properties such as the size distribution due to agglomeration or aggregation of the particles.[239] In addition the toxicity of NMs in solution or suspension may be caused by the soluble species released from the nanomaterial. The need for reference NMs is indicated to allow the assessment of fate, behavior as well as effects that could be related to the properties and characteristics.[239] From the characterization to safety evaluation, the challenges are the absence of well-defined parameters to measure and standardize test protocols for the identifica-tion of reference material for production.

8.6 THE NMs INTELLECTUAL PROPERTY PERSPECTIVE

When a new technology emerges that is completely different from what is famil-iar and known to most, the patent offices are faced with problems. They receive patent applications covering the new field but there are not enough people with the experience and knowledge to examine them. These result in delays, dissatis-fied patent authors, and a lot of overlaps that lead to controversies which either leads to litigations or are accepted by the market.[240]

The patent landscape in nanotechnology is very broad because NMs and the corresponding related processes can be applied to almost any manufactured product across potentially all industry sectors. Thus, control and ownership of nanotechnology is vital for all governments and civil entities. Intellectual prop-erty (IP) will control the nanotechnology market and the price of the NMs and the nano-enabled products. IP will dictate innovations that affect multiple sec-tors from electronics, energy, sports, mining, defense, aviation, health, medi-cine, pharmaceuticals, and agriculture.

The current state of intellectual property related to nanotechnology is in chaos. Because it was and still is an emerging technology that is different from existing technologies, broad patents on NMs, tools, and processes have been granted too early. The flooding of new patent applications has led to rejections of valid claims and the issuance of broad-overlapping claims. The chaos and other challenges in nanotechnology patents may be attributed to several factors.

(1) Due to the lack of in-depth and complete knowledge of nanotechnology, patent examiners may not have the tools necessary to understand the com-plexities of the field.

(2) Because nanotechnology is in its infancy, there is a lack of available prior art, which could allow patent claims to be overly broad allowing stakehold-ers to lock up huge areas of the technology. At the same time, this can lead to overlapping patents.

In 2004, the USPTO has classified nanotechnology in class 977[241] under 35 USC §8 (Classification of Patents), the European Patent Office (EPO) has placed a Y01N for nanotechnology, and the. International Patent Classification has given it under the B82B class.[242] For a patent to be issued, it has to possess the following: 1) novelty, 2) inventive step, and 3) industrial application.[242] Existing knowledge is known as the state of the art and novelty assumes that the invention is not a part of- or cannot be derived from the state of the art in its field. To satisfy the inventive step, the invention must not logically follow from what is already known. The industrial application requirement refers to the applicability of the invention to satisfy a need in a particular industry sector.

The Japan Patent Office (JPO) has also made efforts to improve their classification systems to collect all nanotechnology-related patents in one single patent class: they have created the JPO created ZNM.[243] Because the identification of nanotechnology patents requires elaborate work, a nanotechnology working group (NTWG) was created in 2003 at the EPO. This group first worked on the definition of nanotechnology and appropriate keywords to be able to distinguish an application in the area.[244] This led to the analysis of patent applications from 15 countries or organizations and were analyzed resulting in the identification of about 90,000 patent or non-patent literature documents out of 20M documents belonging to class Y01N.[244] The patent applications submitted directly to the EPO or filled via the Patent Cooperation Treaty (PCT) were used to create the database that included citation information[245] that are very useful for exploring trajectories of technological development and the influence of technologies on successive inventive activities.[246]

The nanotechnology patent applications worldwide showed a steady increase in the United States and the European Union, showing an average annual increase of 12% between 1986 and 1996; and in 1977, it went to 18% for the US and 19% for the EU applications that was mainly due to Germany.[243] Japan showed a steady increase until late 1980s, followed by a decline of about 6% a year between 1990 and 1994 which was the period of the collapse of the Japanese asset price bubble.[243] From 1995, growth in nanotechnology patent applications growth rate was recorded at 12% which is still lower than that of US and EU applications. Korea has shown an average annual growth rate from 1999 to 2001 that is approximately 40% which are seen in registrations at the USPTO.[247] From 1996 to 2003, the number of world nanotechnology-related patents registered with USPTO has increased by 217% while the increase of the number of patents in all fields has increased only by 57%.[247] The nanotechnology patents of US origin accounts for by an additional 3700 nanotechnology patents per year, or by 230% that may be attributed to the upsurge in the US nanotechnology R&D budget from $116M in 1997 to $270M in 2000 and $960M in 2004.[247] In 2003, the biggest number of patents in nanotechnology was held by US (61% of the total of 8630), followed by Japan (10.9%), Germany (8.1%), Canada (2.9%), and France (2.2%) with substantial activities from Korea, Netherlands, Ireland, and China.[247]

The medical applications of nanotechnology are under development or nearing commercialization.[248,249] The US National Science Foundation (NSF) has predicted that the annual global market for nano-related products and services will reach \$1 T that will make it one of the fastest-growing industries.[248,250] In the US, passage of the 21st Century Nanotechnology Research and Development Act infused \$3.7 B in US federal funding from 2005 through 2008 to support nanotechnology R&D that resulted in the creation of the National Nanotechnology Coordination Office. This office is responsible for the funding of various federal nanotechnology initiatives and the creation of R&D centers.

A market research report[251] wrote that sales of products incorporating emerging nanotechnology will increase from <0.1% of global manufacturing output today to 15% in 2014, totaling \$2.6 T. This figure almost equals the size of the information technology and telecom industries combined and will be 10 times larger than biotechnology revenues. Additionally, the NMs like carbon nanotubes and quantum dots will total \$13 B in 2014. Thus, nanotechnology's economic effect will come from the application of NMs and not the raw NMs. The same report projects that 16% of health care and life sciences will incorporate nanotechnologies by 2014. With the diversity of NMs applications in medicine and the life sciences, potential investment activity will upsurge causing the need for patents to be in place. Patents in the applications of NMs in medicine are vital to realize its promising potential and to move beyond academic research.

8.7 CONCLUSION

To date, various governments have become more aware of the possible benefits as well as the dangers of exposure to NMs in various consumer products. This awareness has led to various guidelines worldwide.[236–239] The need to properly establish the various properties of the NMs have also been recognized as essential for the evaluation of the possible effects on health and environmental safety.

The limitations in the risk assessment of NMs are still preventing proper evaluations, and probably, also the possible adoption of strict regulations. The lack of high quality exposure and dose related data for humans and the environment is one of the major drawbacks in adopting regulations for NMs use and applications. There is also the difficulty in determining the presence of NMs and reproducibly quantifying them on a routine basis in various substrates that results from the lack of reliable and standardized measurement techniques. These must first be overcome before regulations for screening/monitoring of nanoscale particles in sensitive work areas can be implemented. The biggest challenges lie on the measurement of NMs in the air, water, and land. This consequently holds as well for food and food products that come from water and land.

Currently, the knowledge on the presence of NMs relies on information provided by manufacturers. The detection of NMs in consumer products suffers from the difficulty in discriminating between the background signals and added NMs. This is also complicated by the coating proteins and other biomolecules on NMs exposed to biological matrix. In addition, exposure estimation is also hampered by lack of information on product use and the use of multiple products containing NMs.

The health and environmental hazards of NMs have been demonstrated by various research groups[48,51,52,55,95,98,131,168,170,178,185,187,189,195] for a variety of manufactured NMs that may be toxic to humans and the environment. But, there is a need for NM hazard identification. While such as paradigm is not yet in place, a case by case approach is still the only approach available for the risk assessment of NMs.

The patent landscape in nanotechnology is gaining much attention because of the projected market and impact in the health and life sciences. Market projections outweigh a lot of existing industries creating investment interest of exorbitant quantities. Much more research and specifications in nanotechnology needs to be in place in order that faster reviews of patents with less overlap can be issued. A lot of activities are going worldwide as shown in the unprecedented increase in patents from various parts of the world with the US leading the pack.

REFERENCES

1. Bakry, R.; Vallant, R. M.; Najam-ul-hag, M.; Rainer, M.; Szabo, Z.; Huck, C. W.; Bonn, G. K. Medicinal Applications of Fullerenes. *Int. J. Nanomed.* **2007**, *2,* 639–649.

2. Jan, E.; Kotov, N. A. Successful Differentiation of Mouse Neural Stem Cells on Layer-by-layer Assembled Single-walled Carbon Nanotube Composite. *Nano. Lett.* **2007**, *7,* 1123–1128.

3. Nasibulin, A. G.; Moisala, A.; Jiang, H.; Kauppinen, E. I. Carbon Nanotube Synthesis by a Novel Aerosol Method. *J. Nanopart. Res.* **2006**, *8,* 465–475.

4. Aguilar, Z.; Aguilar, Y.; Xu, H.; Jones, B.; Dixon, J.; Xu, H.; Wang, A. Nanomaterials in Medicine. *Electrochem. Soc. Trans.* **2010**, *33,* 69–74.

5. Aguilar, Z.; Xu, H.; Jones, B.; Dixon, J.; Wang, A. Semiconductor Quantum Dots for Cell Imaging. *Mater. Res. Soc. Proc.* **2010**, *1237,* 1237-TT1206-1201.

6. Geiber, D.; Charbonnière, L. J.; Ziessel, R. F.; Butlin, N. G.; Löhmannsröben, H.; Hildebrandt, N. Quantum Dot Biosensors for Ultrasensitive Multiplexed Diagnostics. *Angew. Chem. Int. Ed.* **2010**, *49,* 1–6.

7. Juzenas, P.; Chen, W.; Sun, Y. P.; Coelho, M. A. N.; Genralov, R.; Genralova, N.; Christensen, I. L. Quantum dots and nanoparticles for photodynamic and radiation therapies of cancer. *Adv. Drug Deliv. Rev.* **2008,** *60.*

8. Khawaja, A. M. Review: The Legacy of Nanotechnology: Revolution and Prospects in Neurosurgery. *Int. J. Surg.* **2011,** 9(8), 608–614.

9. Smith, A. M.; Duan, H.; Mohs, A. M. Bioconjugated Quantum Dots for In vivo Molecular and Cellular Imaging. *Adv. Drug Deliv. Rev.* **2008,** *60.*

10. Su, H.; Xu, H.; Gao, S.; Dixon, J.; Aguilar, Z. P.; Wang, A.; Xu, H.; Wang, J. Microwave Synthesis of Nearly Monodisperse Core/Multishell Quantum Dots with Cell Imaging Applications. *Nanoscale Res. Lett.* **2010**, *5,* 625–630.

11. Xu, H.; Aguilar, Z.; Dixon, J.; Jones, B.; Wang, A.; Wei, H. Breast Cancer Cell Imaging using Semiconductor Quantum Dots. *Electrochem. Soc. Trans.* **2009**, *25,* 69–77.

12. Xu, H.; Aguilar, Z.; Waldron, J.; Wei, H.; Wang, Y. Application of Semiconductor Quantum Dots for Breast Cancer Cell Sensing, 2009 Biomedical Engineering and Informatics. *IEEE Comp. Soc. BMEI* **2009**, *1,* 516–520.

13. Xu, H.; Aguilar, Z.; Wang, A. Quantum Dot-based Sensors for Proteins. *ECS Trans.* **2010,** *25,* 1–10.

14. Pusic, K.; Xu, H.; Stridiron, A.; Aguilar, Z.; Wang, A. Z.; Hui, H. Blood Stage Merozoite Surface Protein Conjugated to Nanoparticles Induce Potent Parasite Inhibitory Antibodies. *Vaccine* **2011,** *29,* 8898–8908.

15. Xu, H.; Aguilar, Z. P.; Yang, L.; Kuang, M.; Duan, H.; Xiong, Y.; Wei, H.; Wang, A. Y. Antibody Conjugated Magnetic Iron Oxide Nanoparticles for Cancer Cell Separation in Fresh Whole Blood. *Biomaterials* **2011,** *32,* 9758–9765.

16. Yang, L.; Cao, Z.; Sajja, H.; Mao, H.; Wang, L.; Geng, H.; Xu, H.; Jiang, T.; Wood, W.; Nie, S.; Wang, A. Development of Receptor Targeted Iron Oxide Nanoparticles for Efficient Drug Delivery and Tumor Imaging. *J. Biomed. Nanotech.* **2008,** *4,* 1–11.

17. Yang, L.; Peng, X.; Wang, Y.; Wang, X.; Cao, Z.; Ni, C.; Karna, P.; Zhang, X.; Wood, W.; Gao, X.; Nie, S.; Mao, H. Receptor-targeted Nanoparticles for In vivo Imaging of Breast Cancer. *Clin. Cancer Res.* **2009,** *15,* 4722–4732.

18. Jin, S.; Ye, K. Nanoparticle-mediated Drug Delivery and Gene Therapy. *Biotechnol. Prog.* **2007,** *23,* 32–41.

19. Kamps, J. A.; Scherphof, G. L. Receptor versus Non-receptor Mediated Clearance of Liposomes. *Adv. Drug Deliv. Rev.* **1998,** *32,* 81–97.

20. Moghimi, S. M.; Szebeni, J. Stealth Liposomes and Long Circulating Nanoparticles: Critical Issues in Pharmacokinetics, Opsonization and Protein-binding Properties. *Prog. Lipid. Res.* **2003,** *42,* 463–478.

21. Morgen, M.; Lu, G. W.; Dub, D.; Stehle, R.; Lembke, F.; Cervantes, J.; Ciotti, S.; Haskell, R.; Smithey, D.; Haley, K.; Fan, C. Targeted Delivery of a Poorly Water-soluble Compound to Hair Follicles Using Polymeric Nanoparticle Suspensions. *Int. J. Pharm.* **2011,** *416,* 314–322.

22. Pastorino, F.; Brignole, C.; Marimpietri, D.; Sapra, P.; Moase, E. H.; Allen, T. M.; Ponzoni, M. Doxorubicin-loaded Fab' Fragments of Anti-disialoganglioside Immunoliposomes Selectively Inhibit the Growth and Dissemination of Human Neuroblastoma in Nude Mice. *Cancer Res.* **2003,** *63,* 86–92.

23. Tiwari, S. B.; Amiji, M. M. A Review of Nanocarrier-based CNS Delivery Systems. *Curr. Drug Del.* **2006,** *3,* 219–232.

24. Tobio, M.; Sanchez, A.; Vila, A.; Soriano, I.; Evora, C.; Vila-Jato, J. L.; Alonso, M. J. Investigation of Lectin-modified Insulin Liposomes as Carriers for Oral Administration. *Colloids Surf. B* **2000,** *18,* 315–323.

25. Torchilin, V. P.; Shtilman, M. I.; Trubetskoy, V. S.; Whiteman, K.; Milstein, A. M. Amphiphilic Vinyl Polymers Effectively Prolong Liposome Circulation Time In vivo. *Biochim. Biophys. Acta* **1994,** *1195,* 181–184.

26. Zhang, N.; Ping, Q. N.; Huang, G. H.; Xu, W. F. Investigation of Lectin-Modified Insulin Liposomes as Carriers for Oral Administration. *Int. J. Pharm.* **2005,** *294,* 247–259.

27. Topoglidis, E. A.; Cass, E., et al. Protein Adsorption on Nanocrystalline TiO_2 Films: An Immobilization Strategy for Bioanalytical Devices. *Anal. Chem.* **1998,** *70,* 5111–5113.

28. Connor, E. E.; Mwamuka, J.; Gole, A.; Murphy, C. J.; Wyatt, M. D. Gold Nanoparticles are Taken Up by Human Cells but do not Cause Acute Cytotoxicity. *Small* **2005,** *1,* 325.

29. Xu, H.; Qu, F.; Xu, H.; Lai, W.; Wang, Y. A.; Aguilar, Z. P.; Wei, H. Role of Reactive Oxygen Species in the Antibacterial Mechanism of Silver Nanoparticles on *E. coli* O157:H7. *Biometals* **2012,** *25,* 45–53.

30. Loeschner, K.; Hadrup, N.; Qvotrup, K.; Larsen, A.; Gao, X.; Vogel, U.; Mortensen, A.; Lam, H. R.; Larsen, E. H. Distribution of Silver in Rats Following 28 Days of Repeated Oral Exposure to Silver Nanoparticles or Silver Acetate. *Part. Fibre Toxicol.* **2011,** *8,* 18.

31. Schneider, O. D.; Loher, S.; Brunner, T. J.; Schmidlin, P.; Stark, W. J. Flexible, Lilver Containing Nanocomposites for the Repair of Bone Defects: Antimicrobial Effect Against E. coli Infection and Comparison to Tetracycline Containing Scaffolds. *J. Mater. Chem.* **2008**, *18*, 2679–2684.

32. Portilla-Arias, J. P.; Garcia-Alvarez, M.; Galbis, J. A.; Munoz-Guerra, S. Biodegradable Nanoparticles of Partially Methylated Fungal Poly(beta-l-malic acid) as a Novel Protein Delivery Carrier. *Macromol. Biosci.* **2008**, *8*, 551–559.

33. Lacerda, L.; Soundararajan, A.; Singh, R.; Pastorin, G.; Al-Jamal, K. T.; Turton, J., et al. Dynamic Imaging of Functionalized Multi-walled Carbon Nanotube Systemic Circulation and Urinary Excretion. *Adv. Mater.* **2008**, *20*, 225–230.

34. Klippstein, R.; Pozo, D. Nanotechnology-based Manipulation of Dendritic Cells for Enhanced Immunotherapy Strategies. *Nanomed. Nanotechnol. Biol. Med.* **2010**, *6*, 523–529.

35. de Jong, S.; Chikh, G.; Sekirov, L.; Raney, S.; Semple, S.; Klimuk, S., et al. Encapsulation in Liposomal Nanoparticles Enhances the Immunostimulatory, Adjuvant and Anti-tumor Activity of Subcutaneously Administered CpG ODN. *Cancer Immunol. Immunother.* **2007**, *56*, 1251–1264.

36. Goyal, A. K.; Khatri, K.; Mishra, N.; Mehta, A.; Vaidya, B.; Tiwari, S., et al. Aquasomes-a Nanoparticulate Approach for the delivery of Antigen. *Drug Dev. Ind. Pharm.* **2008**, *34*, 1297–1305.

37. Kortylewski, M.; Swiderski, P.; Herrmann, A.; Wang, L.; Kowolik, C.; Kujawski, M., et al. In vivo Delivery of siRNA to Immune Cells by Conjugation to a TLR9 Agonist Enhances Antitumor Immune Responses. *Nat. Biotechnol.* **2009**, *27*, 925–932.

38. O'Hagan, D. T.; Singh, M. Microparticles as Vaccine Adjuvants and Delivery Systems. *Expert Rev. Vaccines* **2003**, *2*, 269–283.

39. Van Der Lubben, I. M.; Konings, F. A.; Borchard, G.; Verhoef, J. C.; Junginger-He, C. In vivo Uptake of Chitosan Microparticles by Murine Peyer's Patches: Visualization Studies Using Confocal Laser Scanning Microscopy and Immunohistochemistry. *J. Drug Target.* **2001**, *9*, 39–47.

40. Kreuter, J.; Ramge, P.; Petrov, V.; Hamm, S.; Gelperina, S. E.; Engelhardt, B.; Alyautdin, R.; von Briesen, H.; Begley, D. J. Direct Evidence that Polysorbate-80-coated Poly(butylcyanoacrylate) Nanoparticles Deliver Drugs to the CNS via Specific Mechanisms Requiring Prior Binding of Drug to the Nanoparticles. *Pharm. Res.* **2003**, *20*.

41. Hoet, P. H.; Bruske-Hohfeld, I.; Salata, O. V. Nanoparticles -Known and Unknown Health Risks. *J. Nanobiotechnol.* **2004**, *2*, 12.

42. Nel, A.; Xia, T.; Madler, L.; Li, N. Tox Potential of Materials at the Nanolevel. *Science* **2006**, *311*, 622–627.

43. Colvin, V. L. The Potential Environmental Impact of Engineered Nanomaterials. *Nat. Biotechnol.* **2003**, *21*, 1166–1170.

44. Lovric, J.; Bazzi, H. S.; Cuie, Y.; Fortin, G. R.; Winnik, F. M.; Maysinger, D. Differences in Subcellular Distribution and Toxicity of Green and Red Emitting CdTe Quantum Dots. *J. Mol. Med.* **2005**, *83*, 377–385.

45. Hardman, R. A Toxicologic Review of Quantum Dots: Toxicity Depends on Physicochemical and Environmental Factors. *Environ. Health Perspect.* **2006**, *114*, 165–172.

46. Borm, P. J.; Kreyling, W. Toxicological Hazards of Inhaled Nanoparticles-potential Implications for Drug Delivery. *J. Nanosci. Nanotech.* **2004**, *4*, 521–531.

47. Portney, N. G.; Ozkan, M. Nano-oncology: Drug Delivery, Imaging, and Sensing. *Anal. Bioanal. Chem.* **2006**, *384*, 620–630.

48. Eun, H. C.; Chung, J. H.; Jung, S. Y.; Cho, K. H.; Kim, K. H. A Comparative Study of the Cytotoxicity of Skin Irritants on Cultured Human Oral and Skin Keratinocytes. *Br. J. Dermatol.* **1994**, *130*, 24–28.

49. Lee, J. K.; Kim, D. B.; Kim, J. I.; Kim, P. Y. In vitro Cytotoxicity Tests on Cultured Human Skin Fibroblasts to Predict Skin Irritation Potential of Surfactants. *Toxicol. In Vitro* **2000,** *14,* 345–349.

50. Allen, D. A.; Riviere, J. E.; Monteiro-Riviere, N. A. Identification of Early Biomarkers of Inflammation Produced by Keratinocytes Exposed to Jet Fuels. *J. Biochem. Mol. Toxicol.* **2000,** *14,* 231–237.

51. Monteiro-Riviere, N. A.; Inman, A. O. Challenges for Assessing Carbon Nanomaterial Toxicity to the Skin. *Carbon* **2006,** *44,* 1070–1078.

52. Monteiro-Riviere, N. A.; Inman, A. O.; Zhang, L. W. Limitations and Relative Utility of Screening Assays to Assess Engineered Nanoparticle Toxicity in a Human Cell Line. *Toxicol. Appl. Pharmacol.* **2009,** *234,* 222–235.

53. Katz, J.; Nanotechnology Boom Expected by 2015: New report forecasts major growth spurt in next seven years. July 22, 2008. Available from: www.industryweek.com

54. Sun, L. F.; Liu, Z. Q.; Katz, J.; Ma, X. C.; Zhong, Z. Y.; Tang, S. B.; Xiong, Z. T., et al. Growth of Carbon Nanotube Arrays Using the Existing Array as a Substrate and their Raman Characterization. *Chem. Phys. Lett.* **2001,** *340,* 222–226.

55. Castranova, V. Overview of Current Toxicological Knowledge of Engineered Nanoparticles. *J. Occup. Environ. Med.* **2011,** *53,* S14–S17.

56. Schrand, A. M.; Rahman, M. F.; Hussain, S. M.; Schlager, J. J.; Smith, D. A.; Syed, A. F. Metal-based Nanoparticles and Their Toxicity Assessment. *Wiley Interdiscip. Rev. Nanomed. Nanobiotechnol.* **2010,** *2,* 544–568.

57. Guldi, D. M.; Prato, M. Excited-state Properties of C(60) Fullerene Derivatives. *Acc. Chem. Res.* **2000,** *33,* 695–703.

58. Jin, C. H.; Wang, J. Y.; Chen, Q.; Peng, L. M. In Situ Fabrication and Graphitization of Amorphous Carbon Nanowires and Their Electrical Properties. *J. Phys. Chem. B* **2006,** *110,* 5423–5428.

59. Treacy, M. M. J.; Ebbesen, T. W.; Gibson, J. M. Exceptionally High Young's Modulus Observed for Individual Carbon Nanotubes. *Nature* **1996,** *381,* 678–680.

60. Lee, C. J.; Park, J.; Kang, S. Y.; Lee, J. H. Growth and Field Electron Emission of Vertically Aligned Multiwalled Carbon Nanotubes. *Chem. Phys. Lett.* **2000,** *326,* 175–180.

61. Armentano, I.; Alvarez-Pérez, M. A.; Carmona-Rodríguez, B.; Gutiérrez-Ospina, I.; Kenny, J. M.; Arzate, H. Analysis of the Biomineralization Process on SWNTCOOH and F-SWNT Films. *Mater. Sci. Eng. C* **2008,** *28,* 1522–1529.

62. Koruga, D.; Matija, L.; Misic, N.; Rakin, P. Fullerene C_{60}: Properties and Possible Applications. *Trans. Tech. Publ. Mat. Sci. Forum* **1996,** *214,* 49–56.

63. Dai, H.; Shim, M.; Chen, R. J.; Li, Y.; Kam, N. W. S. Functionalization of Carbon Nanotubes for Biocompatibility and Biomolecular Recognition. *Nano Lett.* **2002,** *2,* 285–288.

64. Gao, X. P.; Qin, X.; Wu, F.; Liu, H.; Lan, Y.; Fan, S. S.; Yuan, H. T.; Song, D. Y.; Shen, P. W. Synthesis of Carbon Nanotubes by Catalytic Decomposition of Methane Using $LaNi_5$ Hydrogen Storage Alloy as Catalyst. *Chem. Phys. Lett.* **2000,** *327,* 271–276.

65. Iijima, S.; Brabec, C.; Maiti, A.; Bernholc, J. Structural Flexibility of Carbon Nanotubes. *J. Chem. Phys.* **1996,** *104,* 2089–2092.

66. Lovat, V.; Pantarotto, D.; Lagostena, L.; Cacciari, B.; Grolfo, M.; Righi, M., et al. Nanotube Substrates Boost Neuronal Electrical Signaling. *Nano Lett.* **2005,** *5,* 1107–1110.

67. Osawa, E. C_{60}: Buckminsterfullerene. *Kagaku* **1970,** *25,* 854.

68. Nasibulin, A. G.; Pikhitsa, P. V.; Jiang, H.; Brown, D. P.; Krasheninnikov, A. V.; Anisimov, A. S.; Queipo, P.; Moisala, A.; Gonzalez, D.; Lientschnig, G.; Hassanien, A.; Shandakov, S. D.; Lolli, G.; Resasco, D. E.; Choi, M.; Tomanek, D.; Kauppinen, E. I. A Novel Hybrid Carbon Material. *Nat. Nanotechnol.* **2007,** *2,* 156–161.

69. Mamedov, A. A.; Kotov, N. A.; Prato, M.; Guldi, D. M.; Wicksted, J. P.; Hirsch, A. Molecular Design of Strong Single-wall Carbon Nanotube/Polyelectrolyte Multilayer Composites. *Nat. Mater.* **2002,** *1,* 190–194.

70. Kerman, K.; Morita, Y.; Takamura, Y.; Tamiya, E. *Escherichia coli* Single-strand Binding Protein–DNA Interactions on Carbon Nanotube-modified Electrodes from a Label-free Electrochemical Hybridization Sensor. *Anal. Bioanal. Chem.* **2005,** *381,* 1114–1121.

71. Yang, R.; Jin, J.; Chen, Y.; Shao, N.; Kang, H.; Xiao, Z.; Tang, Z.; Wu, Y.; Zhu, Z.; Tan, W. Carbon Nanotube-quenched Fluorescent Oligonucleotides: Probes that Fluoresce upon Hybridization. *JACS* **2008,** *130,* 8351–8358.

72. Mwenifumbo, S.; Shaffer, M. S.; Stevens, M. M. Exploring Cellular Behaviour with Multi-walled Carbon Nanotube Constructs. *J. Mater. Chem.* **2007,** *17,* 1894–1902.

73. Tran, P. A.; Zhang, L.; Webster, T. J. Carbon Nanofibers and Carbon Nanotubes in Regenerative Medicine. *Adv. Drug Deliv. Rev.* **2009,** *61,* 1097–1114.

74. Correa-Duarte, M. A.; Wagner, N.; Rojas-Chapana, J.; Morsczeck, C.; Thie, M.; Giersig, M. Fabrication and Biocompatibility of Carbon Nanotube-based 3dnetworks as Scaffolds for Cell Seeding and Growth. *Nano Lett.* **2004,** *4,* 2233–2236.

75. Mattson, M. P.; Haddon, R. C.; Rao, A. M. Molecular Functionalization of Carbon Nanotubes and Use as Substrates for Neuronal Growth. *J. Mol. Neurosci.* **2000,** *14,* 175–182.

76. Zagal, J. H.; Griveau, Z.; Nyokong, T.; Bedioui, F. Carbon Nanotubes, Phthalocyanines and Porphyrins: Attractive Hybrid Materials for Electrocatalysis and Electroanalysis. *J. Nanosci. Nanotech.* **2009,** *9,* 2201–2214.

77. Poland, C. A.; Duffin, R.; Kinloch, I.; Maynard, A.; Wallace, W. A. H.; Seaton, A.; Stone, V.; Brown, S., et al. Carbon Nanotubes Introduced into the Abdominal Cavity of Mice Show Asbestos-like Pathogenicity in a Pilot-study. *Nat. Nanotech.* **2008,** *3,* 423.

78. Martel, R.; Derycke, V.; Lavoie, C.; Appenzeller, J.; Chan, K. K.; Tersoff, J. Ambipolar Electrical Transport in Semiconducting Single-wall Carbon Nanotubes. *Phys. Rev. Lett.* **2001,** *87,* 256805.

79. Shvedova, A. A.; Kisin, E. R.; Porter, D.; Schulte, P.; Kagan, V. E.; Fadeel, B.; Castranova, V. Mechanisms of Pulmonary Toxicity nd Medical Applications of Carbon Nanotubes. *Pharm. Ther.* **2009,** *121,* 192–204.

80. Porter, A.; Gass, M.; Muller, K.; Skepper, J. N.; Midgley, P. A.; Welland, M. Direct Imaging of Single-walled Carbon Nanotubes in Cells. *Nat. Nanotech* **2007,** *2,* 713–717.

81. Zumwalde, R.; Hodson, L. *Approaches to Safe Nanotechnology: Managing the Health and Safety Concerns Associated with Engineered Nanomaterials.* 2009.

82. Lam, C. W.; James, J. T.; McCluskey, R.; Arepalli, S.; Hunter, R. L. A Review of Carbon Nanotube Toxicity and Assessment of Potential Occupational and Environmental Health Risks. *Crit. Rev. Toxicol.* **2006,** *36,* 189–217.

83. Kolosnjaj, J.; Szwarc, H.; Mousa, F. Toxicity Studies of Carbon Nanotubes. *Adv. Exp. Med. Biol.* **2007,** *620,* 181–204.

84. Zhao, X.; Liu, R. Recent Progress and Perspectives on the Toxicity of Carbon Nanotubes at Organism, Organ, Cell, and Biomacromolecule Levels. *Environ. Int.* **2012,** *40,* 244–255.

85. Deguchi, S.; Alargova, R. G.; Tsujii, K. Stable Dispersions of Fullerenes, C_{60} and C_{70}, in Water. Preparation and Characterization. *Langmuir* **2001,** *17,* 6013–6017.

86. Sayes, C. M.; Fortner, J. D.; Guo, W.; Lyon, D.; Boyd, A. M.; Ausman, K. D.; Tao, Y. J.; Sitharaman, B.; Wilson, L. J.; Hughes, J. B.; West, J. L.; Colvin, V. L. The differential Cyto-toxicity of Water-soluble Fullerenes. *Nano Lett.* **2004,** *4,* 1881–1887.

87. Oberdorster, E.; Zhu, S.; Blickley, T. M.; McClellan-Green, P.; Haasch, M. L. Ecotoxicology of Carbon-based Engineered Nanoparticles: Effects of Fullerene (C_{60}) on Aquatic Organisms. *Carbon* **2006,** *44,* 1112–1120.

88. Oberdorster, E. Manufactured Nanomaterials (Fullerenes, C_{60}) Oxidative Stress in the Brain of Juvenile Largemouth Bass. *Environ. Health Perspect.* **2004,** *1112,* 1058–1062.

89. Isakovic, A.; Markovic, Z.; Nikolic, N.; Todorovic-Markovic, B.; Vranjes-Djuric, S.; Harhaji, L.; Raicevic, N.; Romcevic, N.; Vasiljevic-Radovic, D.; Dramicanin, M.; Trajkovic, V. Inactivation of Nanocrystalline C_{60} Cytotoxicity by Gamma-irradiation. *Biomaterials* **2006,** *27,* 5049–5058.

90. Sayes, C. M.; Marchione, A. A.; Reed, K. L.; Warheit, D. B. Comparative Pulmonary Toxicity Assessments of C_{60} Water Suspensions in Rats: Few Differences in Fullerene Toxicity in Vivo in Contrast to In vitro Profiles. *Nano Lett.* **2007,** *7,* 2399–2406.

91. Sayes, C. M.; Gobin, A. M.; Ausman, K. D.; Mendez, J.; West, J. L.; Colvin, V. L. Nano-C_{60} Cytotoxicity is Due to Lipid Peroxication. *Biomaterials* **2005,** *26,* 7587–7595.

92. Jia, G.; Wang, H.; Yan, L.; Wang, X.; Pei, R.; Yan, T.; Zhoa, Y.; Guo, X. Cytotoxicity of Carbon Nanomaterials: Single-wall Nanotube, Multi-wall Nanotube, and Fullerene. *Environ. Sci. Technol.* **2005,** *39,* 1378–1383.

93. Inman, A. O.; Sayes, C. M.; Colvin, V. L.; Monteiro-Riviere, N. A. NanoC$_{60}$ and Derivatized C_{60} Toxicity in Human Epidermal Keratinocytes. *Soc. Toxicol.* **2006,** *90,* 167.

94. Zhang, L. W.; Zeng, L.; Barron, A. L.; Monteiro-Riviere, N. A. Biological Interactions of Functionalized Single-Wall Carbon Nanotubes in Human Epidermal Keratinocytes. *Int. J. Toxicol.* **2007,** *26,* 103–113.

95. Monteiro-Riviere, N. A.; Nemanich, R. A.; Inman, A. O.; Wang, Y. Y.; Riviere, J. E. Multiwalled Carbon Nanotube Interactions with Human Epidermal Keratinocytes. *Toxicol. Lett.* **2005,** *155,* 377–384.

96. Chan, W. C. W. In *Bio-applications of Nanoparticles*; Springer Science + Business Media: New York, 2007.

97. Flahaut, E.; Durrieu, M. C.; Remy-Zolghadri, M.; Bareille, R.; Baquey, C. Investigation of the Cytotoxicity of CCVD Carbon Nanotubes Towards Human Umbilical Vein Endothelial Cells. *Carbon* **2006,** *44,* 1093–1099.

98. Pulskamp, K.; Diabate, S.; Krug, H. F. Carbon Nanotubes Show No Sign of Acute Toxicity but Induce Intracellular Reactive Oxygen Species in Dependence on Contaminants. *Toxicol. Lett.* **2007,** *168,* 58–74.

99. Chlopek, J.; Czajkowska, B.; Szaraniec, B.; Frackowiak, E.; Szostak, K.; Beguin, F. In vitro Studies of Carbon Nanotubes Biocompatibility. *Carbon* **2006,** *44,* 1106–1111.

100. Panessa-Warren, B. J.; Warren, J. B.; Wong, S. S.; Misewich, J. A. Biological Cellular Response to Carbon Nanoparticle Toxicity. *J. Phys. Condens. Matter* **2006,** *18,* S2185–S2201.

101. Belyanskaya, L.; Weigel, S.; Hirsch, C.; Tobler, U.; Krug, H. F.; Wick, P. Effects of Carbon Nanotubes on Primary Neurons and Glial Cells. *Neurotoxicology* **2009,** *30,* 702–711.

102. Casey, A.; Herzog, E.; Davoren, M.; Lyng, F. M.; Byrne, H. J.; Chambers, G. Spectroscopic Analysis Confirms the Interactions between Single Walled Carbon Nanotubes and Various Dyes Commonly Used to Assess Cytotoxicity. *Carbon* **2007,** *45,* 1425–1432.

103. Koyama, S.; Kim, Y. A.; Hayashi, T.; Takeuchi, K.; Fujii, C.; Kuroiwa, N., et al. In vivo Immunological Toxicity in Mice of Carbon Nanotubes with Impurities. *Carbon* **2009,** *47,* 1365–1372.

104. Murray, A. R.; Kisin, E.; Leonard, S. S.; Young, S. H.; Kommimeni, C.; Kagan, V. E., et al. In vivo Immunological Toxicity in Mice of Carbon Nanotubes with Impurities. *Toxicology* **2009,** *257,* 161–171.

105. Crouzier, D.; Follot, S.; Gentilhomme, E.; Flahaut, E.; Arnaud, R.; Dabouis, V., et al. Carbon nanotubes Induce Inflammation but Decrease the Production of Reactive Oxygen Species in Lung. *Toxicology* **2010,** *272,* 39–45.

106. Elgrabli, D.; Abella-Gallart, S.; Robidel, F.; Rogerieux, F.; Boczkowski, J.; Lacroix, G. Induction of Apoptosis and Absence Of Inflammation in Rat Lung After Intratracheal Instillation of Multiwalled Carbon Nanotubes. *Toxicology* **2008**, *253*, 131–136.

107. Ryman-Rasmussen, J. P.; Cesta, M. F.; Brody, A. R.; Shipley-Phillips, J. K.; Everitt, J. I.; Tewksbury, E. W., et al. Inhaled Carbon Nanotubes Reach the Subpleural Tissue in Mice. *Nat. Nanotechnol.* **2009**, *4*, 747–751.

108. Hirano, S.; Kanno, S.; Furuyama, A. Multi-walled Carbon Nanotubes Injure the Plasma Membrane of Macrophages. *Toxicol. Appl. Pharmacol.* **2008**, *232*, 244–251.

109. Zhu, Y.; Li, W. X.; Li, Q. N.; Li, Y. G.; Li, Y. F.; Zhang, X. Y., et al. Multi-walled Carbon Nanotubes Injure the Plasma Membrane of Macrophages. *Carbon* **2009**, *47*, 1351–1358.

110. Michalet, X.; Pinaud, F. F.; Bentolila, L. A.; Tsay, J. M.; Doose, S.; Li, J. J., et al. Quantum dots for Live Cells, *In vivo* Imaging, and Diagnostics. *Science* **2005**, *307*, 538–544.

111. Byers, R.; Hitchman, E. Quantum Dots Brighten Biological Imaging. *Prog. Histochem. Cytochem.* **2011**, *45*, 201–237.

112. Cai, W.; Shin, D.; Chen, K.; Gheysens, O.; Cao, Q.; Wang, S. X.; Gambhir, S. S.; Chen, X. Peptide-Labeled Near-Infrared Quantum Dots for Imaging Tumor Vasculature in Living Subjects. *Nano Lett.* **2006**, *6*, 669–676.

113. Dennis, A. M.; Bao, G. Quantum Dot-Fluorescent Protein Pairs as Novel Fluorescence Resonance Energy Transfer Probes. *Nano Lett.* **2008**, *8*, 1439–1445.

114. Jiang, W.; Mardyani, S.; Fischer, H.; Chan, W. Design and Characterization of Lysine Cross-Linked Mercapto-acid Biocompatible Quantum Dots. *Chem. Mater.* **2006**, *18*, 872–878.

115. Lidke, D. S.; Nagy, P.; Heintzmann, R.; Arndt-Jovin, D. J.; Post, J. N.; Grecco, H. E.; Jares-Erijman, E. A.; Jovin, T. M. Quantum Dot Ligands Provide New Insights into erbB/HER Receptor-mediated Signal Transduction. *Nat. Biotechnol.* **2004**, *22*, 198–203.

116. Somers, R.; Bawendi, M.; Nocera, D. CdSe Nanocrystal Based Chem-/Bio- Sensors. *Chem. Soc. Rev.* **2007**, *36*, 579–591.

117. Susumu, K.; Uyeda, H.; Medintz, I.; Pons, T.; Delehanty, J.; Mattoussi, H. Enhancing the Stability and Biological Functionalities of Quantum Dots via Compact Multifunctional Ligands. *JACS* **2007**, *129*, 13987–13996.

118. Vaidya, S.; Gilchrist, M.; Maldarelli, C.; Couzis, A. Spectral Bar Coding of Polystyrene Microbeads Using Multicolored Quantum Dots. *Anal. Chem.* **2007**, *79*, 8520–8530.

119. Dubertret, B.; Skourides, P.; Norris, D. J.; Noireaux, V.; Brivanlou, A. H.; Libchaber, A. In vivo Imaging of Quantum Dots Encapsulated in Phospholipid Micelles. *Science* **2002**, *298*, 1759–1762.

120. Ballou, B.; Lagerholm, B. C.; Ernst, L. A.; Bruchez, M. P.; Waggoner, A. S. Noninvasive Imaging of Quantum Dots in Mice. *Bioconjugate Chem.* **2004**, *15*, 79–86.

121. Xiao, Y.; Barker, P. Semiconductor Nanocrystal Probes for Human Metaphase Chromosomes. *Nucleic Acids Res.* **2004**, *32*, e28.

122. Chan, C.; Nie, S. Quantum Dot Bioconjugates for Ultrasensitive Nonisotopic Detection. *Science* **1998**, *281*, 2016–2018.

123. Chen, N.; He, Y.; Su, Y.; Li, X.; Huang, Q.; Wang, H.; Zhang, X.; Tai, R.; Fan, C. The Cytotoxicity of Cadmium-based Quantum Dots. *Biomaterials* **2012**, *33*, 1238–1244.

124. Lewinski, N.; Colvin, V.; Drezek, R. Labelling of Cells with Quantim Dots. *Small* **2008**, *4*, 26–49.

125. Derfus, A. M.; Chan, W. C. W.; Bhatia, S. N. Probing the Cytotoxicity of Semiconductor Quantum Dots. *Nano Lett.* **2004**, *4*, 11–18.

126. Kirchner, C.; Liedl, T.; Kudera, S.; Pellegrino, T.; Javier, A. M.; Gaub, H. E., et al. Cytotoxicity of Colloidal CdSe and CdSe/ZnS Nanoparticles. *Nano Lett.* **2005**, *5*, 331–338.

127. Parak, W. J.; Pellegrino, T.; Plank, C. Labelling of Cells with Quantum Dots. *Nanotechnology* **2005,** *16,* R9–R25.

128. Su, Y.; Hu, M.; Fan, C.; He, Y.; Li, Q.; Li, W., et al. The Cytotoxicity of CdTe Quantum Dots and the Relative Contributions from Released Cadmium Ions and Nanoparticle Properties. *Biomaterials* **2010,** *31,* 4829–4834.

129. Su, Y. Y.; Peng, F.; Jiang, Z. Y.; Zhong, Y. L.; Lu, Y. M., et al. In vivo Distribution, Pharmacokinetics, and Toxicity of Aqueous Synthesized Cadmium-containing Quantum Dots. *Biomaterials* **2011,** *32,* 5855–5862.

130. Aguilar, Z.; Xu, H.; Dixon, J.; Wang, A. Blocking Non-specific Uptake of Engineered Nanomaterials. *Electrochem. Soc. Trans.* **2010,** *25,* 37–48.

131. Aguilar, Z. P.; Xu, H.; Dixon, J. D.; Wang, A. W. *Nanomaterials for Enhanced Antibody Production.* 2012, [Small business innovations research for the National Science Foundation].

132. Aguilar, Z. P.; Wang, Y. A.; Xu, H.; Hui, G.; Pusic, K. M. *Nanoparticle Based Immunological Stimulation 2012.* January 19 2012, US Patent App: 13/350,849.

133. Green, M.; Howman, E. Semiconductor Quantum Dots and Free Radical Induced DNA Nicking. *Chem. Commun.* **2005,** *1,* 121–123.

134. Ipe, B. I.; Lehnig, M.; Niemeyer, C. M. On the Generation of Free Radical Species from Quantum Dots. *Small* **2005,** *1,* 706–709.

135. Gobe, G.; Crane, D. Mitochondria, Reactive Oxygen Species and Cadmium Toxicity in the Kidney. *Toxicol. Lett.* **2010,** *198,* 49–55.

136. Cho, S. J.; Maysinger, D.; Jain, M.; Roder, B.; Hackbarth, S.; Winnik, F. M. Long-term Exposure to CdTe Quantum Dots Causes Functional Impairments in Live Cells. *Langmuir* **2007,** *23.*

137. Chan, W. H.; Shiao, N. H.; Lu, P. Z. CdSe Quantum Dots Induce Apoptosis in Human Neuroblastoma Cells via Mitochondrial-dependent Pathways and Inhibition of Survival Signals. *Toxicol. Lett.* **2006,** *167,* 191–200.

138. Pelley, J. L.; Daar, A. S.; Saner, M. A. State of Academic Knowledge on Toxicity and Biological Fate of Quantum Dots. *Toxicol. Sci.* **2009,** *112,* 276–296.

139. Bottrill, M.; Green, M. Some Aspects of Quantum Dot Toxicity. *Chem. Commun.* **2011,** *47,* 7039–7050.

140. Zhang, L. W.; Baumer, W.; Monteiro-Riviere, N. A. Cellular Uptake Mechanisms and Toxicity of Quantum Dots in Dendritic Cells. *Nanomed. UK* **2011,** *6,* 777–791.

141. Faraday, M. The Bakerian Lecture: Experimental Relations of Gold (and other metals) to LIGHT. *Philos. Trans. R. Soc. London* **1857,** *147,* 145–181.

142. Gagner, J. E.; Lopez, M. D.; Dordick, J. S.; Siegel, R. W. Effect of Gold Nanoparticle Morphology on Adsorbed Protein Structure and Function. *Biomaterials* **2011,** *32,* 7241–7252.

143. Carbó-Argibay, E.; Rodríguez-González, B.; Pastoriza-Santos, I.; Pérez-Juste, J.; Liz-Marán, L. M. Growth of pentatwinned Gold Nanorods into Truncated Decahedra. *Nanoscale* **2010,** *2,* 2377–2383.

144. Sau, T. K.; Murphy, C. J. Room Temperature, High-yield Synthesis of Multiple Shapes of Gold Nanoparticles in Aqueous Solution. *JACS* **2004,** *126,* 8648–8649.

145. Kimlong, J.; Maier, M.; Okenve, B.; Kotaidis, V.; Ballot, H.; Turkevich, P. A. Method for Gold Nanoparticle Synthesis Revisited. *J. Phys. Chem. B* **2006,** *110,* 15700–15707.

146. Jain, P. K.; Lee, K. S.; El-Sayed, I. H.; El-Sayed, M. A. Calculated Absorption and Scattering Properties of Gold Nanoparticles of Different Size, Shape, and Composition: Applications in Biological Imaging and Biomedicine. *J. Phys. Chem. B* **2006,** *110,* 7238–7248.

147. Han, G.; Ghosh, P.; Rotello, V. M. Multi-functional Gold Nanoparticles for Drug Delivery. *Adv. Exp. Med. Biol.* **2007,** *620,* 48–56.

148. Ghosh, P. S.; Kim, C. -K.; Han, G.; Forbes, N. S.; Rotello, V. M. Efficient Gene Delivery Vectors by Tuning the Surface Charge Density of Amino Acid-functionalized Gold Nanoparticles. *ACS Nano* **2008**, *2*, 2213–2218.

149. Ruoslahti, E.; Bhatia, S. N.; Sailor, M. J. Targeting of Drugs and Nanoparticles to Tumors. *J. Cell. Biol.* **2010**, *188*, 759–768.

150. Huang, X.; El-Sayed, I. H.; Qian, W.; El-Sayed, M. A. Cancer Cell Imaging and Photothermal Therapy in the Near-infrared Region by Using Gold Nanorods. *JACS* **2006**, *128*, 2115–2120.

151. Murphy, C. J.; Gole, A. M.; Hunyadi, S. E.; Stone, J. W.; Sisco, P. N.; Alkilany, A., et al. Chemical Sensing and Imaging with Metallic Nanorods. *Chem. Commun.* **2008**, *5*, 544–557.

152. von Maltzahn, G.; Park, J. H.; Agrawal, A.; Bandaru, N. K.; Das, S. K.; Sailor, M. J., et al. Computationally Guided Photothermal Tumor Therapy Using Long-circulating Gold Nanorod Antennas. *Cancer Res.* **2009**, *69*, 3892–3900.

153. Park, J. -H.; von Maltzahn, G.; Xu, M. J.; Fogal, V.; Kotamraju, V. R.; Ruoslahti, E., et al. Cooperative Nanomaterial System to Sensitize, Target, and Treat Tumors. *PNAS USA* **2010**, *107*, 981–986.

154. Cedervall, T.; Lynch, I.; Foy, M.; Berggard, T.; Donnely, S. C.; Cagney, G., et al. Detailed Identification of Plasma Proteins Adsorbed on Copolymer Nanoparticles. *Angew. Chem. Int. Ed.* **2007**, *119*, 5856–5858.

155. De Paoli Lacerda, S. H.; Park, J. J.; Meuse, C.; Pristinski, D.; Becker, M. L.; Karim, A., et al. Interaction of Gold Nanoparticles with Common Human Blood Proteins. *ACS Nano* **2010**, *4*, 365–379.

156. Roker, C.; Potzl, M.; Zhang, F.; Parak, W. J.; Nienhaus, G. U. RA Quantitative Fluorescence Study of Protein Monolayer Formation on Colloidal Nanoparticles. *Nat. Nanotechnol.* **2009**, *4*, 577–580.

157. Mukherjee, P.; Bhattacharya, R.; Wang, P.; Wang, L.; Basu, S.; Nagy, J. A.; Atala, A.; Mukhopadhyay, D.; Soker, S. Antiangiogenic Properties of Gold Nanoparticles. *Clin Cancer Res.* **2005**, *11*, 3530–3534.

158. Sabuncu, A. C.; Grubbs, J.; Qian, S.; Abdel-Fattah, T. M.; Stacey, M. W.; Beskok, A. Probing Nanoparticle Interaction in Cell Culture Media. *Colloids Surf. B* **2012**, *95*, 96–102.

159. Han, M.; Gao, X.; Su, J.; Nie, S. Quantum Dot Tagged Microbead for Multiplexed Coding of Biomolecules. *Nat. Biotechnol.* **2001**, *19*, 631–635.

160. Bulte, J. W.; Kraitchman, D. L. Iron Oxide MR Contrast Agents for Molecular and Cellular Imaging. *NMR Biomed.* **2004**, *17*, 484–499.

161. Kamikawa, T. L.; Mikolajczyk, M. G.; Kennedy, M.; Zhang, P.; Wang, W.; Scott, D. E.; Alocilja, E. C. Nanoparticle-based Biosensor for the Detection of Emerging Pandemic Influenza Strain. *Biosens. Bioelectron.* **2010**, *26*, 1346–1352.

162. Moore, A.; Weissleder, R.; Bogdanov, A., Jr. Uptake of Dextran-coated Monocrystalline Iron Oxides in Tumor Cells and Macrophages. *J. Magn. Reson. Imaging* **1997**, *7*, 1140–1145.

163. Sajja, H.; East, M.; Mao, H.; Wang, Y.; Nie, S.; Yang, L. Development of Multifunctional Nanoparticles for Targeted Drug Delivery and Noninvasive Imaging of Therapeutic Effect. *Curr. Drug Discov. Technol.* **2009**, *6*, 43–51.

164. Xie, J.; Peng, S.; Brower, N.; Pourmand, N.; Wang, S. X.; Sun, S. One-pot Synthesis of Monodisperse Iron Oxide Nanoparticles for Potential Biomedical Applications. *Pure Appl. Chem.* **2006**, *78*, 1003–1014.

165. Mahmoudi, M.; Sant, S.; Wang, B.; Laurent, S.; Sen, T. Superparamagnetic Iron Oxide Nanoparticles (SPIONs): Development, Surface Modification and Applications in Chemotherapy. *Adv. Drug Deliv. Rev.* **2011**, *63*, 24–46.

166. Kodama, R. H. Magnetic Nanoparticles. *J. Magn. Magn. Mat.* **1999**, *200*, 359–372.

167. Hans, M. L.; Lowman, A. M. Biodegradable Nanoparticles for Drug Delivery and Targeting. *Curr. Opin. Solid State Mater. Sci.* **2002,** *6,* 319–327.

168. Goon, I. Y.; Lai, L. M. H.; Lim, M.; Munroe, P.; Gooding, J. J.; Amal, R. Fabrication and Dispersion of Gold-shell-protected Magnetite Nanoparticles: Systematic Control Using Polyethyleneimine. *Chem. Mater.* **2009,** *21,* 673–681.

169. Jaffrezic-Renault, N.; Martelet, C.; Chevolot, Y.; Cloarec, J. Biosensors and Bio-bar Code Assays Based on Biofunctionalized Magnetic Microbeads. *Sensors* **2007,** *7,* 589–614.

170. Kim, J.; Piao, T.; Hyeon, T. Multifunctional Nanostructured Materials for Multimodal Imaging, and Simultaneous Imaging and Therapy. *Chem. Soc. Rev.* **2009,** *38,* 372–390.

171. Philipse, A. P.; Vanbruggen, M. P. B.; Pathmamanoharan, C. Magnetic Silica Dispersions — Preparation and Stability of Surface-modified Silica Particles with a Magnetic Core. *Langmuir* **1994,** *10,* 92–99.

172. Raynal, I.; Prigent, P.; Peyramaure, S.; Najid, A.; Rebuzzi, C.; Corot, C. Macrophage Endocytosis of Superparamagnetic Iron Oxide Nanoparticles: Mechanisms and Comparison of Ferumoxides and Ferumoxtran-10. *Invest. Radiol.* **2004,** *39,* 56–63.

173. Wang, Y.; Wong, J. F.; Teng, X. W.; Lin, X. Z.; Yang, H. Pulling Nanoparticles into Water: Phase Transfer of Oleic Acid Stabilized Monodisperse Nanoparticles into Aqueous Solutions of Alpha-cyclodextrin. *Nano Lett.* **2003,** *3,* 1555–1559.

174. Zhao, X.; Harris, J. M. Novel Degradable Poly(ethylene glycol) Hydrogels for Controlled Release of Protein. *J. Pharm. Sci.* **1998,** *87,* 1450–1458.

175. Tartaj, P.; Sema, C. J. Synthesis of Monodisperse Superparamagnetic Fe/Silica Nanospherical Composites. *JACS* **2003,** *125,* 15754–15755.

176. Zhang, Y.; Kohler, M.; Zhang, M. Surface Modification of Superparamagnetic Magnetite Nanoparticles and their Interacellular Uptake. *Biomaterials* **2002,** *23,* 9.

177. Teja, A. S.; Koh, P. Y. Synthesis, Properties, and Applications of Magnetic Iron Oxide Nanoparticles. *Progr. Cryst. Growth Char. Mater.* **2009,** *55,* 22–45.

178. Sahoo, Y.; Pizem, H.; Fried, T.; Golodnitsky, D.; Burstein, L.; Sukenik, C. N.; Markovich, G. Alkyl Phosphonate/phosphate Coating on Magnetite Nanoparticles: A Comparison with Fatty Acids. *Langmuir* **2001,** *17,* 7907–7911.

179. Pellegrino, T.; Manna, L.; Kudera, S.; Liedl, T.; Koktysh, D.; Rogach, A.; Keller, S.; Raıdler, J.; Natile, G.; Parak, W. *Hydrophobic Nanocrystals Coated with an Amphiphilic Polymer Shell: A General Route to Water Soluble Nanocrystals* **2004,** *4,* 703–707.

180. Moghimi, S. M.; Hunter, A. C.; Murray, J. C. Long-circulating and Target-Specific Nanoparticles: Theory to Practice. *Pharmacol. Rev.* **2003,** *53,* 283–318.

181. Moghimi, S. M.; Hunter, A. C.; Murray, J. C. Long-circulating and Target-specific Nanoparticles: Theory to Practice. *Pharmacol. Rev.* **2001,** *53,* 283–318.

182. Lee, H.; Lee, E. J.; Kim, D. K.; Jang, N. K.; Jeong, Y. Y.; Jon, S. Antibiofouling Polymer-coated Superparamagnetic Iron Oxide Nanoparticles as Potential Magnetic Resonance Contrast Agents for In vivo Cancer Imaging. *JACS* **2006,** *128,* 7383–7389.

183. Gupta, A. K.; Gupta, M. Synthesis and Surface Engineering of Iron Oxide Nanoparticles for Biomedical Applications. *Biomaterials* **2005,** *26,* 3995–4021.

184. Osaka, T.; Nakanishi, T.; Shanmugam, S.; Takahama, S.; Zhang, H. Effect of Surface Charge of Magnetite Nanoparticles on their Internalization into Breast Cancer and Umbilical Vein Endothelial Cells. *Colloids Surf. B* **2009,** *71,* 325–330.

185. Mahmoudi, M.; Shokrgozar, M. A.; Simchi, A.; Imani, M.; Milani, A. S.; Stroeve, P.; Vali, H.; Hafeli, U. O.; Bonakdar, S. Multiphysics Flow Modeling and In vitro Toxicity of Iron Oxide Nanoparticles Coated with Poly(vinyl alcohol). *J. Phys. Chem. C* **2009,** *113,* 2322–2331.

186. Karlsson, H. I.; Cronholm, P.; Gustafsson, J.; Muller, L. Copper Oxide Nanoparticles are Highly Toxic: A Comparison Between Metal Oxide Nanoparticles and Carbon Nanotubes. *Chem. Res. Toxicol.* **2008**, *21,* 1726–1732.

187. Mahmoudi, M.; Simchi, A.; Imani, M.; Shokrgozar, M. A.; Milani, A. S.; Hafeli, U.; Stroeve, P. A New Approach for the In vitro Identification of the Cytotoxicity of Superparamagnetic Iron Oxide Nanoparticles. *Colloids Surf. B* **2010**, *75,* 300–309.

188. Lynch, I.; Dawson, K. A. Protein–nanoparticle Interactions. *Nano Today* **2008**, *3,* 40–47.

189. Mahmoudi, M.; Simchi, A.; Imani, M.; Milani, A. S.; Stroeve, P. An In vitro Study of Bare and Poly(ethylene glycol)-co-fumarate-coated Superparamagnetic Iron Oxide Nanoparticles: A New Toxicity Identification Procedure. *Nanotechnology* **2009**, *20,* 40–47.

190. Nel, A.; Madler, L.; Velegol, D.; Xia, T.; Hoek, E. M. V.; Somasundaran, P.; Klaessig, F.; Castranova, V.; Thompson, M. Understanding Biophysicochemical Interactions at the Nano-bio Interface. *Nat. Mater.* **2009**, *8,* 543–557.

191. Cedervall, T.; Lynch, I.; Lindman, S.; Nilsson, H.; Thulin, E.; Linse, S.; Dawson, K. A. Understanding Biophysicochemical Interactions at the Nano-bio Interface. *PNAS* **2007**, *104,* 2050–2055.

192. Lynch, I.; Cedervall, T.; Lundqvist, M.; Cabaleiro-Lago, C.; Linse, S.; Dawson, K. A. The Nanoparticle-protein Complex as a Biological Entity; A Complex Fluids and Surface Science Challenge for the 21st Century. *Adv. Colloid Interface Sci.* **2007**, *134–135,* 167–174.

193. Walczyk, D.; Bombelli, F. B.; Monopoli, M. P.; Lynch, I.; Dawson, K. A. What the Cell "sees" in Bionanoscience. *JACS* **2010**, *132,* 5761–5768.

194. Douziech-Eyrolles, L.; Marchais, H.; Herve, K.; Munnier, E.; Souce, M.; Linasier, C.; Dubois, P.; Chourpa, I. Nanovectors for Anticancer Agents Based on Superparamagnetic Iron Oxide Nanoparticles. *Int. J. Nanomed.* **2007**, *2,* 541–550.

195. Lubbe, A. S.; Begemann, C.; Brock, J.; McClure, D. G. Physiological Aspects in Magnetic Drug-targeting. *J. Magn. Magn. Mat.* **1999**, *194,* 7.

196. Jones, S.; Bowler, P.; Walker, M.; Parsons, D. Controlling Wound Bioburden with a Novel Silver©\Containing Hydrofiber(R) Dressing. *Wound Repair Reg.* **2004**, *12,* 288–294.

197. Zhao, G.; Stevens, S. Multiple Parameters for the Comprehensive Evaluation of the Susceptibility of *Escherichia coli* to the Silver Ion. *Biometals* **1998**, *11,* 27–32.

198. Gong, P.; Li, H.; He, X.; Wang, K.; Hu, J.; Tan, W.; Zhang, S.; Yang, X. Preparation and Antibacterial Activity of Fe_3O_4@ Ag Nanoparticles. *Nanotechnology* **2007**, *18,* 285604.

199. Jain, P.; Pradeep, T. Potential of Silver Nanoparticle-coated Polyurethane Foam as an Antibacterial Water Filter. *Biotechnol. Bioeng.* **2005**, *90,* 59–63.

200. Tian, J.; Wong, K.; Ho, C.; Lok, C.; Yu, W.; Che, C.; Chiu, J.; Tam, P. Topical Delivery of Silver Nanoparticles Promotes Wound Healing. *Chem. Med. Chem.* **2007**, *2,* 129–136.

201. Morones, J.; Elechiguerra, J.; Camacho, A.; Holt, K.; Kouri, J.; Ramírez, J.; Yacaman, M. The Bactericidal Effect of Silver Nanoparticles. *Nanotechnology* **2005**, *16,* 2346.

202. Dror-Ehre, A.; Mamane, H.; Belenkova, T.; Markovich, G.; Adin, A. Silver Nanoparticle-*E. coli* Colloidal Interaction in Water and Effect on *E. coli* Survival. *J. Colloid Interface Sci.* **2009**, *339,* 521–526.

203. Li, W.; Xie, X.; Shi, Q.; Zeng, H.; OU-Yang, Y.; Chen, Y. Antibacterial Activity and Mechanism of Silver Nanoparticles on *Escherichia coli*. *Appl. Microbiol. Biotechnol.* **2010**, *85,* 1115–1122.

204. Sondi, I.; Salopek-Sondi, B. Silver Nanoparticles as Antimicrobial Agent: A Case Study on *E. coli* as a Model for Gram-negative Bacteria. *J. Colloid Interface Sci.* **2004**, *275,* 177–182.

205. Lok, C.; Ho, C.; Chen, R.; He, Q.; Yu, W.; Sun, H.; Tam, P.; Chiu, J.; Che, C. Proteomic Analysis of the Mode of Antibacterial Action of Silver Nanoparticles. *J. Proteome Res.* **2006,** *5,* 916–924.

206. Kim, K.; Sung, W.; Suh, B.; Moon, S.; Choi, J.; Kim, J.; Lee, D. Antifungal Activity and Mode of Action of Silver Nano-particles on *Candida albicans*. *Biometals* **2009,** *22,* 235–242.

207. Shrivastava, S.; Bera, T.; Roy, A.; Singh, G.; Ramachandrarao, P.; Dash, D. Characterization of Enhanced Antibacterial Effects of Novel Silver Nanoparticles. *Nanotechnology* **2007,** *18,* 225103.

208. Marambio-Jones, C.; Hoek, E. M. V. A Review of the Antibacterial Effects of Silver Nanomaterials and Potential Implications for Human Health and the Environment. *J. Nanopart. Res.* **2010,** *12,* 1531–1551.

209. Bilberg, K.; Døving, K. B.; Beedholm, K.; Baatrup, E. Silver Nanoparticles Disruptolfaction in Crucian carp (*Carassius carassius*) and Eurasian perch (*Perca fluviatilis*). *Aquat. Toxicol.* **2011,** *104,* 145–152.

210. Drake, P. L.; Hazelwood, K. J. Exposure-related Health Effects of Silver and Silver Compounds: A Review. *Ann. Occup. Hyg.* **2005,** *49,* 575–585.

211. Foldbjerg, R.; Dang, D. A.; Autrup, H. Cytotoxicity and Genotoxicity Of Silver Nanoparticles in the Human Lung Cancer Cell Line, A549. Nanoparticles in the Human Lung Cancer Cell Line. *Arch. Toxicol.* **2011,** *85,* 743–750.

212. Kawata, K.; Osawa, M.; Okabe, S. In vitro Toxicity of Silver Nanoparticles at Noncytotoxic Doses to Hepg2 Human Hepatoma Cells. *Environ. Sci. Technol.* **2009,** *43,* 6046–6051.

213. Kim, S.; Choi, J. E.; Choi, J.; Chung, K. H.; Park, K.; Yi, J.; Ryu, D. Y. Oxidative Stressdependent Toxicity of Silver Nanoparticles in Human Hepatoma Cells. *Toxicol. In Vitro* **2009,** *23,* 1076–1084.

214. Mudunkotuwa, I. A.; Grassian, V. H. The Devil is in the Details (or the surface): Impact of Surface Structure and Surface Energetics on Understanding the Behavior of Nanomaterials in the Environment. *J. Environ. Monit.* **2011,** *13,* 1135–1144.

215. Bian, S. W.; Mudunkotuwa, I. A.; Rupasinghe, T.; Grassian, V. H. Aggregation and Dissolution of 4 nm ZnO Nanoparticles in Aqueous Environments: Influence of pH, Ionic strength, Size, and Adsorption of Humic Acid. *Langmuir* **2011,** *27,* 6059–6068.

216. Navarro, E.; Piccapietra, F.; Wagner, B.; Marconi, F.; Kaegi, R.; Odzak, N.; Sigg, L.; Behra, R. Toxicity of Silver Nanoparticles to *Chlamydomonas reinhardtii*. *Environ. Sci. Technol.* **2008,** *42,* 8959–8964.

217. Beer, C.; Foldbjerg, R.; Hayashi, Y.; Sutherland, D. S.; Autrup, H. Toxicity of Silver Nanoparticles-Nanoparticle or Silver Ion?. *Toxicol. Lett.* **2012,** *208,* 286–292.

218. Studer, A. M.; Limbach, L. K.; Van Duc, L.; Krumeich, F.; Athanassiou, E. K.; Gerber, L. C.; Moch, H.; Stark, W. J. Nanoparticle Cytotoxicity Depends on Intracellular Solubility: Comparison of Stabilized Copper Metal and Degradable Copper Oxide Nanoparticles. *Toxicol. Lett.* **2010,** *197,* 169–174.

219. Lovric, J.; Cho, S.; Winnik, F.; Maysinger, D. Unmodified Cadmium Telluride Quantum Dots Induce Reactive Oxygen Species Formation Leading to Multiple Organelle Damage and Cell Death. *Chem. Biol.* **2005,** *12,* 1227–1234.

220. EPA *Chemical Information Overview Assembly at.* Available from:: 2010http://www.dtsc. ca.gov/PollutionPrevention/Chemical_Call_In.cfm.

221. Hart; Research; Associate. *Nanotechnology, Synthetic Biology, & Public Opinion.* 2009. Available from: http://www.nanotechproject.org/process/assets/files/8286/nano_synbio.pdf.

222. Arianna, F.; Alfred, N. *Reconfiguring Responsibility: Lessons for Nanoethics (Part 2 of the Report on Deepening Debate on Nanotechnology).* 2009.

223. Davies, S.; Macnaghten, P.; Kearnes, M. *Reconfiguring Responsibility: Lessons for Public Policy (Part 1 of the report on Deepening Debate on Nanotechnology)*. 2009.

224. Commission, E. *Commission Recommendation on A Code of Conduct for Responsible Nanosciences and Nanotechnologies Research & Council Conclusions on Responsible Nanosciences and Nanotechnologies Research*. 2008. Available from: http://ec.europa.eu/research/research-eu.

225. Bowman, D.; Hodge, G. Nanotechnology: Mapping the Wild Regulatory Frontier. *Futures* **2006,** *38,* 1060–1073.

226. Society, R. *Nanoscience and Nanotechnologies: Opportunities and Uncertainties*. 2004. Available from: http://www.nanotec.org.uk/finalReport.htm.

227. Mee, W.; Katz, E.; Solomon, F.; Lovel, R. In PATH conference: Australia, 2006.

228. Dietrich, H.; Schibeci, R. *Beyond Public Perceptions of Gene Technology: Community Participation in Public Policy in Australia* **2003,** *12.*

229. Marchant, G.; Syvester, D. Transnational Models for Regulation of Nanotechnology. *J. Law Med. Ethics* **2006,** *34,* 714–725.

230. TGA *Safety of Sunscreens Containing Nanoparticles of Zinc Oxide or Titanium Dioxide*. 2006.

231. Faunce, T. A.; Nasu, H.; Murray, K.; Bowman, D. Sunscreen Safety: The Precautionary Principle, The Australian Therapeutic Goods Administration and Nanoparticles in Sunscreens. *Nanoethics* **2008,** *2,* 231–240.

232. Barker, P. J.; Branch, A. The Interaction of Modern Sunscreen Formulations with Surface Coatings. *Progr. Organic Coatings* **2008,** *62,* 313–320.

233. Vines, T.; Faunce, T. A. Assessing the Safety and Cost-effectiveness of Early Nanodrugs. *J. Law Med.* **2007,** *16,* 822–845.

234. Faunce, T. A. Policy Challenges of Nanomedicine for Australia's PBS. *Aust. Health Rev.* **2009,** *33,* 258–267.

235. Faunce, T. A. Toxicological and Public Good Considerations for the Regulation of Nanomaterial-containing Medical Products. *Expert. Opin. Drug. Safety* **2008,** *7,* 103–106.

236. USFDA *FDA Issues Draft Guidance on Nanotechnology Documents Address Use of Nanotechnology by Food and Cosmetics Industries*. 2012. Available from: http://www.fda.gov/Cosmetics/GuidanceComplianceRegulatoryInformation/GuidanceDocuments/ucm300886.htm.

237. USFDA Cosmetics: Draft Guidance for Industry. *Saf. Nanomat. Cosmet. Prod.* 2012. Available from: http://www.fda.gov/Cosmetics/GuidanceComplianceRegulatoryInformation/GuidanceDocuments/ucm300886.htm.

238. USFDA *Draft Guidance for Industry: Assessing the Effects of Significant Manufacturing Process Changes, Including Emerging Technologies, on the Safety And Regulatory Status of Food Ingredients and Food Contact Substances, Including Food Ingredients that are Color Additives*. 2012.

239. SCENIHR. Risk Assessment of Products of Nanotechnologies, 2009. Directorate General for Health Consumers, European Commision, pp. 71.

240. Wild, J. Patent Challenges for Nanotech Investors. *Intellectual Asset Management* **2003,** 29–32.

241. USPTO. *Class 977 Nanotechnology Cross-reference Art Collection*. Accessed on June 24, 2012. Available from: http://www.uspto.gov/patents/resources/classification/class_977_nanotechnology_cross-ref_art_collection.jsp.

242. Koosha, A.; Ahmadi, M.; Nazifi, A.; Mousazadeh, R. Intellectual Property Rights of Nano-Biotechnology in Trade Related Aspects of Intellectual Property Agreement (TRIPS). *Indian J. Sci. Tech.* **2012,** *5,* 2436–2442.

243. Igami, M.; Okazaki, T., DSTI/DOC, Eds.; Organisation for Economic Co-operation and Development: Paris, 2007, Vol. 4, pp 52.

244. Scheu, M.; Veefkind, V.; Verbandt, Y.; Molina Galan, E.; Absalom, R.; Forster, W. Mapping Nanotechnology Patents: The EPO Approach. *World Patent Inf.* **2006,** *28,* 204–211.

245. Webb, C.; Dernis, H.; Harhoff, D.; Hoisl, K. *Analysing European and International Patent Citations: A Set of EPO Patent Database Building Blocks*; STI Working Paper 2005/9OECD; Directorate for Science, Technology, and Industry, 2005.

246. von Warburg, I.; Teichert, T.; Rost, K. Clustering the Science Citation Index using Co-citations. II. Mapping Science. *Scintometrics* **2005,** *8,* 321–340.

247. Huang, Z.; Chen, H.; Chen, Z. K.; Roco, M. C. International Nanotechnology Development in 2003: Country, Institution, and Technology Field Analysis Based on USPTO Patent Database. *J. Nanopart. Res.* **2004,** *6,* 325–354.

248. Bawa, R.; Bawa, S. R.; Maebius, S. B.; Flynn, T.; Wei, C. Commercialization: Protecting New Ideas in Nanomedicine with Patents. *Nanomed. Nanotechnol. Biol. Med.* **2005,** *1.*

249 Baker, S.; Aston, A. The Business of Nanotech. *Business Week* **2005** February 14.

250. Regalado, A. Nanotechnology Patents Surge as Companies Vie to Stake Claim. *Wall Street J.* **2004 June 18.**

251. *Sizing Nanotechnology's Value Chain*; Lux Research, 2004.

Conclusions

Chapter Outline

9.1 INTRODUCTION

Nanomaterials (NMs) have structural features and properties in between those of single atoms/molecules and continuous bulk materials and have at least one dimension in the nanometer range (1 nm = 1×10^{-9} m). They include clusters,[1] nanoparticles,[2–9] quantum dots (QDs),[2,10–21] nanotubes,[22–45] as well as the collection or organization of these individual structures into two- and three-dimensional assemblies. The nanoscale dimensions of NMs bring optical,[46–50] electronic,[39,51] magnetic,[52–65] catalytic and other properties that are distinct from those of atoms/molecules or bulk materials. In order to exploit the special properties that arise due to the nanoscale dimensions of materials, researchers must control and manipulate the size, shape, and surface functional groups[66–70] of NMs and structure them into periodically ordered assemblies to create new products, devices and technologies or improve existing ones. The science of controlling, manipulating, or engineering the properties and utilizing these NMs for the purpose of building microscopic machinery is termed as nanotechnology.[5,71–79]

NMs are directly relevant to medicine because of the role of nanoscale phenomena such as enzyme action, cell cycle, cell signaling, and cell repair.[80] NMs can be used to create tools for analyzing the structure of cells and tissues from the atomic and cellular levels and to design and create biocompatible materials on the nanoscale for therapies, diagnostics, and replacements.[5,6,72,75,79,81–87]

Nanomaterials for Medical Applications. http://dx.doi.org/10.1016/B978-0-12-385089-8.00009-1

NMs can be used to create precisely targeted drugs that are engineered to locate and sit on specific proteins and nucleic acids associated with the disease and/or disorders.[6,10,53,54,61,64,66,88–110]. These NMs can also be used to deliver small organic molecules and peptides at effective sites of action to carry out their function more effectively, protected from degradation, immune attack, and shielded to pass through barriers that block the passage of large molecules.

At present, nanoparticles are being tested for various biomedical applications to learn if they can help facilitate sensitive and accurate medical diagnostics as well as for effective therapeutics. More specifically for drug delivery purposes, the use of nanoparticles is attracting increasing attention due to their unique capabilities and their negligible side effects not only in cancer therapy but also in the treatment of other ailments. Among all types of nanoparticles, biocompatible superparamagnetic iron oxide nanoparticles (SPIONs) with proper surface architecture and conjugated targeting ligands/proteins have attracted a great deal of attention for drug delivery applications.

Chapter 1 introduced the various chapters of the book with the intention to help the reader discover, manipulate, and understand the unique properties of matter at the nanoscale level in order to inspire creativity toward the development of new NMs and new capabilities for potential applications across all fields of science, engineering, technology, and medicine. The book is intended to inspire new innovations that will bring about the realization of the much potential of nanoscale science and technology that are predicted to have an enormous potential economic impact specifically in the various areas of medicine.

9.2 MARKET POTENTIAL

As described, nanotechnology has continued to show enormous growth and has encompassed various fields of research and industry. The research activities involving NMs have seen unsurpassed growth over the past few years. Thousands of nano-enabled products are now enjoying a huge impact in the global market and it continues to grow with a global nanomedicine market that reached $63.8 B in 2010 and $72.8 B in 2011.[111] The BCC research also predicted that this NMs market is expected to grow to $130.9 B by 2016 at compound annual growth rate (CAGR) of 12.5% in 2011–2016. The applications of NMs for the central nervous system alone are expected to reach $46.7 B by 2016 at a CAGR of 10.8% in 2011–2016 according to the same report.[111]

Many nano-enabled medical products have entered the market to date and as the applications grow and infiltrate complicated diseases such as all kinds of cancer, cardiac, and neurodegenerative disorders, infection, tissue engineering etc., the market is predicted to reach considerable growth in the near future. This has been shown in the application of nanoparticles in biomedical sciences that posted a year-on-year growth of over 37% in 2009.[112] In 2013, this area is expected to close at US$ 750 M with a CAGR of over 30% since 2010.[112] The

US leads the nanotechnology market and accounts for an estimated share of around 35% of the global nanotechnology market.[112]

In January, 2012, Cientifica tracked the growth of government funding to a total of \$67.5 B from 2000 to 2011.[112] They have indicated that nano-enabled drug delivery therapeutics will grow from a current value of \$2.3 B to \$136 B by the year 2021 and will represent approximately 15% of the global nano-technology market in 2021.[112] It is the healthcare sector that offers the greatest opportunity to add value to NMs with China as the fastest-growing market sector. [112] The drug and pharmaceutical industry benefit from the formulation of nano-enabled drugs because this enables the extension of patents maintaining if not increasing their existing revenue sources. By 2021, the global growth in the drug delivery market will be led by Asia with a compound annual growth rate (CAGR) of 32.5%.[112] The largest Asian market for nano-based drug delivery systems will be China that will have a worth more than \$18 B and representing 43% of the Asian market.[112] In other countries, France is forecast to surpass Japan as a drug delivery market within 10 years.[112]

BCC research, on the other hand reported that the global nanomedicine market reached \$63.8 B in 2010 and \$72.8 B in 2011.[111] They predicted that the market is expected to grow to \$130.9 B by 2016 at CAGR of 12.5% in 2011–2016. In their report, the central nervous system (CNS) products market reached \$11.7 B in 2010 and \$14.0 B in 2011 and expects this market to grow to \$29.5 B by 2016 with a CAGR of 16.1% in 2011–2016 while the anticancer products market reached \$25.2 B in 2010 and \$28.0 B in 2011.[111] It is expected to reach \$46.7 B by 2016 at a CAGR of 10.8% in 2011–2016 they said in the report.[111]

9.3 SYNTHESIS OF VARIOUS NMs

In Chapter 2, overviews of the various NMs that are currently very useful in nanomedicine were presented. Several processes for the synthesis of some of the most common NMs such as QDs, Magnetic nanoparticles (MNPs), Gold nanoparticles (AuNPs), Silver nanoparticles (AgNPs), liposomes, polymers (polylactic glycolic acid (PLGA) and polylactic acid (PLA)), chitosan, carbon nanotubes (CNTs), micelles, and dendrimers were provided with protocols that are easy to follow and carry out in an academic or small laboratory setting. Many NMs that are at their infancy were not included because these require more intense testing of the method and the protocols before their full potential in medicine can be realized. A selected group of well established nanomaterials with multiple references from multiple laboratories indicating a more advanced status in their medical applications were given greater attention.[5,62,71,113,114] A few of the common current NMs characterization techniques were included to provide an overview of how the properties of NMs are established. Techniques for characterizing NMs that are at the infancy of development were not included in the chapter. Instruments that are useful for NMs topography, chemical composition, size, and shape analytical techniques of particular benefit to nanomaterial characterization were discussed. The instruments include, TEM, DLS, ATR-FTIR, XPS, Time of Flight SIMS, Colorimetry, AFM, and the Zeta sizer.[8,9,38,39,46–48,77,83,108,113,115–127] The introduction of the scanning tunneling microscopy (STM) in the early 1980s allowed the manipulation of individual atoms, that significantly contributed in the rapid discovery and development of fullerenes (carbon 60 molecules), CNTs, and semiconductor QDs.[2,10–13,16,18,21–27,29,31,32,36,37,43,47,75,88,118,119,128–146] At the current status of NMs characterization, novel high-resolution imaging and analytical tools that will allow easy sample preparation and *in situ* monitoring are still needed for a better understanding of NMs and their interactions with biological systems for medical applications.

9.4 NMs SURFACE MODIFICATION AND FUNCTIONALIZATION

In Chapter 3, the focus was on the modification and functionalization of NMs. Most of the commercially available NMs are synthesized in organic solvent.[38,143,147–153] As a result, the products are hydrophobic and are not compatible with biological molecules. In order that the physical, electronic, chemical, and optical properties of NMs can be exploited to benefit medicine the hydrophobic nature has to be converted to hydrophilic state.[2,13,114,131,143,145,154–156] However, at the nanometer scale, the quantum mechanical effects that emerge leading to various and unexpected physicochemical properties that make them useful for medical applications may be disrupted during conversion from hydrophobic to hydrophilic status. In order to harness the novel and unique properties that can provide promising solutions for nanomedicine, much care has to be taken in the conversion of organic soluble to water-soluble NMs.[2,14,17,20,21,26–28,44,69,77,88,124,129,137,145,156–161] Chapter 3 is mainly focused on the various techniques such as ligand exchange, encapsulation, and polymer coating for the preparation of water-soluble NMs. The water-soluble NMs that are commercially available contain functional groups making them easy to manipulate and functionalize with various biomolecules including low molecular weight drugs for various medical applications. The thiols and other functional groups that are introduced during conversion into the water-soluble form and are anchored on the surface of the NMs provide reactive sites for subsequent bioconjugation reactions. NMs with various functional groups such as sulfhydryl –SH, carboxyl –COOH, amine –NH$_2$, hydroxyl –OH and others that allows attachment of biomolecules through various bioconjugation or crosslinking chemistry are now commercially available. Linkers for the water-soluble NMs are carbodiimide, succinimide, maleidiimide and bifunctional crosslinkers; through direct attachment (hydrophobic or electrostatic interactions) and sometimes, through the use of the strong biotin–avidin system.[114,155,161–166] These various methods of conjugating biomolecules or drugs to NMs have unique qualities and properties that serve various needs for different applications.[114,155,161–166]

One of the most important challenges in the medical applications of NMs is surface modification that allows for biocompatibility and functionaliza-tion.[2,3,5,10,12,23,24,47,52–56,71,81,82,88–93,95,97,99,126,130,133,134,138,147–149,151,167–182] Effec-tive surface modifications as well as highly controlled surface conjugation strategies are needed to incorporate specific biomolecules on the surface or inside the NMs.[20,21,40,44,50,61,63–65,68,69,77–80,106,108,109,116,123,124,143–145,154,156,183–200] How-ever, success in functionalization depends on many factors that include NMs size, shape, charge, chemistry, and surface modification. These factors are often dif-ficult to vary independently, so the contribution of each is difficult to generalize.

The nanoscale sizes of NMs that approach the atomic level, more often than not, defy the governing rules at the macroscopic level. Quantum mechanical effects begin to emerge at the nanoscale dimensions leading to varied and unexpected physicochemical   properties.[10,14,15,19,47,48,67,69,75,77,119,124,128,130,145,155,190,201,202] Theoretical calculations, molecular modeling, and indirect methods are fre-quently employed to investigate the intricate interactions and properties of the materials at the nanoscale. These novel and unique properties enable nanotech-nology to provide powerful solutions and alternative to various medical con-cerns and problems.

The QDs are among the most fascinating NMs that have ever been devel-oped.[135,143,203,204] The core QDs are usually prepared in high-temperature solvents that involves a mixture of organic chemicals (trioctyl phosphine and trioctyl phosphine oxide (TOP/TOPO)), followed by a layer of wide-bandgap semiconductor materials that is coated on the surface of the QD core creating the shell.[15,16,19,51,119,124,135,137,139,141,143,155,160,203–207] These QDs are either used as hydrophobic nanocrystals or are made water-soluble by ligand exchange or by adsorption of heterofunctional organic coating on the QD surface that give functionality to the QD surface. These coating materi-als include thiols, silanes/silanols, bidentate thiols, amine box dendrimers, oligomeric phosphines, phosphatidyl compounds, amphiphilic saccha-rides, proteins and peptides, etc.[5,11–13,71–73,130,190,208–223] In the same man-ner, other NMs including iron oxide magnetic nanoparticles (IOMNPs) and other magnetic nanoparticles can be modified like the QDs to make them biocompatible.[60,68,161,183,224–232]

In addition to the recognition moiety, NMs can be equipped with a coating that allows membrane transport or easy cell-internalization, and/or an enzymatic function.[3–5,24,47,89,147,151,167,168,233–235] Peptide or protein coating or amphiphilic polymer coating produce biocompatible NMs that can penetrate membrane sur-faces without damaging the cells.[127,224,225,236–242]

9.5 NANOBIOSENSORS

NMs have also now been used for biosensors development.[190,208–211] Biosensors challenges in medicine include rapid and accurate measurement of molecular entities such as protein biomarkers, genes, cells, and pathogens in biological samples. A growing number of new diagnostic platforms involving dimensions in the nanometer scale, the nanobiosensors,[50,156,193,208,237,243,244] are rapidly surfacing in the literature to detect and measure biomolecules and cells with high sensitivity. A homogeneous nanobiosensor occurs in solution and does not have a phase separation. Chapter 4 is focused mainly on heterogeneous nanobiosensor which involve a solid platform that serves to anchor the analyte being detected. The solid capture platform can in itself be the nanomaterial as in the case of IOMNPs which can be easily separated through strong magnets.[88] In most cases, the NMs are used not to capture but to generate the signals because these allow for improved sensitivities.[2,12,14,47,48,50,71,73,81,90,113,117,118,124,145,156,167,172,173,176,181,190,201,237,243,245–255]

Nanobiosensors are easier to use, faster, and more inexpensive in comparison with conventional diagnostics methods. In addition, inexpensive instrumentation that accompanies these NM based biosensors is also currently being developed and is the focus of Chapter 4. The small dimensions of NMs allow their assembly into barcodes and high-density arrays to detect multiple analytes using miniature hand held sensing devices that may only need light emitting diodes as power source.[64,65,68]

Recent advances in nanoscience and nanotechnology have led to various shifts in biosensing technology. Biosensors find applications not only in the environment and industries; it also has a wide arena of applications in disease monitoring and diagnostics. The use of nanoparticles in diagnostics promises enhanced sensitivity, shorter turn-around-time, and possibly cost-effectiveness. Thus, NMs based diagnostics schemes may surpass current gold standard techniques such as PCR and ELISA. Despite the fact that there are pending regulatory, safety, and intellectual property issues, and the technologies themselves still need further optimization, nanoparticles are primed to transform the field of clinical diagnostics.

The application of NMs for medical biosensors makes use of their unique physicochemical properties for the improvement of the sensing performance. Nanobiosensor is not a field of its own but is a combination of various disciplines such as material sciences, physics, chemistry, biochemistry, engineering, and biology at the nanoscale. The sensitivity, accuracy, reproducibility and reliability of nanobiosensors that are attributed to the unique physicochemical properties of NMs holds promise in monitoring diseases that are difficult to diagnose except in the later stages of the disease where treatment is close to being impossible.[237,256,257]

In the area of nanobiosensors especially in imaging sensors and diagnosis, inorganic semiconductor QDs have emerged as novel fluorescent labels to replace the conventional organic fluorophores.[2,14,19–21,47,69,88,145,156,172,249,251,258,259] This is attributed to the properties of QDs which include broad excitation profiles, narrow and symmetric emission spectra, high photostability and high-quantum efficiency,[208] and multiplexed sensing possibilities.[260,261] QDs with various sizes that, therefore, have different emission wavelengths can be excited by a single excitation source which is a unique characteristics that allows multiple analyte sensing capability in one sample and in one sensor strip or chip.[124,261] In contrast, organic dyes with different emission wavelengths must be excited by different excitation sources, which do not allow multiple analyte sensing capability.[47,139,258,262,263] The need for simultaneous detection of multiple targets in single assay drives the development of inorganic nanocrystal-based fluorescent probes to replace organic fluorophores especially for diagnosing diseases with symptoms that are similar to many different kinds of diseases and health conditions. With QDs-based nanobiosensors, it is less of a challenge to integrate the transducers with the molecular recognition probes that recognize the binding events and actively transduce sensing signals simultaneously.

By far, most of the publications in the literature to date research on nanostructured biosensors are proof-of-concept work that demonstrated the advantages of NMs and nanostructures. Only a few nanobiosensors have entered the market for specific medical applications to date (Table 9.1). However, to achieve a status that is similar to the nano-enabled drugs that are already in the market, more efforts need to be made to move the proof-of-concept studies to the applications of biosensors to real-world samples. Since the signature of nanobiosensors is small, integration with microfluidics to form lab-on-chip devices is not an issue. Studies to integrate the nanostructured sensors with signal-processing instruments to build portable devices for on-site measurement of analytes or for on-time (real-time) monitoring targets of interest and rapid assessment of risks are currently on-going. Among these are point-of-care devices that are easy to use and now has an increasing commercial demand.

Various analytes such as proteins, DNA, and whole cell are presented.[42,117,122,127,175,194,253,262,264–281] Protein analyte may be found in a cell, in which case, the whole cell will be captured on the solid surface. The concept of using NMs in biosensors is similar to an ordinary ELISA except that the signal is not attributed to an enzyme but the NM which may be a QD that emits bright fluorescent light or AuNP that can be detected due to their Raman signals. Because

TABLE 9.1 Commercially Available Nanomaterial Bases Biosensors for Medical Applications

Nanoparticle	Application	Brand	Manufacturer
Gold	Pregnancy test	Clear Blue Easy	Unipath Diagnostics
Gold	Pregnancy test	First Response	First Response
Gold	Pregnancy test	Clear View	Cytodiagnostics
Gold	HIV test	Oraquick	Ora Sure Technologies

NMs can be detected at very low concentrations, the sensitivity of nanobiosensors is expected to be in the low picogram and down to the femtogram levels.[272] As such, especially with QDs that may allow single molecule detection, nanobiosensors hold promise for early disease detection that can provide valuable insights into the medical biology at the atomic level.[15,47,137,172,176,258,282–284]

NMs exhibit unique size-tunable as well as shape-dependent physicochemical properties that do not resemble those of bulk materials.[207,282,285,286] Recent advances in NMs open new avenues to develop various novel biosensors.[2,209,210] These NMs-based nanobiosensors, make use of electrochemical and optical properties of NMs to demonstrate improved limit of detection, sensitivity, ease of use, portability, low cost, portability, and selectivity.[47,50,88,113,156,193,208,237,243,244,249,287,288] The small dimensions of NMs that are comparable to the dimensions of biomolecular probes and to biological analytes make them excellent components of biosensors that are candidates from miniaturization.

Nanobiosensors for detection of various biomolecules that are useful in the clinical diagnosis of different types of diseases are discussed in Chapter 4. These diseases may be genetic, metabolic, or caused by infectious disease causing agents. Various types of NMs based nanobiosensors will be presented and a few protocols will be discussed.

The development of NMs has revolutionized the technologies for disease diagnosis, treatment, and prevention. It has been envisioned that the new nanotechnological innovations have the potential to provide extensive benefit for patients. Nanoparticles can mimic and alter biological processes owing to their size that is comparable to the size of biomolecules. Thus, to date, various NMs are being developed for targeted drug delivery.

9.6 NMs FOR DRUG DELIVERY

Over the past few years, NMs have been studied as drug delivery systems called NMs drug carriers or simply nanocarriers.[406,447] Enormous focus is being directed toward developing nanoparticles for drug delivery for controlling the release of drugs, stabilizing labile molecules (e.g. proteins, peptides, or DNA) from degradation, and site-specific drug targeting.[6,53,88,89,95,98,99,101,103,104,137,169,289–306]. In the late 1969s and early 1979s, the literature experienced the advent of polyacrylamide micelle polymerization along with other polymers that are now components of nano-enabled drugs that are sold in the market.[66,90,94,100,289,307–311] This generation of nano-enabled drugs is mainly dependent on the small size of the particles to increase the surface area to enhance the bioavailability of poorly soluble drugs and to improve the structure of the particles for delayed release. In the USA, the commercial nano-enabled drugs include Rapamune®/Pfizer, Emend®/Merck, INVEGA® SUSTENNA®/Janssen, all based on Elan's NanoCrystal® technology; Abraxane®/Abraxis Bioscience and Triglide™/Sciele Pharma.[312] The NMs in these drugs introduced improved functionalities that are useful for diagnosis, targeting, drug delivery, and enhanced transport and uptake properties.

One of the most promising applications of biocompatible NMs is drug delivery. Today, a number of nano-enabled drugs are commercially available for various applications.[312] Aside from the use of NMs for MRI contrast agents and drug encapsulation, some are also being studied for vaccine delivery.[64,91,197,229,313] Pusic and her group focused on the use of the semiconductor nanoparticles, in particular QDs, as an alternative vaccine delivery platform.[154] For the delivery of peptide vaccines, they used <15 nm QDs with a crystal shell of alternating cationic and anionic layers, being the most widely used CdSe/ZnS. Their results indicated that the QDs they used were nonimmunogenic, stable, and when coated with an organic layer allowed for an array of proteins, DNA, and other biomolecules to be conjugated to their 60 surfaces. Leveraging on the small size and surface modification, the QDs were conjugated with vaccine candidates against malaria.[154] The QDs served as a delivery platform for protein antigens and also activated key immune cells to further increase the immunogenicity of the vaccine. The in vivo tests demonstrated no immediate toxic effects but the system uses QDs that contain Cd which are not compatible for human use. The toxicity of the CdSe/ZnS QDs was contained by coating the core with a shell layer of ZnS that is further coated with an amphiphilic polymer.[12,18,144,202,406,447] Currently, because of the possibility of eventual polymer and nanoparticle degradation, thereby releasing the toxic Cd, attempts is currently being made to develop cadmium free QD nanoparticles as well as the use of other nanoparticles that do not contain Cd such as IOMNPs and AuNPs.

The delivery of drugs to manage incurable diseases such as cancer, tumor, other diseases of similar nature, and those which currently have no cure such as AIDS and HIV are important to optimize the effect of drugs and to reduce toxic side effects.[75,117,314] To date, several nanotechnologies, mostly based on NMs can facilitate drug delivery to these diseases. These NMs have to be carefully and meticulously engineered to provide a design that allows efficient performance of the intended functions. Excellent candidates as drug nanocarriers must be small (less than 100 nm), nontoxic, biodegradable, biocompatible, do not aggregate, avoids the RES and escapes opsonization, noninflammatory, supports prolonged circulation time, and cost effective.[73,77,88,110,119,124,125,138,176,240,271,294,315–321] Many drugs in the market that are now available for human use are already nano-enabled. The ability of these drugs to minimize the side effects that are normally observed in conventional drugs open doors for applications of NMs as safer alternatives to drug delivery.

Aside from the physical and chemical properties including drug-loading to effectively deliver drugs using the NM carrier systems other challenges need further attention. More studies need to focus on the interaction of NMs with their hosts in terms of biodistribution, organ accumulation, degradation while in circulation, damage of cellular structures or inflammatory foreign body effects, and genetic damage. Aggregation or precipitation upon contact with biological fluids in animals or human hosts must be carefully evaluated and its prevention be established to prevent adverse effects. Preliminary studies on possible aggregation in fresh human whole blood and in animals have indicated that some NMs loaded with drugs do not aggregate nor precipitate when the NMs are properly coated with amphiphilic polymer as indicated in Chapter 5. Without the proper coating, the NMs aggregate upon exposure to fresh human whole blood. Such observations need to be prevented if the NMs are to be used for in vivo applications.

Prior to use for in vivo studies, the toxicology of NMs need to be investigated including the possibility of adverse effects if these are to be used as drug nanocarriers.[12,18,25,144,201,202,246,247,322–335] The current level of research and development of some NMs for drug delivery system is still its infancy that more studies need to be conducted very thoroughly. Research on the absorption, distribution, metabolism and elimination (ADME), and drug metabolism and pharmacokinetics (DMPK) must be further elucidated on nanomaterial drug delivery systems in the future before these can be fully trusted and launch for human use.

Depending on their functionalization, biodegradable drug nanocarriers can take a number of different paths within tissues during drug delivery.[144,146,188,290,295,325,336–345] The pharmacokinetics and excretion routes of these nanocarriers demand exhaustive research to clear the path for their human applications. The path that the nano-enabled drugs take after entry into the living system depends on many factors which were discussed in this Chapter 5. Imaging properties may be the most useful characteristics of some NMs for elucidating their ADME and PK during drug delivery. Further investigations on these properties and other modes of detection are important as the NMs enter the realm of human consumption.

NMs are now found as components of FDA approved drugs that are already sold in the market.[312] They are used for easy and efficient delivery of drugs with enhanced therapeutic effects. A few of these examples were discussed Chapter 4, Chapter 5, and in Chapter 7. Drugs that are coated polymer NMs and iron oxide NMs coated with dextran have emerged as very sensitive contrast agents for magnetic resonance imaging (MRI).[6,10,53,54,58,66,90–95,97,102–104,120,137,161,169,183,227,289–295,299,307,312,313,325,346–352] Additionally, several studies in clinical the trials indicate that cancer drugs have also been loaded in nanoparticles for ease of delivery.[56,240,276,350] More studies are underway for the specific targeting of these drugs so that effect on healthy cells can be minimized while focusing the unloading of the drugs on the sick cells such as cancer cells. Other studies have also focused on the use of NMs for eradicating viral infections which have been one of the most difficult challenges of the human population during the last century and into the millennium.[290,295,303,306,309,312] Studies on the use of NMs for the delivery of vaccines especially those diseases that have no existing vaccines in the market have also began to be noticed in the literature.[76,89,114,154,174,196,353]

9.7 NANOMEDICAL DEVICES

NMs when properly combined with biomolecules have found a wide spectrum of applications such as to create novel tissue substitutes, nanorobots, and nanodevices with significantly improved performances.[39,115,187,255,315,354–356] In

Chapter 6, the focus is on the applications of NMs as components or as additives in the design and make-up of various medical devices led to improved biocompatibility and functionality as nanorobots, novel nanochips and nanoimplants serving as tissue substitutes, tissue regeneration, prostheses, tissue engineering, and cell repair.[35,75,80,115,130,148,164,315,354,356-365] Nanosurgery is expected to bring a revolutionary change in terms of neighboring tissue/cell damage during surgery.[75,187,366,367] Nanorobots bring hope to early diagnosis and targeted drug delivery for early cancer treatment. Improvements in implants can reduce cost and provide ease of use to patients while minimizing swelling, toxicity and other side effects. Integration of NMs in implants also allows durability beyond the conventional materials that are currently in use.

Nanorobots are composed of nanoscale or molecular components.[115,315,354,356,357] These devices are injectable in the patient to perform diagnosis or treatment on a cellular level. Treatments with nanorobots involve alterations in structure and composition in the molecular or submolecular level. Nanorobots are used for early diagnosis and targeted drug delivery for cancer therapeutics, nanosized biomedical instrument for surgery, pharmacokinetics, disease monitoring, and improving the affectivity and efficiency of health care.[75,187,366,367]These potential areas of applications leverage the unique nanoscale dimensions of NMs and their various engineering versatilities to be manipulated in order to serve for specific functions. Continued development of more prototypes and more extensive research are necessary to harness the full potential of NMs as medical devices.

Many different kinds of NMs are currently being developed for various nanochips, nanoimplants, and even for stem cell regeneration.[39,75,115,116,187,255,315,354-356,368] These various applications of nanomedical devices hold promise for better diagnosis and improved therapeutics that ultimately benefit the quality of life. Although majority of these applications of NMs in medicine are still in the laboratory, a few are already in full blast clinical use. Some prostheses being used by amputees, scaffolds for tissue regeneration, and some implants currently contain nanomaterial composites. NMs including polymeric NMs, nanocomposites and natural NMs have also been studied for cartilage regeneration. Human cartilage cells attached and proliferated well on hydroxyapatite nanocrystals that were homogeneously dispersed in poly-lactic acid nanocomposites.[39,45,73,123,148,152,162,189,198,359,360,363,365-367,369-373] Titanium NMs with nanometer sized-pores exhibited increased chondrocyte adhesion and migration.[247,355,374,375]

Nanoparticles can be engineered to diagnose conditions and recognize pathogens; identify ideal pharmaceutical agents to treat the condition or pathogens; fuel high-yield production of matched pharmaceuticals (potentially in vivo); locate, attach or enter target tissue, structures or pathogens; and dispense the ideal mass of matched biological compound to the target regions.[6,50,59,77,177,312,376]

An era of advances in the development of processes to integrate nanoscale components into devices at a repeatable, reliable, and at a low cost process needs to emerge.[5,6,39,72,75,77,79,81–87,115,187,196,255,315,354–356,377,378] Large-scale techniques for manufacturing fault-tolerant devices and equivalent lots of NMs will have to be invented. The current widespread medical and nonmedical applications of nanotechnology, we project that its societal impact may be many times greater than that of the microelectronics and computer revolution.

At the rate the rapid research is going, the full potential of nanomedical devices may emerge in the very near future, 5–10 years from now, when the design to construct artificial nanorobots with nanometer-scale is completed. These nanorobots will be prepared through molecular or atomic level assembly and manufacturing techniques to build a molecular device in a structural level by level configuration assembly. This molecular process will involve a repetitious process of layer by layer molecular stacking until the final product is fully assembled. Such a process is yet to be developed and reported in the near future. A few molecular level manufacturing techniques have been demonstrated in the laboratory to date and majority of these apply to NMs synthesis, many of which are still in small-scale level. [143,149,151–153] A few more years is predicted before large-scale processes for QDs, iron oxide, and other NMs can be mastered to reproducibly fabricate stable, uniform, and inexpensive NMs that to appreciably bring the costs down. Lowering the costs of NMs will be followed by more research and faster developments in its medical applications.

9.8 NANOPHARMACOLOGY

The application of nanotechnology for drug design and drug delivery to selected targets for improved pharmacodynamics and kinetic profiles toward safer and effective treatment is the area today that is known as nanopharmacology. It encompasses proper drug engineering design, development, and manufacture of the nanostructured drug or drug carrier for nanoscale molecular targets, drug formulation, and drug release.[9,58,66,77,90,107,169,292,294,308,312,318,379–381] Nanotechnology promises to revolutionize the area of pharmacology owing to the unique size and properties of NMs.

NMs hold promise in improving the curative abilities of various conventional drugs. Nanopharmacology is complicated by the need to establish the behavior of nanoparticles such as QDs, CNTs, AuNPS, IOMNPs, and many more within the traditional pharmacological parameters of absorption, distribution, metabolism and excretion (ADME).[10,58,61,68,89,92,95,97,102,106,108,125,161,169,290,291,298,303,304,306,325,327,346–350,352,357,382] Nanoconstructs, in many cases, have limited metabolism and excretion and persist in biological systems, which gains importance when containing toxic atoms such as cadmium.[18,141,282] This poses a need to carefully examine our common ADME parameters and revise them if necessary.

Absorption into the host system is generally the first hurdle to be overcome which are dependent on route of delivery. Research has established that various nanoparticles can enter an organism through skin absorption, inhalation, oral delivery, and parenteral administration.[9,58,66,77,90,107,169,292,294,308,312,318,379–381] For QDs, the most important route of delivery at present appears to be systemic distribution through parenteral delivery, although occupational and environmental exposures via dermal and inhalation routes are also possible.[12,134,201,202,383] What few studies are available on QD absorption at the organism level primarily utilize parenteral intra-venous (iv) delivery.[12,14,18,134,144,154,200–202,206,207,332,383] QD targeting studies have shown that QDs with targeting functional groups can be accumulated in selected target tissues upon intravenous administration. However, distribution to nontarget tissues in an organism has not been examined and is an area where information is critically needed. Due to the high fluorescence of QDs and the metallic cores, particle deposition within an organism should be readily measurable.

During the past decade, there have been more than 26 FDA approved anticancer drugs for clinical use and other therapeutic agents for various conditions from cardiovascular disease to inflammation.[312] Conventional drugs exhibit therapeutic potential but various limitations hinder clinical translation and disease treatment success. These limitations include the physicochemical properties of the agents that prevent them from being efficiently administered in the molecular form. Majority of the drugs are polycyclic making them insoluble in water. Paclitaxel and dexamethasone have low water solubility (0.0015 mg/mL and 0.1 mg/mL, respectively) making them unacceptable for aqueous intravenous injection.[92,290,295,303,382] A major obstacle that prevents these drugs from reaching their target is the unspecific distribution with only 1 in 10,000 to 1 in 100,000 molecules reaching their intended site of action.[137,213] Hence, a much higher concentration or dosage needs to be administered to attain the desired therapeutic effect with the danger of reaching too close to the toxic level which can therefore, cause toxicity.[12,18,134,144,201,202,332,383] With these factors in mind, it is desirable to alter the drug to include features that would pharmacologically guarantee increased stability, solubility, and specific targeting to the site of action which can be accomplished with engineered NMs. Owing to their unique size and properties, NMs hold promise in improving the therapeutic abilities of various conventional drugs.

The area of medicine in which nanotechnology has contributed the most in the last 15 years is oncology. Liposomes were the most prominent nanocarriers in the treatment of cancer being the first commercially available drug nanocarrier for injectable therapeutics.[102,108,301,347,352,384–393] Liposomal doxorubicin was granted with FDA approval for use against Kaposi's sarcoma in 1990 and was later approved for metastatic breast cancer and recurrent ovarian cancer therapy.[347,394,395] A great variety of nanocarrier based drug delivery systems with various compositions, physicochemical characteristics, geometry and surface functionalizations have been generated and are in different stages of development today.[307,384,385,387,389,391,392,396,397]

Quite a number of nanocarriers for specific drugs are currently undergoing development. These nanocarriers reach the disease through either passive or active mechanisms.[77,107] The liposomes follow the passive mechanism because they utilize the enhanced permeability of the neovasculature to localize into the disease site through enhanced permeation and retention (EPR) mechanism.[93,107,187,360,363,380,386,398–402]

Extravasation of NMs is favored because of the presence of large (several hundred nanometers) vascular fenestrations on newly formed angiogenic vessels. The NMs can have surface modifications with materials such as a polyethylene glycol (PEG) that make the nanocarriers "stealth" eluding uptake by the RES; achieving sufficient prolonged circulation time that improves the chances of reaching and attacking the tumor.[3,4,10,52,71,89,93,167,235,289,290,346,384,403-407] Success in chemistry and materials science yielded several other NMs for drug delivery that includes polymer conjugates, polymer micelles, and dendrimers.[66,82,86,95,97,102,110,154,192,293,303,306,319,352,377,380,399,408,409] Hence, at the onset of NMs applications as drug delivery systems, no active mechanisms of disease site location and therapy were involved. The second generation involves nanodrug delivery systems that are equipped with targeting functionality through careful combination of engineering, protein chemistry, and molecular biology. The active mechanism may result from 1) targeting moiety on the nanocarriers through the presence of specific molecular recognition molecules to receptors that are overexpressed on the tumor cells or adjacent blood vessels (such as Ab conjugated NMs) or 2) a possibility for active/triggered release of the payload at the diseased location (e.g. magnetic nanoparticles).[64,65] Thus, the current NMs for drug delivery are superior to their precursors through the use of targeting moieties, possibility of remote activation, and environmentally sensitive components, bringing additional degrees of sophistication in design that promises increased success in accomplishing the intentions. The presence of logic embedded vectors (LEVs) add further assurance for optimum accomplishment of the intended applications.[410] LEVs are specifically engineered to avoid biological barriers, where the functions of biorecognition, cytotoxicity, and no susceptibility to biobarrier are eliminated through careful manipulation and efficient engineering.[411] By design, the LEV is a drug delivery system that will be able to go through the vasculature after intravenous administration, to reach the desired tumor site at full dosage of the drug, and to selectively kill cancer cells with the loaded drugs and at the same time have minimal harmful side effects.[412-414] These LEVs are, theoretically as of now, useful also for advanced therapy and imaging with immense potential for enhanced drug delivery that will bear a high impact on the future of personalized medicine that is one of the priorities of nanopharmacology.

As all other areas of medicine that had been so far discussed, pharmacology has been revolutionized by this nanotechnology era that sprouted at the end of the twentieth century and has boomed toward the beginning of the twenty-first century. Nanomaterial research and development continue to be engineered in various was to diagnose disease and health conditions; to recognize pathogenic infections; to locate, attach, and penetrate target tissue or structures or pathogens; and dispense the payload of drugs or biological compound to the targeted regions of the body-the area now known as nanopharmacology.

Nanopharmacology, although still in its early stages, has witnessed an overhauling of the conventional pharmacology.[10,89,95-97,120,161,296,297,311,341,346,408] This overhaul are manifested through drug engineering design and development, manufacture of nano-enabled drug or drug carriers, and the application of nanoscale molecular species in drug formulations and drug release. The nanomaterial engineering concepts and processes are geared toward achieving the promises in improving the therapeutic effects of conventional drugs as well as to harness the diagnostic efficacy of modern diagnostic instruments.[6,50,59,77,177,312,376] Multiple NMs have been complexed to drugs and various biomolecules with the goal of improving the diagnostic and therapeutic capabilities for various diseases.[9,58,66,77,90,107,169,294,308,312,318,380]

A section of nanopharmacology that recently emerged as a result of the versatility of some NMs is the area of "theranostics" that refers to the combination of diagnostics and therapeutics.[415,416] The multifunctional capabilities of NMs allows for a combination of detection and therapeutic functions in a single nanoparticle. This integration can make use of imaging detection of therapeutic delivery as well as perform informed observation to assess the treatment efficacy. The NMs that are already used as imaging agents can be readily adopted into the theranostics agents' category by loading therapeutic agents and/or diagnostic functions on them.[2,64,65,68,116,120,143,224] Combining both the targeting and therapeutic requirements in single specially designed and engineered NMs brings both treatment and monitoring of treatment efficacy closer together that will eventually bring benefit to the patient.

9.9 NANOTOXICOLOGY

Nanotoxicology is a new area of study that deals with the toxicological profiles of NMs.[12,18,24,25,31,33,44,118,133,134,146,185,186,188,246,247,322,323,325,329–331,333,335,337,339, 341,342,349,417–424] Compared with the larger counterparts, the quantum size effects and large surface area to volume ratio brings NMs their unique properties that may or may not be toxic to living things.[12,18,24,25,31,33,44,118,133,134,146,185,186,188,246, 247,322,323,325,329–331,333,335,337,339,341,342,349,417–424] It is nanotoxicology that will deal with elucidating how different NMs affect living systems because inert elements like gold can become active at nanoscale dimensions.[55,186,336,425] Nanotoxicity studies are intended to determine whether and to what extent the properties of gold and other materials in the nanoscale dimensions may pose a threat to the environment and to living things.

Chapter 8 is one of the most important chapters of this book because it focuses on the safety and toxicity of the various NMs. Governments awareness of the possible benefits as well as the dangers of exposure to NMs from consumer products have led to various guidelines worldwide.[121] Characterization of the various properties of the NMs have been recognized as essential for the evaluation of the possible effects on health and environmental safety.

The nanotechnology industry has shown an industrial revolution over the last few years, a trend which is more than likely to continue into the future. Unfortunately, the exponential progress in nanotechnology has exceeded the advances of research on the impact of NMs on living systems especially on human health. To date, we have barely scratched the lessons to learn and to comprehend the effects of these tiny molecules on cells, tissues, and whole organisms.

To complete existing knowledge about the interactions between the NMs and the biological systems, nanotoxicology deals with the study of their toxic or biological effects. Because NMs belong to a new class of materials, progress in this new discipline relies largely on developing methodology to characterize NMs in biological samples, quantify them in living systems, study their uptake, translocation, biodistribution, accumulation, and chemical status in vitro and in vivo.[18,24,31,33,134,144,146,186,201,246,322,323,328,329,331,333–335,337,340–342,349,419] In addition, the biochemical pathways and biomolecules that are directly or indirectly affected by their presence in a living system need to be established both short term and long term in order to understand possible consequences when they are used for medical applications. Appropriate analytical techniques and their application to the study of the toxicological activities of NMs need to be developed to provide appropriate and powerful means for characterizing the toxic effects or biological behaviors in biological systems.

Nanotoxicology addresses the toxicology profiles of NMs which appear to have unusual toxicity effects that are not observed with larger particles. The NMs of interest in this book are those which are deliberately produced for medical applications such as engineered CNTs, QDs, iron oxide magnetic nanoparticles, liposomes, titanium oxide, and many more. A few of these NMs such as gold, silver, titanium dioxide, alumina, metal oxides, liposomes, polymers, and CNTs have been studied in terms of toxicity in a limited manner. Some NMs exhibit size dependent pathogenic effects that are different from larger particles. NMs have larger surface area to mass ratios which may be responsible for ease of penetration of cells and tissues or cells that in some cases may lead to the release of immune response.[18,44,144,146,186,188,332–335,345,420,421,423,424] Some NMs exhibit the ability to translocate from solution into cells or even transcend the blood brain barrier.[238,426] This accelerated the studies on nanoparticle toxicology study in the brain, blood, liver, skin, and gut.[58,72,88,91,128,161,169,289,297,307,313,346,351–353,427]

The rapid growth of medical applications of NMs calls for concerns about the potential health and environmental risks related to the use and widespread production required by the demands to support this outburst in nanotechnology. Multiple areas of concern related with the usage of NMs including the deposition and clearing, biocompatibility, systemic translocation and body distribution of NPs, intestinal tract involvement, and direct effects on the central nervous system have been studied so far. The different physicochemical and structural properties of NMs that result from their nanoscale size can be sued to account for a number of material interactions that can lead to toxic effects. Studies have shown that NMs can have pronounced environmental effects even at very low aqueous concentrations.[113] As an example, the use of CdSe QDs in humans may be limited because these contains the heavy metals cadmium which are reportedly toxic to cells at concentrations as low as 10 ug/mL.[12,14,18,129,134,144,201,202,332] The various properties of the QD such as its size, charge, concentration, capping material, functional groups, and mechanical stability have been studied as possible determining factors in toxicity.

Some NMs have been demonstrated to possess health and environmental hazards.[12,24,33,44,55,118,134,144,146,185,186,188,201,202,224,242,246,247,323,330,336,337,419,420,423,424,428,429] Hence, there is a need for NM hazard identification process. But, the process for such identification is not yet in place therefore, a case by case approach is still the only approach available for the risk assessment of NMs.

9.10 GOVERNMENT NANOTOXICITY REGULATIONS

In as much as NMs can bring enormous benefits to medicine, various governments have also become more aware of the possible dangers of exposure to NMs that are found in various consumer products.[74,376] This awareness has led to the creation or drafting of various regulatory guidelines worldwide. This has also led to the awareness for the need to properly establish the various properties and toxicity profiles of NMs as essential conditions for the evaluation of possible effects on health and environmental safety.

To date, knowledge on the presence of NMs in any commercial package rely only on the information provided by the manufacturers. There is still no set-standard in detecting or quantifying the presence of NMs that are shipped from one place to another or from one country to another. In addition, the detection of NMs that are added as components of consumer products suffers from the difficulty in discriminating between the background signals and added NMs. This is also complicated by the coating proteins and other biomolecules on NMs that are exposed to biological matrix. In addition, exposure estimation is also hampered by lack of information on product use and use of multiple products containing NMs.

Different regulatory bodies such as the United States Environmental Protection Agency (US EPA), the Food and Drug Administration (US FDA), and the Health and Consumer Protection Directorate of the European Commission have initiated action regarding the potential risks from NMs.[74] The challenge for regulation is whether a standard system of evaluating the risk to NMs can be developed to identify NMs and the toxicity of their formulations.[229] Currently, there is no authorized body to regulate nanotech-based products and there are also no nanotoxicity standards to follow or toxicity regulations in place to enforce.[430] There are non-nanotechnology specific regulatory agencies that cover some products and processes under existing regulations which are insufficient for the regulation of NMs and nano-enabled products.[431–434]An example is titanium dioxide (TiO_2) that is used in sunscreen. The US FDA reviewed the immediate health effects of exposure to this NM but did not review its impacts for aquatic ecosystems when the sunscreen rubs off, nor did the EPA, or any other agency.[435–438] Similarly, the Australian Therapeutic Goods Administration (TGA) approved the use of nanoparticles in sunscreens (without imposing its inclusion in the package label). Short sighted decision of this type do not consider prolonged use that may or may not be appropriate at this point in time because of our lack of knowledge about the long term impacts of NMs to the environment and to biological systems.

In April 20, 2012, the US FDA addressed the use of NMs in food and cosmetics.[435-438] The two draft guidance documents are entitled "Guidance for Industry: Assessing the Effects of Significant Manufacturing Process Changes, including Emerging Technologies, on the Safety and Regulatory Status of Food Ingredients and Food Contact Substances, Including Food Ingredients that are Color Additives" and "Guidance for Industry: Safety of Nanomaterials in Cosmetic Products." The draft on food outlines the factors that should be considered when determining whether changes in manufacturing processes such as nanotechnology will result in a significant change that may affect the identity of the food substance, affect the safety of the use of the food substance, affect the regulatory status of the use of the food substance, or needs a regulatory submission to FDA. This was similarly done on the draft guidance on cosmetics with legal requirements for nanomaterial-based cosmetics that are the same as those for conventional cosmetics. The draft suggests the modification of existing methods or the development of new methods of safety assessments of cosmetic products containing NMs. The US FDA is investing in an FDA-wide nanotechnology regulatory science program to enhance its scientific capabilities and to develop necessary data and tools to identify properties of NMs as well as to assess possible impacts on products.

In January of 2009, the European Commission Directorate General for Health and Consumers released their report which recognized the current infancy of the procedures for assessing the potential risks of engineered NMs on humans and the environment.[439] Like the FDA draft guidances, the EC recognized the importance of proper characterization of NMs to gather information that can be used as the basis for the safety evaluation and the material safety data sheet (MSDS).[435-438,440] The need for reference NMs is indicated to allow the assessment of fate, behavior as well as effects, that could be related to the properties and characteristics.

With governments adopting draft guidance on their way to regulations for NMs use and applications, challenges still exist in their implementations. The need to characterize and establish the presence of NMs in consumer products has to be addressed. From nanomaterial and nano-enabled products characterization to safety evaluation, the challenges that need to be properly addressed are the absence of well-defined parameters to measure and standardize test protocols for the identification of reference materials that will be used as standards to carry out the evaluations. The health and environmental hazards of NMs have been demonstrated for a variety of manufactured NMs that may be toxic to humans and the environment. But, the knowledge on the presence of NMs in a container currently relies only on information provided by the manufacturers. The detection of NMs in consumer products suffers from the difficulty in discriminating between the background signals and added NMs which is further complicated by the coating proteins and other biomolecules after these are exposed to biological matrix. Ultimately, estimation of human exposure is hampered by lack of information on product use and the use of multiple products containing NMs. Thus, there is an urgent need for consumer product evaluation of NMs content to be rapidly detected and its hazard easily identified. To date, a case by case approach is still the only approach available for the risk assessment of NMs.

9.11 PATENT LANDSCAPE

With the projected market and impact in the health and life sciences, the patent landscape in nanotechnology is gaining much attention worldwide.[441–444] Market projections for NMs outweigh a lot of existing conventional industries creating investment interest of exorbitant quantities. Much more research and specifications in nanotechnology needs to be in place in order that faster reviews of patents with less overlap can be issued. Various activities are soaring worldwide as shown in the unprecedented increase in patents from different parts of the world with the US leading the pack.

As in any new and emerging technology, the current state of intellectual property related to nanotechnology is in chaos. It is very different from existing technologies that broad patents on NMs, tools, and processes have been granted too early. New patent applications have led to rejections of valid claims and the issuance of broad-overlapping claims. These have been due to several factors that are discussed in Chapter 8.

The identification of a new class of patents specifically assigned to nanotechnology in 2004, USPTO class 977 under 35 USC §8 (Classification of Patents), the European Patent Office (EPO) has placed a Y01 N for nanotechnology, and the International Patent Classification has given it under the B82B class has improved the patent scenario.[441–444] The Japan Patent Office (JPO) have also made efforts to improve their classification systems to collect all nanotechnology-related patents in one single patent class under the JPO created ZNM.[441] Databases have also been created that contains keywords that are used by reviewers to relate the patent applications to nanotechnology.

To date, the nanotechnology patent applications worldwide showed a steady increase in the United States and the European Union.[441] The nanotechnology patents of US origin accounts for additional 3700 nanotechnology patents per year, or by 230% that may be attributed to the upsurge in the US nanotechnology R&D budget from \$116 M in 1997 to \$270 M in 2000 and \$960 M in 2004.[441] In 2003, the biggest number of patents in nanotechnology is held by US (61% of the total of 8630), followed by Japan (10.9%), Germany (8.1%), Canada (2.9%) and France (2.2%) with substantial activities from Korea, Netherlands, Ireland, and China.[441]

As predicted by a market research report wrote that sales of products incorporating emerging nanotechnology will increase from <0.1% of global manufacturing output today to 15% in 2014, totaling \$2.6 T.[112,445,446] These predictions indicates that nanotechnology's economic effect will come from the application of NMs and not the raw NMs. The report projects that 16% of health care and life sciences will incorporate nanotechnologies by 2014.[112,445,446] With the diversity of NMs applications in medicine and the life sciences, potential investment activity will upsurge causing the need for patents to be in place.

Patents in the applications of NMs in medicine are vital to realize its promising potential and to move beyond academic research.

REFERENCES

1. Shang, L.; Dong, S. Sensitive Detection of Cysteine Based Fluorescent Silver Clusters. *Biosens. Bioelectron.* **2009,** *24,* 1569–1573.
2. Aguilar, Z.; Xu, H.; Jones, B.; Dixon, J.; Wang, A. Semi Conductor Quantum Dots for Cell Imaging. *Mater. Res. Soc. Symp. Proc.* **2010,** *1237,* 1237-TT1206-1201.
3. Aqil, A.; Qiu, H.; Greish, J.; Jerome, R.; De Pauw, E.; Jerome, C. Coating of Gold Nanoparticles by Thermosensitive Poly (*N*-isopropylacrylamide) End-capped by Biotin. *Polymer* **2008,** *49,* 1145–1153.
4. Arnedo, A.; Irache, J. M.; Merodio, M.; Espuelas, M.; Millan, S. Albumin Nanoparticles Improved the Stability, Nuclear Accumulation and Anticytomegaloviral Activity of a Phosphodiester Oligonucleotide. *J. Control. Release* **2004,** *94,* 217–227.
5. Bharali, D.; Khalil, M.; Gurbuz, M.; Simone, T.; Mousa, S. Nanoparticles and cancer therapy: a concise review with emphasis on dendrimers. *Int. J. Nanomedicine* **2009,** *4,* 1–7.
6. Brigger, I.; Dubernet, C.; Couvreur, P. Nanoparticles in Cancer Therapy and Diagnosis. *Adv. Drug Deliv. Rev.* **2002,** *54,* 631–651.
7. Li, J.; Zhao, X.; Zhao, Y.; Gu, Z. Quantum-Dot-Coated Encoded Silica Colloidal Crystals Beads for Multiplex Coding. *Chem. Commun.* **2009,** 2329–2331.
8. Moghimi, S. M.; Hunter, A. C.; Murray, J. C. Nanomedicine: Current Status and Future Prospects. *FASEB J.* **2005,** *19,* 311–330.
9. Mueller, R. H.; Schwarz, C.; Mehnert, W.; Lucks, J. S. Production of Solid Lipid Nanoparticles (SLN) for Controlled Drug Delivery. *Proc. Int. Symp. Control. Release Bioact. Mater.* **1993,** *20,* 480–481.
10. Akerman, M. E.; Chan, W. C.; Laakkonen, P.; Bhatia, S. N.; Ruoslahti, E. Nanocrystal Targeting In Vivo. *Proc. Natl. Acad. Sci. USA* **2002,** *99,* 12617–12621.
11. Ballou, B.; Lagerholm, B. C.; Ernst, L. A.; Bruchez, M. P.; Waggoner, A. S. Noninvasive Imaging of Quantum Dots in Mice. *Bioconjug. Chem.* **2004,** *15,* 79–86.
12. Bottrill, M.; Green, M. Some Aspects of Quantum Dot Toxicity. *Chem. Commun.* **2011,** *47,* 7039–7050.
13. Byers, R.; Hitchman, E. Quantum Dots Brighten Biological Imaging. *Prog. Histochem. Cytochem.* **2011,** *45,* 201–237.
14. Parak, W. J.; Pellegrino, T.; Plank, C. Labelling of Cells with Quantum Dots. *Nanotechnology* **2005,** *16,* R9–R25.
15. Peng, X.; Manna, L.; Yang, W.; Wickham, J.; Scher, E.; Kadavanich, A.; Alivisatos, A. P. Shape Control of CdSe Nanocrystals. *Nature* **2000,** *404,* 59–61.
16. Resch-Genger, U.; Grabolle, M.; Cavaliere-Jaricot, S.; Nitschke, R.; Nann, T. Quantum Dots Versus Organic Dyes as Fluorescent Labels. *Nat. Methods* **2008,** *5,* 763–775.
17. Smith, A. M.; Gao, X.; Nie, S. Quantum Dot Nanocrystals for *in vivo* Molecular and Cellular Imaging. *Photochem. Photobiol.* **2004,** *80,* 377–385.
18. Su, Y.; Hu, M.; Fan, C.; He, Y.; Li, Q.; Li, W., et al. The Cytotoxicity of CdTe Quantum Dots and the Relative Contributions from Released Cadmium Ions and Nanoparticle Properties. *Biomaterials* **2010,** *31,* 4829–4834.
19. Willard, D.; Carillo, L.; Jung, J.; van Orden, A. CdSe–ZnS Quantum Dots as Resonance Energy Transfer Donors in A Model Protein–Protein Binding Assay. *Nano Lett.* **2001,** *1.*

20. Xu, H.; Aguilar, Z.; Waldron, J.; Wei, H.; Wang, Y. Application of Semiconductor Quantum Dots for Breast Cancer Cell Sensing, 2009 Biomedical Engineering and Informatics. *IEEE Comput. Soc. BMEI* **2009**, *1*, 516–520.

21. Xu, H.; Aguilar, Z.; Wang, A. Quantum Dot-Based Sensors for Proteins. *ECS Trans.* **2010**, *25*, 1–10.

22. Armentano, I.; Alvarez-Pérez, M. A.; Carmona-Rodríguez, B.; Gutiérrez-Ospina, I.; Kenny, J. M.; Arzate, H. Analysis of the Biomineralization Process on SWNTCOOH and F-SWNT Films. *Mater. Sci. Eng. C* **2008**, *28*, 1522–1529.

23. Bakry, R.; Vallant, R. M.; Najam-ul-hag, M.; Rainer, M.; Szabo, Z.; Huck, C. W.; Bonn, G. K. Medicinal Applications of Fullerenes. *Int. J. Nanomedicine* **2007**, *2*, 639–649.

24. Belyanskaya, L.; Weigel, S.; Hirsch, C.; Tobler, U.; Krug, H. F.; Wick, P. Effects of Carbon Nanotubes on Primary Neurons and Glial Cells. *Neurotoxicology* **2009**, *30*, 702–711.

25. Chan, W. C. W. In *Bio-Applications of Nanoparticles*; Springer Science + Business Media: New York, 2007.

26. Correa-Duarte, M. A.; Wagner, N.; Rojas-Chapana, J.; Morsczeck, C.; Thie, M.; Giersig, M. Fabrication and Biocompatibility of Carbon Nanotube-Based 3D Networks as Scaffolds for Cell Seeding and Growth. *Nano Lett.* **2004**, *4*, 2233–2236.

27. Dai, H.; Shim, M.; Chen, R. J.; Li, Y.; Kam, N. W. S. Functionalization of Carbon Nanotubes for Biocompatibility and Biomolecular Recognition. *Nano Lett.* **2002**, *2*, 285–288.

28. Dumortier, H.; Lacotte, S.; Pastorin, G.; Marega, R.; Wu, W.; Bonifazi, D., et al. Functionalized Carbon Nanotubes are Non-Cytotoxic and Preserve the Functionality of Primary Immune Cells. *Nano Lett.* **2006**, *6*, 1522–1528.

29. Gao, X. P.; Qin, X.; Wu, F.; Liu, H.; Lan, Y.; Fan, S. S.; Yuan, H. T.; Song, D. Y.; Shen, P. W. Synthesis of Carbon Nanotubes by Catalytic Decomposition of Methane using LaNi$_5$ Hydrogen Storage Alloy as Catalyst. *Chem. Phys. Lett.* **2000**, *327*, 271–276.

30. Guldi, D. M.; Prato, M. Excited-state Properties of C(60) Fullerene Derivatives. *Acc. Chem. Res.* **2000**, *33*, 695–703.

31. Hirano, S.; Kanno, S.; Furuyama, A. Multi-walled Carbon Nanotubes Injure the Plasma Membrane of Macrophages. *Toxicol. Appl. Pharmacol.* **2008**, *232*, 244–251.

32. Iijima, S.; Brabec, C.; Maiti, A.; Bernholc, J. Structural Flexibility of Carbon nanotubes. *J. Chem. Phys.* **1996**, *104*, 2089–2092.

33. Kolosnjaj, J.; Szwarc, H.; Mousa, F. Toxicity Studies of Carbon Nanotubes. *Adv. Exp. Med. Biol.* **2007**, *620*, 181–204.

34. Koruga, D.; Matija, L.; Misic, N.; Rakin, P. Fullerene C60: Properties and Possible Applications. *Trans. Tech. Publ. Mat. Sci. Forum* **1996**, *214*, 49–56.

35. Mamedov, A. A.; Kotov, N. A.; Prato, M.; Guldi, D. M.; Wicksted, J. P.; Hirsch, A. Molecular Design of Strong Single-Wall Carbon Nanotube/Polyelectrolyte Multilayer Composites. *Nat. Mater.* **2002**, *1*, 190–194.

36. Mattson, M. P.; Haddon, R. C.; Rao, A. M. Molecular Functionalization of Carbon Nanotubes and use as Substrates for Neuronal Growth. *J. Mol. Neurosci.* **2000**, *14*, 175–182.

37. Mwenifumbo, S.; Shaffer, M. S.; Stevens, M. M. Exploring Cellular Behaviour with Multi-Walled Carbon Nanotube Constructs. *J. Mater. Chem.* **2007**, *17*, 1894–1902.

38. Nasibulin, A. G.; Moisala, A.; Jiang, H.; Kauppinen, E. I. Carbon Nanotube Synthesis By a Novel Aerosol Method. *J. Nanopart. Res.* **2006**, *8*, 465–475.

39. Sun, L. F.; Liu, Z. Q.; Ma, X. C.; Zhong, Z. Y.; Tang, S. B.; Xiong, ZT., et al. Growth of Carbon Nanotube Arrays using the Existing Array as a Substrate and their Raman Characterization. *Chem. Phys. Lett.* **2001**, *340*, 222–226.

40. Tokudome, H.; Miyauchi, M. Electrochromism of Titanate-Based Nanotubes. *Angew Chem. Int. Ed.* **2005,** *44,* 1974–1977.

41. Tran, P. A.; Zhang, L.; Webster, T. J. Carbon Nanofibers and Carbon Nanotubes in Regenerative Medicine. *Adv. Drug. Deliv. Rev.* **2009,** *61,* 1097–1114.

42. Yang, R.; Jin, J.; Chen, Y.; Shao, N.; Kang, H.; Xiao, Z.; Tang, Z.; Wu, Y.; Zhu, Z.; Tan, W. Carbon Nanotube-Quenched Fluorescent Oligonucleotides: Probes that Fluoresce upon Hybridization. *J. Am. Chem. Soc.* **2008,** *130,* 8351–8358.

43. Zagal, J. H.; Griveau, Z.; Nyokong, T.; Bedioui, F. Carbon Nanotubes, Phthalocyanines and Porphyrins: Attractive Hybrid Materials for Electrocatalysis and Electroanalysis. *J. Nanosci. Nanotechnol.* **2009,** *9,* 2201–2214.

44. Zhang, L. W.; Zeng, L.; Barron, A. L.; Monteiro-Riviere, N. A. Biological Interactions of Functionalized Single-Wall Carbon Nanotubes In Human Epidermal Keratinocytes. *Int. J. Toxicol.* **2007,** *26,* 103–113.

45. Zhang, X.; Liu, T.; Sreekumar, T. V.; Kumar, S.; Moore, V. C.; Hauge, RH., et al. Poly(Vinylalcohol)/SWNT Composite Film. *Nano Lett.* **2003,** *3,* 1285–1288.

46. Doering, W. E.; Piotti, M. E.; Natan, M. J.; Freeman, R. G. SERS as a Foundation for Nanoscale, Optically Detected Biological Labels. *Adv. Mater.* **2007,** *19,* 3100–3108.

47. Geiber, D.; Charbonnière, L. J.; Ziessel, R. F.; Butlin, N. G.; Löhmannsröben, H.; Hildebrandt, N. Quantum Dot Biosensors for Ultrasensitive Multiplexed Diagnostics. *Angew Chem. Int. Ed.* **2010,** *49,* 1–6.

48. Jin, T.; Fujii, F.; Sakata, H.; Tamura, M.; Kinjo, M. Amphiphilic Psulfonatocalix[4]arene-coated Quantum Dots for the Optical Detection of the Neurotransmitter Acetylcholine. *Chem. Commun.* **2005,** 4300–4302.

49. Wang, Z.; Levy, R.; Fernig, D.; Brust, M. Kinase-catalyzed Modification of Gold Nanoparticles: A New Approach to Colorimetric Kinase Activity Screening. *J. Am. Chem. Soc.* **2006,** *128,* 2214–2215.

50. Yun, Y.; Eteshola, E.; Bhattacharya, A.; Dong, Z.; Shim, J.; Conforti, L.; Kim, D.; Schulz, M.; Ahn, C.; Watts, N. Tiny Medicine: Nanomaterial-Based Biosensors. *Sensors* **2009,** *9,* 9275–9299.

51. Efros, A. L.; Rosen, M. The Electronic Structure of Semiconductor Nanocrystals. *Ann. Rev. Mater. Sci.* **2000,** *30,* 475–521.

52. Arruebo, M.; Fernandez-Pacheco, R.; Ricardo-Ibarra, M.; Santamaria, J. Magnetic Nanoparticles for Drug Delivery. *Nanoday* **2007,** *2,* 22–32.

53. Cao, H.; Gan, J.; Wang, S., et al. Novel Silica-Coated Iron–Carbon Composite Particles and their Targeting Effect as a Drug Carrier. *J. Biomed. Mater. Res.* **2008,** *86,* 671–677.

54. Gang, J.; Park, S. B.; Hyung, W.; Choi, E. H.; Wen, J.; Kim, H. S.; Shul, Y. G.; Haam, S.; Song, S. Y. Magnetic Poly Epsilon-Caprolactone Nanoparticles Containing Fe_3O_4 and Gemcitabine Enhance Anti-Tumor Effect in Pancreatic Cancer Xenograft Mouse Model. *J. Drug. Target.* **2007,** *15,* 445–453.

55. Goon, I. Y.; Lai, L. M. H.; Lim, M.; Munroe, P.; Gooding, J. J.; Amal, R. Fabrication and Dispersion of Gold-Shell-Protected Magnetite Nanoparticles: Systematic Control using Polyethyleneimine. *Chem. Mater.* **2009,** *21,* 673–681.

56. Haun, J. B.; Yoon, T.; Lee, H. J.; Weissleder, R. Magnetic Nanoparticle Biosensors. *Wiley Interdiscip. Rev. Nanomed. Nanobiotechnol.* **2010,** *2,* 291–304.

57. Klostergaard, J.; Bankson, J.; Woodward, W.; Gibson, D.; Seeney, C. Magnetically Responsive Nanoparticles for Vectored Delivery of Cancer Therapeutics. *AIP Conf. Proc.* **2011,** *1311,* 382–387.

58. Mejias, R.; Perez-Yague, S.; Gutierez, L.; Cabrera, L. I.; Spada, R.; Acedo, P.; Serna, C. J.; Lazaro, F. J.; Villanueva, A.; Morales, M. P.; Barber, D. F. Dimercaptosuccinic Acid-Coated Magnetite Nanoparticles for Magnetically Guided In Vivo Delivery of Interferon Gamma for Cancer Immunotherapy. *Biomaterials* **2011,** *32,* 2938–2952.

59. Osterfeld, S. J.; Yu, H.; Gaster, R. S.; Caramuta, S.; Xu, L.; Han, S.; Hall, D. A.; Wilson, R. J.; Sun, S.; White, R. L.; Davis, R. W.; Pourmand, N.; Wang, S. X. Multiplex Protein Assays Based on Real-Time Magnetic Nanotag Sensing. *Proc. Nat. Acad. Sci. USA* **2008,** *105,* 20637–20640.

60. Philipse, A. P.; Vanbruggen, M. P. B.; Pathmamanoharan, C. Magnetic Silica Dispersions — Preparation and Stability of Surface-Modified Silica Particles with a Magnetic Core. *Langmuir* **1994,** *10,* 92–99.

61. Tietze, R.; Schreiber, E.; Lyer, S.; Alexiou, C. Mitoxantrone Loaded Superparamagnetic Nanoparticles for Drug Targeting: A Versatile and Sensitive Method for Quantification of Drug Enrichment in Rabbit Tissues using HPLC–UV. *J. Biomed. Biotechol.* **2010.**

62. Wilhelm, C.; Gazeau, F. Universal Cell Labelling with Anionic Magnetic Nanoparticles. *Biomaterials* **2008,** *29,* 3161–3174.

63. Xu, H.; Aguilar, Z. P.; Yang, L.; Kuang, M.; Duan, H.; Xiong, Y.; Wei, H.; Wang, A. Y. Antibody Conjugated Magnetic Iron Oxide Nanoparticles for Cancer Cell Separation in Fresh Whole Blood. *Biomaterials* **2011,** *32,* 9758–9765.

64. Yang, L.; Cao, Z.; Sajja, S.; Mao, H.; Wang, L.; Geng, H.; Xu, H.; Jiang, T.; Wood, W.; Nie, S.; Wang, A. Development of Receptor Targeted Iron Oxide Nanoparticles for Efficient Drug Delivery and Tumor Imaging. *J. Biomed. Nanotechol.* **2008,** *4,* 1–11.

65. Yang, L.; Peng, X.; Wang, Y.; Wang, X.; Cao, Z.; Ni, C.; Karna, P.; Zhang, X.; Wood, W.; Gao, X.; Nie, S.; Mao, H. Receptor-Targeted Nanoparticles for In Vivo Imaging of Breast Cancer. *Clin. Cancer Res.* **2009,** *15,* 4722–4732.

66. Govender, T.; Stolnik, S.; Garnett, M. C.; Illum, L.; Davis, S. S. PLGA Nanoparticles Prepared by Nanoprecipitation: Drug Loading and Release Studies of A Water Soluble Drug. *J. Control. Release* **1999,** *57,* 171–185.

67. Mitchell, G.; Mirkin, C.; Letsinger, R. Programmed Assembly of DNA Functionalized Quantum Dots. *J. Am. Chem. Soc.*1999, *121,* 8122–8123.

68. Sajja, H.; East, M.; Mao, H.; Wang, Y.; Nie, S.; Yang, L. Development of Multifunctional Nanoparticles for Targeted Drug Delivery and Noninvasive Imaging of Therapeutic Effect. *Curr. Drug. Discov. Technol.* **2009,** *6,* 43–51.

69. Susumu, K.; Uyeda, H.; Medintz, I.; Pons, T.; Delehanty, J.; Mattoussi, H. Enhancing the Stability and Biological Functionalities of Quantum Dots via Compact Multifunctional Ligands. *J. Am. Chem. Soc.* **2007,** *129,* 13987–13996.

70. Xie, J.; Peng, S.; Brower, N.; Pourmand, N.; Wang, S. X.; Sun, S. One-pot Synthesis of monodisperse Iron Oxide Nanoparticles for Potential Biomedical Applications. *Pure Appl. Chem.* **2006,** *78,* 1003–1014.

71. Barrett, T.; Ravizzini, G.; Choyke, P.; Kobayashi, H. Dendrimers in Medical Nanotechnology. *IEEE Eng. Med. Biol. Mag.* **2009,** *28,* 12–22.

72. Battah, S.; Balaratnam, S.; Casas, A.; O'Neill, S.; Edwards, C.; Batlle, A.; Dobbin, P.; Mac-Robert, A. Macromolecular Delivery of 5-aminolaevulinic Acid for Photodynamic Therapy using Dendrimer Conjugates. *Mol. Cancer Ther.* **2007,** *6,* 876.

73. Esumi, K.; Matsumoto, T.; Seto, Y.; Yoshimura, T. Preparation of Goldgold/Silver dendrimer Nanocomposites in the Presence of Benzoin in Ethanol by UV Irradiation. *J. Colloid Interface Sci.* **2005,** *284,* 199.

74. Jia, L. Global Government Investments in Nanotechnologies. *Curr. Nanosci.* **2005,** *1,* 263–266.

75. Khawaja, A. M. Review: The Legacy of Nanotechnology: Revolution and Prospects in Neurosurgery. *Int. J. Surg.* **2011,** *9,* 608–614.

76. Peek, L. J.; Middaugh, C. R.; Berkland, C. Nanotechnology in Vaccine Delivery. *Adv. Drug. Deliv. Rev.* **2008,** *60,* 915–928.

77. Surendiran, A.; Sandhiya, S.; Pradhan, S. C.; Adithan, C. Novel Applications of Nanotechnology in Medicine. *Indian J. Med. Res.* **2009,** *130,* 689–701.

78. Tekade, R.; Kumar, P.; Jain, N. Dendrimers in Oncology: An Expanding Horizon. *Chem. Rev.* **2009,** *109,* 49–87.

79. van Nostrum, C. Polymeric Micelles to Deliver Photosensitizers for Photodynamic Therapy. *Adv. Drug Deliv. Rev.* **2004,** *56,* 9–12.

80. Wang, S.; Cai, L. *Polymers for Fabricating nerve Conduits.* 2010, June 16 2012 [cited 2010].

81. de Jong, S.; Chikh, G.; Sekirov, L.; Raney, S.; Semple, S.; Klimuk, S., et al. Encapsulation in Liposomal Nanoparticles Enhances the Immunostimulatory, Adjuvant and Anti-Tumor Activity of Subcutaneously Administered CpG ODN. *Cancer Immunol. Immunother.* **2007,** *56,* 1251–1264.

82. Goyal, A. K.; Khatri, K.; Mishra, N.; Mehta, A.; Vaidya, B.; Tiwari, S., et al. Aquasomes-a Nanoparticulate Approach for the Delivery of Antigen. *Drug. Dev. Ind. Pharm.* **2008,** *34,* 1297–1305.

83. Klippstein, R.; Pozo, D. Nanotechnology-based Manipulation of Dendritic Cells for Enhanced Immunotherapy Strategies. *Nanomedicine* **2010,** *6,* 523–529.

84. Kortylewski, M.; Swiderski, P.; Herrmann, A.; Wang, L.; Kowolik, C.; Kujawski, M., et al. In Vivo Delivery of siRNA to Immune cells by Conjugation to a TLR9 Agonist Enhances Antitumor Immune Responses. *Nat. Biotechnol.* **2009,** *27,* 925–932.

85. O'Hagan, D. T.; Singh, M. Microparticles as Vaccine Adjuvants and Delivery Systems. *Expert Rev. Vaccines* **2003,** *2,* 269–283.

86. Pandey, R. S.; Sahu, S.; Sudheesh, M. S.; Madan, J.; Kumar, M.; Dixit, V. K. Carbohydrate Modified Ultrafine Ceramic Nanoparticles for Allergen Immunotherapy. *Int. Immunopharmacol.* **2011,** *11,* 925–931.

87. Van Der Lubben, IM.; Konings, F. A.; Borchard, G.; Verhoef, J. C.; Junginger-He, C. In Vivo Uptake of Chitosan Microparticles by Murine Peyer's Patches: Visualization Studies using Confocal Laser Scanning Microscopy and Immunohistochemistry. *J. Drug Target.* **2001,** *9,* 39–47.

88. Aguilar, Z.; Aguilar, Y.; Xu, H.; Jones, B.; Dixon, J.; Xu, H.; Wang, A. Nanomaterials in Medicine. *Electrochem. Soc. Trans.* **2010,** *33,* 69–74.

89. Akagi, T.; Wang, X.; Uto, T.; Baba, M.; Akashi, M. Protein Direct Delivery to Dendritic Cells using Nanoparticles Based on Amphiphilic Poly(amino acid) Derivatives. *Biomaterials* **2007,** *28,* 3427–3436.

90. Calvo, P.; Remuñan-López, C.; Vila-Jato, J. L.; Alonso, M. J. Chitosan and Chitosan/Ethylene Oxide-propylene Oxide Block Copolymer Nanoparticles as Novel Carriers for Proteins and Vaccines. *Pharm. Res.* **1997,** *14,* 1431–1436.

91. Chertok, B.; Moffat, B. A.; David, A. E.; Yu, F.; Bergemann, C.; Ross, B. D.; Yang, V. C. Iron Oxide Nanoparticles as a Drug Delivery Vehicle for MRI Monitored Magnetic Targeting of Brain Tumors. *Biomaterials* **2008,** *29,* 486–496.

92. Cho, H. S.; Dong, Z.; Pauletti, G. M., et al. Fluorescent, Superparamagnetic Nanospheres for Drug Storage, Targeting, and Imaging: A Multifunctional Nanocarrier System for Cancer Diagnosis and Treatment. *ACS Nano.* **2010,** *4,* 5398–5404.

93. Fang, T.; Sawa, X.; Maeda, H., Eds.; *Factors and Mechanism of "EPR" Effect and the Enhanced Antitumor Effects of Macromolecular Drugs Including SMANCS Book Series Advances in Experimental Medicine and Biology*; SpringerLink Netherlands: Dordrecht, Netherlands, 2004.

94. Fresta, M.; Puglisi, G.; Giammona, G.; Cavallaro, G.; Micali, N.; Furneri, P. M. Pefloxacine Mesilate- and Ofloxacin-Loaded Polyethylcyanoacrylate Nanoparticles: Characterization of the Colloidal Drug Carrier Formulation. *J. Pharm. Sci.* **1995,** *84,* 895–902.

95. Hu, C.; Feng, H.; Zhu, C. Preparation and Characterization of Rifampicin-PLGA Microspheres/Sodium Alginate In Situ Gel Combination Delivery System. *Colloids Surf. B: Biointerfaces* **2012,** *96,* 162–169.

96. Hu, Y.; Jiang, X.; Ding, Y.; Ge, H.; Yuan, Y.; Yang, C. Synthesis and Characterization of Chitosan–Poly(acrylic acid) Nanoparticles. *Biomaterials* **2002,** *23,* 3193–3201.

97. Jain, G. K.; Pathan, S. A.; Akhter, S.; Jayabalan, N.; Talegaonkar, S.; Khar, R. K.; Ahmad, F. J. Microscopic and Spectroscopic Evaluation of Novel PLGA-Chitosan Nanoplexes as an Ocular Delivery System. *Colloids Surf. B: Biointerfaces* **2011,** *82,* 397–403.

98. Jain, K. K. Use of Nanoparticles for Drug Delivery in Glioblastome Multiforme. *Expert. Rev. Neurother.* **2007,** *7,* 363–372.

99. Jin, S.; Ye, K. Nanoparticle-Mediated Drug Delivery and Gene Therapy. *Biotechnol. Prog.* **2007,** *23,* 32–41.

100. Magenheim, B.; Levy, M. Y.; Benita, S. A New In Vitro Technique for the Evaluation of Drug Release Profile from Colloidal Carriers-Ultrafiltration Technique at Low Pressure. *Int. J. Pharm.* **1993,** *94,* 115–123.

101. Moghimi, S. M.; Hunter, A. C.; Murray, J. C. Long-Circulating and Target-Specific Nanoparticles: Theory to Practice. *Pharmacol. Rev.* **2001,** *53,* 283–318.

102. Morgen, M.; Lu, G. W.; Dub, D.; Stehle, R.; Lembke, F.; Cervantes, J.; Ciotti, S.; Haskell, R.; Smithey, D.; Haley, K.; Fan, C. Targeted Delivery of a Poorly Water-Soluble Compound to Hair Follicles using Polymeric Nanoparticle Suspensions. *Int. J. Pharm.* **2011,** *416,* 314–322.

103. Muller, R. H.; Mader, K.; Gohla, S. Solid Lipid Nanoparticles (SLN) for Controlled Drug Delivery ± A Review of the State of the Art. *Eur. J. Pharm. Biopharm.* **2000,** *50,* 161–177.

104. Panyam, J.; Labhasetwar, V. Biodegradable Nanoparticles for Drug and Gene Delivery to Cells and Tissue. *Adv. Drug Deliv. Rev.* **2003,** *55.*

105. Redhead, H. M.; Davis, S. S.; Illum, L. Drug Delivery in Poly(lactide-co-glycolide) Nanoparticles Surface Modified with Poloxamer 407 and Poloxamine 908: In Vitro Characterisation And In Vivo Evaluation. *J. Control. Release* **2001,** *70,* 353–363.

106. Ruenraroengsak, P.; Cook, J. M.; Florence, A. T. Nanosystem Drug Targeting: Facing up to Complex Realities. *J. Control. Release* **2010,** *141,* 265–276.

107. Sahoo, S. K.; Sawa, T.; Fang, J.; Tanaka, S.; Miyamoto, Y.; Akaike, T.; Maeda, H. Pegylated Zinc Protoporphyrin: A Water-soluble Heme Oxygenase Inhibitor with Tumor-Targeting Capacity. *Bioconjug. Chem.* **2002,** *13,* 1031–1038.

108. Tiwari, S. B.; Amiji, M. M. A Review of Nanocarrier-based CNS Delivery Systems. *Curr. Drug Deliv.* **2006,** *3,* 219–232.

109. Ueno, Y.; Futagawa, H.; Takagi, Y.; Ueno, A.; Mizushima, Y. Drug-Incorporating Calcium Carbonate Nanoparticles for a New Delivery System. *J Control Release* **2005,** *103,* 93–98.

110. Vauthier, C.; Dubernet, C.; Chauvierre, C.; Brigger, I.; Couvreur, P. Drug Delivery to Resistant Tumors: The Potential of Poly(alkyl cyanoacrylate) Nanoparticles. *J. Control. Release* **2003,** *93,* 151–160.

111. BCC Research *Nanotechnology in Medical Applications.* 2012 Available from: http://www.bccresearch.com/report/nanotechnology-medical-applications-global-market-hlc069b.html.

112. Cientifica *Nanotech Drug Delivery.* 2012 Available from: http://www.pitchengine.com/cientificaltd/nanotech-drug-delivery-will-be-15-of-global-nanotechnology-market-by-2021.

113. Didenko, Y.; Suslick, K. Chemical Aerosol Flow Synthesis of Semiconductor Nanoparticles. *J. Am. Chem. Soc.* **2005,** *127,* 12196–12197.

114. Mottram, P. L.; Leong, D.; Crimeen-Irwin, B.; Gloster, S.; Xiang, S. D.; Meanger, J.; Ghildyal, R.; Vardaxis, N.; Plebanski, M. Type 1 and 2 Immunity Following Vaccination is Influenced by Nanoparticle Size: Formulation of a Model Vaccine for Respiratory Syncytial Virus. *Mol. Pharm.* **2007,** *4,* 73–84.

115. Martel, S.; Felfoul, O.; Mohammadi, M. 2008; 264–269.

116. Ricles, L. M.; Nam, S. Y.; Sokolov, K.; Emelianov, S. Y.; Suggs, L. J. Function of Mesenchymal Stem Cells Following Loading of Gold Nanotracers. *Int. J. Nanomedicine* **2011,** *6,* 407–416.

117. Hassen, W.; Chaix, C.; Abdelghani, A.; Bessueille, F.; Leonard, D.; Jaffrezic-Renault, N. An Impedimetric DNA Sensor Based on Functionalized Magnetic Nanoparticles for HIV and HBV Detection. *Sens. Actuators B* **2008,** *134,* 755–760.

118. Deguchi, S.; Alargova, R. G.; Tsujii, K. Stable Dispersions of Fullerenes, C60 and C70, in Water. Preparation and Characterization. *Langmuir* **2001,** *17,* 6013–6017.

119. Juzenas, P.; Chen, W.; Sun, Y. P.; Coelho, M. A. N.; Genralov, R.; Genralova, N.; Christensen, I. L. Quantum Dots and Nanoparticles for Photodynamic and Radiation Therapies of Cancer. *Adv. Drug Deliv. Rev.* **2008,** *60.*

120. Kateb, B.; Chiu, K.; Black, K.; Yamamoto, V.; Khalsa, B.; Ljubimova, J.; Ding, H.; Patil, R.; Portilla-Arias, J.; Modo, M.; Moore, D.; Farahani, K.; Okun, M.; Prakash, N.; Neman, J.; Ahdoot, D.; Grundfest, W.; Nikzad, S.; Heiss, J. Nanoplatforms for Constructing New Approaches to Cancer Treatment, Imaging, and Drug Delivery: What Should be the Policy?. *NeuroImage* **2011,** *54,* S106–S124.

121. Martel, R.; Derycke, V.; Lavoie, C.; Appenzeller, J.; Chan, K. K.; Tersoff, J. Ambipolar Electrical Transport in Semiconducting Single-Wall Carbon Nanotubes. *Phys. Rev. Lett.* **2001,** *87,* 256805.

122. Merkoci, A.; Aldavert, M.; Tarrasón, G.; Eritja, R.; Alegret, S. Toward an ICPMS-Linked DNA Assay Based on Gold Nanoparticles Immunoconnected through Peptide Sequences. *Anal. Chem.* **2005,** *77,* 6500–6503.

123. Rai, M.; Yadav, A.; Gade, A. Recently, a Variety of Nanocomposites Based on Polyester and Carbon Nanostructures have been Explored for Potential use as Scaffold Materials. *Biotechnol. Adv.* **2009,** *27,* 76–83.

124. Smith, A. M.; Duan, H.; Mohs, A. M. Bioconjugated Quantum Dots for In Vivo Molecular and Cellular Imaging. *Adv. Drug Deliv. Rev.* **2008,** *60.*

125. Chertok, B.; Cole, A. J.; David, A. E.; Yang, V. C. Comparison of Electron Spin Resonance Spectroscopy and Inductively-Coupled Plasma Optical Emission Spectroscopy for Biodistribution Analysis of Iron-Oxide Nanoparticles. *Mol. Pharm.* **2010,** *7,* 375–385.

126. Herr, J. K.; Smith, J. E.; Medley, C. D.; Shangguan, D.; Tan, W. Aptamer-Conjuagted Nanoparticcles for Selective Collection and Detection of Cancer Cells. *Anal. Chem.* **2007,** *78,* 2918–2924.

127. Hutter, E.; Pileni, M. P. Detection of DNA Hybridization by Gold Nanoparticle Enhanced Transmission Surface Plasmon Resonance Spectroscopy. *J. Phys. Chem. B* **2003,** *107,* 6497–6499.

128. Aguilar, Z. P.; Wang, Y. A.; Xu, H.; Hui, G.; Pusic, K. M. Nanoparticle Based Immunological Stimulation 2012 January 19 2012 US Patent App: 13/350,849]

129. Aguilar, Z. P.; Xu, H.; Dixon, J. D.; Wang, A. W. *Nanomaterials for Enhanced Antibody Production*; Small Business Innovations Research for the National Science Foundation, 2012.

130. Bulte, J. W.; Douglas, T.; Witwer, B.; Zhang, S. C.; Strable, E.; Lewis, BK., et al. Magneto-dendrimers Allow Endosomal Magnetic Labeling and In Vivo Tracking of Stem Cells. *Nat. Biotechnol.* **2001,** *19,* 1141–1147.

131. Cai, W.; Shin, D.; Chen, K.; Gheysens, O.; Cao, Q.; Wang, S. X.; Gambhir, S. S.; Chen, X. Peptide-Labeled Near-Infrared Quantum Dots for Imaging Tumor Vasculature in Living Subjects. *Nano Lett.* **2006,** *6,* 669–676.

132. Casey, A.; Herzog, E.; Davoren, M.; Lyng, F. M.; Byrne, H. J.; Chambers, G. Spectroscopic Analysis Confirms the Interactions between Single Walled Carbon Nanotubes and Various Dyes Commonly used to Assess Cytotoxicity. *Carbon* **2007,** *45,* 1425–1432.

133. Cherukuri, P.; Bachilo, S. M.; Litovsky, S. H.; Weisman, R. B. Near-Infrared Fluorescence Microscopy of Single-Walled Carbon Nanotunes in Phagocytic Cells. *J. Am. Chem. Soc.* **2004,** *126,* 15638–15639.

134. Cho, S. J.; Maysinger, D.; Jain, M.; Roder, B.; Hackbarth, S.; Winnik, F. M. Long-term Exposure to CdTe Quantum Dots causes Functional Impairments in Live Cells. *Langmuir* **2007,** *23.*

135. Dabbousi, B. O.; Rodríguez-Viejo, J.; Mikulec, F. V.; Heine, J. R.; Mattoussi, H.; Ober, R.; Jensen, K. J.; Bawendi, M. G. (CdSe)ZnS Core-Shell Quantum Dots: Synthesis and Characterization of a Size Series of Highly Luminescent Nanocrystallites. *J. Phys. Chem. B* **1997,** *101,* 9463–9475.

136. Dennis, A. M.; Bao, G. Quantum Dot-Fluorescent Protein Pairs as Novel Fluorescence Resonance Energy Transfer Probes. *Nano Lett.* **2008,** *8,* 1439–1445.

137. Gao, X.; Cui, Y.; Levenson, R. M.; Chung, L. W. K.; Nie, S. In Vivo Cancer Targeting and Imaging with Semiconductor Quantum Dots. *Nat. Biotechnol.* **2004,** *22,* 969–976.

138. Jin, T.; Fujii, F.; Sakata, H.; Tamura, M.; Kinjo, M. Calixarene-Coated Water-Soluble CdSe-ZnS Semiconductor Quantum Dots that are Highly Fluorescent and Stable in Aqueous Solution. *Chem. Commun.* **2005,** 2829–2831.

139. Lidke, D. S.; Nagy, P.; Heintzmann, R.; Arndt-Jovin, D. J.; Post, J. N.; Grecco, H. E.; Jares-Erijman, E. A.; Jovin, T. M. Quantum Dot Ligands Provide New Insights into erbB/HER Receptor-Mediated Signal Transduction. *Nat. Biotechnol.* **2004,** *22,* 198–203.

140. Lovat, V.; Pantarotto, D.; Lagostena, L.; Cacciari, B.; Grolfo, M.; Righi, M., et al. Nanotube Substrates Boost Neuronal Electrical Signaling. *Nano Lett.* **2005,** *5,* 1107–1110.

141. Pradhan, N.; Battaglia, D. M.; Liu, Y.; Peng, X. Efficient, Stable, Small, and Water Soluble Doped ZnSe Nanocrystal Emitters as Non-Cadmium Based Biomedical Labels. *Nano Lett.* **2007,** *7,* 312–317.

142. Pulskamp, K.; Diabate, S.; Krug, H. F. Carbon Nanotubes Show no Sign of Acute Toxicity but Induce Intracellular Reactive Oxygen Species in Dependence on Contaminants. *Toxicol. Lett.* **2007,** *168,* 58–74.

143. Su, H.; Xu, H.; Gao, S.; Dixon, J.; ZP, A.; Wang, A.; Xu, J.; Wang, J. Microwave Synthesis of Nearly Monodisperse Core/Multishell Quantum Dots with Cell Imaging Applications. *Nanoscale Res. Lett.* **2010,** *5,* 625–630.

144. Su, Y. Y.; Peng, F.; Jiang, Z. Y.; Zhong, Y. L.; Lu, Y. M., et al. In Vivo Distribution, Pharmacokinetics, and Toxicity of Aqueous Synthesized Cadmium-Containing Quantum Dots. *Biomaterials* **2011,** *32,* 5855–5862.

145. Xu, H.; Aguilar, Z.; Wei, H.; Wang, A. Development of Semiconductor Nanomaterial Whole Cell Imaging Sensor on Silanized Microscope Slides. *Front. Biosci.* **2011,** *E3,* 1013–1024.

146. Zhu, Y.; Li, W. X.; Li, Q. N.; Li, Y. G.; Li, Y. F.; Zhang, X. Y., et al. Multi-Walled Carbon Nanotubes Injure the Plasma Membrane of Macrophages. *Carbon* **2009,** *47,* 1351–1358.

147. Ahmad, M. B.; Shameli, K.; Darroudi, M.; Yunus, W.; Ibrahim, N. A. Synthesis and Characterization of Silver/Clay Nanocomposites by Chemical Reduction Method. *Am. J. Appl. Sci.* **2009,** *6,* 1909–1914.

148. Borum-Nicholas, L.; Wilson, J. O. C. Surface Modification of Hydroxyapatite. Part I. Dodecyl Alcohol. *Biomaterials* **2003,** *24,* 367–369.

149. Carbó-Argibay, E.; Rodríguez-González, B.; Pastoriza-Santos, I.; Pérez-Juste, J.; Liz-Marán, L. M. Growth of Pentatwinned Gold Nanorods into Truncated Decahedra. *Nanoscale* **2010,** *2,* 2377–2383.

150. Ebbesen, T. W.; Ajayan, P. M. Large-scale Synthesis of Carbon Nanotubes. *Nature* **1992,** *358,* 220–222.

151. Huang, C.; Zusing Yang, Z.; Lee, K.; Chang, H. Synthesis of Highly Fluorescent Gold Nanoparticles for Sensing Mercury(II). *Angew Chem. Int. Ed.* **2007,** *46,* 6824–6828.

152. Li, J.; Lu, X. L.; Zheng, Y. F. Effect of Surface Modified Hydroxyapatite on the Tensile Property Improvement of HA/PLA Composite. *Appl. Surf. Sci.* **2008,** *255,* 494–497.

153. Webster, T. J.; Ergun, C. D.; Siegel, R. W.; Bizios, R. Enhanced Functions of Osteoclast-like Cells on Nanophase Ceramics. *Biomaterials* **2001,** *22,* 1327–1333.

154. Pusic, K.; Xu, H.; Stridiron, A.; Aguilar, Z.; Wang, A. Z.; Hui, H. Blood Stage Merozoite Surface Protein Conjugated to Nanoparticles Induce Potent Parasite Inhibitory Antibodies. *Vaccine* **2011,** *29,* 8898–8908.

155. Jiang, W.; Mardyani, S.; Fischer, H.; Chan, W. C. W. Design and Characterization of Lysine Cross-Linked Mercapto-Acid Biocompatible Quantum Dots. *Chem. Mater.* **2006,** *18,* 872–878.

156. Xu, H.; Aguilar, Z.; Dixon, J.; Jones, B.; Wang, A.; Wei, H. Breast Cancer Cell Imaging using Semiconductor Quantum Dots. *Electrochem. Soc. Trans.* **2009,** *25,* 69–77.

157. Lacerda, L.; Soundararajan, A.; Singh, R.; Pastorin, G.; Al-Jamal, K. T.; Turton, J., et al. Dynamic Imaging of Functionalized Multi-Walled Carbon Nanotube Systemic Circulation and Urinary Excretion. *Adv. Mater.* **2008,** *20,* 225–230.

158. Shvedova, A. A.; Kisin, E. R.; Porter, D.; Schulte, P.; Kagan, V. E.; Fadeel, B.; Castranova, V. Mechanisms of Pulmonary Toxicity nd Medical Applications of Carbon Nanotubes. *Pharm. Ther.* **2009,** *121,* 192–204.

159. Singh, R.; Pantarotto, D.; Lacerdo, L.; Pastorin, G.; Klumpp, C.; Prato, M.; Bianco, A.; Kostarelos, K. Tissue Biodistribution and Blood Clearance Rates of Intravenously Administered Carbon Nanotube Radiotracers. *Proc. Natl. Acad. Sci. USA* **2006,** *103,* 3357–3362.

160. Slotkin, J. R.; Chakrabarti, L.; Dai, H. N.; Carney, R. S.; Hirata, T.; Bregman, B. S.; Gallicano, G. I.; Corbin, J. G.; Haydar, T. F. In Vivo Quantum Dot Labeling of Mammalian Stem and Progenitor Cells. *Dev. Dyn.* **2007,** *236,* 3393–3401.

161. Mahmoudi, M.; Sant, S.; Wang, B.; Laurent, S.; Sen, T. Superparamagnetic Iron Oxide Nanoparticles (SPIONs): Development, Surface Modification and Applications in Chemotherapy. *Adv. Drug Deliv. Rev.* **2011,** *63,* 24–46.

162. Freed, L. E.; Novakovic, G. V.; Biron, R. J.; Eagles, D. B.; Lesnoy, D. C.; Barlow, SK., et al. Biodegradable Polymer Scaffolds for Tissue Engineering. *Biotechnology* **1994,** *12,* 689–693.

163. Gilding, D. K.; Reed, A. M. Biodegradable Polymers for use in Surgery-Polyglycolic/Poly (lactic acid) Homo- and Copolymers: 1. *Polymer* **1979,** *20,* 1459–1464.

164. Langer, R.; Vacanti, J. P. Tissue Engineering. *Science* **1993,** *260,* 9220–9926.

165. Loo, C.; Hirsch, I.; Lee, M. H.; Chang, E.; West, J. L.; Halas, N. J., et al. Gold Nanoshell Bioconjugates for Molecular Imaging in Living Cells. *Opt. Lett.* **2005,** *30,* 1012–1014.

166. Sekhon, B.; Kamboj, S. Inorganic Nanomedicine: Part 1. *Nanomedicine* **2010,** *6,* 516–522.

167. Ambrosi, A.; Castaneda, M.; Killard, A.; Smyth, M.; Alegret, S.; Merkoci, A. Double-Codified Gold Nanolabels for Enhanced Immunoanalysis. *Anal. Chem.* **2007,** *79,* 5232–5240.

168. Atiyeh, B. S.; Costagliola, M.; Hayek, S. N.; Dibo, S. A. Effect of Silver on Burn Wound Infection Control and Healing: Review of the Literature. *Burns* **2007,** *33,* 139–148.

169. Bu, H. Z.; Gukasyan, H. J.; Goulet, L.; Lou, X. -J.; Xiang, C.; Koudnakova, T. Ocular Dispo-sition, Pharmacokinetics, Efficay and Safety of Nanoparticle-Formulated Ophthalmic Drugs. *Curr. Drug Metab.* **2007,** *8,* 91–107.

170. Chen, G.; Shen, B.; Zhang, F.; Wu, J.; Xu, Y.; He, P.; Fang, Y. A new Electrochemically Active-Inactive Switching Aptamer Molecular Beacon to Detect Thrombin Directly in Solution. *Biosens. Bioelectron,* **2010,** *25,* 2265–2269.

171. Chu, X.; Duan, D.; Shen, G.; Yu, R. Amperometric Glucose Biosensor Based on Electrodepo-sition of Platinum Nanoparticles onto Covalently Immobilized Carbon Nanotube Electrode. *Talanta* **2007,** *71,* 2040–2047.

172. Dixit, S.; Goicochea, N.; Daniel, M.; Murali, A.; Bronstein, L.; De, M.; Stein, B.; Rotello, V.; Kao, C.; Dragnea, B. Quantum Dot Encapsulation in Viral Capsids. *Nano Lett.* **2006,** *6,* 1993–1999.

173. Escosura-Miniz, A. d.; Diaz-Freitas, B.; Sanchez-ESpinel, C.; Gonzalez-Fernandez, A.; Merkoci, A. Rapid Identification and Quantification of Tumour Cells using a Novel Electro-catalytic Method Based in Gold Nanoparticles. *Anal. Chem.* **2009,** *81,* 10268–10274.

174. Fifis, T.; Gamvrellis, A.; Crimeen-Irwin, B.; Pietersz, G. A.; Li, J.; Mottram, P. L.; McKenzie, I. F.; Plebanski, M. Size-Dependent Immunogenicity: Therapeutic and Protective Properties of Nano-Vaccines Against Tumors. *J. Immunol.* **2004,** *173,* 3148–3154.

175. Fujiwara, M.; Yamamoto, F.; Okamoto, K.; Shiokawa, K.; Nomura, R. Adsorption of Duplex DNA on Mesoporous Silicas: Possibility of Inclusion of DNA into their Mesopores. *Anal. Chem.* **2005,** *77,* 8138–8145.

176. Ge, Y.; Zhang, Y.; He, S.; Nie, F.; Teng, G.; Gu, N. Fluorescence Modified Chitosan-Coated Mag-netic Nanoparticles for High-Efficient Cellular Imaging. *Nanoscale Res. Lett.* **2009,** *4,* 287–295.

177. Gong, J.; Liang, Y.; Huang, Y.; Chen, J.; Jiang, J.; Shen, G.; Yu, R. Ag/SiO(2) Core-Shell Nanoparticle-Based Surface-Enhanced Raman Probes for Immunoassay of Cancer Marker using Silica-Coated Magnetic Nanoparticles as Separation Tools. *Biosens. Bioelectron.* **2006,** *22,* 1501–1507.

178. Guo, W. Z.; Li, J. J.; Wang, Y. A.; Peng, X. G. Conjugation Chemistry and Bioapplications of Semiconductor Box Nanocrystals Prepared via Dendrimer Bridging. *Chem. Mater.* **2003,** *15,* 3125–3133.

179. Hessel, C. M.; Rasch, M. R.; Hueso, J. L.; Goodfellow, B.; Akhavan, V. A.; Puvanakrishnan, P.; Tunnel, J. W.; Korgel, B. A. Alkyl Passivation and Amphiphilic Polymer Coating of Silicon Nanocrystals for Diagnostic Imaging. *Small* **2010,** *6,* 2026–2034.

180. Hu, L.; Kim, H.; Lee, J.; Peumans, P.; Cui, Y. Scalable Coating and Properties of Transparent, Flexible, Silver Nanowire Electrodes. *ACS Nano.* **2010,** *4,* 2955–2963.

181. Huang, C. C.; Chiang, C. K.; Lin, Z. H.; Lee, K. H.; Chang, H. T. Bioconjugated Gold Nanodots and Nanoparticles for Protein Assays Based on Photoluminescence Quenching. *Anal. Chem.* **2008,** *80,* 1497–1504.

182. Jaffrezic-Renault, N.; Martelet, C.; Chevolot, Y.; Cloarec BiosensorsBio-Bar Code, J. Assays Based on Biofunctionalized Magnetic Microbeads. *Sensors* **2007,** *7,* 589–614.

183. Raynal, I.; Prigent, P.; Peyramaure, S.; Najid, A.; Rebuzzi, C.; Corot, C. Macrophage Endocy-tosis of Superparamagnetic Iron Oxide Nanoparticles: Mechanisms and Comparison of Feru-moxides and Ferumoxtran-10. *Invest. Radiol.* **2004,** *39,* 56–63.

184. Roy, R.; Hohng, S.; Ha, T. A Practical Guide to Single-Molecule FRET. *Nat. Methods* **2008,** *5,* 507–516.

185. Ryman-Rasmussen, J. P.; Cesta, M. F.; Brody, A. R.; Shipley-Phillips, J. K.; Everitt, J. I.; Tewksbury, E. W., et al. Inhaled Carbon Nanotubes Reach the Subpleural Tissue in Mice. *Nat. Nanotechnol.* **2009,** *4,* 747–751.

186. Sabuncu, A. C.; Grubbs, J.; Qian, S.; Abdel-Fattah, T. M.; Stacey, M. W.; Beskok, A. Probing Nanoparticle Interaction in Cell Culture Media. *Colloids Surf. B: Biointerfaces* **2012**, *95,* 96–102.

187. Saini, R.; Saini, S. Nanotechnology and Surgical Neurology. *Surg. Neurol. Int.* **2010**, *1,* 57.

188. Sayes, C. M.; Marchione, A. A.; Reed, K. L.; Warheit, D. B. Comparative Pulmonary Toxicity Assessments of C60 Water Suspensions in Rats: Few Differences in Fullerene Toxicity in Vivo in Contrast to in Vitro Profiles. *Nano Lett.* **2007**, *7,* 2399–2406.

189. Schneider, O. D.; Loher, S.; Brunner, T. J.; Schmidlin, P.; Stark, W. J. Flexible, Silver Containing Nanocomposites for the Repair of Bone Defects: Antimicrobial Effect against *E. coli* Infection and Comparison To Tetracycline Containing Scaffolds. *J. Mater. Chem.* **2008**, *18,* 2679–2684.

190. Somers, R.; Bawendi, M.; Nocera, D. CdSe Nanocrystal Based Chem-/Bio- Sensors. *Chem. Soc. Rev.* **2007**, *36,* 579–591.

191. Vaidya, S.; Gilchrist, M.; Maldarelli, C.; Couzis, A. Spectral Bar Coding of Polystyrene Microbeads using Multicolored Quantum Dots. *Anal. Chem.* **2007**, *79,* 8520–8530.

192. Vidal, G.; Delord, B.; Neri, W.; Gounel, S.; Roubeau, O.; Bartholome, C.; Ly, I.; Poulin, P.; Labrugere, C.; Sellier, E.; Durrieu, M. -C.; Amedee, J.; Salvetat, J. -P. The Effect of Surface Energy, Adsorbed RGD Peptides and Fibronectin on the Attachment and Spreading of Cells on Multiwalled Carbon Nanotube Papers. *Carbon* **2011**, *49,* 2318–2333.

193. Wang, J. Nanomaterial-Based Electrochemical Biosensors. *Analyst* **2005**, *130,* 421–426.

194. Wang, L.; Liu, X.; Hu, X.; Song, S.; Fan, C. Unmodified Gold Nanoparticles as a Colorimetric Probe for Potassium DNA Aptamers. *Chem. Commun.* **2006**, 3780–3782.

195. Webster, T. J.; Ejiofor, J. U. Increased Osteoblast Adhesion on Nanophase Metals: Ti, Ti_6Al_4V, and CoCrMo. *Biomaterials* **2004**, *25,* 4731–4739.

196. Xiang, S. d.; Scalzo-Inguanti, K.; Minigo, G.; Park, A.; Hardy, C. L.; Plebanski, M. Promising Particle-Based Vaccines in Cancer Therapy. *Expert Rev. Vaccines* **2008**, *7,* 1103–1119.

197. Xie, J.; Zhang, F.; Aronova, M.; Zhu, L.; Lin, X.; Quan, Q.; Liu, G.; Zhang, G.; Choi, K. Y.; Kim, K.; Sun, X.; Lee, S.; Sun, S.; Leapman, R.; Chen, X. Manipulating the Power of an Additional Phase: A Flower-like Au–Fe_3O_4 Optical Nanosensor for Imaging Protease Expressions In Vivo. *ACS Nano.* **2011**, *5,* 3043–3051.

198. Xu, X.; Yang, Q.; Bai, J.; Lu, T.; Li, Y.; Jing, X. Fabrication of Biodegradable Electrospun Poly(L-lactide-co-glycolide) Fibers with Antimicrobial Nanosilver Particles. *J. Nanosci. Nanotechnol.* **2008**, *8,* 5066–5070.

199. Zauner, W.; Farrow, N. A.; Haines, A. M. In Vitro Uptake of Polystyrene Microspheres: Effect of Particle Size, Cell Line and Cell Density. *J. Control. Release* **2001**, *71,* 39–51.

200. Zhang, L. W.; Baumer, W.; Monteiro-Riviere, N. A. Cellular Uptake Mechanisms and Toxicity of Quantum Dots in Dendritic Cells. *Nanomed.-UK* **2011**, *6,* 777–791.

201. Derfus, A. M.; Chan, W. C. W.; Bhatia, S. N. Probing the Cytotoxicity of Semiconductor Quantum Dots. *Nano. Lett.* **2004**, *4,* 11–18.

202. Kirchner, C.; Liedl, T.; Kudera, S.; Pellegrino, T.; Javier, A. M.; Gaub, H. E., et al. Cytotoxicity of Colloidal CdSe and CdSe/ZnS Nanoparticles. *Nano. Lett.* **2005**, *5,* 331–338.

203. Manna, L.; Scher, E.; Alivisatos, A. Synthesis of Soluble and Processable Rod-, Arrow-, Teardrop-, and Tetrapod-shaped CdSe Nanocrystals. *J. Am. Chem. Soc.* **2000**, *122,* 12700–12706.

204. Murray, C.; Norris, D.; Bawendi, M. Synthesis and Characterization of Nearly Monodisperse CdE (E = sulfur, selenium, tellurium) Semiconductor Nanocrystallites. *J. Am. Chem. Soc.* **1993**, *115,* 8706–8715.

205. Wolcott, A.; Gerion, D.; Visconte, M.; Sun, J.; Schwartzberg, A.; Chen, S.; Zhang, J. Z. Silica-coated CdTe Quantum Dots Functionalized with Thiols for Bioconjugation fot IgG Proteins. *J. Phys. Chem. B* **2006**, *110,* 5779–5789.

206. Brus, L. E. Electron-Electron and Electron-hole Interaction in Small Semiconductor Crystallines–the Size Dependence of the Lowest Excited Electronic State. *J. Chem. Phys.* **1984,** *80,* 4403–4409.

207. Norris, D. J.; Sacra, A.; Murray, C. B.; Bawendi, M. G. Measurement of the Size-Dependent Hole Spectrum in CdSe Quantum Dots. *Phys. Rev. Lett.* **1994,** *72.*

208. Medintz, I.; Clapp, A.; Mattoussi, H.; Goldman, E.; Fisher, B.; Mauro, J. Self-Assembled Nanoscale Biosensors Based on Quantum Dot FRET Donors. *Nat. Mater.* **2003,** *2,* 630–638.

209. Medintz, I. L.; Uyeda, H. T.; Goldman, E. R.; Mattoussi, H. Quantum Dot Bioconjugates for Imaging, Labeling and Sensing. *Nat. Mater.* **2005,** *4,* 435–446.

210. Michalet, X.; Pinaud, F. F.; Bentolila, L. A.; Tsay, J. M.; Doose, S.; Li, J. J.; Sundaresan, G.; Wu, A. M.; Gambhir, S. S.; Weiss, S. Quantum Dots for Live Cells, *In Vivo* Imaging, and Diagnostics. *Science* **2005,** *307,* 538–544.

211. So, M. K.; Xu, C.; Loening, A. M.; Gambhir, S. S.; Rao, J. Self-Illuminating Quantum Dot Conjugates for In Vivo Imaging. *Nat. Biotechnol.* **2006,** *24,* 339–343.

212. Bhadra, D.; Bhadra, S.; Jain, P; Jain, N. K. Pegnology: A Review of PEG-ylated Systems. *Pharmazie* **2002,** *57,* 5–29.

213. Alivisatos, A. P.; Gu, W.; Larabell, C. Quantum Dots as Cellular Probes. *Annu. Rev. Biomed. Eng.* **2005,** *7,* 55–76.

214. Iyer, G.; Weiss, S.; Pinaud, F.; Tsay, J. M. Solubilization of Quantum Dots with a Recombinant Peptide from *Escherichia coli. Small* **2007,** *3,* 793–798.

215. Jamieson, T.; Bakhshi, R.; Petrova, D.; Pocock, R.; Seifalian, A. M. Biological Applications of Quantum Dots. *Biomaterials* **2007,** *28,* 4717–4732.

216. Liu, W.; Howarth, M.; Greytak, A. B.; Zheng, Y.; Nocera, D. G.; Ting, A. Y., et al. Compact Biocompatible Quantum Dots Functionalized for Cellular Imaging. *J. Am. Chem. Soc.* **2008,** *130,* 1274–1284.

217. Carion, O.; Mahler, B.; Pons, T.; Dubertret, B. Synthesis, Encapsulation, Purification and Coupling of Single Quantum Dots in Phospholipid Micelles for their use in Cellular and *In Vivo* Imaging. *Nat. Protoc.* **2007,** *2,* 2383–2390.

218. Pinaud, F.; King, D.; Moore, H. P.; Weiss, S. Bioactivation and Cell Targeting of Semiconductor CdSe/ZnS Nanocrystals with Phytochelatin-Related Peptides. *J. Am. Chem. Soc.* **2004,** *126,* 6115–6123.

219. Dufes, C.; Uchegbu, I.; Schatzlein, A. Dendrimers in Gene Delivery. *Adv. Drug Deliv. Rev.* **2005,** *57,* 2177.

220. Hecht, S.; Frechet, J. Dendritic Encapsulation of Function: Applying Nature's Site Isolation Principle from Biomimetics to Materials Science. *Angew Chem. Int. Ed.* **2001,** *40,* 74.

221. Lai, P.; Lou, P.; Peng, C.; Pai, C.; Yen, W.; Huang, M.; Young, T.; Shieh, M. Doxorubicin Delivery by Polyamidoamine Dendrimer Conjugation and Photochemical Internalization for Cancer Therapy. *J. Control. Release* **2007,** *122,* 39.

222. Satoh, K.; Yoshimura, T.; Esumi, K. Effects of Various Thiol Molecules Added on Morphology of Dendrimer-Gold Nanocomposites. *J. Colloid Interface Sci.* **2002,** *255,* 312.

223. Tomalia, D.; Reyna, L.; Svenson, S. Dendrimers as Multi-Purpose Nanodevices for Oncology Drug Delivery and Diagnostic Imaging. *Biochem. Soc. Trans.* **2007,** *35,* 61.

224. Kim, J.; Piao, T.; Hyeon, T. Multifunctional Nanostructured Materials for Multimodal Imaging, and Simultaneous Imaging and Therapy. *Chem. Soc. Rev.* **2009,** *38,* 372–390.

225. Lee, H.; Lee, E. J.; Kim, D. K.; Jang, N. K.; Jeong, Y. Y.; Jon, S. Antibiofouling Polymer-coated Superparamagnetic Iron Oxide Nanoparticles as Potential Magnetic Resonance Contrast Agents For In Vivo Cancer Imaging. *J. Am. Chem. Soc.* **2006,** *128,* 7383–7389.

226. Mahmoudi, M.; Simchi, A.; Imani, M.; Milani, A. S.; Stroeve, P. An In Vitro Study of Bare and Poly(Ethylene glycol)-Co-Fumarate-Coated Superparamagnetic Iron Oxide Nanoparticles: A New Toxicity Identification Procedure. *Nanotechnol.* **2009,** *20,* 40–47.

227. Moore, A.; Weissleder, R.; Bogdanov, A., Jr. Uptake of Dextran-Coated Monocrystalline Iron Oxides in Tumor Cells and Macrophages. *J. Magn. Reson. Imaging* **1997,** *7,* 1140–1145.

228. Osaka, T.; Nakanishi, T.; Shanmugam, S.; Takahama, S.; Zhang, H. Effect of Surface Charge of Magnetite Nanoparticles on their Internalization into Breast Cancer and Umbilical Vein Endothelial Cells. *Colloids Surf. B: Biointerfaces* **2009,** *71,* 325–330.

229. Runge, V. M. *Contrast Agents Safety Profile.* 2008 June 18, 2012. Available from: http://www.clinical-mri.com/pdf/Contrast%20Agents/Contrast%20Agents%20-%20Safety%20Profile%20amended%20table.pdf.

230. Sahoo, Y.; Pizem, H.; Fried, T.; Golodnitsky, D.; Burstein, L.; Sukenik, C. N.; Markovich, G. Alkyl Phosphonate/Phosphate Coating on Magnetite Nanoparticles: A Comparison with Fatty Acids. *Langmuir* **2001,** *17,* 7907–7911.

231. Teja, A. S.; Koh, P. Y. Synthesis, Properties, and Applications of Magnetic Iron Oxide Nanoparticles. *Prog. Cryst. Growth Charact. Mater.* **2009,** *55,* 22–45.

232. Wang, Y.; Wong, J. F.; Teng, X. W.; Lin, X. Z.; Yang, H. Pulling" Nanoparticles into Water: Phase Transfer of Oleic Acid Stabilized Monodisperse Nanoparticles into Aqueous Solutions of Alpha-Cyclodextrin. *Nano Lett.* **2003,** *3,* 1555–1559.

233. Alfinito, E.; Millithaler, J. F.; Pennett, C.; Reggiani, L. A Single Protein Based Nanobiosensor for Odornat Recognition. *Microelectron. J.* **2010,** *41,* 718–722.

234. Baker, K. N.; Rendall, M. H.; Patel, A.; Boyd, P.; Hoare, M.; Freedman, R. B.; James, D. C. Rapid Monitoring of Recombinant protein products: A Comparison of Current Technologies. *Trends Biotechnol.* **2002,** *20,* 149–156.

235. Gelperina, S. E.; Khalansky, A. S.; Skidan, I. N.; Smirnova, Z. S.; Bobruskin, A. I.; Severin, S. E.; Turowski, B.; Zanella, F. E.; Kreuter, J. Toxicological Studies of Doxorubicin Bound to Polysorbate 80-coated Poly(butyl cyanoacrylate) Nanoparticles in Healthy Rats and Rats with Intracranial Glioblastoma. *Toxicol. Lett.* **2002,** *126,* 131–141.

236. Huang, S.; Chen, Y. Ultrasensitive Fluorescence Detection of Single Protein Molecules Manipulated Electrically on Au Nanowire. *Nano Lett.* **2008,** *8,* 2829–2833.

237. Khanna, V. K. New-Generation Nano-engineered Biosensors, Enabling Nanotechnologies and Nanomaterials. *Sens. Rev.* **2008,** *28,* 39–45.

238. Kreuter, J.; Ramge, P.; Petrov, V.; Hamm, S.; Gelperina, S. E.; Engelhardt, B.; Aly-autdin, R.; von Briesen, H.; Begley, D. J. Direct Evidence that Polysorbate-80-Coated Poly(butylcyanoacrylate) Nanoparticles Deliver Drugs to the CNS Via Specific Mechanisms Requiring Prior Binding of Drug to the Nanoparticles. *Pharm. Res.* **2003,** *20,* 409–416.

239. Kularatne, B.; Lorigan, P.; Browne, S.; Suvarna, S.; Smith, M.; Lawry, J. Monitoring Tumour Cells in the Peripheral Blood of Small Cell Lung Cancer Patients. *Cytometry* **2002,** *50,* 160–167.

240. Lee, H.; Yoon, T.; Figueiredo, J.; Swirski, F. K.; Weissleder, R. Rapid Detection and Profiling of Cancer Cells in Fine-Needle Aspirates. *Proc. Natl. Acad. Sci. USA* **2009,** *106,* 12459–12464.

241. Lee, J.; Cho, E. C.; Cho, K. Incorporation and Release Behavior of Hydrophobic Drug in Functionalized Poly(D, L-lactide)-Block-Poly(Ethylene Oxide) Micelles. *J. Control. Release* **2004,** *94,* 323–335.

242. Lee, J. K.; Kim, D. B.; Kim, J. I.; Kim, P. Y. In Vitro Cytotoxicity Tests on Cultured Human Skin Fibroblasts to Predict Skin Irritation Potential of Surfactants. *Toxicol In Vitro* **2000,** *14,* 345–349.

243. Li, M.; Li, R.; Li, C. M.; Wu, N. Electrochemical and Optical Biosensors Based on Nanomaterials and Nanostructures: A Review. *Front in Biosci.* **2011,** *S3,* 1308–1331.

244. Xiao, Y.; Patolsky, F., et al. Plugging into Enzymes: Nanowiring of Redox Enzymes by a Gold Nanoparticle. *Science* **2003,** *299,* 1877–1881.

245. Baselt, D. R.; Lee, G. U.; Natesan, M.; Metzger, S. W.; Sheehan, P. E.; Colton, R. J. A Biosensor Based on Magnetoresistance Technology. *Biosens. Bioelectron.* **1998,** *13,* 731–749.

246. Beer, C.; Foldbjerg, R.; Hayashi, Y.; Sutherland, D. S.; Autrup, H. Toxicity of Silver Nanoparticles-Nanoparticle or Silver Ion?. *Toxicol. Lett.* **2012,** *208,* 286–292.

247. Brunner, T. J.; Wick, P.; Manser, P.; Spohn, P.; Grass, R. N.; Limbach, L. K.; Bruinink, A.; Stark, W. J. In Vitro Cytotoxicity of Oxide Nanoparticles: Comparison to Asbestos, Silica, and the Effect of Particle Solubility. *Environ. Sci. Technol.* **2006,** *40,* 4374–4381.

248. Demers, L.; Mirkin, C.; Mucic, R.; Reynolds, R.; Letsinger, R.; Elghanian, R.; Viswanadham, G. A Fluorescence-Based Method for Determining the Surface Coverage and Hybridization Efficiency of Thiol-Capped Oligonucleotides Bound to Gold Thin Films and Nanoparticles. *Anal. Chem.* **2000,** *72,* 5535–5541.

249. Dyadyusha, L.; Yin, H.; Jaiswal, S.; Brown, T.; Baumberg, J.; Booye, F.; Melvin, T. Quenching of CdSe Quantum Dot Emission, a New Approach for Biosensing. *Chem. Commun.* **2005,** 3201–3203.

250. Feng, J.; Ding, S. Y.; Tucker, M. P.; Himmel, M. E.; Kim, Y. H.; Zhang, S. B.; Keyes, B. M.; Rumbles, G. Cyclodextrin Driven Hydrophobic/Hydrophilic Transformation of Semiconductor Nanoparticles. *Appl. Phys. Lett.* **2005,** *86,* 033108.

251. Gill, R.; Willner, I.; Shweky, I.; Banin, U. Fluorescence Resonance Energy Transfer in CdSe/ZnS-DNA Conjugates: Probing Hybridization and DNA Cleavage. *J. Phys. Chem. B* **2005,** *109,* 23715–23719.

252. Jaiswal, J.; Mattoussi, H.; Mauro, J.; Simon, S. Long-Term Multiple Color Imaging of Live Cells using Quantum Dot Bioconjugates. *Nat. Biotechnol.* **2003,** *21,* 47–51.

253. Liu, J.; Lu, Y. A Colorimetric Lead Biosensor Using DNAzyme-Directed Assembly of Gold Nanoparticles. *J. Am. Chem. Soc.* **2003,** *125,* 6642–6643.

254. Merkoci, A. Electrochemical Biosensing with Nanoparticles. *FEBS J.* **2007,** *274,* 310–316.

255. Vaseashta, A.; Dimova-Malinovska, D. Nanostructured and Nanoscale Devices, Sensors and Detectors. *Sci. Technol. Adv. Mat.* **2005,** *6,* 312–318.

256. Fan, X.; White, I. M.; Shopova, S. I.; Zhu, H.; Suter, J. D.; Sun, Y. Sensitive Optical Biosensors for Unlabeled Targets: A Review. *Anal. Chim. Acta* **2008,** *620,* 8–26.

257. Velasco, M. N. Optical Biosensors for Probing at the Cellular Level: A Review of Recent Progress and Future Prospects. *Semin. Cell Dev. Biol.* **2009,** *20,* 27–33.

258. Chan, C.; Nie, S. Quantum Dot Bioconjugates for Ultrasensitive Nonisotopic Detection. *Science* **1998,** *281,* 2016–2018.

259. Clapp, A.; Medintz, I.; Mauro, J.; Fisher, B.; Bawendi, M.; Mattoussi, h Fluorescence Resonance Energy Transfer Between Quantum Dot Donors and Dye-Labeled Protein Acceptors. *J. Am. Chem. Soc.* **2004,** *126,* 301–310.

260. Bruchez, M., Jr.; Moronne, M.; Gin, P.; Weiss, S.; Alivisatos, A. P. Semiconductor Nanocrystals as Fluorescent Biological Labels. *Science* **1998,** *281,* 2013–2016.

261. Rzigalinski, B. A.; Strobl, J. S. Cadmium-Containing Nanoparticles: Perspectives on Pharmacology and Toxicology of Quantum Dots in New Insights into the Mechanisms of Cadmium Toxicity – Advances in Cadmium Research. *Toxicol. Appl Pharmacol.* **2009,** *238,* 280–288.

262. Cai, H.; Shang, C.; Hsing, I. M. Sequence-Specific Electrochemical Recognition of Multiple Species using Nanoparticle labels. *Anal. Chim. Acta* **2004,** *523,* 61–68.

263. Freeman, R.; Tali Finder, T.; Bahshi, L.; Willner, I. β-Cyclodextrin-Modified CdSe/ZnS Quantum Dots for Sensing and Chiroselective Analysis. *Nano Lett.* **2009,** *9,* 2073–2076.

264. Abad-Valle, P.; Fernandez-Abedul, M. T.; Costa-Garcia, A. Genosensor on Gold Films with Enzymatic Electrochemical Detection of a SARS Virus Sequence. *Biosens. Bioelectron.* **2005,** *20,* 2251–2260.

265. AValle, P.; FAbedul, M. T.; Costa-Garcia, A. Genosensor on Gold films with Enzymatic Eletcrochemical Detection of a SARS virus sequence. *Biosens. Bioelectron.* **2005,** *20,* 2251–1160.

266. Cao, Y.; Jin, R.; Mirkin, C. Nanoparticles with Raman spectroscopic fingerprints for DNA and RNA detection. *Science* **2002,** *297,* 1536–1540.

267. Carpini, G.; Lucarelli, F.; Marazza, G.; Mascini, M. Oligonucleotide-Modified Screen-printed Gold Electrodes for Enzyme-Amplified Sensing of Nucleic Acids. *Biosens. Bioelectron.* **2004,** *20,* 167–175.

268. Dai, Q.; Liu, X.; Coutts, J.; Austin, L.; Huo, Q. A One-Step Highly Sensitive Method for DNA Detection using Dynamic Light Scattering. *J. Am. Chem. Soc.* **2008,** *130,* 8138–8139.

269. Fritzsche, W.; Taton, T. A. Metal Nanoparticles as Labels for Heterogeneous, Chip-based DNA Detection. *Nanotechnology* **2003,** *14,* R63–R73.

270. Glynou, K.; Loannou, P. C.; Christopoulos, T. K.; Syriopoulou, V. Oligonucleotide-Functionalized Gold Nanparticles as Probes in a Dry-Reagent Strip Biosensor for DNA Analysis by Hybridization. *Anal. Chem.* **2003,** *75,* 4155–4160.

271. Huber, M.; Wei, T. F.; Muller, U. R.; Lefebvre, O. A.; Marla, S. S.; Bao, Y. P. Gold nanoparticle Probe-Based Gene Expression Analysis with Unamplified Total Human RNA. *Nat. Biotechnol.* **2004,** *32,* e137.

272. Li, L.; Li, X.; Li, L.; Wang, J.; Jin, W. Ultrasensitive DNA Assay Based on Single-Molecule Detection Coupled with Fluorescent Quantum Dot-Labeling and its Application to Determination of Messenger RNA. *Anal. Chim. Acta* **2011,** *685,* 52–57.

273. Liu, J.; Lu, Y. Adenosine-Dependent Assembly of Aptazyme-Functionalized Gold Nanoparticles and its Application as a Colorimetric Biosensor. *Anal. Chem.* **2004,** *76,* 1627–1632.

274. Mao, X.; Liu, G. Nanomaterial Based Electrochemical DNA Biosensors and Bioassays. *J. Biomed. Nanotechnol.* **2008,** *4,* 419–431.

275. Maruccio, G.; Primiceri, E.; Marzo, P.; Arima, V.; Torre, A. D.; Rinaldi, R.; Pellegrino, T.; Krahne, R.; Cingolani, R. A nanobiosensor to Detect Single Hybridization Events. *Analyst* **2009,** *134,* 2458–2461.

276. Merkoci, A. Nanoparticles-based Strategies for DNA, Protein and Cell Sensors. *Biosens. Bioelectron.* **2010,** *26,* 1164–1177.

277. Park, S. -J.; Taton, T. A.; Mirkin, C. A. Array-based Electrical Detection of DNA with Nanoparticle Probes. *Science* **2002,** *295,* 1503–1506.

278. Storhoff, J. J.; Marla, S. S.; Bao, P.; Hagenow, S.; Mehta, H.; Lucas, A.; Garimella, V.; Patno, T. J.; Buckingham, W.; Cork, W. H., et al. Gold Nanoparticle-based Detection of Genomic DNA Targets on Microarrays using a Novel Optical Detection System. *Biosens. Bioelectron.* **2004,** *19,* 875–883.

279. Wang, J. Nanoparticle-based Electrochemical DNA Detection. *Anal. Chim. Acta* **2003,** *500,* 247–257.

280. Wang, W.; Chen, C.; Qian, M.; Zhao, X. Aptamer Biosensor for Protein Detection using Gold Nanoparticles. *Anal. Biochem.* **2008,** *373,* 213–219.

281. Wark, A. W.; Lee, H. J.; Qavi, A. J.; Corn, R. M. Nanoparticle-Enhanced Diffraction Gratings for Ultrasensitive Surface Plasmon Biosensing. *Anal. Chem.* **2007,** *79,* 6697–6701.

282. Han, M.; Gao, X.; SU, J.; Nie, S. Quantum Dot Tagged Microbead for Multiplexed Coding of Biomolecules. *Nat. Biotechnol.* **2001,** *19,* 631–635.

283. Parak, W.; Gerion, D.; Pellegrino, T.; Zanchet, D.; Micheel, C.; Williams, S.; Boudreau, R.; Le Gros, M.; Larabell, C.; Alivisatos, A. Biological Applications of Colloidal Nanocrystals. *Nanotechnology* **2003**, *14*, R15–R27.

284. Niemeyer, C. Nanoparticles, Proteins, and Nucleic Acids: Biotechnology Meets Materials Science. *Angew Chem. Int. Ed.* **2001**, *40*, 4128–4158.

285. Barbosa, S.; Agrawal, A.; Rodríguez-Lorenzo, L.; Pastoriza-Santos, I.; Alvarez-Puebla, R. A.; Kornowski, A.; Weller, H.; Liz-Marzan, L. M. Tuning Size and Sensing Properties in Colloidal Gold Nanostars. *Langmuir* **2010**, *26*, 14943–14950.

286. Hu, J.; Li, L.; Yang, W.; Manna, L.; Wang, L.; Alivisatos, A. P. Linearly Polarized Emission from Colloidal Semiconductor Quantum Rods. *Science* **2001**, *292*, 2060–2063.

287. Grieshaber, D.; MacKenzie, R.; Voros, J.; Reimhult, E. Electrochemical Biosensors-Sensor Principles and Architectures. *Sensors* **2008**, *8*, 1400–1458.

288. Tothill, I. T. Review: Biosensors for Cancer Markers Diagnostics. *Semin. Cell Dev. Biol.* **2009**, *20*, 55–62.

289. Aspden, T. J.; Mason, J. D.; Jones, N. S. Chitosan as a Nasal Delivery System: The Effect of Chitosan Solutions on In Vitro and In Vivo Mucociliary Transport Rates in Human Turbinates and Volunteers. *J. Pharm. Sci.* **1997**, *86*, 509–513.

290. Blum, J. L.; Savin, M. A.; Edelman, G.; Pippen, J. E.; Robert, N. J.; geister, B. V.; Kirby, R. L.; Clawson, A.; O'shaughnessy, J. A. Phase II Study of Weekly Albumin-bound Paclitaxel for Patients with Metastatic Breast Cancer Heavily Pretreated with Taxanes. *Clin. Breast. Cancer* **2007**, *7*, 850–856.

291. El-Sayed, I. H. Nanotechnology in Head and Neck Cancer: The Race is on. *Curr. Oncol. Rep.* **2010**, *12*, 121–128.

292. Ge, H.; Hu, Y.; Jiang, X.; Cheng, D.; Yuan, Y.; Bi, H.; Yang, C. Preparation, Characterization, and Drug Release Behaviors of Drug Nimodipine-Loaded Poly(epsilon-caprolactone)-Poly(ethylene oxide)-Poly(epsilon-caprolactone) Amphiphilic Triblock Copolymer Micelles. *J. Pharm. Sci.* **2002**, *91*, 1463–1473.

293. Gelderblom, H.; Verweij, J.; Nooter, K.; Sparreboom, A. Cremophor EL: The Drawbacks and Advantages of Vehicle Selection for Drug Formulation. *Eur. J. Cancer* **2001**, *37*, 1590–1598.

294. Govender, T.; Riley, T.; Ehtezazi, T.; Garnett, M. C.; Stolnik, S.; Illum, L.; Davis, S. S. Defining the Drug Incorporation Properties of PLA-PEG Nanoparticles. *Int. J. Pharm.* **2000**, *199*, 95–110.

295. Gradishar, W. J.; Tjulandin, S.; Davidson, N.; Shaw, H.; Desai, N.; Bhar, P.; Hawkins, M.; O'Shaughnessy, J. Phase III Trial of Nanoparticle Albumin-Bound Paclitaxel Compared with Polyethylated Castor Oil-Based Paclitaxel in Women with Breast Cancer. *J. Clin. Oncol.* **2005**, *23*, 7794–7803.

296. Hans, M. L.; Lowman, A. M. Biodegradable Nanoparticles for Drug Delivery and Targeting. *Curr. Opin. Solid State Mater. Sci.* **2002**, *6*, 319–327.

297. La, S. B.; Okano, T.; Kataoka, K. Preparation and Characterization of Micelle-Forming Polymeric Drug Indomethacin-Incorporated Poly(Ethylene oxide)–Poly(β-benzyl l-aspartate) Block Copolymer Micelles. *J. Pharm. Sci.* **1996**, *85*, 85–90.

298. Lamprecht, A.; Ubrich, N.; Yamamoto, H.; Schäfer, U.; Takeuchi, H.; Maincent, P.; Kawashima, Y.; Lehr, C. M. Biodegradable Nanoparticles for Targeted Drug Delivery in Treatment of Inflammatory Bowel Disease. *J Pharmacol. Exp. Ther.* **2001**, *299*, 775–781.

299. Mamot, C.; Drummond, D. C.; Hong, K.; Kirpotin, D. B.; Park, J. W. Liposome-based Approaches to Overcome Anticancer Drug Resistance. *Drug Resist. Updat.* **2003**, *6*, 271–279.

300. Miller, D. W.; Batrakova, E. V.; Kabanov, A. V. Inhibition of Multidrug Resistance-Associated Protein (MRP) Functional Activity with Pluronic Block Copolymers. *Pharm. Res.* **1999**, *16*, 396–401.

301. Moghimi, S. M.; Szebeni, J. Stealth Liposomes and Long Circulating Nanoparticles: Critical Issues in Pharmacokinetics, Opsonization and Protein-Binding Properties. *Prog. Lipid. Res.* **2003,** *42,* 463–478.

302. Paciotti, G. F.; Myer, L.; Weinreich, D.; Goia, D.; Pavel, N.; McLaughlin, E.; Tamarkin, L. Colloidal Gold: A Novel Nanoparticle Vector for Tumor Directed Drug Delivery. *Drug Deliv.* **2004,** *11,* 169–183.

303. Parveen, S.; Sahoo, S. K. Long Circulating Chitosan/PEG Blended PLGA Nanoparticle for Tumor Drug Delivery. *Eur. J. Pharm.* **2011,** *670,* 372–383.

304. Patil, Y. B.; Swaminathan, S. K.; Sadhukha, T.; Panyam, J. The Use of Nanoparticle-Mediated Gene Silencing and Drug Delivery to Overcome Tumor Drug Resistance. *Biomaterials* **2010,** *31,* 358–365.

305. Portilla-Arias, J. P.; Garcia-Alvarez, M.; de Ilarduya, A. M.; Holler, E.; Galbis, J. A.; Munoz-Guerra, S. Synthesis, Hydrodegradation and Drug Releasing Properties of Methyl Esters of Fungal Poly(β, 1-malic acid). *Macromol. Biosci.* **2008,** *8,* 540–550.

306. Seju, U.; Kumar, A.; Sawani, K. K. Development and Evaluation of Olanzapine-Loaded PLGA Nanoparticles for Nose-to-Brain Delivery: In Vitro and In Vivo Studies. *Acta Biomater.* **2011,** *7,* 4169–4176.

307. Chonn, A.; Semple, S. C.; Cullis, P. R. Association of Blood Proteins with Large Unilamellar Liposomes In Vivo. Relation to Circulation Lifetimes. *J. Biol. Chem.* **1992,** *267,* 18759–18765.

308. Linhardt, R. J. In *Controlled Release of Drugs*; Rosoff, M., Ed.; VCH Publishers: New York, 1989; pp 53–95.

309. Westesen, K.; Bunjes, H.; Koch, M. H. J. Physicochemical Characterization of Lipid Nanoparticles and Evaluation of their Drug Loading Capacity and Sustained Release Potential. *J. Control. Release* **1997,** *48,* 223–236.

310. Yang, S.; Zhu, J.; Lu, Y.; Liang, B.; Yang, C. Body Distribution of Camptothecin Solid Lipid Nanoparticles after Oral Administration. *Pharm. Res.* **1999,** *16,* 751–757.

311. *Nanoparticles*; Kreuter, J., Ed.; M. Dekker: New York, 1994.

312. Panagiotou, T.; Fisher, R. J. Enhanced Transport Capabilities via Nanotechnologies: Impacting Bioefficacy, Controlled Release Strategies, and Novel Chaperones. *J. Drug Deliv.* **2011,** *2011,* 1–14.

313. Bulte, J. W.; Kraitchman, D. L. Iron Oxide MR Contrast Agents for Molecular and Cellular Imaging. *NMR Biomed.* **2004,** *17,* 484–499.

314. Gourley, P. L. Brief Overview of BioMicroNano Technologies. *Biotechnol. Prog.* **2005,** *21,* 2–10.

315. Berna, J.; Leigh, D. A.; Lubomska, M.; Mendoza, S. M.; Perez, E. M.; Rudolf, P., et al. Macroscopic Transport by Synthetic Molecular Machines. *Nat. Mater.* **2005,** *4,* 704–710.

316. Bonham, A. J.; Braun, G.; Pavel, I.; Moskovits, M.; Reich, N. Detection of Sequence-Specific Protein-DNA Interactions Via Surface Enhanced Resonance Raman Scattering. *J. Am. Chem. Soc.* **2007,** *129,* 14572–14573.

317. Garcia, J. T.; Farina, J. B.; Munguia, O.; Llabres, M. Comparative Degradation Study of Biodegradable Microspheres of Poly(DL-lactide-co-glycolide) with Poly(ethyleneglycol) Derivates. *J. Microencapsul.* **1999,** *16,* 83–94.

318. Panyam, J.; Williams, D.; Dash, A.; Leslie-Pelecky, D.; Labhasetwar, V. Solid-state Solubility Influences Encapsulation and Release of Hydrophobic Drugs from PLGA/PLA Nanoparticles. *J. Pharm. Sci.* **2004,** *93,* 1804–1814.

319. Soma, C. E.; Dubernet, C.; Bentolila, D.; Benita, S.; Couvreur, P. Reversion of Multidrug Resistance by Co-encapsulation of Doxorubicin and Cyclosporin A in Polyalkylcyanoacrylate Nanoparticles. *Biomaterials* **2000,** *21,* 1–7.

320. Wang, M.; Mi, C.; Wang, W.; Liu, C.; Wu, Y.; Xu, Z.; Mao, C.; Xu, S. Immunolabeling and NIR-Excited Fluorescent Imaging of HELA Cells by using NaYF4:Yb, Er Upconversion Nanoparticles. *ACS Nano.* **2009,** *3,* 1580–1586.

321. Wilson, R. The use of Gold Nanoparticles in Diagnostics and Detection. *Chem. Soc. Rev.* **2008,** *37,* 2028–2045.

322. Bilberg, K.; Døving, K. B.; Beedholm, K.; Baatrup, E. Silver Nanoparticles Disruptolfaction in Crucian carp (Carassius carassius) and Eurasian perch (Perca fluviatilis). *Aquat. Toxicol.* **2011,** *104,* 145–152.

323. Castranova, V. Overview of Current Toxicological Knowledge of Engineered Nanoparticles. *J. Occup. Environ. Med.* **2011,** *53,* S14–S17.

324. Cedervall, T.; Lynch, I.; Lindman, S.; Nilsson, H.; Thulin, E.; Linse, S.; Dawson, K. A. Understanding Biophysicochemical Interactions at the Nano-bio Interface. *Proc. Natl. Acad. Soc. USA* **2007,** *104,* 2050–2055.

325. Das, S.; Jagan, L.; Isiah, R.; Rajech, B.; Backianathan, S.; Subhashini, J. Nanotechnology in Oncology: Characterization and *In Vitro* Release Kinetics of Cisplatin-Loaded Albumin Nanoparticles: Implications in Anticancer Drug Delivery. *Indian J. Pharmacol.* **2011,** *43,* 409–413.

326. Eun, H. C.; Chung, J. H.; Jung, S. Y.; Cho, K. H.; Kim, K. H. A Comparative Study of the Cytotoxicity of Skin Irritants on Cultured Human Oral and Skin Keratinocytes. *Br. J. Dermatol.* **1994,** *130,* 24–28.

327. Hagens, W. I.; Oomen, A. G.; de Jong, W. H.; Cassee, F. R.; Sips, A. What do we (need to) Know About the Kinetic Properties of Nanoparticles in the Body?. *Regul. Toxicol. Pharmacol.* **2007,** *49,* 217–229.

328. Isakovic, A.; Markovic, Z.; Nikolic, N.; Todorovic-Markovic, B.; Vranjes-Djuric, S.; Harhaji, L.; Raicevic, N.; Romcevic, N.; Vasiljevic-Radovic, D.; Dramicanin, M.; Trajkovic, V. Inactivation of Nanocrystalline C60 Cytotoxicity by Gamma-Irradiation. *Biomaterials* **2006,** *27,* 5049–5058.

329. Koyama, S.; Kim, Y. A.; Hayashi, T.; Takeuchi, K.; Fujii, C.; Kuroiwa, N., et al. In Vivo Immunological Toxicity in Mice of Carbon Nanotubes with Impurities. *Carbon* **2009,** *47,* 1365–1372.

330. Mahmoudi, M.; Simchi, A.; Imani, M.; Shokrgozar, M. A.; Milani, A. S.; Hafeli, U.; Stroeve, P. A New Approach for the In Vitro Identification of the Cytotoxicity of Superparamagnetic Iron Oxide Nanoparticles. *Colloids Surf. B: Biointerfaces* **2010,** *75,* 300–309.

331. Marambio-Jones, C.; Hoek, E. M. V. A Review of the Antibacterial Effects of Silver Nanomaterials and Potential Implications for Human Health and the Environment. *J. Nanopart. Res.* **2010,** *12,* 1531–1551.

332. Pelley, J. L.; Daar, A. S.; Saner, M. A. State of Academic Knowledge on Toxicity and Biological Fate of Quantum Dots. *Toxicol. Sci.* **2009,** *112,* 276–296.

333. Schrand, A. M.; Rahman, M. F.; Hussain, S. M.; Schlager, J. J.; Smith, D. A.; Syed, A. F. Metal-based Nanoparticles and their Toxicity Assessment. *Wiley Interdiscip. Rev. Nanomed. Nanobiotechnol.* **2010,** *2,* 544–568.

334. Xu, H.; Qu, F.; Xu, H.; Lai, W.; Wang, Y. A.; Aguilar, Z. P.; Wei, H. Role of Reactive Oxygen Species in the Antibacterial Mechanism of Silver Nanoparticles on Ecoli O157:H7. *Biometals* **2012,** *25,* 45–53.

335. Zhao, X.; Liu, R. Recent Progress and Perspectives on the Toxicity of Carbon Nanotubes at Organism, Organ, Cell, and Biomacromolecule Levels. *Environ. Int.* **2012,** *40,* 244–255.

336. Connor, E. E.; Mwamuka, J.; Gole, A.; Murphy, C. J.; Wyatt, M. D. Gold Nanoparticles are Taken up by Human Cells but do not Cause Acute Cytotoxicity. *Small* **2005,** *1,* 325.

337. Crouzier, D.; Follot, S.; Gentilhomme, E.; Flahaut, E.; Arnaud, R.; Dabouis, V., et al. Carbon Nanotubes Induce Inflammation but Decrease the Production of Reactive Oxygen Species in Lung. *Toxicology* **2010,** *272,* 39–45.

338. Ehrenberg, M.; Friedman, A.; Finkelstein, J.; Oberdorster, G.; McGrath, J. The Influence of Protein Adsorption on Nanoparticle Association with Cultured Endothelial Cells. *Biomaterials* **2009,** *30,* 603–610.

339. Elgrabli, D.; Abella-Gallart, S.; Robidel, F.; Rogerieux, F.; Boczkowski, J.; Lacroix, G. Induction of Apoptosis and Absence of Inflammation in Rat Lung after Intratracheal Instillation of Multiwalled Carbon Nanotubes. *Toxicology* **2008,** *253,* 131–136.

340. Jia, G.; Wang, H.; Yan, L.; Wang, X.; Pei, R.; Yan, T.; Zhoa, Y.; Guo, X. Cytotoxicity of Carbon Nanomaterials: Single-wall Nanotube, Multi-wall Nanotube, and Fullerene. *Environ. Sci. Technol.* **2005,** *39,* 1378–1383.

341. Kreyling, W. G.; Möller, W.; Semmler-Behnke, M.; Oberdörster, G. In *Particle Toxicology*; Born, D. K., Ed.; CRC Press: Boca Raton, 2007.

342. Lam, C. W.; James, J. T.; McCluskey, R.; Arepalli, S.; Hunter, R. L. A Review of Carbon Nanotube Toxicity and Assessment of Potential Occupational and Environmental Health Risks. *Crit. Rev. Toxicol.* **2006,** *36,* 189–217.

343. Lubbe, A. S.; Begemann, C.; Brock, J.; McClure, D. G. Physiological Aspects in Magnetic Drug-Targeting. *J. Magn. Magn. Mater.* **1999,** *194,* 7.

344. Muller, R. H.; Maassen, S.; Weyhers, H.; Mehnert, W. Phagocytic Uptake and Cytotoxicity of Solid Lipid Nanoparticles (SLN) Sterically Stabilized with Poloxamine 908 and Poloxamer 407. *J. Drug Target.* **1996,** *4,* 161–170.

345. Zhang, Y.; Kohler, M.; Zhang, M. Surface Modification of Superparamagnetic Magnetite Nanoparticles and their Interacellular Uptake. *Biomaterials* **2002,** *23,* 9.

346. Alexiou, C.; Arnold, W.; Klein, R. J., et al. Locoregional Cancer Treatment with Magnetic Drug Targeting. *Cancer Res.* **2006,** *60,* 6641–6648.

347. Allen, T. M.; Mumbengegwi, D. R.; Charrois, G. J. Anti-CD19-targeted Liposomal Doxorubicin Improves the Therapeutic Efficacy in Murine B-cell Lymphoma and Ameliorates the Toxicity of Liposomes with Varying Drug Release Rates. *Clin. Cancer Res.* **2005,** *11,* 3567–3573.

348. Bertholon, I.; Ponchel, G.; Labarre, D.; Couvreur, P.; Vauthier, C. Bioadhesive Properties of Poly(alkylcyanoacrylate) Nanoparticles Coated with Polysaccharide. *J. Nanosci. Nanotechnol.* **2006,** *6,* 3102–3109.

349. Beyerle, A.; Merkel, O.; Stoeger, T.; Kissel, T. PEGylation Affects Cytotoxicity and Cell-compatibility of Poly(ethylene imine) for Lung Application: Structure Function Relationships. *Toxicol. Appl. Pharmacol.* **2010,** *242,* 146–154.

350. Lübbe, A. S.; Alexiou, C.; Bergemann, C. Clinical Applications of Magnetic Drug Targeting. *J. Surg. Res.* **2001,** *95,* 200–206.

351. Mykhaylyk, O. M.; Dudchenko, N. O.; Dudchenko, A. K. Pharmacokinetics of the Doxorubicin Magnetic Nanoconjugate in Mice Effects of the Nonuniform Stationary Magnetic Field. *Ukr Biokhim Zh* **2005,** *77,* 80–92.

352. Nguyen, S.; Hiorth, M.; Rykke, M.; Smistad, G. The Potential of Liposomes as Dental Drug Delivery Systems. *Eur. J. Pharm. Biopharm.* **2011,** *77,* 75–83.

353. Mingo, G.; Scholzen, A.; Tang, C. K.; Hanley, J. C.; Kalkainidis, M.; Pietersz, G. A.; Apostolopoulos, V.; Plebanski, M. Poly-L-Lysine-Coated Nanoparticles: A Potent Delivery System to Enhance DNA Vaccine Efficacy. *Vaccine* **2007,** *25,* 1316–1327.

354. Ferber, D. Microbes made to order. *Science* **2004,** *303,* 158–161.

355. Topoglidis, E. A.; Cass, E., et al. Protein Adsorption on Nanocrystalline TiO_2 Films: An Immobilization Strategy for Bioanalytical Devices. *Anal. Chem.* **1998,** *70,* 5111–5113.

356. *Nanoelectronics*; Wang, S. Y.; Williams, R. S., Eds.; Springer: New York, 2005.

357. Andrianantoandro, E.; Basu, S.; Karig, D. K.; Weiss, R. Synthetic biology: new engineering rules for an emerging discipline. *Mol. Syst. Biol.* **2006,** *2,* E1–E14, msb4100073.

358. Armentano, I.; Dottori, M.; Fortunati, E.; Mattioli, S.; Kenny, J. M. Biodegradable Polymer Matrix Nanocomposites for Tissue Engineering: A Review. *Polym. Degrad. Stabil.* **2010,** *95,* 2126–2146.

359. Hong, Z. K.; Zhang, P.; He, C.; Qiu, X.; Liu, A.; Chen, L., et al. Nano-Composite of Poly (L-lactide) and Surface Grafted Hydroxyapatite: Mechanical Properties and Biocompatibility. *Biomaterials* **2005,** *26,* 6296–6304.

360. Otsuka, H.; Nagasaki, Y.; Kataoka, K. Dynamic Wettability Study on the Functionalized PEGylated Layer on a Polylactide Surface Constructed by Coating of Aldehyde-ended Poly(Ethylene Glycol) (PEG)/Polylactide (PLA) Block Copolymer. *Sci. Technol. Adv. Mater.* **2000,** *1,* 21–29.

361. Paiva, M. C.; Zhou, B.; Fernando, K. A. S.; Lin, Y.; Kennedy, J. M.; Sun, Y. P. Mechanical and Morphological Characterization of Polymere Carbon Nanocomposites from Functionalized Carbon Nanotubes. *Carbon* **2004,** *42,* 2849–2854.

362. Pattison, M. A.; Wurster, S.; Webster, T. J.; Haberstroh, K. M. Three-Dimensional, Nano-Structured PLGA Scaffolds for Bladder Tissue Replacement Applications. *Biomaterials* **2005,** *26,* 2491–2500.

363. Tang, Z. G.; Black, R. A. Surface Properties and Biocompatibility of Solvent-Cast Poly[3-caprolactone] Films. *Biomaterials* **2004,** *25,* 4741–4748.

364. Wu, D.; Wu, L.; Sun, Y.; Zhang, M. Rheological Properties and Crystallization Behavior of Multi-walled Carbon Nanotube/Poly(3-caprolactone) Composites. 2007, *25,* 3137–3147.

365. Xiao, G. Solvent-Induced Changes on Corona-Discharge-Treated Polyolefin Surfaces Probed by Contact Angle Measurement. *J. Colloid Interface Sci.* **1995,** *171,* 200–204.

366. Klein, C. P. A.T.; Driessen, A. A.; de Groot, K.; van den Hooff, A. Biodegradation Behaviour of Various Calcium Phosphate Materials in Bone Tissue. *J Biomed. Mater. Res.* **2004,** *17,* 769–784.

367. Rezwan, K.; Chen, Q. Z.; Blaker, J. J.; Boccaccini, A. R. Biodegradable and Bioactive Porous Polymer/Inorganic Composite Scaffolds for Bone Tissue Engineering. *Biomaterials* **2006,** *27.*

368. Jan, E.; Kotov, N. A. Successful Differentiation of Mouse Neural Stem Cells on Layer-by-layer Assembled Single-walled Carbon Nanotube Composite. *Nano Lett.* **2007,** *7,* 1123–1128.

369. Ferraz, M. P.; Monteriro, F. J.; Manuel, C. M. Hydroxyapatite Nanoparticles: A Review of Preparation Methodologies. *J. Appl. Biomater. Biomech.* **2004,** *2,* 74–80.

370. Hench, L. L.; Polak, J. M. Third-Generation Biomedical Materials. *Science* **2002,** *295,* 1014–1017.

371. Kretlow, J. D.; Mikos, A. G. Review: Mineralization of Synthetic Polymer Scaffolds for Bone Tissue Engineering. *Tissue Eng.* **2007,** *13,* 927–938.

372. Lee, J. Y.; Nagahata, J. L. R.; Horiuchi, S. Effect of Metal Nanoparticles on Thermal Stabiliza-tion Of Polymer/Metal Nanocomposites Prepared by a One-step Dry Process. *Polymer* **2006,** *47,* 7970–7979.

373. Woodard, R.; Hilldore, A. J.; Lan, S. K.; Park, C. J.; Morgan, A. W.; Eurell, J. A. C., et al. The Mechanical Properties and Osteoconductivity of Hydroxyapatite Bone Scaffolds With Multi-Scale Porosità. *Biomaterials* **2007,** *28,* 45–54.

374. Imanaka, N.; Masui, T.; Hirai, H.; Adachi, G. Do Nanoparticles and Sunscreens mix?. *Chem Mater* **2003,** *15,* 2289–2291.

375. Webster, T. J.; Siegel, R. W.; Bizios, R. Osteoblast Adhesion on Nanophase Ceramics. *Bioma-terials* **1999,** *20,* 1221–1227.

376. Wagner, W.; Dullaart, A.; Bock, A. K.; Zweck, A. The Emerging Nanomedicine Landscape. *Nat. Biotechnol.* **2006**, *24,* 1211–1217.

377. Kwong, B.; Liu, H.; Irvine, D. J. Induction of Potent Anti-Tumor Responses while Eliminating Systemic Side Effects via Liposome-Anchored Combinatorial Immunotherapy. *Biomaterials* **2011**, *32,* 5134–5147.

378. tenTije, A. J.; Verweij, J.; Loos, W. J.; Sparreboom, A. Pharmacological Effects of Formulation Vehicles: Implications for Cancer Chemotherapy. *Clin. Pharmacokinet.* **2003**, *42,* 665–685.

379. Krishnadas, A.; Rubinstein, I.; Onyuksel, H. Sterically Stabilized Phospholipid Mixed Micelles: In Vitro Evaluation as a Novel Carrier for Water-Insoluble Drugs. *Pharm. Res.* **2003**, *20,* 297–302.

380. Maeda, H. The Enhanced Permeability and Retention (EPR) Effect in Tumor Vasculature: The Key Role of Tumor-selective Macromolecular Drug Targeting. *Adv. Enzyme Regul.* **2001**, *41,* 189–207.

381. Panyam, J.; Sahoo, S. K.; Prabha, S.; Bargar, T.; Labhasetwar, V. Fluorescence and Electron Microscopy Probes for Cellular and Tissue Uptake of Poly(d, l-lactide-co-glycolide) Nanoparticles. *Int. J. Pharm.* **2003**, *262,* 1–11.

382. Wang, H.; Zhao, Y.; Wu, Y.; Hu, Y.; Nan, K.; Nie, G.; Chen, H. Enhanced Anti-tumor Efficacy by Co-delivery of Doxorubicin and Paclitaxel with Amphiphilic PEG-PLGA Copolymer Nanoparticles. *Biomaterials* **2011**, *32,* 8281–8290.

383. Chan, W. H.; Shiao, N. H.; Lu, P. Z. CdSe Quantum Dots Induce Apoptosis in Human Neuroblastoma Cells via Mitochondrial-dependent Pathways and Inhibition of Survival Signals. *Toxicol. Lett.* **2006**, *167,* 191–200.

384. Drummond, D. C.; Meyer, O.; Hong, K.; Kirpotin, D. B.; Papahadjopoulos, D. Optimizing Liposomes for Delivery of Chemotherapeutic Agents to Solid Tumors. *Pharmacol. Rev.* **1999**, *51,* 691–743.

385. Fetterly, G. J.; Straubinger, R. M. Pharmacokinetics of Paclitaxel-Containing Liposomes in Rats. *AAPS Pharm. Sci.* **2003**, *5,* 1–11.

386. Hoarau, D.; Delmas, P.; David, S.; Roux, E.; Leroux, J. C. Novel Longcirculating Lipid Nanocapsules. *Pharm. Res.* **2004**, *21,* 1783–1789.

387. Kamps, J. A.; Scherphof, G. L. Receptor Versus Non-receptor Mediated Clearance of Liposomes. *Adv. Drug Deliv. Rev.* **1998**, *32,* 81–97.

388. Mattiasson, B.; Borrebaeck, C. In *Enzyme Immunoassay*; Maggio, E. T., Ed.; CRC Press, Inc.: Boca Raton, 1980; pp 295.

389. Papahadjopoulos, D.; Jacobson, K.; Nir, S.; Isac, T. Phase Transitions in Phospholipid Vesicles. Fluorescence Polarization and Permeability Measurements Concerning the Effect of Temperature and Cholesterol. *Biochim. Biophys. Acta* **1973**, *311,* 330–348.

390. Pastorino, F.; Brignole, C.; Marimpietri, D.; Sapra, P.; Moase, E. H.; Allen, T. M.; Ponzoni, M. Doxorubicin-loaded Fab' Fragments of Anti-disialoganglioside Immunoliposomes Selectively Inhibit the Growth and Dissemination of Human Neuroblastoma in Nude Mice. *Cancer Res.* **2003**, *63,* 86–92.

391. Yan, X.; Kuipers, F.; Havekes, L. M.; Havinga, R.; Dontje, B.; Poelstra, K.; Scherpof, G. L.; Kamps, J. A. A.M. The Role of Apolipoprotein E in the Elimination of Liposomes from Blood by Hepatocytes in the Mouse. *Biochem. Biophys. Res. Commun.* **2005**, *328,* 57–62.

392. Zhang, J. A.; Anyarambhatla, G.; Ma, L.; Ugwu, S.; Xuan, T.; Sardone, T.; Ahmad, I. Development and Characterization of a Novel Cremophor® EL free Liposome-based Paclitaxel (LEP-ETU) Formulation. *Eur. J.Pharm. Biopharm.* **2005**, *59,* 177–187.

393. Zhang, N.; Ping, Q. N.; Huang, G. H.; Xu, W. F. Investigation of Lectin-Modified Insulin Liposomes as Carriers for Oral Administration. *Int. J. Pharm.* **2005,** *294,* 247–259.

394. Medina, O. P.; Pillarsetty, N.; Glekas, A.; Punzalan, B.; Longo, V.; Gönen, M.; Zanzonico, P.; Smith-Jones, P.; Larson, S. M. Optimizing Tumor Targeting of the Lipophilic EGFR-binding Radiotracer SKI 243 using Liposomal NANOPARTICLE Delivery System. *J. Control. Release* **2011,** *149,* 292–298.

395. Scadden, D.; Howard, W. W. AIDS-Related Malignancies. *The Oncologist* **1998,** *3,* 119–123.

396. Tobio, M.; Sanchez, A.; Vila, A.; Soriano, I.; Evora, C.; Vila-Jato, J. L.; Alonso, M. J. Investigation of Lectin-modified Insulin Liposomes as Carriers for Oral Administration. *Colloids Surf. B: Biointerfaces* **2000,** *18,* 315–323.

397. Torchilin, V. P.; Shtilman, M. I.; Trubetskoy, V. S.; Whiteman, K.; Milstein, A. M. Amphiphilic Vinyl Polymers Effectively Prolong Liposome Circulation Time. *In Vivo. Biochim. Biophys. Acta* **1994,** *1195,* 181–184.

398. Dabholkar, R. D.; Sawant, R. M.; Mongayt, D. A. Polyethylene Glycol-Phosphatidylethanolamine Conjugate (PEG-PE)-based Mixed Micelles: Some Properties, Loading with Paclitaxel, and Modulation of P-Glycoprotein-Mediated Efflux. *Int. J. Pharm.* **2006,** *315,* 148–157.

399. Geish, K. Enhanced Permeability and Retention Effect of Macromolecular Drugs in Solid Tumors: A Royal Gate for Targeted Anticancer Medicines. *J. Drug Target.* **2007,** *15,* 457–464.

400. Lal, R.; Ramachandran, S.; Arnsdorf, M. F. Multidimensional Atomic Force Microscopy: A Versatile Novel Technology for Nanopharmacology Research. *AAPS J.* **2010,** *12,* 716–728.

401. Palmer, H. M.; Higgins, S. P.; Herring, A. J.; Kingston, M. A. Use of PCR in the Diagnosis of Early syphilis in the United Kingdom. *Sex Transm. Infect.* **2003,** *79,* 479–483.

402. Woodbury, R. G.; Wendin, C.; Clendenning, J.; Melendez, J.; Elkind, J.; Bartholomew, D.; Brown, S.; Furlong, C. E. Construction of Biosensors using a Gold-binding Polypeptide and a Miniature Integrated Surface Plasmon Resonance Sensor. *Biosens. Bioelectron.* **1998,** *13,* 1117–1126.

403. Bergqvist, L.; Sundberg, R.; Ryden, S.; Strand, S. E. The "Critical Colloid Dose" in Studies of Reticuloendothelial Function. *J. Nucl. Med.* **1987,** *28,* 1424–1429.

404. Bradfield, J. W. A New Look at Reticuloendothelial Blockade. *Br. J. Exp. Pathol.* **1980,** *61,* 617–623.

405. Aldana, J.; Wang, Y. A.; Peng, X. G. Photochemical Instability of CdSe Nanocrystals Coated by Hydrophilic Thiols. *J. Am. Chem. Soc.* **2001,** *123,* 8844–8850.

406. Au, J. L.; Jang, S. H.; Zheng, J.; Chen, C. T.; Song, S.; Hu, L.; Wientjes, M. G. Determinants of Drug Delivery and Transport to Solid Tumors. *J. Control. Release* **2001,** *74,* 31–46.

407. Bell, S. E. J.; NarayanaSirimuthu, N. M. S. Surface-Enhanced Raman Spectroscopy (SERS) for Sub-Micromolar Detection of DNA/RNA Mononucleotides. *J. Am. Chem. Soc.* **2006,** *128,* 15580–15581.

408. Herrero-Vanrell, R.; Rincón, A. C.; Alonso, M.; Reboto, V.; Molina-Martinez, I. T.; Rodríguez-Cabello, J. C. Self-assembled Particles of an Elastin-like Polymer as Vehicles for Controlled Drug Release. *J. Control. Release* **2005,** *102,* 113–122.

409. Maeda, H.; Bharate, G. Y.; Daruwalla, J. Polymeric Drugs for Efficient Tumortargeted Drug Delivery Based on EPR Effect. *Eur. J. Pharm. Biopharm.* **2009,** *71,* 409–419.

410. Ferrari, M. Frontiers in Cancer Nanomedicine: Directing Mass Transport through Biological Barriers. *Trends Biotechnol.* **2010,** *786,* 1–8.

411. Sakamoto, J. H.; van de Ven, A. L.; Godin, B.; Blanco, E.; Serda, R. E.; Grattoni, A.; Ziemys, A.; Bouamrani, A.; Hu, T.; Ranganathan, S. I.; De Rosa, E.; Martinez, J. O.; Smid, C. A.; Buchanan, R.; Lee, S. Y.; Srinivasan, S.; Landry, M.; Meyn, A.; Tasciotti, E.; Li, X.; Decuzzi, P.; Ferrari, M. Review: Enabling Individualized Therapy through Nanotechnology. *Pharm. Res.* **2010**, *62*, 57–89.

412. Canal, P.; Gamelin, E.; Vassal, G.; Robert, J. Benefits of Pharmacological Knowledge in the Design and Monitoring of Cancer Chemotherapy. *Pathol. Oncol. Res.* **1998**, *4*, 171–178.

413. Ferrari, M. Cancer Nanotechnology: Opportunities and Challenges. *Nat. Rev. Cancer* **2005**, *5*, 161–171.

414. Tallaj, J. A.; Franco, V.; Rayburn, B. K.; Pinderski, L.; Benza, R. L.; Pamboukian, S., et al. Response of Doxorubicin Induced Cardiomyopathy to the Current Management Strategy of Heart Failure. *J. Heart Lung Transplant* **2005**, *24*, 196–201.

415. Rai, P.; Mallidi, S.; Zheng, X.; Rahmanzadeh, R.; Mir, Y.; Elrington, S.; Khurshid, A.; Hasan, T. Development and Applications of Photo-Triggered Theranostic Agents. *Adv. Drug Deliv. Rev.* **2010**, *62*, 1094–1124.

416. Shubayev, V. I.; Pisanic, T. R.; Jin, S. Magnetic Nanoparticles for Theragnostics. *Adv. Drug Deliv. Rev* **2009**, *61*, 467–477.

417. Borm, P. J.; Kreyling, W. Toxicological Hazards of Inhaled Nanoparticles-Potential Implications for Drug Delivery. *J. Nanosci. Nanotechnol.* **2004**, *4*, 521–531.

418. Colvin, V. L. The Potential Environmental Impact of Engineered Nanomaterials. *Nat. Biotechnol.* **2003**, *21*, 1166–1170.

419. Monteiro-Riviere, N. A.; Inman, A. O.; Zhang, L. W. Limitations and Relative Utility of Screening Assays to Assess Engineered Nanoparticle Toxicity in a Human Cell Line. *Toxicol. Appl. Pharmacol.* **2009**, *234*, 222–235.

420. Murray, A. R.; Kisin, E.; Leonard, S. S.; Young, S. H.; Kommimeni, C.; Kagan, V. E., et al. In vivo Immunological Toxicity in Mice of Carbon Nanotubes with Impurities. *Toxicology* **2009**, *257*, 161–171.

421. Nel, A.; Madler, L.; Velegol, D.; Xia, T.; Hoek, E. M. V.; Somasundaran, P.; Klaessig, F.; Castranova, V.; Thompson, M. Understanding Biophysicochemical Interactions at the Nano-Bio Interface. *Nat. Mater.* **2009**, *8*, 543–557.

422. Oberdorster, E. Manufactured Nanomaterials (fullerenes, C60) Induce Oxidative Stress in the Brain Of Juvenile Largemouth Bass. *Environ. Health Perspect.* **2004**, *1112*, 1058–1062.

423. Oberdorster, E.; Zhu, S.; Blickley, T. M.; McClellan-Green, P.; Haasch, M. L. Ecotoxicology of Carbon-based Engineered Nanoparticles: Effects of Fullerene (C_{60}) on Aquatic Organisms. *Carbon* **2006**, *44*, 1112–1120.

424. Sayes, C. M.; Fortner, J. D.; Guo, W.; Lyon, D.; Boyd, A. M.; Ausman, K. D.; Tao, Y. J.; Sitharaman, B.; Wilson, L. J.; Hughes, J. B.; West, J. L.; Colvin, V. L. The Differential Cytotoxicity of Water-soluble Fullerenes. *Nano Lett.* **2004**, *4*, 1881–1887.

425. Mukherjee, P.; Bhattacharya, R.; Wang, P.; Wang, L.; Basu, S.; Nagy, J. A.; Atala, A.; Mukhopadhyay, D.; Soker, S. Antiangiogenic Properties of Gold Nanoparticles. *Clin. Cancer Res.* **2005**, *11*, 3530–3534.

426. Czerniawska, A. Experimental Investigations on the Penetration of 198Au from Nasal Mucous Membrane into Cerebrospinal Fluid. *Acta Otolaryngol.* **1970**, *70*, 58–61.

427. Iscan, Y. Y.; Hekimoglu, S.; Kas, S.; Hinca, A. A. *Formulation and Characterization of Solid Lipid Nanoparticles for Skin Delivery, Conference Lipid and Surfactant Dispersed Systems*. Moscow, Proceedings Book; , 1999, pp. 163–166.

428. Mahmoudi, M.; Shokrgozar, M. A.; Simchi, A.; Imani, M.; Milani, A. S.; Stroeve, P.; Vali, H.; Hafeli, U. O.; Bonakdar, S. Multiphysics Flow Modeling and in Vitro Toxicity of Iron Oxide Nanoparticles Coated with Poly(vinyl alcohol). *J. Phys. Chem. C* **2009**, *113*, 2322–2331.

429. Monteiro-Riviere, N. A.; Nemanich, R. A.; Inman, A. O.; Wang, Y. Y.; Riviere, J. E. Multi-Walled Carbon Nanotube Interactions with Human Epidermal Keratinocytes. *Toxicol. Lett.* **2005,** *155,* 377–384.
430. Arianna, F.; Alfred, N. *Reconfiguring Responsibility: Lessons for Nanoethics.* (Part 2 of the Report on Deepening Debate on Nanotechnology); , 2009.
431. Faunce, T. A. Toxicological and Public Good Considerations for the Regulation of Nanomaterial-containing Medical Products. *Expert Opin. Drug Safety* **2008,** *7,* 103–106.
432. Faunce, T. A. Policy Challenges of Nanomedicine for Australia's PBS. *Aust. Health Rev.* **2009,** *33,* 258–267.
433. Faunce, T. A.; Nasu, H.; Murray, K.; Bowman, D. Sunscreen Safety: The Precautionary Principle, The Australian Therapeutic Goods Administration and Nanoparticles in Sunscreens. *Nanoethics* **2008,** *2,* 231–240.
434. Vines, T.; Faunce, T. A. Assessing the Safety and Cost-Effectiveness of Early Nanodrugs. *J. Law Med.* **2007,** *16,* 822–845.
435. FDA *FDA and Nanotechnology Products: Frequently Asked Questions.* , 2007.
436. USFDA *FDA Issues Draft Guidance on Nanotechnology Documents Address use of Nanotechnology by Food and Cosmetics Industries.* 2012 Available from: http://www.fda.gov/Cosmetics/GuidanceComplianceRegulatoryInformation/GuidanceDocuments/ucm300886.htm.
437. USFDA *Cosmetics: Draft Guidance for Industry: Safety of Nanomaterials in Cosmetic Products.* 2012 Available from: http://www.fda.gov/Cosmetics/GuidanceComplianceRegulatoryInformation/GuidanceDocuments/ucm300886.htm.
438. USFDA *Draft Guidance for Industry: Assessing the Effects of Significant Manufacturing Process Changes, Including Emerging Technologies, on the Safety and Regulatory Status of Food Ingredients and Food Contact Substances, Including Food Ingredients that are Color Additives.* 2012.
439. Commission, E. *Commission Recommendation on A Code of Conduct for Responsible Nanosciences and Nanotechnologies Research & Council Conclusions on Responsible Nanosciences and Nanotechnologies Research.* 2008 Available from: http://ec.europa.eu/research/research-eu.
440. Kehoe, S.; Zhang, X. F.; Boyd, D. FDA Approved Guidance Conduits and Wraps for Peripheral Nerve Injury: A Review of Materials and Efficacy. *Injury* **2012,** *43,* 553–572.
441. Huang, Z.; Chen, H.; Chen, Z. K.; Roco, M. C. International Nanotechnology Development in 2003: Country, Institution, and Technology Field Analysis Based on USPTO Patent Database. *J. Nanopart. Res.* **2004,** *6,* 325–354.
442. Igami, M.; Okazaki, T. *Capturing Nanotechnology's Current State Of Development Via Analysis Of Patents.* , 2007, DSTI/DOC. pages.
443. Koosha, A.; Ahmadi, M.; Nazifi, A.; Mousazadeh, R. Intellectual Property Rights of Nano-Biotechnology in Trade Related Aspects of Intellectual Property Agreement (TRIPS). *Indian J. Sci. Tech.* **2012,** *5,* 2436–2442.
444. USPTO *Class 977 Nanotechnology Cross-Reference Art Collection.* 2012, June 24, 2012]. Available from: http://www.uspto.gov/patents/resources/classification/class_977_nanotechnology_cross-ref_art_collection.jsp.
445. Sargent, J. F. J. *The National Nanotechnology Initiative: Overview, Reauthorization, and Appropriations Issues.* 2012, [cited 7–5700 RL34401].
446. Sizing Nanotechnology's Value Chain. *Lux.* 2004.
447. Heath, J. R.; Davis, M. E. Nanotechnology and cancer. *Annu Med Rev.* **2008,** 59, 251–265.

Index

Note: Page numbers with "f" denote figures; "t" tables.

W

X

Y

Z

Printed in the United States
By Bookmasters